Cataract and Lens Surgery

Springer Nature More Media App

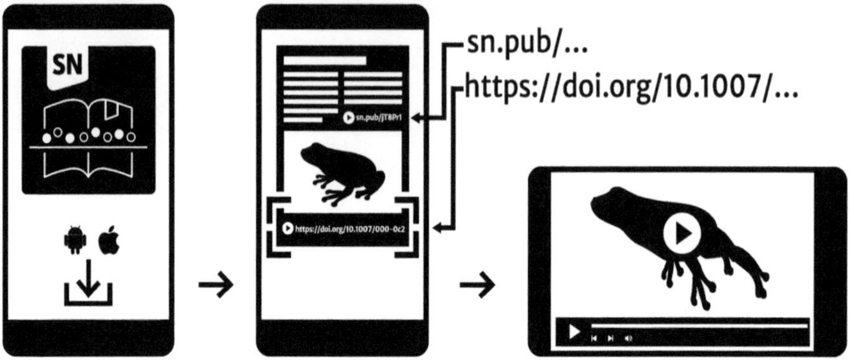

1.
Download

2.
Scan Link

3.
Enjoy Video

Support: customerservice@springernature.com

Mehdi Shajari · Siegfried Priglinger ·
Thomas Kohnen · Thomas C. Kreutzer ·
Wolfgang J. Mayer
Editors

Cataract and Lens Surgery

Springer

Editors
Mehdi Shajari
Department of Ophthalmology
University Hospital Frankfurt
Frankfurt am Main, Germany

Thomas Kohnen
Department of Ophthalmology
University Hospital Frankfurt
Frankfurt am Main, Germany

Wolfgang J. Mayer
Department of Ophthalmology
University Hospital Munich
Munich, Germany

Siegfried Priglinger
Department of Ophthalmology
University Hospital Munich
Munich, Germany

Thomas C. Kreutzer
Department of Ophthalmology
University Hospital Munich
Munich, Germany

This work contains media enhancements, which are displayed with a "play" icon. Material in the print book can be viewed on a mobile device by downloading the Springer Nature "More Media" app available in the major app stores. The media enhancements in the online version of the work can be accessed directly by authorized users.

ISBN 978-3-031-05393-1 ISBN 978-3-031-05394-8 (eBook)
https://doi.org/10.1007/978-3-031-05394-8

Translation from the German language edition: "Katarakt- und Linsenchirurgie" by Mehdi Shajari et al.,

This Springer imprint is published by the registered company Springer Nature Switzerland AG
The registered company address is: Gewerbestrasse 11, 6330 Cham, Switzerland

Written by a team of international authors and dedicated to ophthalmic surgeons around the globe who share our passion for cataract and lens surgery.

Contents

Introduction

Implantation of Artificial Intraocular Lenses—A Brief History

Thomas Neuhann

The very first replacement of an opacified natural lens by a clear artificial lens was performed by Harold Ridley at St. Thomas' Hospital in London on 29 November 1949. The implant was largely modelled after the natural lens, both in shape and size, and was inserted into the capsular bag after extracapsular lens extraction. The circumstances leading up to the event are stuff of legend and surrounded by numerous anecdotes—It is said that Ridley was inspired by a student who watched him perform cataract surgery and naively asked why he did not simply insert a new lens in the place of the old one. The meetings between Ridley and John Pike of Rayner & Keeler, the manufacturer of the first IOL, used to occur huddled together in Harold Ridley's Bentley. Finally, his choice of Perspex PMMA plastic was inspired out of tragedy—during the second world war, Royal Air Force pilots presented with intraocular shards of the material when their aircraft canopies shattered. Ridley observed that despite the damage, the material remained inert inside the eye and could perhaps be shaped into an effective implant.

Like many disruptive, paradigm shifting innovations, the process was extremely controversial in ophthalmology. The initial furious rejection by the establishment however was at least tempered by the fascinated acceptance of a few who also saw the true potential of the intraocular lens.

In the 1950s however, the trend of intracapsular cataract extraction increasingly replaced the previously preferred extracapsular surgery. This left no capsular bag to support an IOL so naturally inhibited the further adoption of the Ridley lens implant. Intraocular lens innovation however did not remain dormant, but in the absence of a capsular bag, a new fixation principle was required. This need led to the introduction of anterior chamber lenses, supported by the chamber angle, and as a result, lens implantation experienced a new upswing at that time. Again, the leading innovators of the time met the similar fierce resistance that had hounded

T. Neuhann (✉)
Group Practice and Eye Department, Red Cross Hospital, Munich, Germany
e-mail: prof@neuhann.de

M. Shajari et al. (eds.), *Cataract and Lens Surgery*,
https://doi.org/10.1007/978-3-031-05394-8_1

Ridley. The lens models of these IOL pioneers; Dannheim and Schreck in Germany, Barraquer in Spain and, last but not least, Choyce in England, to name only the most prominent, helped the new principle in gaining increasing interest, though at that time it was reserved for very selected cases, namely younger patients with unilateral aphakia. Lens implantation as a routine correction of aphakia was not considered to be possible, even then.

The initial enthusiasm of the short-term results was eventually followed by a period of considerable disillusionment as the long-term results and complications began to roll in. Increasing reports of complications due to ingrowth of the haptics into the chamber angle, secondary glaucoma, chronic inflammatory reactions, corneal decompensation—to name only the most important ones—fired the opposition. Those performing IOL implantations were considered to be taking unnecessary risks and were seen to be on the fringe of mainstream ophthalmology. The problem however was not the concept of an IOL itself but rather the limitations in surgical methods and options to treat complications compared to what we have nowadays. As a result, in the late 1960s/early 1970s, lens implantation, the greatest innovation in anterior segment surgery, was widely considered obsolete and irresponsible.

But good ideas are seldom forgotten and fortunately, the official ban from the establishment did not stop some ophthalmologists from advancing IOL development. Peter Choyce refined the principle of the chamber angle fixation with his design to such an extent that the complication rate decreased considerably. In the Netherlands, Cornelius Binkhorst developed a completely new fixation principle, namely to the previously ignored iris, with his 4-loop lens. In the mid to late 1970s, the first surgeons in Germany started testing these new lenses. This was again disruptive and as controversial as in Ridley's time: When I myself moved from Heidelberg, the center of the "never again IOL coalition" to Mainz in 1977, the first Binkhorst 4-loop lenses had just been implanted there. The controversy in German ophthalmology was fierce and the bias was passed on to the younger generations throughout the academic institutions.

This controversy and debate still raged even as the next paradigm shifting development challenged ophthalmology: the rebirth of extracapsular cataract surgery in its modern refined technology. The debate was now to include the choice between Dr. Charles Kelman's new phacoemulsification technique to perform an extracapsular cataract extraction and the "classic" but now microsurgically reliable "large incision" cataract surgery.

The refinement of the extracapsular technique in the late 1970s finally made S. Shearing's introduction of the posterior chamber lens possible and feasible. Its two J-shaped haptics were based on Barraquer's earlier anterior chamber lens—but the lens was now to be placed retroiridially, in the ciliary sulcus. This change in positioning was only fractions of a millimeter more posterior than the anterior chamber placement but a decisive difference. When the refinement of the anterior capsulorhexis technique with a continuous closed edge (capsulorhexis) made secure and permanent fixation in the capsular bag possible in 1984, the circle of lens development—at least up to its current state—was closed. The IOL had returned into the capsular bag, just where Ridley had originally intended it to be.

The beginning of the 1980s was, without exaggeration, turbulent in the field of cataract surgery: ICCE versus ECCE, to perform phacoemulsification or not, to implant a lens or not, and if so, which lens design or fixation method was best....

It is beyond the scope of this brief description to describe the many tortuous ways that the development and the decisions and statements of the professional associations in this context have taken during this time. Where the development has led to in a comparatively short time is more than obvious today. In cataract surgery today, phacoemulsification is the leading surgical technique and—lens implantation is an indisputable standard. The controversy of whether to implant a lens or not is resolved. Discussions today are more related to the optical-refractive properties and refinements of the lenses.—The implants have grown more sophisticated in what they can offer and one of the newer challenges is how to advise patients correctly in this area, which is demanding in terms of both time and understanding the complicated details and physical principles underlying the lens technologies....

It is not an exaggeration to say that Sir Harold Ridley's epochal invention has very significantly improved the quality of life of millions and millions of people. He, fortunately, lived long enough to finally receive the recognition and honors he deserved from the international scientific community from the mid-1980s onwards. In 1999, on the 50th anniversary of the first implantation, the annual meeting of the ESCRS in Vienna payed honor to the man who had long been rejected by the establishment. The elevation to the peerage of Sir Harold Ridley by the Queen of his country in the year 2000—was satisfying and touching.

From someone who has witnessed this development over the last 47 years—and had the opportunity to help shape it a little—I would like to share this appeal.

While what is new is certainly never automatically good—it is also never a priori bad. It may just be ahead of contemporary understanding. One should always remain critical and curious at the same time—and if curiosity prevails a little, it is less harmful and potentially more useful than if "establishment-always-good" arrogance prevails.

In the end, the words of my revered mentor and friend Richard Kratz remain valid:

Do not talk too much—do good work—and be available.

Bibliography

1. Apple, DJ, Mamalis, N, Olson, RJ, Kincaid, MC. Intraocular lenses. In: Evolution, Designs, Complications, and Pathology. Baltimore: Williams & Wilkins;1998.
2. Apple DJ, Sims J. Harold Ridley and the invention of the intraocular lens. Surv Ophthalmol. 1996;40(4):279–92.
3. Neuhann Th. The development of modern cataract surgery in Germany. Ophthalmic Surg. 2019;31(2):98–106.

Epidemiology

Lukas Bisorca-Gassendorf and Martin Wenzel

In March 2020 there were 7.7 billion people in the world, 1.2% (95 million) of whom suffer from advanced cataract.

According to the "Global estimates of visual impairment: 2010" report by the WHO [1] the number of people visually impaired worldwide was estimated to be 285 million, of whom 39 million were considered to be blind. While lens opacities ranked as the second major cause of visual impairment (33% of cases), this was just behind uncorrected refractive errors (43% of cases). It is also worth noting that cataract was defined as the leading cause of blindness worldwide, accounting for more than half (51%) of all cases. In 2020 the report of the "Lancet Global Health Commission on Global Eye Health: vision beyond 2020" [2] showed that these rankings did not change. The leading causes of blindness remained cataract with around 17 million cases, and lens opacities were still the second major cause of "moderate and severe vision impairment" (MSVI, defined as Snellen VA between 6/18 and 3/60) affecting around 83.5 million people globally. While cataract is a curable disease in most parts of the world, the access to safe surgical procedures for cataract extraction still varies throughout the globe. Unfortunately, there are few reliable figures on the global frequency of cataract and most reports are based on estimates. This is partly because it often occurs with other age-related diseases and the contribution of lens opacity to vision impairment is difficult to assess. Secondly, the surgeries are performed by different national health care frameworks in different countries, whose data may be difficult to combine.

Recently, a review article published by Hashemi et al. [3] attempted to address the gap of scarce epidemiological data. Its aim was to estimate regional and global prevalence of the disease and consisted of a comprehensive systemic review and

L. Bisorca-Gassendorf · M. Wenzel (✉)
Petrisberg Eye Clinic, Trier, Germany
e-mail: martin.wenzel@augenklinik-petrisberg.de

L. Bisorca-Gassendorf
e-mail: lukas.bisorca@augenklinik-petrisberg.de

M. Shajari et al. (eds.), *Cataract and Lens Surgery*,
https://doi.org/10.1007/978-3-031-05394-8_2

meta-analysis of 9922 articles and 45 studies, resulting in a sample size of over 160,000 of patients from all around the world. The study concluded that out of 1000 randomly chosen people, between 133 and 210 people were expected to have cataract (CI = 95%), increasing at ages above 60 years, unsurprisingly. A WHO-Region subgroup analysis conducted, with six distinctive regions, highlighted the geographic heterogeneity of the disease. The highest rate of "age-standardized pooled prevalence estimate" (ASPPE), which the authors used as the main index for comparison, was 37% in southeast Asia. Prevalence of cataract in the Eastern Mediterranean region was reported to be 6% higher in comparison with the Americas or southeast Asia in contrast to Europe.

The aforementioned report by the Lancet Global Health Commission [3] confirmed the higher prevalence of cataract in Oceania, south and southeast Asia. As might be expected, in these regions the prevalence of cataract blindness is also remarkably elevated. Lens opacities are responsible for roughly half of all-cause blindness. Both economic factors, reflected in reduced access to surgery, and environmental factors, such as UV radiation combined with higher levels of outdoor activity, are believed to be responsible for this increased prevalence. Racial and ethnic variances may also contribute to this interregional dissimilarity. Despite increasing numbers of cataract procedures worldwide, the global ASPPE is expected to rise further, primarily due to demographic changes.

Twenty-five million cataract surgeries are performed worldwide every year. While the population demographics for developed countries shifts to older life expectancies, the number of patients living with cataract has not increased in recent years due to increased surgical activity. Overall, the numbers denote a high burden of treatable and preventable cases of visual impairment and blindness. Being a major global health issue, cataract needs to be addressed continuously, despite or especially because it is treatable.

A key factor influencing a countries operation rate is the indication of when to operate. In more developed countries where many seniors drive their own car, visual acuity of 6/9 may be an indication for surgery [4]. In such countries, the surgery rate may be more than 12 per thousand. If a cutoff of 6/18 is used as an indication for cataract surgery, only 3 per thousand inhabitants are operated [5]. Taking Germany as an example, the annual surgery rate is 15 operations per 1000 inhabitants. In 5% of all cataract procedures, special lenses are implanted (60,000 per year), half of which are toric and half multifocal, with half of those again being toric-multifocal. An emerging trend is that in some situations, the lens extraction is performed on clear lenses, before the appearance of cataract or on "near-clear" lenses. This is primarily performed from refractive purposes. Approximately 30,000 of these refractive lens exchanges are performed annually in Germany [6].

In recent years there have been initiatives to centralize and register cataract procedures on a continental level, the most established of which is the "European Registry of Quality Outcomes for Cataract and Refractive Surgery" (EUREQUO). Unfortunately, from an epidemiological point of view we are still far from being able to assess the exact incidence or prevalence of the disease, since not all procedures are being reported. Despite this, during a 10 year period (from January

2008 to December 2017), over 2.7 million cataract surgeries were recorded. However, Lundström et al. [7] were able to show that certain parameters, such as mean age (from 74.5 to 73.0 years) or the proportion of women (from 60.6 to 57.2%), also changed over the decade.

References

1. Pascolini D, Mariotti SP. Global estimates of visual impairment: 2010. Br J Ophthalmol. 2012;96(5):614–8.
2. Burton MJ, Ramke J, Marques AP, Bourne RRA, Congdon N, Jones I, et al. The *lancet global health* commission on global eye health: vision beyond 2020. The Lancet Global Health;2021.
3. Hashemi H, Pakzad R, Yekta A, Aghamirsalim M, Pakbin M, Ramin S, et al. Global and regional prevalence of age-related cataract: a comprehensive systematic review and meta-analysis. Eye (Lond). 2020;34(8):1357–70.
4. McCarty CA, Keeffe JE, Taylor HR. The need for cataract surgery: projections based on lens opacity, visual acuity, and personal concern. Br J Ophthalmol. 1999;83(1):62–5.
5. Taylor HR. Cataract: how much surgery do we have to do? Br J Ophthalmol. 2000;84(1):1–2.
6. Wenzel M, Dick B, Scharrer A, Schayan K, Agostini H, Reinhard T. Ambulante und stationäre Intraokularchirurgie 2019: Ergebnisse der aktuellen Umfrage von BDOC, BVA DGII und DOG. Ophthalmo-Chirurgie. 2020;32:341–50.
7. Lundstrom M, Dickman M, Henry Y, Manning S, Rosen P, Tassignon MJ, et al. Changing practice patterns in European cataract surgery as reflected in the European registry of quality outcomes for cataract and refractive surgery 2008–2017. J Cataract Refract Surg. 2020.

2008 to December 2017), over 2.7 million cataract surgeries were recorded. However, Lundström et al. [7] were able to show that certain parameters, such as mean age (from 74.5 to 73.0 years) or the proportion of women (from 60.6 to

Anatomy and Physiology of the Anterior Segment

Andreas Ohlmann

The human eye is anatomically composed of three layers. The outermost layer, which includes both the sclera and cornea, forms the tough outer tunic of the eye and is comprised of dense connective tissue, which is derived embryonically from migrated neuroectodermal tissue. The middle layer, the uvea, comprises the iris, the ciliary body and the choroid. The innermost layer of the eye consists of the retina and the retinal pigment epithelium, both of which emerges embryologically from the tissue of the optic cup. Clinically, the eye is classified into the anterior and posterior segments, which are separated by the ciliary processes, the zonular fibers and the posterior lens capsule. Furthermore, there are three anatomical cavities defined in the eye; (1) the anterior chamber, between the cornea, iris and lens; (2) the posterior chamber, between the posterior surface of the iris, ciliary body, zonular fibers and the anterior lens capsule; and (3) the vitreous chamber (Fig. 1). The anatomy and physiology of the anterior segment are the most relevant for cataract surgery and are therefore the focus of this chapter.

Cornea

The cornea transitions into the sclera at the limbus, and sits like a watch glass over the rest of the globe due to its steeper curvature. The cornea begins to develop after the lens vesicle detaches from the ectoderm. A cell-free layer forms between the lens and the ectoderm, which later gives rise to the corneal epithelium. As the development progresses, neural crest-derived mesenchymal cells migrate into the space between ectoderm and lens vesicle and differentiate into the corneal

A. Ohlmann (✉)
Department of Ophthalmology, Ludwig Maximilian University of Munich, Munich, Germany
e-mail: andreas.ohlmann@med.uni-muenchen.de

M. Shajari et al. (eds.), *Cataract and Lens Surgery*,
https://doi.org/10.1007/978-3-031-05394-8_3

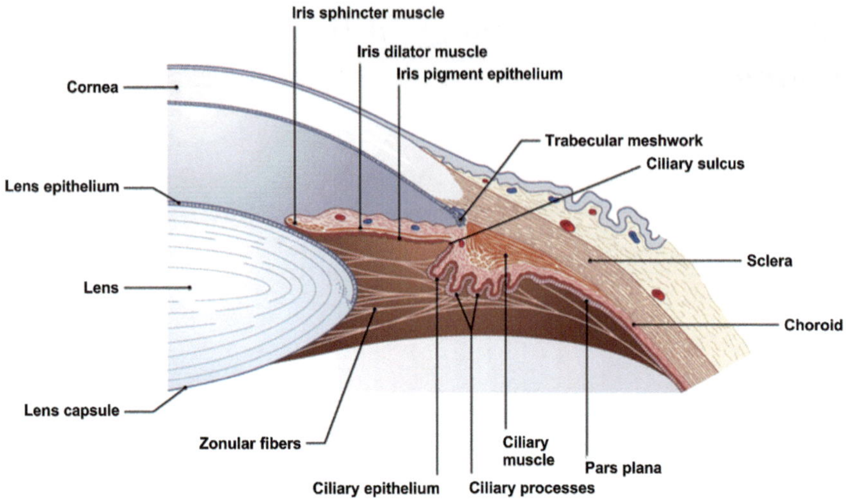

Fig. 1 Schematic drawing of the anterior eye segment, part of a horizontal section (modified from [1])

endothelium. In a second wave of migration, mesenchymal cells migrate between corneal epithelium and endothelium to develop into the corneal stroma.

Histologically, the cornea is composed of five different layers. The corneal epithelium, which is the outer layer of the cornea, is a non-keratinized stratified squamous epithelium. The epithelium is highly proliferative, but also has a short life-span of only about 6–7 days (Fig. 2a; [2]). The corneal epithelium is continuously regenerated by stem cells, which are located at the corneoscleral limbus, nourished by a dense limbal vessel plexus [3]. The acellular Bowman's membrane is located under the corneal epithelium, which connects the basal membrane of the epithelium to the corneal stroma (Fig. 2a). The layer beneath that, the corneal stroma, accounts for approximately 90% of the corneal thickness. It consists of keratocytes, collagen fibrils, proteoglycans and glycosaminoglycans, which are organized into extremely regular layers known as lamellae (Fig. 2a). Within these lamellae, the collagen fibrils, in contrast to the sclera, are aligned parallel to one another, which is a basic prerequisite for the transparency of the cornea. The collagen fibrils of each layer are arranged at right angles relative to fibers in adjacent lamellae, conferring a high degree of stability [4]. Proteoglycans are located between the individual layers, and have the same refractive index as the collagen fibrils, when water homeostasis is balanced. Keratocytes are the predominant cell type in the corneal stroma and are located between the collagen fibrils. Keratocytes are connected to each other via thin cellular processes thereby forming a functional syncytium. In 2013, Dua and colleagues described another corneal layer, which they termed the Dua's Layer, and described as being between the corneal stroma and the Descemet membrane [5]. The rationale for naming it as a new entity is that it shows some mechanical properties useful to know in corneal

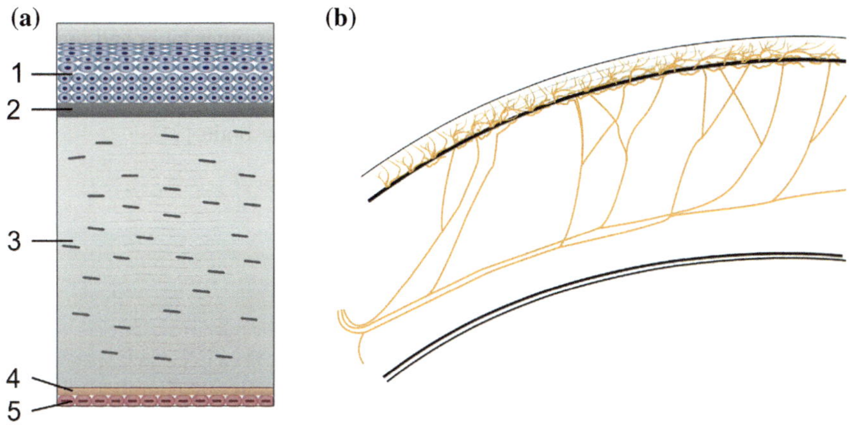

Fig. 2 **a** Schematic drawing of the cornea with the corneal epithelium (1), Bowman's membrane (2), the corneal stroma (3), Descemet membrane (4) and the corneal endothelium (5). **b** Schematic representation of corneal nerves and their plexus formation in the anterior human cornea

lamellar surgeries. Whether this is actually a separate corneal layer or just the innermost layer of the corneal stroma is still under discussion.

Note

The Descemet membrane is the strongest basal membrane in the body, which is formed by the endothelial cells of the cornea, and has a thickness of 7–10 μm in adults (Fig. 2a).

The next layer lining the corneal stroma is the Descemet membrane which itself is composed of 2 layers. The outer banded layer of the Descemet membrane is about 3 μm thick and is formed by corneal endothelial cells before birth. The inner non-banded layer is a homogeneous layer, which increases in thickness during life. In the periphery of the cornea, the Descemet membrane fuses with the trabecular meshwork at region known as the Schwalbe's line. The corneal endothelium is a single layer of flat, hexagonal cells, which maintain water homeostasis of the cornea via their Na^+/K^+-ATPase channels (Fig. 2a). Healthy adults have a corneal endothelial cell density of about 3000–4000 cells/mm^2 that decreases throughout life to 2600 cells/mm^2 in the eighth decade [4]. Even though the corneal endothelium has only a low regenerative potential, studies in recent years suggest that the corneal endothelium could have precursor cells at its transition zone to the trabecular meshwork [6].

The cornea is one of the most densely innervated tissues in the body. Corneal nerves arise from the ophthalmic nerve of the trigeminal nerve, which innervates the cornea via its long ciliary nerves of the nasociliary nerve. Approximately 70 nerve bundles enter the peripheral stroma of the cornea at the limbus and extend towards the central cornea (Fig. 2b). In the corneal stroma the nerves branch and extend to the anterior stroma to form the subepithelial nerve plexus beneath

Bowman's membrane (Fig. 2b). From there, nerve fibers penetrate Bowman's membrane and form the subbasal nerve plexus between its outer layer and the basal cells of the epithelium. From the subbasal nerve plexus, free nerve endings extend between epithelial cells, to release trophic molecules to maintain the homeostasis of the corneal epithelium and to transmit nociception to the brain [7].

Aqueous Humor Outflow

Keypoint

The trabecular meshwork is located in the angle of the anterior chamber which is formed by the iris and the cornea. The conventional outflow pathway of the aqueous humor drains approximately 85% of the aqueous humor via the trabecular meshwork into the Schlemm's canal. The remaining 15% of the aqueous humor exits the eye via the ciliary muscle, the supraciliary pathway and through the suprachoroidal space which are known as unconventional outflow pathways [8].

The trabecular meshwork extends circularly between the Schwalbe's line and the scleral spur, the ciliary muscle, and the outermost peripheral iris. From the inside out, the trabecular meshwork consists of three layers. The two inner parts are composed of a trabecular network and is arranged in a lamellar pattern. The uveal meshwork forms the innermost part, which consists of one to three layers, and extends between the proximal ciliary body and the Schwalbe's line (Fig. 3). The 8–15 trabecular lamellae of the corneoscleral part, which is adjacent to the uveal part, develop from the scleral spur and are thicker than the uveoscleral trabeculae (Fig. 3). The outermost, juxtacanalicular portion of the trabecular meshwork consists of a thin plate of loose connective tissue which lies directly over the endothelium of Schlemm's canal (Fig. 3; [9]). The lumen of Schlemm's canal is kept open, even when the intraocular pressure increases, via connections between the lamellae of the trabecular meshwork and the juxtacanalicular plate. Schlemm's canal is a circular endothelial tube that drains approximately 85% of the aqueous humor into the venous system of the sclera, episclera and conjunctiva via collector channels. The flow of the aqueous humor through the uveo- and corneoscleral trabecular meshwork has only a minor influence on outflow resistance of the chamber angle. The juxtacanalicular part of the trabecular meshwork provides most outflow resistance to the aqueous humor, which must diffuse through the loose extracellular matrix. From here, the aqueous humor passes through pores and transcellular channels of the endothelium of Schlemm's canal into its lumen [9].

In addition to the trabecular meshwork, the aqueous humor can be drained from the anterior chamber of the eye via the uveoscleral route. In this alternative route, the fluid enters the uvea, the ciliary body and the ciliary muscle via fissures, and drains into the venous system of choroid and sclera [10].

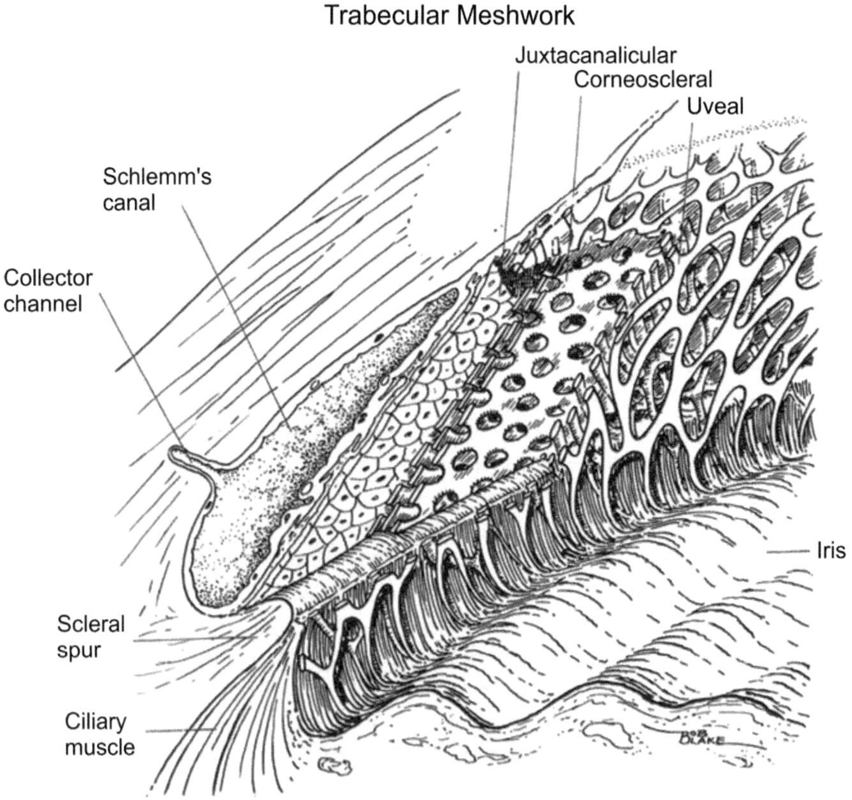

Fig. 3 The three layers of the trabecular meshwork (shown in a cutaway illustration): (1) uveal, (2) corneoscleral and (3) juxtacanalicular (modified from [11])

Iris

The iris inserts into the anterior part of the ciliary body and, together with the lens, separates the anterior from the posterior chamber. The inner edge of the iris defines the pupil, which can have a diameter of 0.5–9 mm [8].

The iris has two layers, the stroma and the pigment epithelium. The stroma consists of loose connective tissue, in which fine collagen bundles are arranged in a series of arcs, extending from the iris root to the pupil, to form a grid [2]. In addition to fibroblasts, the iris stromal layer contains melanocytes, which are largely located at the anterior surface. The pigment epithelium of the iris is composed of a double epithelial layer that arises from the anterior part of the optic cup. The anterior epithelial layer is a myoepithelium with long basal processes extending from the pupil to the iris root, like muscle fibers. These processes form the dilator muscle of the iris and receive sympathetic innervation. The posterior layer of the pigment epithelium is formed by cuboidal epithelial cells, which are densely loaded with pigment granules. The iris sphincter muscle is a ring of smooth muscle cells located at the pupillary border, which is predominantly innervated by the parasympathetic component of the oculomotor nerve. The vasculature of the iris is supplied by the long posterior and anterior ciliary arteries, which form the major arterial circle at the iris root. Radial vessels run from the major arterial circle to the pupil margin, where the minor arterial circle is formed.

Ciliary Body

The ciliary body is the anterior continuation of the choroid, the retina and the retinal pigment epithelium. Macroscopically, it can be subdivided into the anterior pars plicata with its approx. 70–80 ciliary processes and the posterior pars plana [2].

The inner surface of the ciliary body is covered with zonular fibers (fibers of Zinn), which have a longitudinal orientation in the pars plana. In the pars plicata, the zonular fibers insert between the ciliary processes and, together with the longitudinal fibers of the pars plana, extend towards the lens capsule. The ciliary processes themselves are free of zonular fibers and their primary function is to produce aqueous humor [12]. The anterior surface of the ciliary body and the posterior surface of the iris base form a circular groove, the ciliary sulcus (Fig. 1). The inner surface of the ciliary body is lined by two layers of epithelium; an unpigmented inner ciliary epithelium derived from the inner layer of the optic cup, and a pigmented outer epithelium that arises from the outer layer of the optic cup. Epithelial cells of the unpigmented ciliary epithelium are connected by apical tight junctions, which allow only molecules with a low-molecular weight to diffuse from the ciliary body into the aqueous humor (blood-aqueous barrier). Furthermore, the pigmented and unpigmented ciliary epithelium form a functional syncytium by gap junctions, located between the cells.

The ciliary muscle is a ring of smooth muscle cells, which is located beneath the anterior sclera. It is innervated by parasympathetic fibers of the oculomotor nerve. Within the ciliary muscle, three different fibers of muscle cells can be distinguished. On the outer side of the muscle, longitudinal fibers run parallel to the sclera in a V-shape from their base at the scleral spur into the choroid with their tip. On the inside, radial muscle fibers are attached to scleral spur, which also have a V-shape and insert with their tip at the base of the ciliary processes. The very innermost part of the ciliary muscle is formed by circular muscle fibers forming a sphincter-like ring muscle [13]. The ciliary muscle adjoins the base plate of the ciliary body, which consists of loose connective tissue with a large number of capillaries elongating into the processes of the ciliary body and elastic fibers which radiate into Bruch's membrane.

The aqueous is formed by the ciliary epithelium through active and passive secretion. Blood plasma is filtrated from the fenestrated capillaries into the stroma of the ciliary processes. Transport molecules of the two-layer ciliary epithelium secrete water-soluble substances, such as glucose molecules, into the posterior chamber of the eye creating an osmotic gradient and subsequent passively diffusing water into the posterior chamber. The secretion of aqueous humor is controlled by the sympathetic nervous system. Activation of β2-receptors increases the production of aqueous humor, whereas α2-activation reduces its secretion.

Lens

Keypoint

In adults, the biconvex lens has a smaller radius at the posterior lens surface (6.12–7.54 mm) than at the anterior surface (10.27–14.14 mm), and has an equatorial diameter of approximately 9 mm [8].

The development of the lens starts when the optic vesicle comes into contact with the embryonic ectoderm, inducing local proliferation and invagination of the epithelium (Fig. 4). As it grows, the lens placode translocates into the loose connective tissue of the eye cup and finally separates from the surface ectoderm. At this stage of development, the lens vesicle has an inner, cell-free cavity, and is known as the lens vesicle (Fig. 4). To fill this vesicle, the columnar epithelial cells of the posterior lens transform into lens fibers, and elongate towards the anterior lens surface, resulting in a homogeneous embryonic lens nucleus [14]. Crystalline proteins accumulate in the cytoplasm as well as the nucleus and most of the other cell organelles are removed, which improves the optical properties of the lens fibers [15].

As the lens continues to grow, the lens epithelial cells, located under the anterior lens capsule, proliferate and migrate to the equator of the lens, where they differentiate into elongated lens fibers. The lens fibers arrange themselves parallel to their

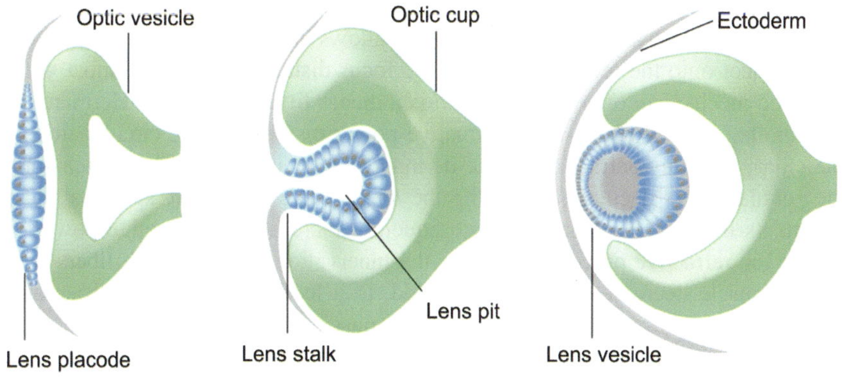

Fig. 4 The development of the optic vesicle is associated with the induction and the invagination of the lens placode towards the optic cup and subsequent the development of the lens vesicle (modified from [14])

longitudinal axis to form meridional rows extending from the anterior to the posterior pole. Lens fibers that do not have contact with the anterior or posterior pole, form tight interdigitating seams with their adjacent cells, which are known as Y-sutures [14]. The growth of the lens continues throughout life leading to an average increase in lens diameter of approximately 0.023 mm per year [8].

Keypoint

The lens epithelial cells and fibers are surrounded by the lens capsule, which anatomically represents a modified basement membrane. At the anterior pole and the equator, the lens capsule is significantly thicker (approx. 7–20 μm) and thus more stable than at the posterior pole of the lens (2–4 μm) [8].

Like the entire lens, the lens capsule also increases in thickness throughout life. In the posterior chamber, the lens is fixed via zonular fibers that radiate from the pars plicata of the ciliary body into the anterior and posterior lens capsule.

Lens Transparency and Accommodation

The major function of the lens is to project light onto the retina as sharply as possible. Transparency is an essential to accomplish this function, and this is achieved by various mechanisms. In the lens fibers, many of the intracellular organelles, such as the cell nucleus and endoplasmic reticulum, are lost during differentiation to avoid aberrations. The cytoplasm of the lens fibers is highly enriched with proteins, which consist predominately of crystallines, to keep the refractive index of the lens stable. The parallel arrangement of the lens fibers and the very close juxtaposition of their cell membranes contribute to reduce aberrations of light as well [15].

The lens can change its radius of curvature, which changes its refractive power in a process known as accommodation. This allows the lens to project a clear image of an object onto the retina even when the focus distance varies. The most widely accepted mechanism of accommodation is a theory first proposed by Hermann von Helmholtz [16]. To increase the refractive power of the lens, the circular fibers of the ciliary muscle contract to reduce its inner diameter. As a result, the tension of the zonular fibers decreases, allowing the lens to take on a more spherical shape, due to its inherent elasticity, and subsequently increases its refractive power. To reduce the refractive power of the lens, the innervation of the circular fibers of the ciliary muscle decreases. Elastic fibers and, to a lesser extent, the contraction of radially arranged muscle fibers of the ciliary muscle pull the circular part outwards, causing the zonular fibers to be tensioned, and thus flattening the lens. The range of accommodation is about 14 diopters between the ages of 10 and 19 and decreases continuously throughout life [8].

References

1. Zilles K, Tillmann BN. Anatomie. Berlin Heidelberg: Springer-Verlag; 2010.
2. Rohen JW. Morphologie und Embryologie des Sehorgans. In: FJuH F, editor. Augenheilkunde in Klinik und Praxis. Stuttgart Thieme; 1977.
3. Li W, Hayashida Y, Chen YT, Tseng SC. Niche regulation of corneal epithelial stem cells at the limbus. Cell Res. 2007;17(1):26–36.
4. DelMonte DW, Kim T. Anatomy and physiology of the cornea. J Cataract Refract Surg. 2011;37(3):588–98.
5. Dua HS, Faraj LA, Said DG, Gray T, Lowe J. Human corneal anatomy redefined: a novel pre-Descemet's layer (Dua's layer). Ophthalmology. 2013;120(9):1778–85.
6. Van den Bogerd B, Dhubhghaill SN, Koppen C, Tassignon MJ, Zakaria N. A review of the evidence for in vivo corneal endothelial regeneration. Surv Ophthalmol. 2018;63(2):149–65.
7. Marfurt CF, Cox J, Deek S, Dvorscak L. Anatomy of the human corneal innervation. Exp Eye Res. 2010;90(4):478–92.
8. Bergua A. Das menschliche Auge in Zahlen. Berlin, Heidelberg: Springer; 2017.
9. Tamm ER. The trabecular meshwork outflow pathways: structural and functional aspects. Exp Eye Res. 2009;88(4):648–55.
10. Johnson M, McLaren JW, Overby DR. Unconventional aqueous humor outflow: a review. Exp Eye Res. 2017;158:94–111.
11. Shields MB, Krieglstein GK. Glaukom. Grundlagen, Differentialdiagnose, Therapie. Springer-Verlag Berlin Heidelberg; 1993.
12. Tamm ER, Lutjen-Drecoll E. Ciliary body. Microsc Res Tech. 1996;33(5):390–439.
13. Remington LA. Clinical anatomy and physiology of the visual system. Edition r: Elsevier Inc.; 2012.
14. Tamm ER, Ohlmann A. Development of the human eye. Ophthalmologe. 2012;109(9):911–28.
15. Hejtmancik JF, Shiels A. Overview of the lens. Prog Mol Biol Transl Sci. 2015;134:119–27.
16. Helmholtz H. Ueber die Accommodation des Auges. Archiv für Ophthalmologie. 1855;1 (2):1–74.

Cataract Forms and Grading

Christopher Wirbelauer

Cataract Types

Partial or complete opacification of the lens is called cataract and can be diagnosed at the slit lamp (Fig. 1). Cataract can be congenital (approx. 1%) or acquired (approx. 99%). Age-related (senile) cataracts are the most frequent cause of acquired lens opacities.

For a better understanding of lens opacities, the anatomical structure and physiological processes are important [1]. The crystalline lens is enclosed in a lens capsule, which is affixed to the ciliary body by the zonula fibres. Once embryonic development completes, this remains a closed space. The anterior lens capsule, which is about 15 µm thick, is lined by a single-layered cubic lens epithelium. The lens epithelial cells divide in the area of the lens equator, where they gradually migrate posteriorly along the posterior lens capsule, which is about 5 µm thick, transforming into elongated lens fibres, and gradually losing the cellular nucleus. These lens fibres form the majority of the lens substance. New fibre cells are deposited in concentric layers, so that the oldest lens fibres are found in the lens core and the youngest in the cortex. This unopposed growth continues throughout life and the lens becomes increasingly dense as the lens fibres in the nucleus increase and the lens becomes increasingly cloudy (Fig. 2).

The lens has multiple functions; it forms part of the dioptric apparatus (about 15–20 diopters), provides accommodation for near vision, and filters ultraviolet radiation (280–400 nm). The lens also separates the anterior and posterior segments of the eye.

All diseases of the lens lead to a more or less pronounced cataract. Risk factors for lens clouding include age, gender, family history, photooxidative stress caused by UV radiation (sunlight exposure), metabolic disorders, nutritional conditions,

C. Wirbelauer (✉)
Augenklinik Berlin-Marzahn GmbH, Berlin, Germany
e-mail: ch.wirbelauer@augenklinik-berlin.de

M. Shajari et al. (eds.), *Cataract and Lens Surgery*,
https://doi.org/10.1007/978-3-031-05394-8_4

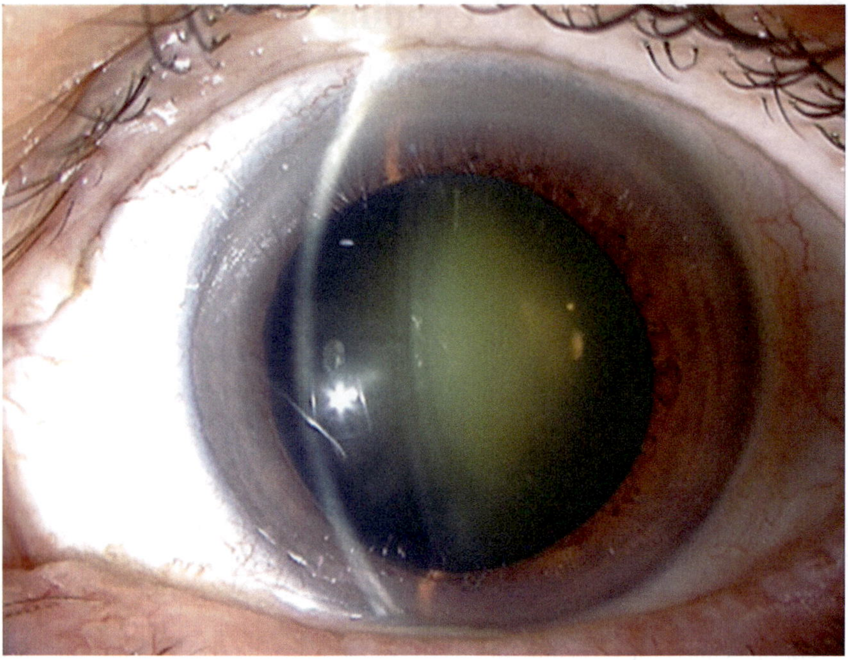

Fig. 1 Nuclear sclerosis in Cat. nuclearis. This form of cataract is very common and can lead to myopia by increasing the central refractive power

alcohol consumption, diabetes mellitus, deficiency of essential amino acids, medications and increased dehydration [1, 2].

The typical symptoms of cataract are a gradual decrease in visual acuity, glare, decrease in contrast vision and monocular double vision [3]. Colour perception may be reduced due to the deposition of chromophores causing a filter effect.

Cataract forms can be classified according to different systems:

(A) temporal occurrence/age (congenital, postnatal, juvenile, senile)
(B) anatomical (nuclear, cortical, subcapsular)
(C) extent (beginning, mature)
(D) etiological (see Table 1 for causes).

(A) Classification of cataract according to age of onset

- congenital—at birth
- postnatal—in the first years of life
- juvenileuntil the age of 30
- senile—all forms associated with increasing age.

In congenital cataracts, heredity and embryonic developmental disorders play the most important role (accounting for approx. 30%) and are usually diagnosed by

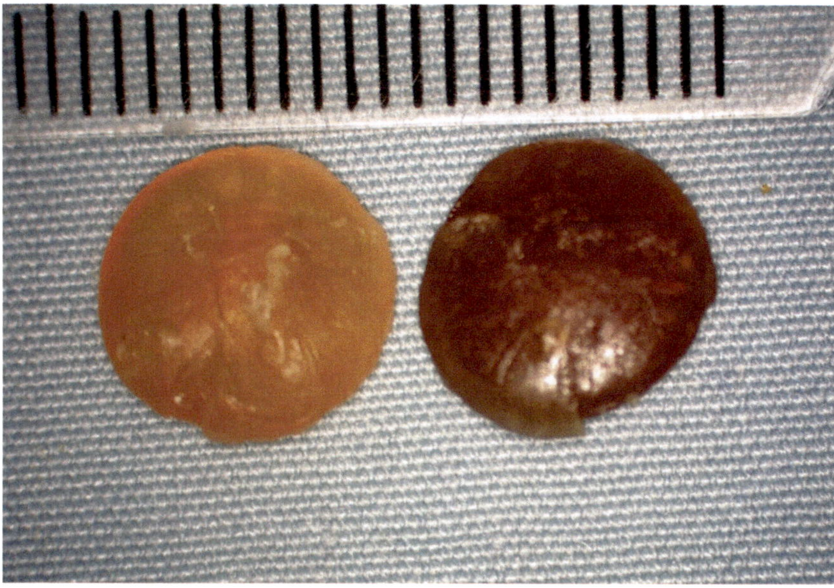

Fig. 2 Brownish discolouration of the lens with increasing clouding. The strong compression in the lens core leads to an increase in the hardness of the lens. These lenses were taken during manual ECCE (left: yellowish-brownish, right: brownish-reddish clouding of the lens)

detecting a leukocoria at screening examinations. Chromosomal causes, as in trisomy 21, and metabolic causes should also be considered (see Table 1). In galactosemia, vacuolisation and swelling of the subcapsular lens fibres occur in the first months of life and are reversible by a diet low in galactose. Furthermore, intrauterine infections, especially in the first 3 months of pregnancy in cases of rubella or toxoplasmosis, are also significant causes of cataract. Rubella infection used to cause cataract more frequently, before the widespread protection by vaccination, as an infection in the first 4 weeks of pregnancy can lead to unilateral or bilateral cataract in up to 50% of cases.

Examples of a congenital cataract are the cataract zonularis/pulverulenta where the clouding of the lens is particularly prominent in the embryonic nucleus (Fig. 3). This risk of severe visual impairment is high due to the dominant heredity and risk of amblyopia (particularly if the cataract is unilateral). Typically, visual acuity improves if the pupil is wide. The more frequent anterior polar cataract is characterized by a central, focal opacity due to a degeneration of the pupillary membrane. A rarer form is the posterior polar cataract (autosomal dominant) with a severe opacity on the rear surface of the lens caused. This is caused by an incomplete regression of the embryonic vitreous vessels (Vasa hyaloidea) or the persistent hyperplastic primary vitreous (PHPV) [1]. Since in many cases the posterior capsule is also defective, there is an increased risk of capsule rupture during cataract surgery in these patients.

Table 1 Rare causes of cataract development

Causes	Type	Features
General	Tetanus	Due to calcium deficiency in hypoparathyroidism occurrence of subcapsular point clouding and radial streaks of the (layered cataract)
	Myotonic dystrophy (Curschmann-Steinert)	Autosomal dominant, dot-like, coloured and white turbidities in the middle cortex, radial spokes, crystallization, rosette figure of the posterior cortex
	Skin diseases (Cat. syndermatotica)	Posterior shell opacity as capsule epithelial cataract in chronic neurodermatitis, more rarely in scleroderma
Metabolism	Diabetes	In type 1 diabetics, there is posterior subcapsular opacity due to metabolic disorders, myopic refraction changes in hyperglycaemia is possible, osmotic changes due to accumulation of sorbitol
	Galactosemia	Galactokinase deficiency, deep posterior cortical opacity due to accumulation of galactite, regression through galactose-free diet
	Wilson's disease	Autosomal recessive, hepatolenticular degeneration in copper storage disease, sunflower cataract due to granular copper deposits in the central lens capsule
Medications	Cortisone	Posterior subcapsular clouding, cataractogenic >10 mg/day for 1 year
Injuries	Siderosis	Brownish opacities due to rust formation (oxidation) of a ferrous intraocular foreign body
	Chalcosis	Sunflower cataract due to greenish intracapsular copper deposits
	Acid-alkaline burns	Different forms of opacities until the lens becomes completely cloudy
Environmental factors	Infrared light	Thermal damage, glass-blowing cataract with fire lamella (true exfoliation on the anterior lens capsule)
	X-rays	Critical dose >2–6 Gy with damage to the epithelium at the equator, clouding of the cortex near the posterior pole after 1–2 years
	Electricity	Vacuoles, axial opacification, anterior, subcapsular

(continued)

Table 1 (continued)

Causes	Type	Features
Syndromes	Down syndrome (trisomy 21)	Cataracta coerulea with flaky cloudiness at the cortex in the equatorial region leads to blue-green colour iridescence
	Patau syndrome (trisomy 13)	Severe ocular malformations with complete opacity of the lens, microphthalmia and coloboma of the uvea
	Alport syndrome	Autosomal dominant, spherophakia due to missing zonula fibres, anterior lenticonus
	Lowe syndrome	X-chromosomal recessive, mikrophakia with small platelike, flattened lens without differentiation of cortex and nucleus (1 mm thickness, 5 mm diameter)
	Fabry disease	Alpha-galactosidase defect, accumulation of glycosphingolipids, Cornea verticillata
Congenital	Coloboma	Indentation at the lens equator inferonasally, missing zonula fibres in this area, usually combined with other coloboma forms of the eye (iris, choroid)
	Spherophakia	
	Microphakia	Lens diameter is reduced and lens thickness increased (spherical lens), refractive myopia, luxation into the pupil with secondary angle block glaucoma (see Weill-Marchesani syndrome)
	Lenticonus/ lentiglobus	Bulging of the anterior or posterior lens pole

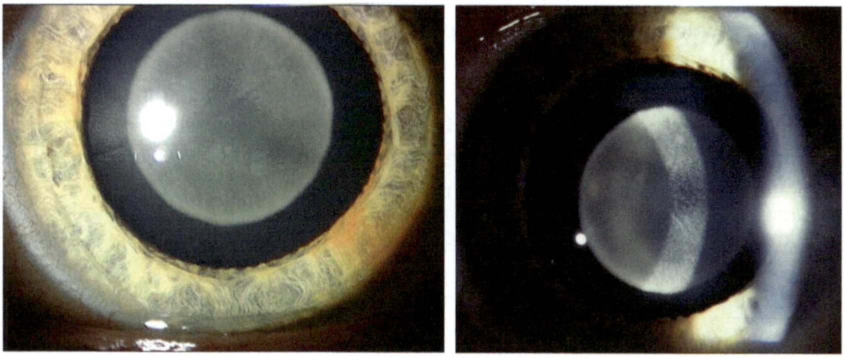

Fig. 3 Cataracta pulverulenta (zonularis) with fine dusty and dot-like opacities and the danger of amblyopia

The most frequent lens opacity in acquired cataracts is the age-related cataract (Cataracta senilis). The development of this form of cataract is multifactorial and can be observed in 5% of patients at 70 years of age increasing to 10% at an age of 80 years. Clouding of the lens in associated with systemic conditions occurs particularly in diabetes mellitus and neurodermatitis. Due to the common embryonic origin of skin and lens from the surface ectoderm, the lens is involved in many dermatological diseases. Iritis/uveitis also leads to a cataract more frequently. Drug-induced cataract occurs mainly during high-dose topical or systemic cortisone therapy. Finally, ocular trauma can also cause cataract.

Note

All diseases of the lens lead to cataract.

(B) Anatomical classification of the cataract

The type of opacity can be assessed using the slit lamp:

- Nuclear opacity (nuclearis) is caused by an increase in the number of lens fibres within the lens, resulting in a significant increase in protein content of up to 30% (Fig. 1). The nuclear opacity leads to a myopic and near vision may again be possible without reading glasses "second sight of the elderly". However, this can be accompanied by monocular double vision and visual acuity may improve at night due to mydriasis.
- Cortical opacity (corticalis) occurs due to wedge-shaped opacities along the lens fibres caused by constant movement during accommodation. Progression is slow in these cases and the symptoms include blurred vision and monocular diplopia. —In posterior subcapsular opacity (subcapsularis posterior), fibrous metaplasia of the lens cells occurs as a result of disturbance in the transformation of the lens fibres from the equatorial zone, i.e. due to metabolic disorders. Rapid progression can occur in these cases and causes severe glare. Near vision in these cases is typically worse than far vision. This form of cataract is common with general diseases, such as diabetes, neurodermatitis and with cortisone therapy.
- Cataracta coronaria (wreath-shaped cataract) with cortical clouding of the cortex
- Cataract coerulea (Blue-dot cataract) with wreath-shaped aquamarine turbidities
- Christmas tree cataract is characterised by colourful, iridescent crystalline clouding due to the inclusion of cholesterol crystals.

(C) Developmental stages of lens opacities

- Cat. incipiens: beginning opacity individual layers.
- Cat. provecta: advanced lens opacity with the indication for cataract surgery
- Cat. intumescens: rapid clouding due to fluid absorption and volume increase, especially in the cortex area with the risk of phacolytic glaucoma if lens proteins escape the capsule.
- Cat. immatura: combination of different anatomical lens opacities (see above).

- Cat. matura: complete opacity of the lens. The lens may be whitish (nivea), brownish (brunescens), reddish (rubra), or black (nigra) in colour (Fig. 2). This classification makes it possible to estimate the hardness of the lens, which can make it difficult to break up the nucleus with phacoemulsification. In cataracta nivea there is often increased intracapsular pressure due to an incipient liquefaction of the lens material with the risk of spontaneous tearing of the entire lens capsule or during capsulorhexis (so-called "Argentinian flag sign").
- Cat. hypermatura (Cat. Morgagni): the lens material is partially liquefied, and the lens core has sunken into the capsular bag, with the risk of phacolytic glaucoma due to tearing of the lens capsule.

(D) Etiological classification of cataract

Although there are many causes for lens opacities, they are particularly common in metabolic disorders (see Table 1).

Cataracta complicata refers to a clouding of the eye lens as a result of intraocular disease or eye surgery, caused by proliferation of lens epithelial cells on the posterior capsule. The most common are anterior uveitis without/with posterior synechia, myopia, and hereditary vitreoretinal diseases, such as retinopathy pigmentosa or untreated retinal detachment. The most common operations are filtrating glaucoma surgery or pars plana vitrectomy, which leads to clouding of the lens in 80–90% of patients in the first 2 years postoperatively.

Other causes of lens opacification occur after injuries (cat. traumatica). Opacities can occur due to blunt trauma (contusio bulbi) in the form of a contusion rosette (Fig. 4a) or opacities in the area of intraocular injuries due to fibrous metaplasia of the lens epithelium. In these cases, the epithelium can be stimulated to unspecific proliferation. These opacities may be partial or complete, and may be associated with swelling of the lens in various degrees with a dangerous increase in intraocular pressure. Occasionally, an intracapsular metallic foreign body can be observed

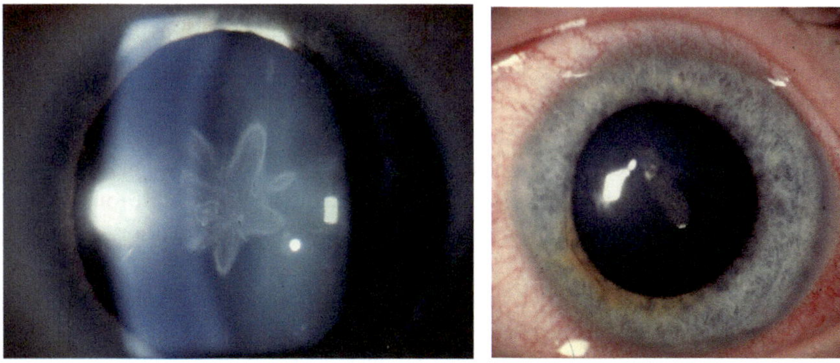

a) b)

Fig. 4 Cat. traumatica with a contusion rosette (**a**) and intracapsular metallic foreign body (**b**)

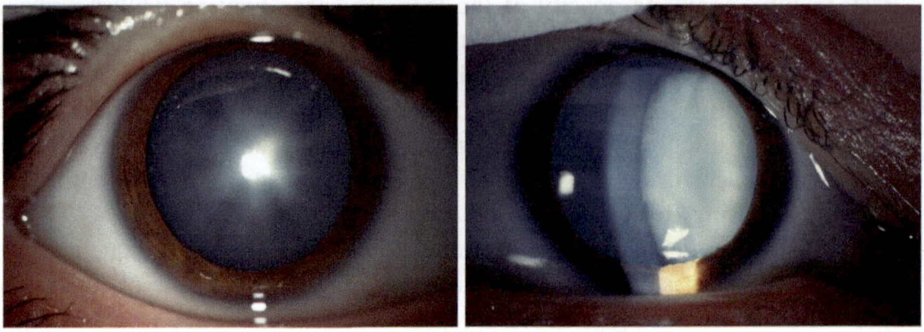

Fig. 5 Cat. electrica with complete opacity of the lens after a high-voltage accident while "surfing the suburban railway"

during slit-lamp examination (Fig. 4b). High-voltage accidents can also lead to a complete opacification of the lens (Fig. 5).

Other eye pathologies

Changes in the shape of the lens (coloboma, spherophakia, microphakia, lenticonus/lentiglobus) are usually due to embryonic malformations (see also Table 1). These can occur as an isolated anomaly or as a result of genetic defects (trisomy 13) or after intrauterine rubella infection in the first months of pregnancy.

Luxations of the lens

In the case of luxations or subluxations of the lens, a lens tremor (lentodonesis) and/or iris tremor (iridodonesis) is noticeable during slit-lamp examination with small eye movements. Typically, monocular double vision is caused by a displacement of the lens edge in the pupil. Causes of lens luxation include aplasias of the zonula fibres, which can be isolated or diffuse. Hereditary causes include Marfan syndrome (autosomal dominant) with typical segmental zonula defects inferiorly, leading to a superotemporal subluxation of the lens. Conversely, in homocystinuria (autosomal recessive/autosomal dominant) the progressive degeneration of the entire zonular apparatus due to cysteine inclusions leads to inferonasal luxation of the lens. Finally, in Weill-Marchesani syndrome (autosomal recessive, cystathionine synthetase decreased) we see a progressive degeneration and elongation of the zonular fibres with anterior and inferior dislocation, which is also associated with microspherophakia. Acquired causes include traumatic damage to the zonular fibres, and high myopia, usually due to diffuse zonular weakness. In the case of complete dislocation from its normal position, the lens may shift to the anterior chamber or drop into the vitreous.

Note

In disorders of the zonula fibers cataract surgery is significantly more difficult.

Pseudoexfoliation syndrome (PEX), is a generalised degenerative process of the extracellular matrix, and can also lead to instability of the suspension apparatus through focal infiltration of the zonula fibres [1]. The presence of PEX at an older age can be easily detected at the slit lamp by the typical circular, whitish deposits of a fine fibrillar protein on the edge of the iris and anterior lens capsule.

Grading of Cataracts

A clinical assessment of lens opacity (grading) is important to document prior to surgery. This is usually carried out at the slit lamp but can be influenced by subjective bias from the examiner observations. In clinical trials, objective assessment methods are preferred to the examiner's own opinions to better classify the patient's symptoms of visual deterioration, glare and double vision.

Since cataracts cause opacity and increased light scattering resulting from disturbed fibre architecture and/or spatial arrangement of protein molecules in the fibre cells [1], a systematic assessment of lens opacity (lens opacity classification system, LOCS) was been proposed [4]. The LOCS-III system can be performed at the slit lamp or by using standardised photographs and has proven particularly useful for scientific comparisons [4, 5]. In this system, three forms of opacification are divided into 5–6 stages and subjectively assessed using a classification system. A distinction is made between opacification of the nucleus (nuclear), the cortex (cortical) and the posterior lens (subcapsular). In the case of nuclear opacities, the extent of the opacity (opalescence) and the colour intensity (colour) are also subdivided.

The further development of imaging techniques has also been useful in the assessment of lens opacity. Optical methods based on the Scheimpflug principle, aberrometry (double-pass technique) and optical coherence tomography (OCT) have all been applied to the problem of objective quantification of lens opacity.

Scheimpflug based imaging techniques use a blue-light emitting diode to display the anterior segments of the eye [6]. With the "Pentacam nucleus staging" (PNS) a cataract classification in steps from 0 (without opacity) to 5 (complete lens opacity) and a lens density from 0 to 100% have been described. A lens density greater than 11% and a PNS greater than 1 are regarded as limits for cataract classification.

Aberrometry involves projecting an infrared laser beam into the eye and recording the light scattering by a camera [7]. In this double-pass technique, an "ocular scatter index" (OSI) is determined, where a higher light scatter of >1 OSI indicates a cataract with a decrease in visual acuity.

Optical coherence tomography (OCT) imaging systems have been applied to examine lens density using both spectral-domain (SD) and swept-source (SS) techniques. Lens density was determined using the older SD-OCT but this has been superseded by automated lens densitometry using SS-OCT (IOL-Master 700, Zeiss) [8, 9]. With the "average lens densitometry" (ALD) a greyscale analysis of the image data points (pixels) can be performed. A higher intensity of the light reflections in the data points was associated with a higher cataract density. A value of >74 units (pixel units) combined with a decrease in visual acuity showed a high sensitivity and specificity for cataract [9].

All methods were reproducible and reliable, but a good agreement with clinical cataract findings was not always seen. However, there was a clear improvement compared over the error-prone photo documentation. In general, the density measurement was more reliable, as the different colouring is not a good indicator of lens opacity, which has been clinically confirmed over time.

In summary, the clinical classification of lens opacity coupled with the typical symptoms is still the cornerstone for the preoperative examination of cataract. The standardised classification procedures (LOCS-III) or the newer imaging techniques can further add to the objectification of the cataract and can be useful in both clinical decision making and scientific comparisons. In the future, lens densitometry could be integrated into optical biometric devices for IOL calculation.

References

1. Schlötzer-Schrehardt U, Naumann GOH. Linse. In: Naumann GOH, editor. Pathologie des Auges. Berlin: Springer; 1997. p. 849–954.
2. Grehn F. Augenheilkunde. 32nd ed. Berlin: Springer-Verlag; 2019. p. 197–227.
3. Auffarth GU, Dick HB. Kataraktchirurgie. In: Augustin AJ, editor. Augenheilkunde. 4th ed. Heidelberg: Kaden-Verlag; 2019. p. 745–71.
4. Chylack LT, Wolfe JK, Singer DM, et al. The lens opacities classification system III. Arch Ophthalmol. 1993;111:831–6.
5. Leske MC, Chylack LT, He Q, et al. Incidence and progression of cortical and posterior subcapsular opacities. Ophthalmololgy. 1997;104:1987–93.
6. Grewal DS, Brar GS, Grewal SP. Correlation of nuclear cataract lens density using Scheimpflug images with lens opacities classification system III and visual function. Ophthalmology. 2009;116:1436–43.
7. Martínez-Roda JA, Vilaseca M, Ondategui JC, et al. Double-pass technique and compensation-comparison method in eyes with cataract. J Cataract Refract Surg. 2016;42:1461–9.
8. Brás JEG, Sickenberger W, Hirnschall N, Findl O. Cataract quantification using swept-source optical coherence tomography. J Cataract Refract Surg. 2019;44:1478–81.
9. Panthier C, de Wazieres A, Rouger H, Moran S, Saad A, Gatinel D. Average lens density quantification with swept-source optical coherence tomography: optimized, automated cataract grading technique. J Cataract Refract Surg. 2019;45:1746–52.

Optical Principles

Kerstin Petermann and Lisa Hinzelmann

Light is an electromagnetic radiation. It can be perceived by the human eye in the range of 380–780 nm. It has properties of both particles and waves and it's dual character becomes easier to understand when looking at the human eye. Light is refracted at the cornea and lens where it acts as a wave. When reaching the retina however, it acts as a particle, a photon, which activates the photoreceptor layer and leads to a biochemical reaction that ultimately results in light perception.

Radiation Optics or Geometrical Optics (GO)

The description of imaging, i.e. the projection of an object point to an image point by means of an optical system, is done in Geometrical Optics (GO) via a simplified notion of light rays, which in turn are the normals of the wave fronts. These are unaffected by diffraction, and propagate in homogeneous media with the same refractive index termed n. The refractive index n is defined as the speed of light in vacuum divided by the speed of light in the medium. For the representation of the imaging ratios, a theoretically, infinitely small space around the optical axis is assumed. In this paraxial Gaussian space, the actually thick lens is simplified to a thin lens with infinitely large radius. The optical axis of imaging systems runs in the GO always as a straight line through the center of curvature. In the eye, this assumption no longer applies, since the center of curvature of the cornea and the

K. Petermann (✉) · L. Hinzelmann
Department of Ophthalmology, Goethe-University, Frankfurt, Germany
e-mail: kerstin.petermann@kgu.de

L. Hinzelmann
e-mail: lisa.hinzelmann@kgu.de

M. Shajari et al. (eds.), *Cataract and Lens Surgery*,
https://doi.org/10.1007/978-3-031-05394-8_5

front and back surfaces of the lens are not located on a straight line. Therefore, only an approximate determination of the optical axis and the application of the optical laws can be made.

Refraction

When light passes between media of different densities, there is a change of direction, which is known as refraction. Refraction always occurs towards the incidence slot of the optically denser medium (Snell's law of refraction).

In order to distribute the incident light to different focal points, a refractive optical system, such as the intraocular lens, either consists of zones with different refractive indices or a surface with different radii of curvature that merge smoothly into one another. In the ocular system, the incident light is projected onto the retina as an image point by changing the refractive power of the natural lens.

Refractive Power D

The refractive power D is defined as the reciprocal of the focal length f and is expressed in diopter [D, dpt], which corresponds to m^{-1}.

$$D = \frac{1}{f}$$

At optically interfaces in paraxial space, the refractive power is calculated from the ratio of the refractive indices (n) of medium 1 in front of the interface (n_1) and medium 2 behind the interface (n_2) as well as the angle of incidence of the light, which in the case of lenses results from the given radius of curvature (r).

$$D = \frac{n_2 - n_1}{r}$$

The refractive index depends on the speed of light as it varies in different media. For the cornea, a refractive index of $n = 1.3672$ is most frequently used but as the cornea is a human tissue there is no standardized n. It is important to acknowledge this fact when working with different devices as they might use different values for n. An adjustment is therefore necessary when using keratometry values of different devices.

Aberration

Aberrations (lat. aberratio meaning deviation) occur outside of paraxial space and depend on the wavelength of light. They prevent a complete unification of rays radiating from the object point into the conjugate image point and impair a true-to-scale, true-color image. A distinction must be made between chromatic aberrations, which are caused by the wavelength dependence of the refractive index, and monochromatic aberrations, in which only one wavelength is considered.

Chromatic aberration occurs because, in most media, short-wavelength light is slowed down more than long-wavelength light, meaning that long-wavelength (red; 640–780 nm) light is refracted less than short-wavelength (blue; 430–490 nm) light. As a result, light is separated and becomes visible in its spectral colors.

Monochromatic aberrations are again divided into lower-order aberrations (spherical and astigmatism) and higher-order aberrations (for example coma, spherical aberration, secondary astigmatism). Lower-order aberrations can be corrected by spectacle lenses which higher-order aberrations cannot.

For refractive procedures and lens surgery, spherical aberration, coma, and astigmatism of oblique bundles are particularly important, as they can significantly influence the image quality (Fig. 1).

One of the most influential higher-order aberrations on image quality is *spherical aberration* (SA). As the height of incidence of a parallel incident light beam increases, the angle of incidence changes. Rays far from the axis are refracted more strongly (positive SA) or more weakly (negative SA) than rays close to the axis, resulting in a circle of confusion instead of a sharp image point. The larger the

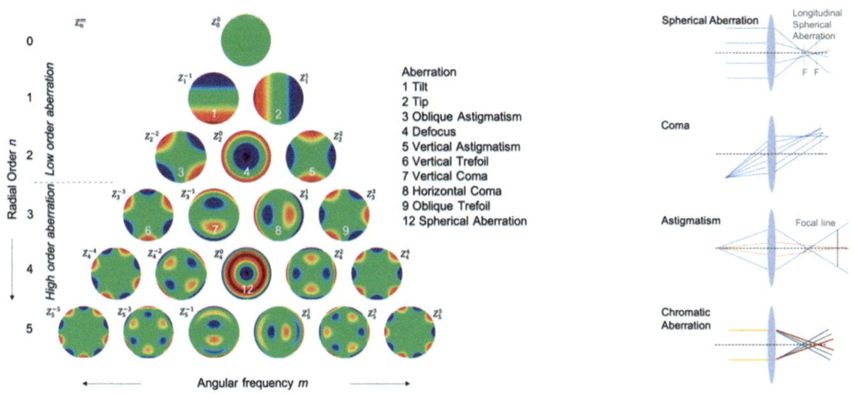

Fig. 1 Representation of the imaging errors: schematically on the right and as Zernike polynomials up to 5th order on the left. The values are given as Z_n^m, where m is the meridional frequency (number of oscillations when orbiting the center) and n is the radial (Zernike) order. With increasing order, the influence on the quality of vision decreases

aperture of the incident beam, the greater the effect of spherical aberration. Aspherical lenses can counteract this as they provide a different radius peripherally than centrally. They can also be used simultaneously to focus an extended depth of field. Their effectiveness here is highly dependent on pupil size and centration of the intraocular implant in the capsular bag.

Coma is perhaps the second most important of the higher order aberrations. It arises at object points that do not lie on the optical axis as an image-side ray bundle with a comet-tail-like, asymmetrical appearance. It is the asymmetric portion of the image superimposed with spherical aberration. Coma is especially seen in eyes with keratoconus, corneal scars after keratoplasty, radial keratotomy or decentered excimer ablation. In astigmatism of oblique bundles, the object point is also located outside of the optical axis and is imaged in two perpendicular image areas, for example due to tilted optics or oblique incident light.

Wave Optics

Light is described in wave optics by a transverse wave with wavelength, amplitude and phase. Since light is an electromagnetic wave, the model of geometrical optics cannot explain all effects. A wave arises when a locally occurring oscillation continues via the coupling of neighboring boundary elements.

Diffraction and Interference

When a wave is deflected by an obstacle, diffraction occurs and new waves are created. The wave can also spread behind the obstacle. According to the Huygens–Fresnel principle, every point of the wave front is a starting point for a new elementary wave. If the oscillations of several waves overlap at a single point, interferences occur. Interference between different elementary waves results in intensity distribution of diffraction, as the amplitudes are enhanced or cancelled. Interference distributions of light can be used to create multifocal optics. In this process, concentric rings with different step heights and distances from each other act on as phase gratings on the intraocular lenses for diffraction of the incident light rays. The light is focused to different focal points for distance, intermediate, and near, with some of the light lost as scattered light. Diffractive systems act independently of the aperture and as a results are not pupil-dependent.

Zernike Polynomials

The description of a wavefront and its aberrations is often done by using Zernike polynomials (Fig. 1). This is a set of polynomials defined on a unit circle. Each polynomial describes the characteristic shape of the error component, and together they represent the total wavefront error. Using polar coordinates, the polynomials result as the product of the angular function and radial polynomials. An infinite number of Zernike polynomials can be used to describe higher order aberration. For the eye, however, only the first twenty (thus up to the 5th order) are really clinically relevant. Aberrations of the 1st and 2nd order are correctable with spectacle lenses and as mentioned previously are often called aberrations of lower order. Accordingly, all aberrations of the 3rd order and higher, such as coma, spherical aberration and trefoil, are considered higher order aberrations.

Lens Design

A greater understanding of these optical principles have resulted in Intraocular lenses (IOL) becoming available in different optical designs. They differ in the number of focal points and the surface progression. The breakdown of lens options can be described as follows: spherical, aspheric and toric mono- and multifocal lenses. Multifocal lenses can be additionally differentiated into rotationally symmetrical refractive or diffractive lenses.

Intraocular lenses are implanted as part of cataract surgery or refractive lens exchange in the capsular bag and replace the natural lens or as a phakic lens in addition to the natural lens. They refract the incident light in one or more focal points.

Monofocal intraocular lenses correct the spherical equivalent (lower order aberrations) and refract the incident light so that it is imaged onto a single focal point. The postoperative target refraction can be set to either distance, intermediate, or near. For example, if distance is selected, the patient will require spectacles lenses for the intermediate and near ranges.

Aspheric intraocular lenses are modified and correct the spherical aberration of the eye. By correcting the aberration, better vision is made possible, especially in twilight when the pupil is wider. The wider the pupil the more of the corneal spherical aberrations influence the image so aspheric lenses can mitigate this effect.

Toric intraocular lenses are used to correct astigmatic eyes. These correct the corneal radii, which are strongly curved at different angles to each other, and thus reproduce the incident light in a pixel on the retina. Toric lenses are available as monofocal or multifocal lenses.

Multifocal IOLs are usually rotationally symmetric and use refractive and/or diffractive optics to image objects at different distances on the retina.

Bibliography

1. Bass M, Decusatis C, Enoch JM et al. Handbook of optics, third edition volume I: geometrical and physical optics, polarized light, components and instruments. New York: McGraw-Hill, Inc;2009.
2. Haferkorn H. Optik: Physikalisch-technische Grundlagen und Anwendungen. Hoboken: Wiley;2008.
3. Hecht E. Optics, global edition, 5th ed. Harlow: Pearson Education Limited;2017.
4. Liftin G. Technische Optik in der Praxis, 3. aktualisierte und erweiterte Aufl. Berlin: Springer Berlin Heidelberg;2005.
5. Velzel C. A course in lens design. Dordrecht: Springer;2014.
6. Yanoff M, Duker J. Ophthalmology. 5th ed. Philadelphia: Mosby, Elsevier;2019.

Digitalization in Lens Surgery

Wolfgang J. Mayer

Introduction

Like all branches of medicine, ophthalmology is seeing more are more digitalization taking place. This can be seen in the increasing adoption of electronic patient records (EMR), the field of diagnostics with management of imaging data, and in the field of research where we are seeing more applications of machine learning and artificial intelligence to reduce to workload and improve accuracy of the clinicians., In ophthalmic surgery, and in lens surgery in particular, digital assistance systems are now helping surgeons to perform surgical steps with greater accuracy and patient safety [1–4].

Digital Working Environment

One prerequisite for a digital working environment is the EMR. Many companies now offer software solutions for this purpose [5, 6]. When choosing an EMR software option it is very important not only to ensure the security and integration of a digital software module in the clinical workflow, but also that diagnostic devices are capable of networking with this system so a much of the patients' clinical information can be centralized and stored where it is most useful.

When choosing a modern diagnostic system, one should ensure that the raw data can be exported in the Digital Imaging and Communications in Medicine (DICOM) format, the international standard for medical data image storage. Exporting in DICOM means that the data can be networked with most EMR software solutions

W. J. Mayer (✉)
Department of Ophthalmology, Ludwig Maximilian University, Munich, Germany
e-mail: wolfgang.j.mayer@med.uni-muenchen.de

M. Shajari et al. (eds.), *Cataract and Lens Surgery*,
https://doi.org/10.1007/978-3-031-05394-8_6

Primary networking of patient data is done via the Health Level 7 interface (HL7). HL7 refers to a set of international standards for the transfer of data between healthcare organizations and their computer systems.

Example of a Digital Workflow Setting in a University Eye Clinic Setting

As of November 2020, over 40 diagnostic systems are in use at the Eye Clinic of the LMU Munich. These devices are mainly connected via the DICOM protocol. Where the export of raw data is not possible, a report-print interface allows the export of screen recordings or generated reports to a central Picture Archiving and Communication System (PACS). The EMR based on I.s.h.-med (SAP/Cerner) serves as a main host. The SAP system is networked with the PACS system from Zeiss (FORUM®). Based on the HL7 interface, the FORUM system is used to process work lists that were placed as clinical orders via the I.s.h-med profile. The FORUM system then retrieves the corresponding diagnostic findings from the devices and stores them in a central server.

The aim here is the paperless exchange of image data and findings, which are available at every workstation. In this way, the clinical workflow from patient registration to diagnostics and findings can be streamlined.

Digital Toric Lens Surgery: From Planning to Surgery

The benefits of a digital ophthalmic surgical workflow can be demonstrated using the example of toric lens surgery using the Zeiss FORUM system networked with the IOL master and the surgical digital Callisto Eye unit on the surgical microscope.

After clinical examination, the patient receives a comprehensive diagnosis with biometry, corneal tomography and refraction. These data are merged into the PACS system (FORUM®). In the FORUM system itself, a virtual working environment (EQ Workplace®) allows planning and calculation of the toric lens.

The advantage of this system is the direct transfer of relevant measurement parameters, such as biometric data from the IOL master, directly into the IOL calculation system. This replaces the laborious manual entry of all data required for calculation and the user only has to verify the data. In addition to the target refraction and the SIA ("surgical induced astigmatism"), the corneal refractive power and the refractive index are also included. For the corneal refractive power, using the total refractive power including the back surface of the cornea is recommended (TK, Total Keratometry).

The lens and the lens formula are then selected. Several formulas can be compared simultaneously. The lens power including the cylinder can also be adjusted manually, depending on the desired spherical equivalent. The next step is the planning of the surgery. In addition to the sitting position of the surgeon, digital assistants can also be planned for use with the Callisto Eye System in the operating theatre.

Example insertion of corneal incisions, capsulorhexis guide line, toric axis for toric IOL alignment.

The planning is then completed and a Zeiss lens can be ordered directly via a created PDF form from the manufacturer, which can be sent by e-mail. The planned data can be transmitted via network directly to the Callisto Eye system in the OR (Fig. 1). This eliminates the need for any paper printout or export to an external storage medium [4].

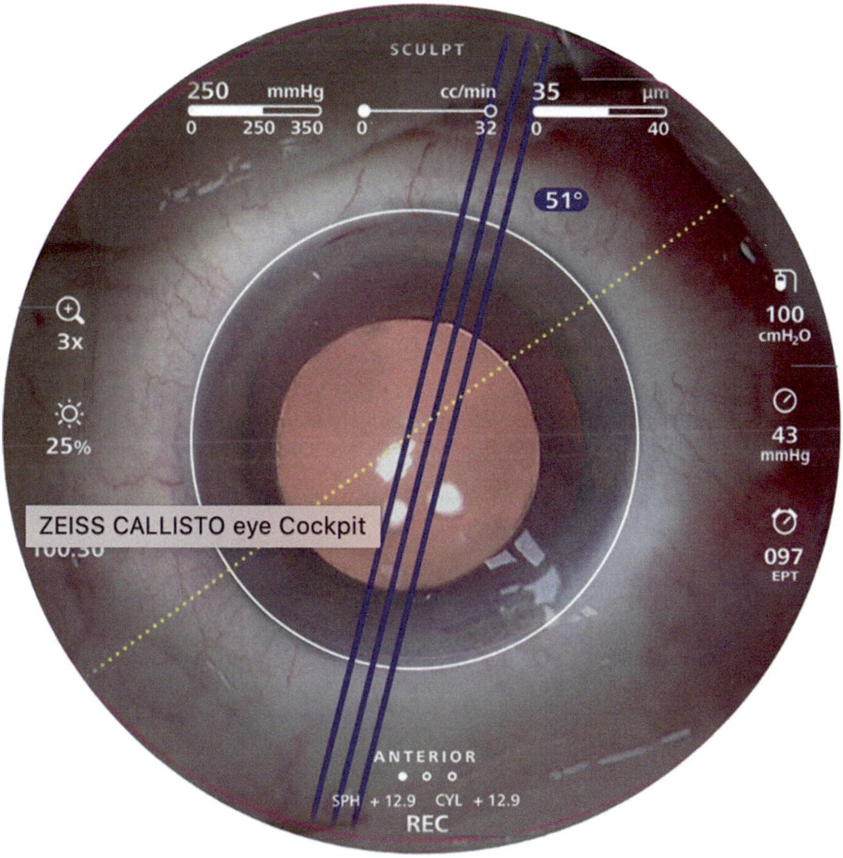

Fig. 1 Digital reflection of the toric axis in the surgical microscope for alignment of the toric intraocular lens after successful adjustment of the reference image for “eye tracking” (Callisto Eye, Zeiss, courtesy of Zeiss Meditec)

Outlook: Artificial Intelligence

In the future, advanced assistance systems based on artificial intelligence will help us to better understand diagnostic findings, but will also be applied to simplify therapy decisions based on "big data" analyses. Several study groups are working in the area with data on both the anterior and posterior segments of the eye. The potential for AI can be seen in the example of intravitreal drug therapy on the basis of OCT findings. AI in ophthalmology is the subject of intensive research in order to gain new insights from large treatment collectives on the one hand, and to increase the efficiency and cost effectiveness of diagnostics and treatment on the other [7–15].

References

1. Luebke J, Boehringer D, Maier P, Reinhard T, Eberwein P. Toric IOL positioning with a no-touch head-up display axis alignment. Int Ophthalmol. 2020;40(3):617–26.
2. Khatib ZI, Haldipurkar SS, Shetty V. Verion digital marking versus smartphone-assisted manual marking and isolated manual marking in toric intraocular lens implantation. Indian J Ophthalmol. 2020;68(3):455–8.
3. Webers VSC, Bauer NJC, Visser N, Berendschot T, van den Biggelaar F, Nuijts R. Image-guided system versus manual marking for toric intraocular lens alignment in cataract surgery. J Cataract Refract Surg. 2017;43(6):781–8.
4. Mayer WJ, Kreutzer T, Dirisamer M, Kern C, Kortuem K, Vounotrypidis E, et al. Comparison of visual outcomes, alignment accuracy, and surgical time between 2 methods of corneal marking for toric intraocular lens implantation. J Cataract Refract Surg. 2017;43 (10):1281–6.
5. Spira-Eppig C, Eppig T, Bischof M, Schiessl G, Milioti G, Kasmann-Kellner B, et al. Work in progress: adaptation of electronic medical records to the requirements of a university eye clinic: individual extensions of the software "FIDUS" at the Department of Ophthalmology of the Saarland University Medical Center UKS. Ophthalmologist. 2019;116(11):1046–57.
6. Alnawaiseh M, Alten F, Huelsken G, Rentmeister G, Lange M, Claes T, et al. Implementation of electronic health records at a tertiary care eye hospital. Ophthalmologist. 2015;112 (4):337–45.
7. Schworm B, Luft N, Keidel LF, Hagenau F, Kern C, Herold T, et al. Response of neovascular central serous chorioretinopathy to an extended upload of anti-VEGF agents. Graefes Arch Clin Exp Ophthalmol. 2020;258(5):1013–21.
8. Scheifelbein J, Muller M, Kern C, Herold T, Liegl R, Fasler K, et al. Gender-related differences in patients treated with intravitreal anti-vascular endothelial growth factor medication for diabetic macular oedema. Eur J Ophthalmol. 2020:1120672119899627.
9. Kern C, Schiefelbein J, Fu DJ, Schworm B, Sim D, Herold T, et al. Two year visual acuity and structural outcomes in patients with diabetic macular oedema treated with intravitreal aflibercept—a retrospective cohort study. Clin Ophthalmol. 2020;14:533–41.
10. Core C, Fu DJ, Kortuem K, Huemer J, Barker D, Davis A, et al. Implementation of a cloud-based referral platform in ophthalmology: making telemedicine services a reality in eye care. Br J Ophthalmol. 2020;104(3):312–7.
11. Fasler K, Fu DJ, Moraes G, Wagner S, Gokhale E, Kortuem K, et al. Moorfields AMD database report 2: fellow eye involvement with neovascular age-related macular degeneration Br J Ophthalmol. 2020; 104(5):684–90.

12. Core C, Kortuem K, Hamilton R, Fasolo S, Cai Y, Balaskas K, et al. Clinical outcomes of a hospital-based teleophthalmology service: what happens to patients in a virtual clinic? Ophthalmol Retina. 2019;3(5):422–8.
13. Rohm M, Tresp V, Muller M, Kern C, Manakov I, Weiss M, et al. Predicting visual acuity by using machine learning in patients treated for neovascular age-related macular degeneration. Ophthalmology. 2018;125(7):1028–36.
14. Kortuem K, Fasler K, Charnley A, Khambati H, Fasolo S, Katz M, et al. Implementation of medical retina virtual clinics in a tertiary eye care referral centre. Br J Ophthalmol. 2018;102 (10):1391–5.
15. Core C, Kortuem K, Wertheimer C, Nilmayer O, Dirisamer M, Priglinger S, et al. Modern corneal eye-banking using a software-based IT management solution. J Ophthalmol. 2018;2018:2645280.

Examination

Medical History

Johannes Burger and Thomas Kreutzer

The medical history should be asked in a personal and individual setting without time pressure.

When taking a clinical history, three goals in particular should be considered:

- Understanding the patient's visual problems
- Clarifying expectations of a possible surgical procedure
- Assessing previous systemic and ophthalmological conditions.

Some patients find it pleasant if relatives or caregivers can be present during this conversation. A joint medical consultation can therefore help to reduce fears, clarify open questions, and create trust in advance. If there is a language barrier, a competent interpreter should be present as well.

A consistent structure should be followed when taking the clinical history, regardless of whether it is a standard cataract procedure or a "clear lens exchange" with possible implantation of a premium IOL. Nevertheless, the focus of the clinical history can shift significantly between refractive lens exchange and therapeutic cataract surgery. In the former, expectations play a particularly important role, whereas in the case of cataract patients, who are generally older, concomitant diseases and medication are the focus.

J. Burger (✉)
Augen MVZ Landshut, ÜBAG Deggendorf, Deggendorf, Germany
e-mail: burger@augenarzt-burger.de

T. Kreutzer
Ludwig Maximilian University of Munich, Munich, Germany
e-mail: thomas.kreutzer@med.uni-muenchen.de

M. Shajari et al. (eds.), *Cataract and Lens Surgery*,
https://doi.org/10.1007/978-3-031-05394-8_7

Author's recommendation

During the interview, the patient's medically relevant history should be asked in a standardized and focused way, but the patient's professional and social aspects should also be examined closely.

The Start of the Conversation

An open question about the current subjective perception of his or her own visual performance is a good initial question. In the course of this initial self-assessment, the patient's motives and motivation for an operation or the patient's level of disability can often be identified during the conversation. Symptoms such as deteriorated vision, blurred vision, glare and changes in refraction and corrections of glasses are usually found in cataract patients, while the refractive patient complains about the need for glasses and contact lenses. While the expectations of the cataract patient often include a restoration of the old visual acuity, the refractive patient wants to see without glasses, and achieve comparable or even better visual acuity and quality of vision.

Ask About Relevant General Medical Conditions

In addition to the family and ophthalmological history, the general medical history taken should, above all, include diseases of the patient that are relevant for the surgery. Even though modern lens surgery is generally possible without any problems even for seriously ill patients due to its minimally invasive approach, multimorbid patients may require an increased level of support from an anaesthesiological team.

Pre-existing arterial hypertension should be treated before planned lens surgery. Even with planned topical anaesthesia, it might be necessary to switch to a para- or retrobulbar anaesthesia procedure if the surgery becomes complex. In this situation, uncontrolled arterial hypertension can significantly increase the occurrence of retrobulbar bleeding and the risk of suprachoroidal bleeding.

Diabetes mellitus (diabetes type/diabetes duration/current setting incl. HbA1c) plays an important role in ophthalmic surgery and has a high prevalence in the general population. Insufficient blood glucose control should be treated before lens surgery if possible. Even in the case of proper diabetic medication, a diabetic patient still has an increased risk of complications during lens surgery and needs to be informed about this [1].

The use of oral anticoagulants should be documented. Pausing intake is not usually necessary for most patients, except for in very complex situations.

Further questions in this regard must be explored where relevant and depending on the individual findings (questions about e.g. myocardial infarction, coagulation disorders, previous vascular occlusion, embolism, thromboses, etc.), as they influence the choice of anaesthesiological surveillance.

Other important areas that should be investigated:

- Allergies (drugs in general and especially antibiotics)
- Rheumatological (rheumatoid arthritis/chronic polyarthritis, Sjögren's syndrome, immunosuppression)
- Pulmonological (asthma/COPD)
- Dermatological (neurodermatitis/psoriasis)
- Infectious diseases (including HIV, hepatitis B and C)
- Colonisation with multi-resistant germs (MRSA, EHEB)
- Neurological diseases (e.g. apoplexy, epilepsy, multiple sclerosis)
- Mental illness (including depression)
- Urological: prostatic hyperplasia (therapy with α1 adrenoceptor (AR) antagonist, e.g. tamsulosin with regard to floppy iris syndrome) [2].

In the case of planned special or multifocal intraocular lenses in particular, the patient's profession must be considered. Professions such as drivers (particularly night driving), and professions with passenger transport and pilots must be clarified or selected with regard to visual night-time side effects.

The patients' leisure activities (hobbies/sport) must also be considered as they might play a role in IOL selection.

Ophthalmologic History

It is advisable to proceed chronologically and start with questions in regards to childhood ophthalmological issues. This includes questions about vision in childhood, glasses in childhood, strabismus, amblyopia and the question of any occlusion therapy or surgery performed in childhood.

This should be followed by questions about known changes, pathologies or traumas of the anterior and posterior segments of the eye.

Traumas should be investigated in greater depth, since contusion traumas are associated with loose zonulae, while penetrating injuries can also cause primary defects of the lens capsule and scarring in the lens capsule and iris. This can make the use of premium IOLs impossible.

Author's recommendation

Without exception, every patient must be asked about previous surgical procedures in the anterior and posterior segment of the eye and, in particular, about any previous corneal surgeries. This is because corneal surgery in particular might have a large impact on biometry and IOL calculation.

All ophthalmologic diagnoses should be queried, especially those that can have an influence on postoperative visual acuity.

Due to the high prevalence of these conditions, they should be inquired about specifically:

- Diabetic retinal disease,
- Age-related macular degeneration (AMD),
- Vascular occlusions in the eye,
- Dry eye disease and
- Glaucoma.

If the patient has glaucoma, changes in the visual field and local medication should be documented. Two drugs in particular can play a role in the surgical outcomes.

The extent to which prostaglandin analogues can be linked to an increased incidence of postoperative cystoid macular edema is still debated but some ophthalmologists prefer to switch to another medication preoperatively.

Pilocarpine, which is occasionally used in chronic narrow-angle glaucoma, is also a particularly relevant medication to discuss prior to lens surgery. Depending on the individual anatomical conditions (anterior chamber depth, chamber angle, hyperopia), the extent to which an iridotomy should be performed preoperatively, and which replacement therapy should be used, must be discussed.

The question of the patient's dry-eye symptoms and the current use of tear substitutes, and the type and dosage of the preparations used should be always asked before any lens surgery is performed. It can be of great importance throughout the entire process of surgical planning, diagnostics, implementation and aftercare.

In a patient with known tear film disorder and blepharitis, errors in both visual fluctuations and measurement inaccuracies in corneal biometry can occur. Chronic blepharitis and keratoconjunctivitis sicca should therefore be sufficiently treated preoperatively and if needed, patients should be asked to return for a repeat preoperative examination.

Refraction/Glasses/Contact Lens

The examination of existing refractive errors or presbyopia within the framework of the medical history and their current correction is also a very important point which can have a decisive influence.

This is an intersection of diagnostics (objective refraction), examination (subjective comparison) and clinical history (do they use glasses? How old/current are the glasses? Are contact lenses used?). Only by considering all of these points can an optimal IOL selection be achieved.

In case of higher ametropias, it is essential to discuss the expected postoperative situation after the treatment of the first eye. Postoperative anisometropias often lead to visual complaints and dissatisfaction, as well as to a prolonged inability to work or a temporary lack of roadworthiness. The possible consequences of a bilateral operation, despite good visual acuity in one eye, should be discussed and documented in advance.

In the case of higher myopia and presbyopia, the habits and requirements of the patient and contact lens wear have to be determined specifically, as these patients are often used to emmetropia with regard to the postoperative target refraction and may also be considered for multifocal optics [3].

In summary, the aim should be to acquire an thorough history that is as standardised as possible but flexible to consider the individual needs and wishes of the patient.

References

1. Peterson SR, Silva PA, Murtha TJ, Sun JK. Cataract surgery in patients with diabetes: management strategies. Semin Ophthalmol. 2018;33(1):75–82.
2. Haridas A, Syrimi M, Al-Ahmar B, Hingorani M. Intraoperative floppy iris syndrome (IFIS) in patients receiving tamsulosin or doxazosin—a UK-based comparison of incidence and complication rates. Graefe's Arch Clin Exp Ophthalmol = Albrecht Graefe's Arch Clin Exp Ophthalmol. 2013;251(6):1541–5.
3. Martiano D, Cochener B. Multifocal IOLs in the high myope, 6-year follow-up. J Fr Ophtalmol. 2014;37(5):393–9.

Testing of Visual Function: Visual Acuity, Refraction, Contrast Sensitivity

Bettina von Livonius and Dan Z. Reinstein

Vision is commonly expressed as visual acuity, but to evaluate visual function not only in terms of quantity but also quality, additional measurements such as contrast sensitivity, color perception, stereopsis and visual fields should be included. In the context of lens surgery, visual acuity, contrast sensitivity, and stereopsis are of particular interest and most informative for testing practical visual function. In this chapter, we consider visual acuity and contrast sensitivity in the context of lens surgery.

The Visual Acuity

The basis of an examination of the visual system is the determination of visual acuity. It is relatively easy to measure, reproducible within a certain range of variation, and comparable between individuals. Depending on the type of visual stimulus, the following types of visual acuity can be determined [1]:

1. Recognition visual acuity (minimum cognoscible) = visual acuity
2. Resolution visual acuity (minimum separable) = grating visual acuity
3. Localization visual acuity (minimum discriminable)
4. Point visual acuity (minimum visible)
5. Reading ability

B. von Livonius (✉) · D. Z. Reinstein
Ludwig Maximilian University of Munich, Munich, Germany
e-mail: bettina.livonius@med.uni-muenchen.de

M. Shajari et al. (eds.), *Cataract and Lens Surgery*,
https://doi.org/10.1007/978-3-031-05394-8_8

Standards of Distance Visual Acuity Determination

In practice, the recognition visual acuity (i.e. the visual acuity), is of particular interest. It is defined as the limit of ability to discriminate points as separate objects and is determined by means of calibrated visual objects (optotypes). The following parameters have been defined for the visual acuity test according to EN ISO 8596:

- Sighting mark: Landolt rings with openings in eight directions.
- Examination distance: at least 4 m if there is no significant visual impairment.
- Test field size: diameter 2.0–5.0°.
- Test field luminance: 160–320 cd/m^2.
- Character contrast: luminance of the optotypes <15% of the luminance of the test field.
- Distance between optotypes: >15′ or more (depending on the visual acuity level).
- Distance of the optotypes from the edge of the test field: 0.5°.
- Termination criteria: A visual level is detected if 60% of the visual signs could be correctly named (e.g., 3 of 5 or 6 of 10 optotypes) [2].

Abbreviations such as "p" or "pp" (in the sense of "partially read"), after the achieved visual acuity level should be avoided, as they can lead to misinterpretations due to a lack of standardized application guidelines. It is also important to motivate the patient to make a statement for each optotype (=principle of Forced choice). Thus, "guessing" the optotypes should be explicitly encouraged when reaching the limit of detection acuity [3]. During visual acuity testing, care should be taken to ensure that the subject is not adversely affected by light sources or reflections. Impairment due to prior diagnostic tests, topical drop application or contact tonometric pressure measurement before determination of visual acuity should also be avoided, as this can lead to false measurements.

Standards of Near Visual Acuity Determination

In addition to recognition visual acuity (distance visual acuity), reading ability is also an important assessment of visual function. In the measurement of distance visual acuity, only about 1° of intact function of the fovea is necessary, whereas for fluent reading, a central visual field of at least 4° horizontally and 2° vertically are required [4]. Therefore, reading visual acuity cannot be extrapolated from distance visual acuity alone. When testing reading visual acuity, it is preferable to use actual text, rather than series of numbers, to better reflect real world scenarios where the spacing between optotypes vary within words. In an attempt to improve interindividual comparability for reading ability, the Commission for Quality

Assurance Systems of the DOG has recommended a defined, logarithmic gradation of character sizes for reading samples. The following reading samples meet these requirements to a large extent: The Colenbrander and the MNread Chart, the OCULUS near vision sample and the RADNER reading chart. In much of the published literature, near visual acuity according to the Jäger optotypes is frequently employed. These Jäger plates are not standardized however, and therefore not optimal for the comparative determination of the near visual acuity.

In everyday practice, a reading level is usually considered to have been reached when the test reading text is read fluently. The objectivity of fluency suffers from the subjective discretion of the examiner. The objectivity can be improved by determining how many words-per-minute are read from a standardized test reading text. For the sentence optotypes of the RADNER reading charts, for example, a stopping criterion of 20 s. is chosen for the block of text to be read (this corresponds to 42 wpm, words-per-minute), considered as the lower threshold for coherent reading ability. Thus, in order to consider a text block level of visual acuity to have been attained, it must be completed in less than 20 s. The visual level is also considered to be unattained if errors are made in a sentence that render the meaning of the sentence as significantly altered or unintelligible. Again, this is a determination that can be affected by subjective interpretation on the part of the examiner [5].

Objective Refraction Determination—Subjective Refraction Determination

The goal of refraction is to determine the optimal sphere magnitude and cylinder vector that optimise distance acuity.

Objective Refraction

Objective refraction is classically determined by examination using a retinoscope or sciascope by a technique known as retinoscopy or sciascopy. With sufficiently translucent ocular media, experienced examiners can obtain an objective refraction with very good accuracy within a fraction of a minute for each eye. However, the use of this technique has declined in many parts of the developed world due to the abundance of devices that perform the same function in an automated fashion. Automated refractometry is thus performed by "autorefractometers". These devices average refraction values by automated sciascopic methods within a defined zone of the pupil area. This zone is conventionally standardized to a diameter of 2.3 mm in most instruments. In retinoscopy the refraction is obtained within the physiologically determined pupil diameter. The decline in the use of retinoscopy has led to the loss of additional very valuable information about light transmission within the optical media (e.g. the detection of posterior sub-capsular cataract) as well as an analog form of wavefront analysis (e.g. the presence of 'scissoring' of the retinoscopic reflex produced by coma, induced by asymmetrical corneal distortion such as in keratoconus). Cycloplegic retinoscopy is still the gold standard for objective refraction determination in children as it can be performed even in conditions of poor cooperation. Furthermore, retinoscopy remains preferable to autorefractometers when examining non-cooperative patients (e.g., dementia) and in individuals who cannot be positioned behind an autorefractometer (e.g., spinal abnormalities).

Subjective Refraction

Optical irregularities of the eye can lead to variable amounts of aberration of the retinal image, and these can be significantly affected by differences in pupil size (optical zone). Spherical aberration in particular can affect the determination of sphere according to pupil analysis zone. Schober et al. measured the pupil area and found refraction differences of up to 1.4 dpt [6]. Thus, it is important to consider control of the lighting conditions present during subjective refraction, rather than only relying on standardized autorefraction.

The standard recommended procedure is to first perform an objective refraction and then to refine the determined values subjectively [7]. **Maximum distance and near vision correction should be used as the examination benchmark**.

When a patient first presents, it is advisable to determine both monocular and binocular "uncorrected visual acuity" for distance and near. This measure of uncorrected visual function is relevant for both legal reasons (e.g. driving standards) but also for the assessment of the patient before a surgical or refractive intervention. In addition, the uncorrected visual acuity allows the patient to appreciate to what extent the visual acuity can be improved by spectacle correction. This is followed by measurement of objective refraction and then, subjective refraction (where possible). It is advisable to refract each eye to the best possible spectacle corrected vision, that is, beyond 20/20 or 0.0 logMAR, where possible. In this way any changes in the distance corrected visual acuity (DCVA) can be monitored over time. For example, a patient may complain of a drop in vision and found to have a visual acuity of 20/20 or 0.00 logMAR, simply because the vision was previously 20/12 (−0.20 logMAR).

Before any surgical intervention, it is worth repeating vision and refraction measurements. In the case of a patient presenting for cataract surgery on the second eye, for example, a week after the first eye, it is recommended that the vision and refraction be documented for both the post-operative eye as well as the eye about to undergo the intervention.

From a medico-legal perspective as well as a functional standpoint, we recommend that distance visual acuity both monocularly and binocularly with and without correction be documented at each visit.

Postoperative Visual Acuity Prognosis in Dense Media Opacities

Measurement of Retinal Visual Acuity by Laser Interference/ Retinometer

If a more precise indication of postoperative visual acuity in nuclear, cortical, and secondary cataracts is required prior to cataract surgery, measurement of retinal visual acuity by retinometer (laser interference measurement) can be useful [8]. It should be noted, however, that prediction becomes less accurate when posterior shell opacity, high myopia, amblyopia, or maculopathies (diabetes and AMD-related) are present [9]. In laser interference measurement, a retinometer is used to project two 0.05 mm diameter light spots into the pupillary plane of the eye being examined. Due to the coherence of the partial beams, a figure of alternating black and red stripes is formed in the overlapping area of both beams, which can be seen by the person under examination. By changing the point spacing, the line density can also be changed and it is correlated to the achievable visual acuity (the thinner the stripes become, the higher the grating visual acuity) (Fig. 1). The stripe patterns are offered in different, randomly selected spatial orientations (horizontal, vertical, diagonal). During the measurement, increasingly closer line spacings (corresponding to higher visual acuity) are projected at different orientations until the patient is only able to provide answers at the level of the guess probability, i.e., less than 3 out of 5. The last reproducibly measured level, where 3 out of 5 orientations of the stripe patterns could be correctly named, corresponds to interference visual acuity. The measurements are largely independent of refraction and can be also be performed through small pupils. In the case of more advanced lens opacification, a dilated pupil can make retinometry easier as the light spots can be projected through different regions of the entrance pupil in order to get around denser lens opacities. It should also be noted that the values obtained are actual grating visual acuity measures, not optotype recognition acuity [1].

Estimation of Retinal Visual Acuity with the Purkinje Choroidal/Retinal Vessel Shadow Figure

In cases where the opacity of the media is so dense that retinometer measurements are not possible, the use of the entoptic phenomenon, where retinal vessel

Fig. 1 Measurement of grating visual acuity with the retinometer. Interference pattern as seen by the patient. The thinner the stripes, whose orientation are correctly detected, the higher the grating visual acuity

shadowing is produced, can be used to grossly assess retinal function. The "Purkinje vascular entoptic test" as it is known, is a test of retinal function which employs a light directed through the sclera, illuminating the fundus. This light casts shadows of retinal blood vessels onto posterior pole photoreceptors. By moving the trans-scleral illumination of the globe, the retinal vessels cast shadows on a constantly changing area of sensory cells producing a "vein map". Inspection of the vein map is best achieved in a dark room. The vein map visualization is produced by shining a small, intense light source trans-sclerally about 5 mm behind the limbus and this light source is moved at a frequency of two to four swings per second (Fig. 2a). Direct illumination of the retina through the pupil should be avoided and the other eye should be covered so that the patient is not distracted by other visual impressions. The range of visible vein figure perception increases when the light source is moved farther from the limbus. The phenomenon disappears immediately when the light is static. The patient's perception of the vein figure is subjectively described very differently, e.g., as branches of a tree or rivers in a landscape (Fig. 2b). The possibility of triggering the vein figure depends very much on the patient's cooperation and understanding. It is recommended to describe the expected image to the patient beforehand. Since it is not always possible to produce the vein figure perception even in healthy eyes, a non-recognition of the vein figure by the patient is no proof of a functional disorder. However, if triggering of the choroidal figure is possible, a postoperative visual acuity of at least 1.0 logMAR can be assumed if the central choroidal figure is complete (the central 20° part of the visual field, forms the center of the vein figure with the enclosing vascular arches). The vein figure is pathologically obliterated in cases of retinal detachments, retinal (especially arterial) vascular occlusions, and severe forms of tapetoretinal degeneration. In central scotomas (neuritis), parts of the figure are not perceived. Overall, as a simple procedure to perform, testing of the vein figure provides a good indication of central visual acuity in cases of severe media opacities and can thus be used as a prognostic factor in upcoming surgery [10].

(a)

(b)

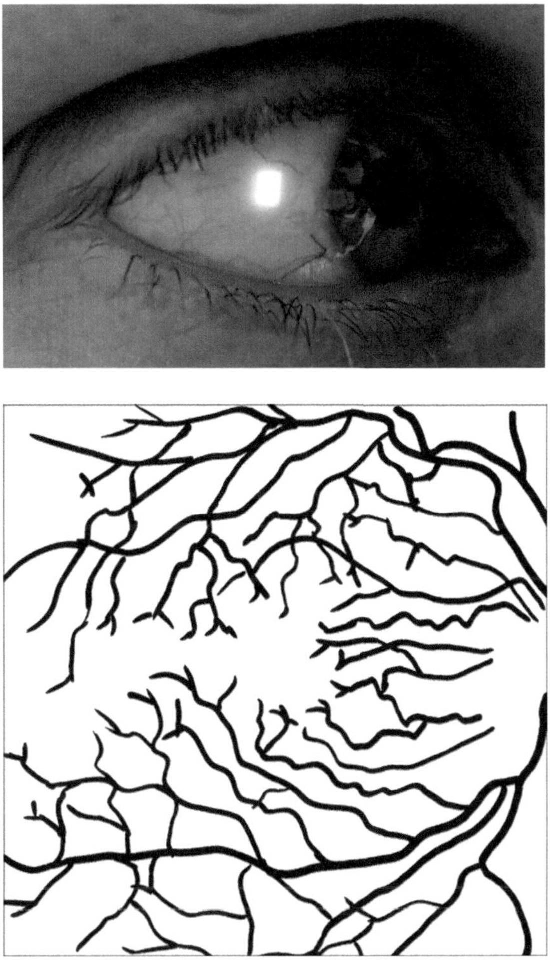

Fig. 2 **a** Testing of the vein figure. The vascular shadow figure of the retina is best evoked by projecting an intense light source onto the sclera near the limbus in the area of the temporal palpebral fissure. The light source must then be moved slowly up and down. The eye of the person being examined is in adduction. **b** Schematic representation of the vessel shadow figure as perceived by the person under examination

Neuronal Functional Testing of the Retina

If severe media opacities are present where no view of the fundus is visible and where no retinometer is available, a flash VEP (visual evoked cortical potentials) can be used to make a global assessment of the entire visual system, up to the visual cortex. However, it should be considered that in the case of pronounced media opacities, it may no longer be possible to elicit a flash VEP. Compared to the pattern VECP, the waveforms of the flash VECP are very variable and therefore only suitable to answer rough questions about whether a signal arrives in the visual cortex at all. For the flash stimulus (with a stroboscopic flash unit), the flash area should be at least 20° of the visual field, and the flash duration should be less than 5 ms. The stimulus should be diffuse and have an intensity of 1.5 to 3 cd s/m^2 (standard flash of the ISCEV-ERG standard) [11].

Contrast Vision

Good contrast vision is particularly important when driving in poor visibility conditions, i.e., in fog, rain or snow, but also for recognizing uneven surfaces, e.g., curbs and steps. Reading different fonts on colored backgrounds or on paper with poor contrast or in poor lighting also requires functional contrast vision [12]. Reduced contrast vision can occur even when visual acuity measured is still good. Causes of a loss in contrast sensitivity can be an opacity of the optical media, such as corneal edema or incipient cataract, or as a consequence of higher order aberrations due to irregularities on the cornea or lens. Normal aging processes can also lead to a decrease in contrast sensitivity. Since contrast is high when visual acuity is determined by visual sign projectors or on optotype charts, contrast sensitivity should be tested separately. The Pelli–Robson test charts or the MARS charts can be used to measure low contrast acuity. Both boards work with large letters that do not change in size but are printed on the boards with increasingly weaker contrast. These charts can be used to test contrast vision under daylight conditions in a readily reproducible form. It is essential however, that standardized illumination (60–120 cd/m^2 or 189 to 377 lx) is maintained for testing. Contrast vision is measured in logCS (the mentioned panels allow testing between 0 and 2.0 logCS). As borderline contrast vision, 1.5 logCS is given in the literature for elderly persons over 60 years of age (instruction manual of the MARS panels). Values lower than 1.5 are considered to have moderate contrast sensitivity limitation and values lower than 0.5 are considered to have massive contrast sensitivity limitation [3].

Contrast sensitivity can also be measured using sine-wave gratings where the luminance of the grating is varied from 0.5% contrast to 90% contrast. The contrast sensitivity is the lowest contrast level that can be detected by the patient. Contrast sensitivity charts present 4–5 rows of 8–10 contrast level gratings, with each row a different spatial frequency of the sinusoidal pattern (i.e. different thickness of the grey stripes, similar to the retinometer gratings). By measuring responses at different spatial frequencies, a contrast sensitivity curve is plotted to show the lowest contrast level a patient can detect for each spatial frequency from low (thick gratings) to high (thin gratings). The spatial frequencies used are usually 1.5, 3, 6, 12, and 18 cycles per degree. An example of this is the CSV-1000 (VectorVision, Greenville, OH), which has been used in the majority of FDA clinical trials for laser refractive surgery and is a fast and efficient test for measuring contrast sensitivity [13].

In lens surgery, it is useful to routinely test contrast vision before surgery as a baseline measurement that can be used to monitor the progression and extent of a cataract. Because it is a more sensitive test than visual acuity, contrast sensitivity may also diagnose visually significant cataract earlier. This is particularly important for the implantation of multifocal lenses, as these can lead to a lower contrast sensitivity, particularly when performing clear lens exchange. Measuring the contrast sensitivity again after surgery can be used as a compelling demonstration of the improvement in quality of vision gained from lens surgery. Postoperatively, contrast sensitivity tests can be used to assess whether a patient might benefit from a YAG treatment for posterior capsule opacification (PCO), and again in demonstrating an improvement following the YAG.

Note

Before any surgical procedure, it is important to perform an objective refraction as a baseline and for surgical planning. Afterwards the distance visual acuity should be determined with the best subjective refraction and then the near visual acuity, if necessary, with an accommodation compensation. An additional determination of the contrast visual acuity is especially interesting before implantation of special lenses.

Objective Measurement of Quality of Vision

Quality of vision can also be assessed using devices that measure higher order aberrations and/or point spread function. Aberrometers are in widespread use in refractive surgery and help in the diagnosis of patients complaining from reduced quality of vision. Spherical aberration and coma are the dominant aberrations linked to patient symptoms. Modern high resolution aberrometers, such as the Osiris (CSO, Florence, Italy), are even able to measure the aberrations within a multifocal IOL. An example of an Osiris scan for an eye implanted with a diffractive multifocal IOL is shown in Fig. 3, where the rings are clearly visible on the scan and correlated with the image drawn by the patient describing their vision with that eye.

Devices measuring optical scatter as a point spread function are also available and can provide an objective measurement to complement the subjective clinical interpretation of cataract progression. In many cases where a lens can appear yellow, the point spread function can still be within normal limits, indicating that a corneal procedure may be the preferred option for a patient with early presbyopia.

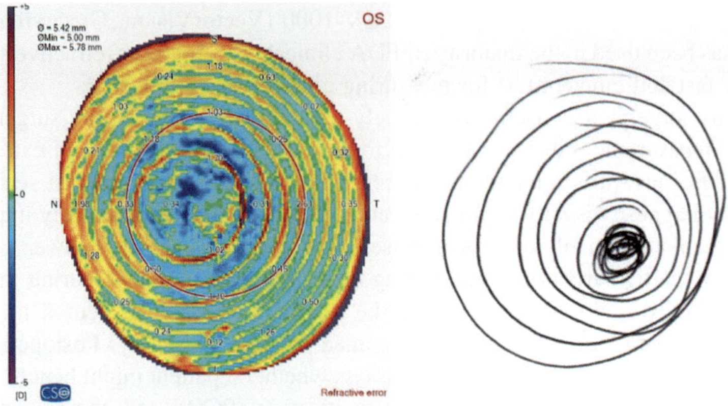

Fig. 3 Osiris refractive error map for an eye implanted with a Symfony multifocal IOL (J&J, New Brunswick, NJ) showing the aberrations due to the diffractive lens design. In this patient, these induced concentric rings around lights (e.g. traffic lights) as drawn by the patient

The HD Analyser (Keeler, Windsor, UK) and iTrace (Tracey Technologies, Houston, TX) are two examples. The HD Analyser provides the optical scatter index (OSI), which grades the point spread function with an OSI of 2 or below within normal limits.

References

1. Kroll P, Küchle M, Küchle HJ. Augenärztliche Untersuchungsmethoden, 3rd ed. New York: Thieme Publishing House;2008.
2. Wesemann W, Schiefer U, Bach M. New DIN norms for determination of visual acuity. Ophthalmologe. 2010;107(9):821–6. https://doi.org/10.1007/s00347-010-2228-2.
3. Maritzen A, Kamps N. Rehabilitation bei Sehbehinderung und Blindheit. Berlin: Springer Publishing House;2013.
4. Diepes H, Krause K, Rohrschneider K. Sehbehinderung. Lévis: DOZ Publishing House;2007.
5. Radner W. Ophthalmologic reading charts: part 2: current logarithmically scaled reading charts. Ophthalmologe. 2016;113(12):1029–35. https://doi.org/10.1007/s00347-015-0175-7.
6. Schober H, Wohletz J, Zolleis F. Monochromatic aberration of the human eye. Klin Monbl Augenheilkd. 1969;155(2):243–57.
7. Friedburg D, Krause K. Subjective refraction assessment II: monocular fine adjustment. Ophthalmologe. 2002;99(8):657–63; quiz 664–5; 667. https://doi.org/10.1007/s00347-002-0671-4.
8. Barrett BT, Davison PA, Eustace PE. Clinical comparison of three techniques for evaluating visual function behind cataract. Eye (Lond). 1995;9(Pt 6):722–7. https://doi.org/10.1038/eye.1995.184.
9. Faulkner W. Laser interferometric prediction of postoperative visual acuity in patients with cataract. Am J Ophthalmol. 1983;95(5):626–36. https://doi.org/10.1016/0002-9394(83)90381-1.
10. Kluxen G. Ungeahnte Bilder. Kaden Publishing House;2007.

11. Bach M, Kellner U. Electrophysiological diagnosis in ophthalmology. Ophthalmologe. 2000;97(12):898–920. https://doi.org/10.1007/s003470070018.
12. Lachenmayr B. Begutachtung in der Augenheilkunde, 3rd ed. Berlin: Springer Publishing House;2019.
13. Wachler BS, Krueger RR. Normalized contrast sensitivity values. J Refract Surg. 1998 Jul–Aug;14(4):463–6.

Assessment of Optical Phenomena

Gernot Steinwender and Sonia H. Yoo

The photopic, high-contrast examination methods for determining visual acuity described in the previous chapter represent only one aspect of visual perception and can only partially explain some visual complaints [1]. In order to be able to assess the visual impression and its influence on the patient's quality of life more comprehensively, additional evaluations are necessary, including light scattering, glare sensitivity, and the assessment of subjective visual quality of life by means of questionnaires.

These examinations are particularly helpful in the management of dissatisfied patients after lens surgery. An analysis of pseudophakic patients with monofocal intraocular lenses (IOL) with very good postoperative visual acuity revealed that, after excluding other ocular pathology, the extent of dysphotopsia (disturbing optical phenomena) was the most important reason for dissatisfaction postoperatively [2].

In principle, dysphotopsias are divided into positive and negative dysphotopsias. **Positive dysphotopsias** include a wide range of bright light phenomena such as arcs, streaks and halos. The incidence of positive dysphotopsias after cataract surgery is almost 50%, although the symptoms are usually self-limiting and persist in only 2.2% of patients [3]. Light scattering induced by the edge of the IOL are assumed to be at least partially responsible for the occurrence of the light phenomena [4]. The cause of **negative dysphotopsias**, mostly dark shadows or crescents in the temporal visual field, is not yet fully understood. Negative dysphotopsias are less common than positive dysphotopsia, affecting about 15% of patients after cataract surgery and persisting in only 2–3% of patients [5].

G. Steinwender (✉)
Medical University of Graz, Graz, Austria
e-mail: steinwender.gernot@gmail.com

S. H. Yoo
University of Miami Miller School of Medicine, Miami, USA
e-mail: syoo@med.miami.edu

M. Shajari et al. (eds.), *Cataract and Lens Surgery*,
https://doi.org/10.1007/978-3-031-05394-8_9

Pronounced differences in the subjective perception of optical phenomena complicate not only the examination but also the treatment of dysphotopsias. Since **questionnaires** allow the measurement not only of visual factors but also psychological factors contributing to an individual's unique perception, they are frequently used in the diagnosis of dysphotopsias. In recent years, a questionnaire developed and validated by McAlinden to measure visual quality has become increasingly applied to this problem [6]. The 10 visual symptoms surveyed in this questionnaire provide an overview about a variety of optical phenomena and include:

- Glare
- Haloes
- Starbursts
- Hazy vision
- Blurred vision
- Distortion
- Double vision
- Fluctuation in vision
- Focusing difficulties
- Depth perception.

As each symptom is evaluated in 3 categories (frequency, severity and bothersomeness of the symptom), the questionnaire includes a total of 30 items per patient. Seven of the visual symptoms are also illustrated on the questionnaire (Fig. 1). Due to the standardized measurement of the subjective visual quality, the test is also very useful for monitoring progress and for comparing pre- and post-operative perception.

In addition to questionnaire-based examinations, visual symptoms can also be measured using **instrumental measurement methods**. One option is to measure straylight induced by light scattering in the eye's optical media that leads to phenomena such as glare, blurred vision and contrast loss. The Straylight meter (C-Quant, Oculus Optikgeräte, GmbH, Wetzlar, Germany) is based on a psychophysical method called compensation comparison, allowing the amount the ocular straylight to be quantified. With this device, the patient is asked to compare the two halves of a test field, one with and one without counter-phase flickering compensation light, and choose the one with higher intensity of flickering [7].

Halometry is another way to quantify optical phenomena. Using a web-based software platform (Halo & Glare Simulator, Eyeland-Design Network, GmbH, Vreden), dysphotopsias observed while driving a car at night can be simulated visually. The optical phenomena can be adjusted by the patient via sliders utilizing a scale for halo intensity, halo size, and furthermore a classification of haloes into 3 subtypes (diffuse halo ring, star burst type and distinct halo ring) [8]. Alternatively, there is also a tablet-based method of halometry (Aston Halometer, Aston Eye-Tech, Ltd, UK). In this method, a small letter is moved centrifugally from a

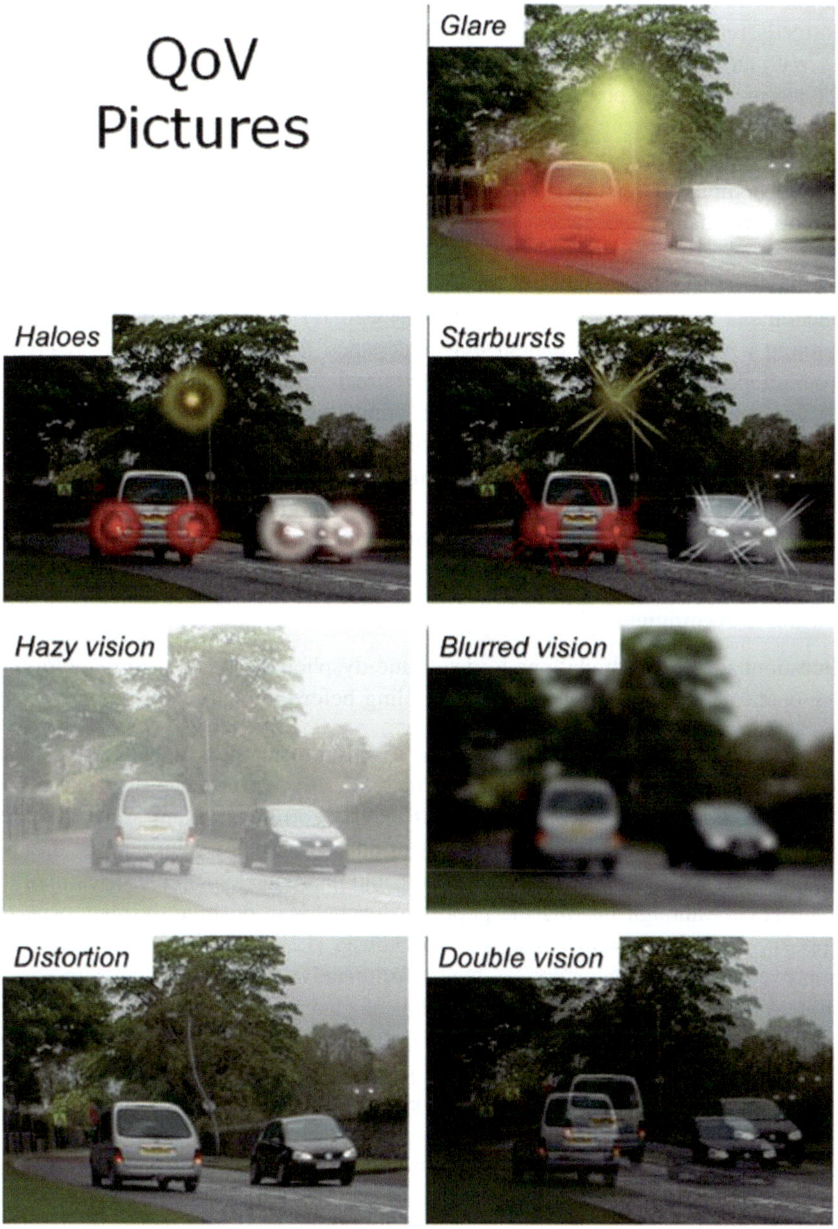

Fig. 1 Illustration of the image quality for the first 7 optical phenomena in the questionnaire developed by McAlinden (courtesy of Colm McAlinden) [6]

bright central light source on the display and the position at which the letter was correctly recognized by the patient is recorded [9].

With an ever-increasing spectrum of presbyopia-correcting IOLs in recent years, the requirements for preoperative **patient counseling** have also increased. Patients need to make important decisions about how they want to see postoperatively in a relatively short period of time during a typical consultation. It is equally demanding for the ophthalmologist to establish a common vocabulary with the patient and to determine whether the patient is flexible enough to make a certain compromise between spectacle independence and optical quality. Nothing can substitute for a thorough conversation, but the above-mentioned methods for measuring optical phenomena can be very helpful in this respect. By filling out a questionnaire or running a simulation, the patient will understand the possibility of postoperative dysphotopsias and thus will be better able to realize the optical compromise for the desired spectacle independence. Vision simulators such as the SimVis Gekko (2eyesvision, Madrid, Spain) can also hold promise for patients soon to be able to try out their premium lenses before committing to having them implanted [10]. Thorough patient education is all the more important prior to refractive lens exchange, since dysphotopsias caused by an incipient cataract may be less pronounced than those that are potentially induced by an IOL with a multifocal optic.

Author's recommendation

Questionnaires and simulations to determine dysphotopsias can also be helpful in pre-operative patient selection and counseling before refractive lens surgery.

The **management of patients with dysphotopsia** after uneventful cataract surgery is challenging and sometimes frustrating. In the presence of positive dysphotopsia, conservative treatment options include correction of any refractive error with glasses or contact lenses, treatment of any coexisting ocular surface disease, treatment of posterior capsule opacification, and pharmacological constriction of the pupil [11]. Although making the pupil smaller helps in positive dysphotopsia, the opposite is the case with negative dysphotopsia [12]. Dilation of the pupil often improves negative dysphotopsia but unfortunately, may not be an appropriate strategy for these patients due to induction of glare.

Surgery for dysphotopsia is discussed only after all possible exacerbating factors are eliminated and the symptoms still persist. Residual refractive error can be corrected with laser refractive surgery or secondary implantation of a piggyback IOL in the ciliary sulcus. Determining the significance of posterior capsule opacification might be challenging, as treatment with posterior capsulotomy can complicate future IOL exchange. While in some circumstances the decision for IOL explantation is obvious, such as in opacified or decentered IOLs, judgment can be very difficult in cases where patients are highly dissatisfied by optical phenomena from a multifocal IOL, which is perfectly centered and clear. In such situations patients should be encouraged to wait at least 6 to 12 months for neural adaption [13]. Then the final decision should be made as otherwise lens exchange may become too difficult due to severe fibrosis of the IOL haptics in the capsular bag. An alternative procedure to a bag-to-bag IOL exchange is removal of the inciting IOL and placement of a 3-piece IOL with the haptics in the ciliary sulcus, allowing an optic capture in cases with an open posterior capsule and adequate integrity of the zonule [14]. An additional technique used primarily in the surgical management of negative dysphotopsia is reverse optic capture [15]. In this procedure, the haptics of a single-piece IOL remain in the capsular bag while the capsulotomy is manipulated to go under the edge of the IOL optic, requiring a well-sized and well-centered anterior capsulotomy. Prior to all these strategies, in-depth counseling regarding possible surgical plans, the purpose of surgery, alternative options, and possible complications is a must.

References

1. Pesudovs K, Marsack JD, Donnelly WJ, Thibos LN, Applegate RA. Measuring visual acuity —mesopic or photopic conditions, and high or low contrast letters? J Refract Surg. 2004;20 (5):S508-14.
2. Kinard K, Jarstad A, Olson RJ. Correlation of visual quality with satisfaction and function in a normal cohort of pseudophakic patients. J Cataract Refract Surg. 2013;39(4):590–7. https://doi.org/10.1016/j.jcrs.2012.11.023.
3. Henderson BA, Geneva II. Negative dysphotopsia: a perfect storm. J Cataract Refract Surg. 2015;41(10):2291–312. https://doi.org/10.1016/j.jcrs.2015.09.002.
4. Hu J, Sella R, Afshari NA. Dysphotopsia: a multifaceted optic phenomenon. Curr Opin Ophthalmol. 2018;29(1):61–8. https://doi.org/10.1097/ICU.0000000000000447.
5. Bournas P, Drazinos S, Kanellas D, Arvanitis M, Vaikoussis E. Dysphotopsia after cataract surgery: comparison of four different intraocular lenses. Ophthalmologica. 2007;221(6):378–83. https://doi.org/10.1159/000107496.
6. McAlinden C, Pesudovs K, Moore JE. The development of an instrument to measure quality of vision: the quality of vision (QoV) questionnaire. Invest Ophthalmol Vis Sci. 2010;51 (11):5537–45. https://doi.org/10.1167/iovs.10-5341.
7. Guber I, Bachmann LM, Guber J, Bochmann F, Lange AP, Thiel MA. Reproducibility of straylight measurement by C-Quant for assessment of retinal straylight using the compensation comparison method. Graefes Arch Clin Exp Ophthalmol. 2011;249(9):1367–71. https://doi.org/10.1007/s00417-011-1704-y.
8. Giers BC, Khoramnia R, Varadi D, Wallek H, Son H-S, Attia MS, et al. Functional results and photic phenomena with new extended-depth-of-focus intraocular lens. BMC Ophthalmol. 2019;19(1):197. https://doi.org/10.1186/s12886-019-1201-3.
9. Buckhurst PJ, Naroo SA, Davies LN, Shah S, Buckhurst H, Kingsnorth A, et al. Tablet App halometer for the assessment of dysphotopsia. J Cataract Refract Surg. 2015;41(11):2424–9. https://doi.org/10.1016/j.jcrs.2015.05.041.
10. Vinas M, Aissati S, Romero M, Benedi-Garcia C, Garzon N, Poyales F, et al. Pre-operative simulation of post-operative multifocal vision. Biomed Opt Express. 2019;10(11):5801. https://doi.org/10.1364/BOE.10.005801.
11. Hood CT, Sugar A. Subjective complaints after cataract surgery: common causes and management strategies. Curr Opin Ophthalmol. 2015;26(1):45–9. https://doi.org/10.1097/ICU.0000000000000112.
12. Holladay JT, Simpson MJ. Negative dysphotopsia: causes and rationale for prevention and treatment. J Cataract Refract Surg. 2017;43(2):263–75. https://doi.org/10.1016/j.jcrs.2016.11.049.

13. Pepin SM. Neuroadaptation of presbyopia-correcting intraocular lenses. Curr Opin Ophthalmol. 2008;19(1):10–2. https://doi.org/10.1097/ICU.0b013e3282f31758.
14. Masket S, Rupnick Z, Fram NR, Kwong S, McLachlan J. Surgical management of positive dysphotopsia: U.S. perspective. J Cataract Refract Surg. 2020;46(11):1474 9. https://doi.org/10.1097/j.jcrs.0000000000000307.
15. Masket S, Fram NR, Cho A, Park I, Pham D. Surgical management of negative dysphotopsia. J Cataract Refract Surg. 2018;44(1):6–16. https://doi.org/10.1016/j.jcrs.2017.10.038.

Slit Lamp Examination

Gernot Steinwender and Andreas Wedrich

Accurate preoperative diagnostics are essential for patient selection and surgical planning. The assessment of the anterior eye segment is of particular importance, as this is the location of the most relevant refractive structures. Even though imaging diagnostics advanced fundamentally in the last decade, the slit-lamp microscope still is an indispensable preoperative instrument.

During preoperative slit-lamp examination, a macroscopic assessment of the **periocular region** should be performed in addition to the microscopic examination. Findings that may potentially complicate the surgical procedure, such as deep-set eyes or prominent brows, can be identified. Eyelid malpositions relevant for lens surgery are described in detail in Chap. "Eyelids". When assessing the **eyelids**, attention should be paid to signs of blepharitis, which should be treated prior to surgery. Even in the presence of meibomian gland dysfunction, preoperative treatment with warm compresses, lid massages and lid scrubs as well as anti-inflammatory therapy may alleviate dry eye symptoms which are typically exacerbated by lens surgery [1].

Disorders of the ocular surface and **tear film** are common in patients presenting for lens surgery. Thus, the assessment should include instillation of fluorescein drops to determine the tear film break-up time (TBUT) and to detect epitheliopathy. Regardless of whether a monofocal or multifocal intraocular lens (IOL) is implanted, the optical quality after lens surgery may be impaired by aggravation of ocular surface disorders in the first postoperative months [2]. For a detailed description of this topic refer to Chap. "Tear Film Analysis". When inspecting the **conjunctiva**, attention should be paid to irregularities of the bulbar conjunctiva (e.g. scars after strabismus or glaucoma surgery, pinguecula), which may lead to

G. Steinwender (✉) · A. Wedrich
Medical University of Graz, Graz, Austria
e-mail: steinwender.gernot@gmail.com

A. Wedrich
e-mail: andreas.wedrich@medunigraz.at

M. Shajari et al. (eds.), *Cataract and Lens Surgery*,
https://doi.org/10.1007/978-3-031-05394-8_10

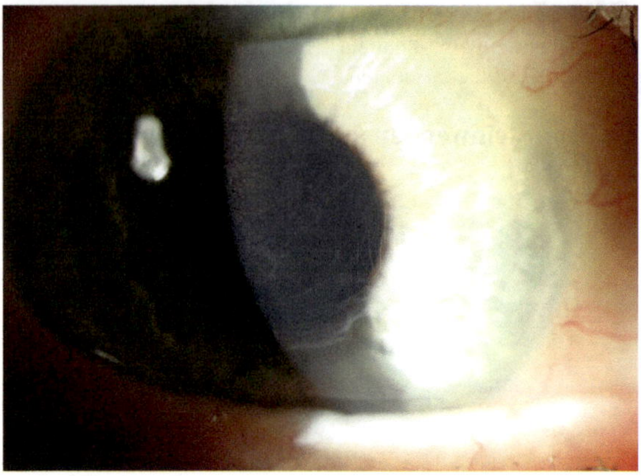

Fig. 1 Epithelial basement membrane dystrophy with fingerprint-like lines and geographic lesions

suction problems when attaching the patient interface to the eye in femtosecond laser-assisted cataract surgery.

The **cornea** as the most important refractive structure should deserve particularly careful examination. Corneal dystrophies, scars or pterygium may have an impact on the visual result after lens surgery. Epithelial basement membrane dystrophy (EBMD) (Fig. 1) can lead to clinically significant changes in keratometry values [3] as well as to fluctuations in postoperative refraction and visual acuity. For these reasons, the use of multifocal IOLs is not recommended in patients with EBMD, as the postoperative result could be severely impaired. Furthermore, toric IOLs should only be considered in EBMD patients if consistent keratometry values can be achieved with different measuring devices over several days. Pre-treatment with phototherapeutic keratectomy (PTK) in symptomatic patients often leads to an alleviation of visual complaints, although the condition may recur [4].

Patients with Fuchs' endothelial dystrophy (Fig. 2) should not be considered eligible for multifocal IOLs, as the optical quality may be impaired even in early stages [5]. It is known that implantation of multifocal IOLs potentially decrease contrast sensitivity in otherwise healthy eyes [6]. Consequently, the reduced optical quality is not likely to be outweighed by the potential benefits of a multifocal IOL in Fuchs' dystrophy, especially considering the progressive course of the disease. When using toric IOLs in patients with Fuchs' endothelial dystrophy, special consideration should be given to potential alterations of corneal astigmatism by a subsequent endothelial keratoplasty [7].

Corneal scars require further diagnostic measures to fully examine location, depth and induced astigmatism. Peripheral asymptomatic scars do not represent a contraindication for multifocal or toric IOL implantation. In the presence of pterygium, active progression should be ruled out and the potential impact on the visual outcome should be reflected in IOL selection.

When assessing the **iris**, attention should be paid to signs of intraocular inflammation (synechiae, iris pigment deposits on anterior lens surface) and pigment dispersion (iris transillumination) (Fig. 3). Patients with iris atrophy have an increased risk of postoperative dysphotopsia (e.g. glare) and zonular instability (caused by previous inflammation) for both multifocal and monofocal IOLs. Phakic

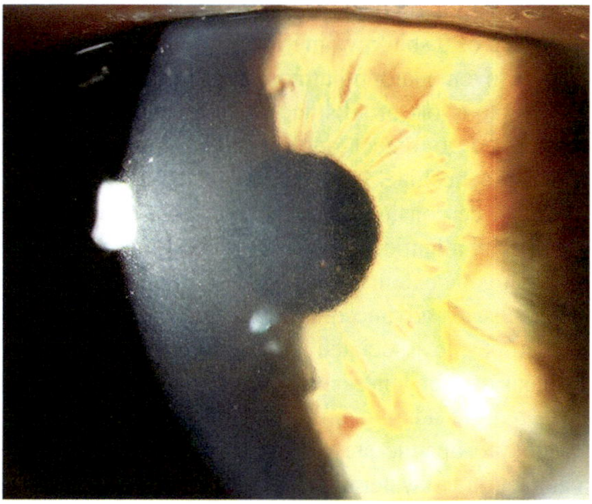

Fig. 2 Fuchs' endothelial corneal dystrophy with guttata on the back of the cornea

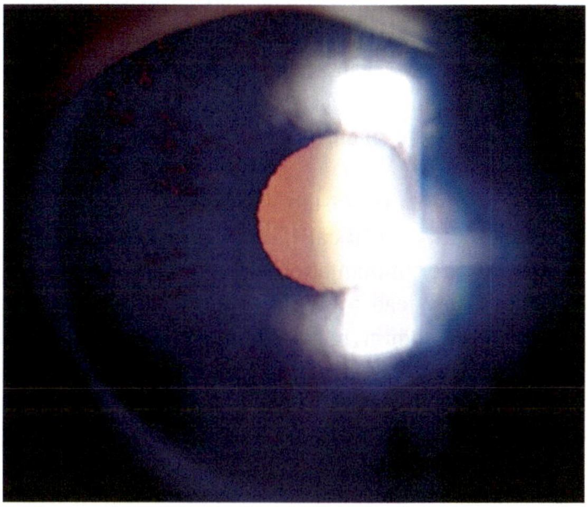

Fig. 3 Iris transillumination due to pigment defects of the iris

IOLs should not be implanted in patients with iris atrophy or pigment dispersion syndrome, as direct contact between the IOL and the iris can potentially induce inflammatory reactions and increased pigment dispersion [8]. Iridodonesis at the margin of the undilated pupil is a sign of reduced zonular integrity and therefore may alter the surgical plan.

A small pupil can lead to difficulties with IOL implantation. Intraoperative application of pupil dilating techniques (e.g. Malyugin ring, iris hooks) can damage the iris sphincter and subsequently lead to iatrogenic mydriasis, which may lead to disturbing reflections and dysphotopsias, especially in multifocal IOLs [6]. More complex pupillary anomalies such as eccentric pupils or iris colobomas are considered a contraindication for multifocal IOLs, since a dislocated capsulorhexis is a risk factor for IOL decentration which may impair IOL function [9].

The depth of the **anterior chamber** should be determined preoperatively, as presence of a shallow anterior chamber might indicate a narrow angle, a very short eye or even nanophthalmos, an intumescent cataract, or ciliary body pathology leading to a forward displacement of the iris-lens diaphragm. Gonioscopy should be performed to detect angle abnormalities like neovascularisations or peripheral anterior synechiae. In presence of a closable angle, removal of a relatively clear lens can also be considered to create more space in the anterior chamber.

Special attention should be paid to the examination of the **lens**. Pupil dilation for assessing the extent of lens opacification is essential prior to lens surgery. Brunescent cataracts are advanced nuclear cataracts that appear brown and opaque but may sometimes be associated with remarkably good visual acuity. Nevertheless, the hard nucleus of such lenses may require a high amount of phacoemulsification energy and may require adaptions of the surgical plan. Advanced cortical cataracts becoming white and opaque are called mature cataracts. Progressive swelling of the cortical cataract due to water up take leads to intumescent cataract, which is associated with a higher risk of complications, particularly during the capsulorhexis. Posterior subcapsular cataracts often appear in patients younger than those presenting with cortical or nuclear cataract and can best be detected by retroillumination.

In the absence of significant lens opacification, the implantation of myopic phakic posterior chamber IOLs represents an interesting alternative to refractive lens exchange, as the manufacturer recently expanded the age range for patients up to 60 years.

Signs of zonular instability should be examined and documented prior to lens surgery. With multifocal IOLs in particular, patient satisfaction is strongly dependent on proper implantation and centration of the IOL. A decentration of as little as 0.75 mm may lead to a significant reduction of postoperative optical quality [10]. The most common reason for IOL decentration is pseudoexfoliation syndrome (PEX) [11] (Fig. 4). In characteristic asymmetrical zonular instability, the IOL shifts away from the weakened area towards the intact fibres. Thus, the stability regarding IOL centration and rotation is not predictable in PEX patients and may change over time. To avoid these issues, multifocal and toric IOLs are not recommended in patients with PEX. The use of a capsular tension ring during lens surgery distributes forces along the equator of the lens capsule more evenly in eyes with modest asymmetrical zonular weakness and therefore has a stabilising effect on the IOL position, though it does not reduce the long term risk of IOL luxation. In eyes at risk, the simultaneous use of a capsular tension ring during implantation of toric or multifocal IOLs significantly improved visual outcomes [12].

Author's recommendation

In the presence of pseudoexfoliation syndrome, the use of multifocal or toric IOLs is not recommended due to an increased risk of subsequent IOL decentration or rotation.

Biomicroscopic examination of the anterior segment should always be followed by dilated fundoscopy to assess the posterior segment prior to lens surgery. This is not only to identify potentially limiting conditions, but also to document random

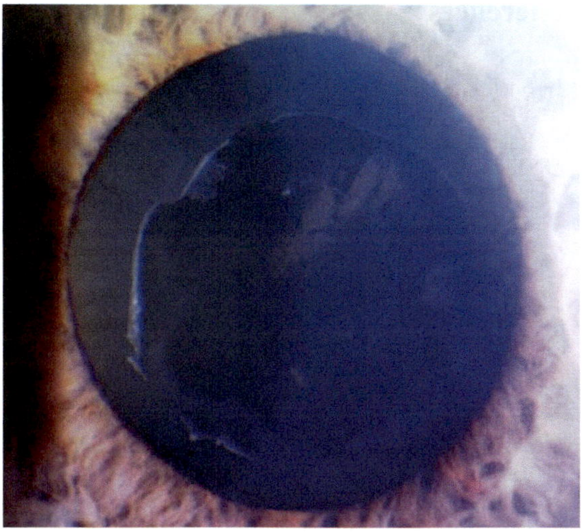

Fig. 4 Pseudoexfoliation syndrome with typical deposits on the anterior lens capsule

findings primarily without causal impact on the visual result, but which can be interpreted by the patient as being causal if problems arise at a later stage.

In the presence of **retinal** disease, the patient selection for multifocal IOL implantation depends primarily on the expected course of the disease. Potential issues that may arise include both a reduced visual outcome for the patient and reduced visualisation of the posterior eye segment for the treating ophthalmologist. While retinitis pigmentosa and Stargardt's disease are classified as absolute contraindications for the use of multifocal IOLs, the more frequent maculopathies, such as diabetic retinopathy, age-related macular degeneration or epiretinal membranes, can have a wide range of presentations which may still be compatible with some multifocal lenses [13, 14]. A crucial criterion for patient selection is the progression of retinal diseases after cataract surgery. These diseases lead to a loss of contrast sensitivity, which can be exacerbated by the further reduction of contrast sensitivity associated with the implantation of multifocal IOLs. Signs of myopic maculopathy should also be documented and discussed with the patient, although good results can be achieved for highly myopic patients after multifocal IOL implantation [15].

Peripheral retinal degenerations are not uncommon in patients (often myopic) prior to lens surgery and should also be documented and discussed. A correlation between such lesions with an increased risk for retinal detachment has not been confirmed [16] and prophylactic laser coagulation should only be performed after individual consideration of all risk factors (patient age, degree of myopia, type of degeneration, presence of vitreous detachment, complication risk of lens surgery).

Anomalies of the **optic nerve** that can potentially limit visual acuity, contrast sensitivity, colour perception or visual field are generally considered as contraindications for the use of multifocal IOLs, particularly in progressive diseases such as glaucoma [17]. The implantation of phakic IOLs is also contraindicated in manifest glaucoma, since (especially in sulcus-fixated models) sporadic increases in intraocular pressure have been described [8].

References

1. Song P, Sun Z, Ren S, Yang K, Deng G, Zeng Q, et al. Preoperative management of MGD alleviates the aggravation of MGD and dry eye induced by cataract surgery: a prospective. Randomized Clinical Trial Biomed Res Int. 2019;2019:2737968.
2. Omes JAP, Azar DT, Baudouin C, Efron N, Hirayama M, Horwath-Winter J, et al. TFOS DEWS II iatrogenic report. Ocul Surf. 2017;15(3):511–38.
3. Goerlitz-Jessen MF, Gupta PK, Kim T. Impact of epithelial basement membrane dystrophy and Salzmann nodular degeneration on biometry measurements. J Cataract Refract Surg. 2019;45(8):1119–23.
4. Germundsson J, Fagerholm P, Lagali N. Clinical outcome and recurrence of epithelial basement membrane dystrophy after phototherapeutic keratectomy a cross-sectional study. Ophthalmology. 2011;118(3):515–22.
5. Watanabe S, Oie Y, Fujimoto H, Soma T, Koh S, Tsujikawa M, et al. Relationship between corneal guttae and quality of vision in patients with mild Fuchs' endothelial corneal dystrophy. Ophthalmology. 2015;122(10):2103–9.
6. de Vries NE, Webers CAB, Touwslager WRH, Bauer NJC, de Brabander J, Berendschot TT, et al. Dissatisfaction after implantation of multifocal intraocular lenses. J Cataract Refract Surg. 2011;37(5):859–65.
7. Shajari M, Kolb CM, Mayer WJ, Agha B, Steinwender G, Dirisamer M, et al. Characteristics of preoperative and postoperative astigmatism in patients having Descemet membrane endothelial keratoplasty. J Cataract Refract Surg. 2019;45(7):1001–6.
8. Kohnen T, Kook D, Morral M, Güell JL. Phakic intraocular lenses: part 2: results and complications. J Cataract Refract Surg. 2010;36(12):2168–94.
9. Montés-Micó R, López-Gil N, Pérez-Vives C, Bonaque S, Ferrer-Blasco T. In vitro optical performance of nonrotational symmetric and refractive-diffractive aspheric multifocal intraocular lenses: impact of tilt and decentration. J Cataract Refract Surg. 2012;38(9):1657–63.
10. Tandogan T, Son HS, Choi CY, Knorz MC, Auffarth GU, Khoramnia R. Laboratory evaluation of the influence of decentration and pupil size on the optical performance of a monofocal, bifocal, and trifocal intraocular lens. J Refract Surg. 2017;33(12):808–12.
11. Walkow T, Anders N, Pham DT, Wollensak J. Causes of severe decentration and subluxation of intraocular lenses. Graefes Arch Clin Exp Ophthalmol. 1998;236(1):9–12.
12. Miyoshi T, Fujie S, Yoshida H, Iwamoto H, Tsukamoto H, Oshika T. Effects of capsular tension ring on surgical outcomes of premium intraocular lens in patients with suspected zonular weakness. PLoS ONE. 2020;15(2):e0228999.
13. Alio JL, Plaza-Puche AB, Férnandez-Buenaga R, Pikkel J, Maldonado M. Multifocal intraocular lenses: an overview. Surv Ophthalmol. 2017;62(5):611–34.
14. Grzybowski A, Kanclerz P, Tuuminen R. Multifocal intraocular lenses and retinal diseases. Graefes Arch Clin Exp Ophthalmol. 2020;258(4):805–13.
15. Steinwender G, Schwarz L, Böhm M, Slavík-Lenčová A, Hemkeppler E, Shajari M, et al. Visual results after implantation of a trifocal intraocular lens in high myopes. J Cataract Refract Surg. 2018;44(6):680–5.
16. Wilkinson CP. Interventions for asymptomatic retinal breaks and lattice degeneration for preventing retinal detachment. Cochrane Database Syst Rev. 2014;(9):CD003170.
17. Kumar BV, Phillips RP, Prasad S. Multifocal intraocular lenses in the setting of glaucoma. Curr Opin Ophthalmol. 2007;18(1):62–6.

Binocular Vision and Motility

Oliver Ehrt

The frequency of diplopia after lens surgery is reported to be as high as 3% [1]. In many cases, this occasionally extremely disturbing complication can be avoided by careful preoperative history, orthoptic examination and an adapted plan for the lens surgery [2–5].

Binocular problems after lens and refractive surgery

Most often, binocular diplopia results from decompensation of a **pre-existing strabismus**. This decompensation can occur by changing the accommodation/convergence tone, fusion disturbance due to altered aniseikonia (see below), postoperative complications (e.g. metamorphopsia in CME), not realising that the patient had been wearing prismatic glasses prior to lens surgery and other errors.

Another cause of diplopia can be the loss of suppression of one eye due to a change in fixation after lens surgery. This can occur, for example, if the amblyopic eye is operated first or in cases of monovision. A dense cataract or uncorrected aphakia can lead to secondary strabismus or loss of fusion if it persists for over 2–3 years.

Patients with a preoperative anisometropia of greater than 3 dioptres are at a particular risk. In these cases, the patient is often accustomed to the prismatic side effect of their glasses, which varies in lateral gaze. If the patient no longer needs to wear glasses after the lens operation, they may suddenly be bothered by double images in lateral gaze. Surgeries that are intended to reduce anisometropia in particular can cause issues. The new aniseikonia can cause diplopia by itself, or as an obstacle to fusion.

Patients with planned monovision or reduction of a pre-existing anisometropia, a preoperative contact lens trial is mandatory unless the cataract is too dense to simulate the postoperative situation.

O. Ehrt (✉)
Ludwig Maximilian University of Munich, Munich, Germany
e-mail: oliver.ehrt@med.uni-muenchen.de

M. Shajari et al. (eds.), *Cataract and Lens Surgery*,
https://doi.org/10.1007/978-3-031-05394-8_11

The timing of lens and strabismus surgeries

If a patient is scheduled for both a lens and an extraocular muscle surgery, surgery should usually be performed in two stages. The lens surgery is typically performed first as an improvement in visual acuity can influence strabismus in both positive and negative ways:

- Improvement of fusion
- More accurate evaluation of strabismus
- Rarely post-operative elevation deficit or binocular complications.

An improvement in fusion after cataract surgery can improve strabismus-related complaints such as diplopia or asthenopia, so that therapy may no longer be necessary, prismatic treatment or only a lower degree of extraocular muscle surgery may be required. Due to the improved visual acuity, strabismus can often also be more accurately examined (squint angle measurement, prism wearing test, better estimation of the postoperative risk of diplopia) and consequent strabismus surgery can be better planned. If new binocular problems arise as a complication of a lens operation (see below), these can be taken into account in the strabismus operation that follows.

In rare cases, it may be useful to perform eye muscle operation before lens operation. In the case of strabismus fixus, in which the eye cannot be moved to the primary position, it is advisable to first bring the eye into primary position so that the lens operation can then be performed more easily and with fewer complications. This extreme situation can occur in severe endocrine orbitopathy, eso-hypotropia in myopia magna ("heavy-eye"), or after orbital injuries. In the case of planned secondary IOL implantation in aphakia and strabismus, an attempt should be made to first test whether diplopia can be eliminated with eye muscle surgery and contact lenses. If no satisfactory field of binocular single vision (BSV) can be achieved, the secondary IOL implantation should not be performed to avoid permanent diplopia.

Simultaneous eye muscle and lens surgery can be considered if no improvement in vision is to be expected from the lens surgery or if there is an increased risk of multiple general anaesthesia in cases where local anaesthesia is not possible. In patients with pronounced nystagmus, no prior eye muscle surgery is needed unless extreme abnormal head position makes biometry more difficult, but good retrobulbar anaesthesia or surgery under general anaesthesia should be considered to immobilise the eyes during lens surgery.

Which eye should be cataract operated on first in case of unilateral amblyopia?

The prevalence of amblyopia is relatively high, seen in approximately 5% of the Caucasian population, so having a plan for managing these patients is valuable. In a patient with unilateral amblyopia and bilateral cataract, the lower relevance of possible complications is in favour of surgery on the amblyopic eye first. However, there is a risk of diplopia if postoperative fixation changes, because the amblyopic eye may become the better eye and suppression may no longer be possible.

Performing surgery on the fixing eye is recommended because it also leads to a faster visual rehabilitation of the patient [6].

Elevation deficit after retrobulbar anaesthesia

One rare complication (1–3/1000) is the myotoxic effect of retrobulbar anaesthesia, which usually leads to an elevation deficit with vertical diplopia. In most cases a good result can be achieved by prism correction or inferior rectus recession.

Conclusion

For each patient, the following points should be considered when planning lens surgery to minimise the risk of postoperative diplopia [2, 3]:

- History: amblyopia, previous occlusion therapy, eye training, strabismus surgery, intermittent diplopia or diplopia in lateral view
- Spectacles: prismatic correction, near addition to treat convergence excess
- Objective refraction, measured in cycloplegia
- Contact lens trial if change of anisometropia >3 dioptres or monovision is planned
- Orthoptic examination: Bagolini test, stereopsis, distance and near cover test.

References

1. Nayak H, Kersey JP, Oystreck DT, Cline RA, Lyons CJ. Diplopia following cataract surgery: a review of 150 patients. Eye (Lond). 2008;22(8):1057–64.
2. Godts D, Tassignon MJ, Gobin L. Binocular vision impairment after refractive surgery. J Cataract Refract Surg. 2004;30(1):101–9.
3. Kushner BJ, Kowal L. Diplopia after refractive surgery: occurrence and prevention. Arch Ophthalmol. 2003;121(3):315–21.
4. Bouffard MA, Cestari DM. Diplopia after cataract extraction. Seminar Ophthalmol. 2018;33 (1):11–6.
5. Sobol EK, Rosenberg JB. Strabismus After Ocular Surgery. J Pediatr Ophthalmol Strabismus. 2017;54(5):272–81.
6. Samuel Williams G, Radwan M, Menon J. Cataract surgery planning in amblyopic patients—which eye first? Awareness of the potential for post-operative diplopia amongst consultant ophthalmic surgeons in Wales. Ulster Med J. 2013;82(2):82–4.

Measurement of Intraocular Pressure

Matthias Nobl and Kaweh Mansouri

The preoperative measurement of intraocular pressure (IOP) is an essential basic test to perform and document prior to cataract surgery. Firstly, basic diseases such as ocular hypertension or glaucoma can be detected and treated, and secondly, important conclusions can be drawn about the intra- and postoperative course of the cataract surgery.

Goldmann applanation tonometry (GAT) is the so-called "gold standard" for measuring IOP. Frequently used alternatives to GAT, which are less reliable than GAT, and not always well-tolerated by all patients, are pneumotonometry (PT) or rebound tonometry (RT). All of these measurement methods mentioned are influenced by the central corneal thickness and other corneo-scleral properties. If the cornea is thicker it presents a higher resistance to deformation and the IOP can be measured incorrectly too high. If the cornea is thinner it presents a lower resistance and can be measured incorrectly too low. This deviation is most pronounced with PT with normal IOP values varying by 0.6 mmHg per 10 μm, and least pronounced with GAT, varying by 0.3 mmHg per 10 μm [1]. Corneal changes such as scars, dystrophies or keratoplasty can also influence IOP measurement. In a study on IOP measurement in corneal lesions, RT was successful in all participants, while GAT was possible in 98.2% of cases [2]. RT can therefore be very helpful in everyday practice to measure IOP in patients with corneal irregularities, although it should be noted that a significant underestimation of the actual IOP can occur [2].

As part of the preliminary examination for cataract surgery, it is important that GAT is only carried out after biometry and corneal topography have been performed. Otherwise, these measurements are distorted by the applanation and

M. Nobl (✉)
Ludwig Maximilians University of Munich, Munich, Germany
e-mail: matthias.nobl@med.uni-muenchen.de

K. Mansouri
University of Colorado School of Medicine, Denver, USA

M. Shajari et al. (eds.), *Cataract and Lens Surgery*,
https://doi.org/10.1007/978-3-031-05394-8_12

fluorescein, which can significantly affect the planning of the most suitable intraocular lens [3].

As already mentioned, important conclusions can be drawn from the preoperative IOP. Browning et al. showed that a higher preoperative IOP, the presence of ocular hypertension or glaucoma are significant risk factors for an IOP of 26 mmHg or higher on the first postoperative day [4]. In addition, cataract surgery is known to have an IOP lowering effect. The higher the preoperative IOP, and the flatter the anterior chamber, the greater the effect [5]. In a study population of 999 patients with preoperative IOP values between 7 and 21 mmHg, the average IOP reduction three months postoperatively was 1.6 mmHg [5].

It is also important to follow IOP measurements postoperatively and be aware that corneal oedema can falsify the measured values. Neuburger et al. showed in an experimental setup with artificial anterior chambers that oedematous donor corneas and manometrically controllable IOP could be measured more accurately with RT than with GAT or PT using an ocular response analyser [6]. With manometrically determined anterior chamber internal pressure of 10, 20, 30, 40 and 50 mmHg, IOP was increasingly measured too low using GAT, with an average deviation of 3.5 mmHg at 20 mmHg up to 14.9 mmHg at 50 mmHg [6].

Author's recommendation

In the presence of postoperative corneal oedema, RT might be a more accurate method to measure IOP.

References

1. Chen M, Zhang L, Xu J, Chen X, Gu Y, Ren Y, et al. Comparability of three intraocular pressure measurement: iCare pro rebound, non-contact and Goldmann applanation tonometry in different IOP group. BMC Ophthalmol. 2019;19(1):225.
2. Rose Treader A, Athanasopoulos A, Shield AM, Lappas A, Course Depths C, Diets TS. Rebound, applanation, and dynamic contour tonometry in pathologic corneas. Cornea. 2013; 32(3):313–8.
3. Rabsilber TM, Bueltmann S, Holzer MP, Auffarth GU. Effect of applanation tonometry on precision of biometry measurements. Der Ophthalmol: J Ger Ophthalmol Soc. 2011; 108(1):52–6.
4. Browning AC, Alwitry A, Hamilton R, Rotchford A, Bhan A, Amoaku WM. Role of intraocular pressure measurement on the day of phacoemulsification cataract surgery. J Cataract Refract Surg. 2002;28(9):1601–6.
5. Yang HS, Lee J, Choi S. Ocular biometric parameters associated with intraocular pressure reduction after cataract surgery in normal eyes. Am J Ophthalmol. 2013;156(1):89-94.e1.
6. Neuburger M, Maier P, Böhringer D, Reinhard T, Jordan FJ. The impact of corneal edema on intraocular pressure measurements using Goldmann applanation tonometry, Tono-Pen XL, iCare, and ORA: an in vitro model. J Glaucoma. 2013; 22(7):584–90.

Eyelids

Christoph Hintschich

When planning a lens operation also some issues with regard to the eyelids should be considered. These conditions include eyelid malformations, eyelid tumors and lacrimal drainage occlusion.

Which eyelid malpositions are relevant in lens surgery?

Both pre-existing eyelid malpositions, which can cause an increased risk of complications and impair the result of lens surgery [1], and malpositions caused or deteriorated secondary to lens surgery [2] are relevant.

Pre-existing Eyelid Malpositions

In the first group we find malpositions that cause impairment of the regular ocular surface, i.e. changes that prevent even and complete moistening of the ocular surface or cause exposure of the ocular surface, thereby leading to surface defects (Ocular Surface Disease—OSD). These include eyelid margin irregularities, trichiasis and distichiasis, entropion of the lower or upper eyelid. Ectropion and eyelid retraction, and generally any form of lagophthalmos in the absence of a Bell′ s phenomenon, can cause OSD. Introducing the term "Meibomian gland inversion" Malhotra [3] has recently described a commonly unnoticed inversion of the meibomian gland exiting in the margin of the eyelid as a cause of persistent ocular surface problems.

Rubbing lashes in entropion and trichiasis/distichiasis, and lagophthalmos i.e. in posttraumatic eyelid retraction, facial palsy or Graves' disease can lead to surface disturbance due to corneal exposure; the same applies to the relatively common age-associated acquired ectropion of the lower lid. Spontaneous nocturnal eversion of the upper eyelid due to a "floppy eyelid syndrome" [4], which is usually asso-

C. Hintschich (✉)
Augenklinik der LMU, Klinikum der Universität München, Campus Innenstadt, Mathildenstr. 8, D-80336 München, Deutschland
e-mail: christoph.hintschich@med.uni-muenchen.de

M. Shajari et al. (eds.), *Cataract and Lens Surgery*,
https://doi.org/10.1007/978-3-031-05394-8_13

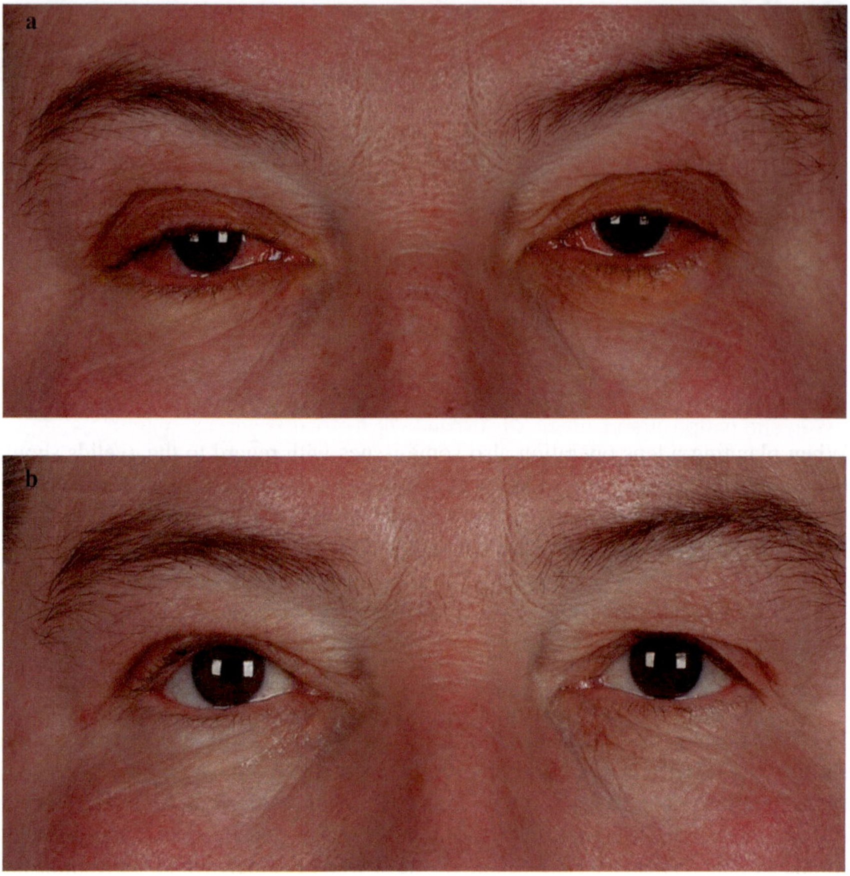

Fig. 1 **a** Patient with bilateral red eye and conjunctival irritation (OSD) due to floppy eyelid syndrome with involutional ptosis. **b** Same patient after bilateral horizontal eyelid shortening and ptosis correction, now white and quiet ocular surface, before lens surgery

ciated with sleep apnoea, leads to red eye with OSD and thus increased risk after lens surgery (Fig. 1).

Special attention and prophylactic measures are indicated in the presence of an ocular pemphigoid. This includes systemic immunosuppression to be administered preoperatively and, if indicated, surgical correction of manifest eyelid malpositions, avoiding any direct conjunctival traumatization [5].

For the correction of relevant eyelid malpositions, well-established surgical techniques such as a lateral canthal sling procedure (Fig. 2), everting or inverting sutures, blepharotomy and numerous other more sophisticated surgical procedures are available; usually they can be performed under local anesthesia.

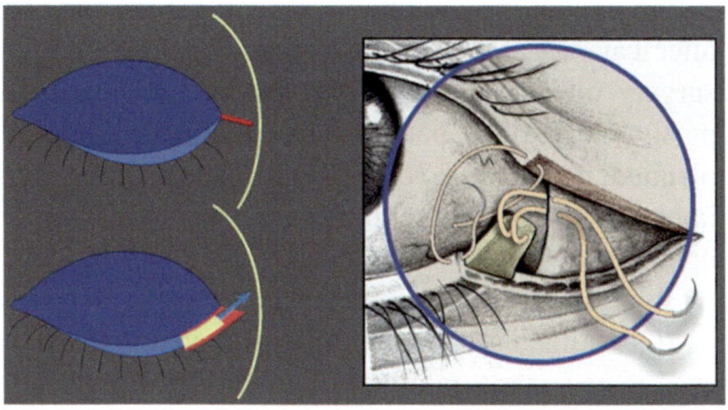

Fig. 2 Lateral canthal sling procedure: periosteal fixation within the inner area of the lateral bony orbital entrance

Author's recommendation

Any eyelid malposition causing disturbance of the ocular surface with conjunctival irritation or keratopathy should be corrected surgically before scheduled lens surgery.

Eyelid Malpositions Caused by Cataract Surgery

The prevalence of persistent upper eyelid ptosis after cataract surgery is a frequently described but ultimately only incompletely understood phenomenon. The frequency is quoted as 3.2% [6] to as high as 33.6% [7], transient postoperative ptosis is much more frequent.

The extent of ptosis on the first post-operative day was found to be a predictor of persistent ptosis after 6 months [8]. Several factors are discussed as causes: Local anesthesia (volume effect and myotoxicity), traction suture, eyelid closure, size and location of the incision, pre-existing dehiscence of the levator aponeurosis, eyelid oedema, experience of the surgeon and duration of surgery [6, 9]. Most of these factors no longer occur in modern cataract surgery. This is also reflected in a lower incidence in recent studies that refer to phacoemulsification without a traction suture under topical anesthesia [6, 10].

Although the incidence is decreasing due to gentler surgical techniques, pre-operative information and counselling of patients is recommended [6]. It is also important to look for signs of pre-existing involutional ptosis before cataract surgery and to document this. These are a reduced or asymmetric vertical eyelid fissure and a high eyelid skin crease in combination with a good levator function. If indicated, the surgical correction of acquired involutional upper eyelid ptosis can reliably be performed under local anesthesia [11].

After a ptosis correction, changes in the corneal topography have been described [12]. However, these very small deviations are usually temporary and of minor relevance in everyday clinical practice [13]. Nevertheless, they are a reason to wait a few months before measuring the refraction before lens surgery; the main reason for a time interval until cataract surgery is, however, the fact that after a ptosis correction, transient sicca symptoms with reduced eyelid closure are also observed [14, 15].

Pre-existing involutional ptosis, on the other hand, will usually be addressed after cataract surgery, not at least because of the possible influence of cataract surgery on eyelid height. Exceptions are possible, especially in cases of severe ptosis and explicit patient request. If lens surgery after ptosis correction is then planned, it should be postponed for at least three months to wait for the spontaneous improvement of the eyelid closure with sicca symptoms that occurs after each ptosis operation.

What to do in the case of eyelid tumors?

If a malignant lesion in the eyelid area is suspected, it should first be diagnosed and, if necessary, removed by a histopathologically controlled surgical excision. This is particularly true in fast-growing tumors such as a squamous cell carcinoma or Merkel cell tumor. Because of possible impairment of eyelid closure and a mechanical instability of the eyelid after reconstruction, lens surgery using an eyelid retractor should then be postponed for 3–6 months.

Rehabilitation of lacrimal duct stenosis—cataract surgery: what first?

A manifest epiphora or a history of recurrent inflammation of the lacrimal duct should always be clarified and, if necessary, surgically repaired before cataract surgery, considering that lacrimal duct stenosis represents a proven risk of complications after cataract surgery, which can lead to endophthalmitis [16].

Author's recommendation

- Do not ignore the eyelids and their role for ocular surface integrity during the pre-op examination for scheduled lens surgery.
- Correct any eyelid malposition with negative impact on the ocular surface before lens surgery; if necessary, introduce the patient to a colleague with oculoplastic experience.
- Document pre-existing upper eyelid ptosis (photo).
- Inform the patient about the risk of deterioration or new occurrence of acquired involutional ptosis after lens surgery.
- Treat malignant eyelid tumors in consultation with the patient before lens surgery (ideally: histologically controlled excision); after reconstruction (lid margin suture) wait 6–12 weeks with cataract extraction (careful with eyelid retractor).
- In the case of epiphora, clarify the flow disturbance of the lacrimal drainage system; if possible, treat manifest causes (lacrimal punctum eversion, lacrimal duct stenosis) before lens surgery.

References

1. Chuang JSK, Chan TC, Wan KH, Jhanji V, Tong L. Preoperative optimisation of ocular surface disease before cataract surgery. J Cataract Refract Surg. 2017;43(12):1596–607.
2. Ahuero AE, Mark H. Eyelid malposition after cataract and refractive surgery. Int Ophthalmol Clin. 2010; 50(1):25–36.
3. Siah WF, Boboridis K, Tan P, Litwin AS, Daya SM, Malhotra R. Meibomian gland inversion: under-recognized entity. Acta Ophthalmol. 2019;97(8):e1116-22.

4. Idowu OOAD, Vagefi MR, Kersten RC, Winn BJ. Floppy eyelid syndrome: ocular and systemic associations. Curr Opin Ophthalmol. 2019;30(6):513–24.
5. Geerling GDJ. Management and outcome of cataract surgery in ocular cicatricial pemphigoid. Graefes Arch Clin Exp Ophthalmol. 2000;238(2):112–8.
6. Kashkouli MB, Abdolalizadeh P, Es'haghi A, Nilforushan N, Aghaei H, Karimi N. Postoperative blepharoptosis after modern phacoemulsification procedure. On J Ophthalmol. 2020;213:17–23.
7. Singh SK, Sekhar GC, Gupta S. Etiology of ptosis after cataract surgery. J Cataract Refract Surg. 1997;23(9):1409–13.
8. Hosal BM, Tekeli O, Gursel E. Eyelid malpositions after cataract surgery. Eur J Ophthalmol. 1998;8(1):12–5.
9. Chaplain LJ, Jaffe NS, Clayman HM. Ptosis and cataract surgery. A multivariant computer analysis of a prospective study. Ophthalmology. 1985; 92(2):237–42.
10. Puvanachandra N, Hustler A, Seah LL, Tyers AG. The incidence of ptosis following extracapsular and phacoemulsification surgery: comparison of two prospective studies and review of the literature. Orbit. 2010;29(6):321–3.
11. Hintschich C. [Ptosis surgery. current aspects]. Ophthalmologist. 2012; 109(5):430–7.
12. Savino G, Battendieri R, Riso M, Traina S, Poscia A, D'Amico G, et al. Corneal topographic changes after eyelid ptosis surgery. Cornea. 2016;35(4):501–5.
13. Holck DE, Dutton JJ, Wehrly SR. Changes in astigmatism after ptosis surgery measured by corneal topography. Ophthalmic Plast Reconstr Surg. 1998;14(3):151–8.
14. Watanabe A, Selva D, Kakizaki H, Oka Y, Yokoi N, Wakimasu K, et al. Long-term tear volume changes after blepharoptosis surgery and blepharoplasty. Invest Ophthalmol Vis Sci. 2014;56(1):54–8.
15. Zloto O, Matani A, Prat D, Leshno A, Ben SG. The effect of a ptosis procedure compared to an upper blepharoplasty on dry eye syndrome. On J Ophthalmol. 2020;212:1–6.
16. Kam JK, Cheng NM, Sarossy M, Allen PJ, Brooks AM. Nasolacrimal duct screening to minimize post-cataract surgery endophthalmitis. Clin Exp Ophthalmol. 2014;42(5):447–51.

Optical Biometry

Oliver Findl and Nino Hirnschall

One of the most important developments in the calculation of IOLs was the introduction of optical biometry [1]. This is followed closely by developments in IOL power calculation formulae [2]. In this chapter, the evolution, fundamentals and latest developments of optical biometry will be discussed.

Partial Coherence Interferometry (PCI)

Before the introduction of optical biometry, the measurement of the eye length was the second largest source of error [3–5]. The introduction of optical biometry to the field was a milestone and took place in Austria, in Vienna at the Institute for Medical Physics specifically. Prof. Fercher [6] was the original pioneer of this method, which was then further developed together with Profs. Hitzenberger and Drexler. The first studies were eventually carried out on cataract patients, in cooperation with Prof. Findl [7]. In the 1980s the concept of partial coherence interferometry was already in clinical use in the measurement of ocular axial length [8] and the first clinical studies for the measurement of the anterior segment and axial length followed in the 1990s [3, 9, 10]. The PCI method had some clear advantages over the ultrasound method. PCI could be performed without touching the globe, so the eye length s not manipulated during the examination. This was a significant advantage over contact ultrasound where the act of touching the globe can induce a dent making the measurement inaccurate. Immersion ultrasound avoids this risk but still requires some manipulation to create the fluid interface.—PCI biometry required no contact with the eye at all, unlike any other type of ultrasound. Some further advantages of optical biometry are that the examination is technician independent and can be carried out much faster and with much higher

O. Findl
VIROS-Vienna Institute for Research in Ocular Surgery, Hanusch hospital, Vienna, Austria

N. Hirnschall (✉)
Department of Ophthalmology and Optometry, Johannes Kepler University, Linz, Austria
e-mail: nino.hirnschall@kepleruniklinikum.at

M. Shajari et al. (eds.), *Cataract and Lens Surgery*,
https://doi.org/10.1007/978-3-031-05394-8_14

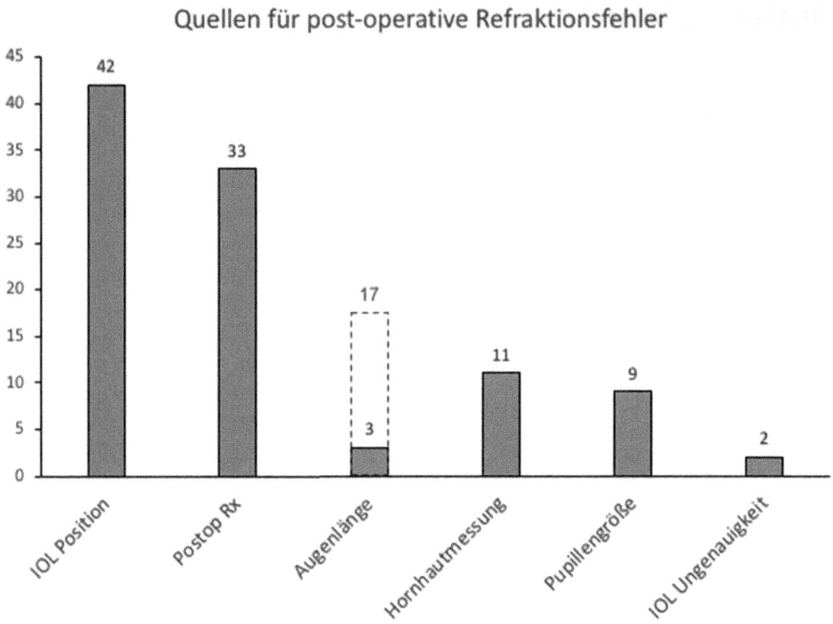

Fig. 1 Sverker Norrbys graphic from 2008 in modified form [5]. The individual bars represent the sources of error. For axial length, the value for contact ultrasound (17%) and for partial coherence interferometry technology (3%) is given—the remaining bars refer to the PCI method. Augenlänge = axial eye length; Hornhautmessung = corneal radii, Pupillengröße = pupil size; IOL Ungenauigkeit = IOL labelling error

precision and resolution than the previous ultrasound devices [11]. Finally, the measurement is based on the fixation axis of the eye, which is not necessarily the case with ultrasound.

Over 10 years ago, Norrby [5] showed that axial length measurement with contact ultrasound accounted for 17% of the total error in the calculation of IOLs. However, when this study is re-evaluated using PCI technology instead of contact ultrasound, the error of the measurement decreases from 17 to 3% (Fig. 1).

While the underlying physical principles of the PCI method are out of the scope of this chapter, basically, a "dual beam" version of the classic Michelson interferometer using a light source with a wavelength of usually 780 nm (Fig. 2) [3]. The measuring distance is another point that should be considered. With classical ultrasound, the measurement is made from the anterior corneal surface to the inner limiting membrane but with PCI procedures the measurement is to the retinal pigment epithelium. This difference was "converted" to ultrasound when optical biometry devices were originally introduced.

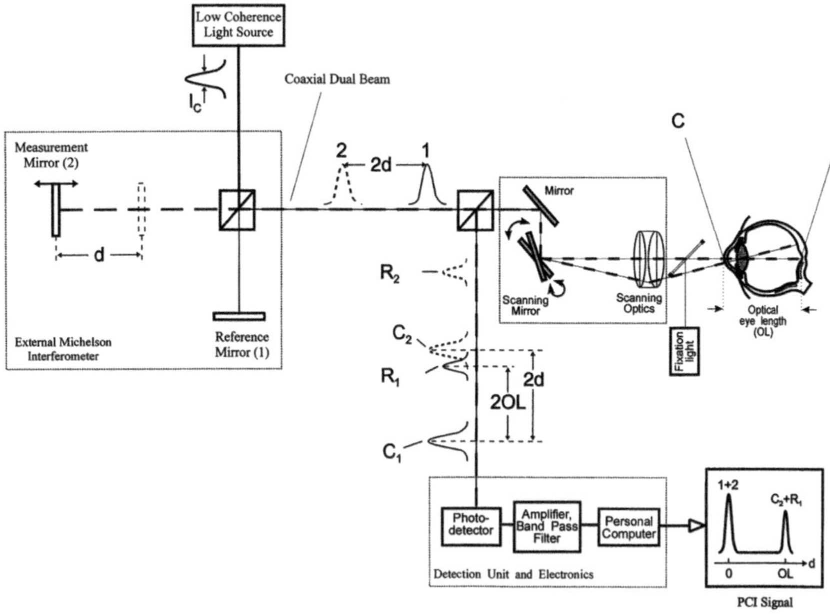

Fig. 2 Representation of partial coherence interferometry (taken over from [3]). The eye is illuminated by means of an external interferometer, which generates a co-axial double beam with a specific wavelength. Important components of the external interferometer are a semitransparent mirror and a reference mirror. Both parts of the double beam have a common time delay which is twice the interferometer length difference (2d). In the eye, the two beam components are changed ("delayed") due to contact with different refractive indices and a partial coherence interferometry signal (PCI signal) is produced. Reflected signals from the eye (in the figure as an example C1, C2, R1 and R2) are detected by a photodetector, whereupon the PCI signal of the axial length is generated as optical distance (OL). A scanning mirror is used for this. Finally, the optical signal has to be corrected according to the refractive indices in the eye (usually a group refractive index) to obtain an anatomical distance

Composite Scan

While PCI technology has many clear advantages, it is not without a disadvantage. If the media is too opacified, optical biometric measurements may not be possible and an ultrasonic measurement should be used. The reason for this is a mixture of different optical phenomena such as absorption, reflection and scattered light (especially Rayleigh scattering) can distort the PCI measurement. There are different approaches to reduce this problem. The first approach, known as composite scanning, was introduced in the IOL master (Carl Zeiss Meditec AG, Jena, Germany) by upgrading the software [12]. Prior to the introduction of the composite scan, each measurement (i.e., each A-scan) was evaluated individually. Each peak of the A-scan was evaluated using the signal to noise ratio (SNR) and if the main peak was not sufficiently distinct from the remaining peaks (noise), the scan was not successful. In the composite scan, the individual scans are superimposed

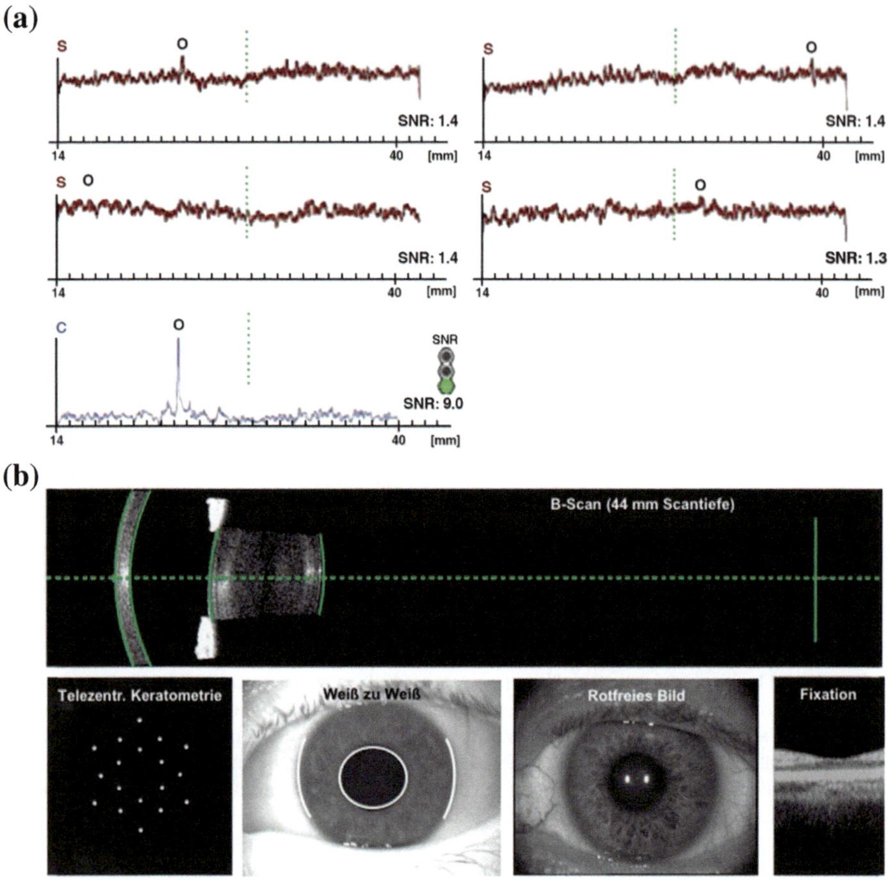

Fig. 3 **a** Four PCI-based A-scans (red) of a patient with dense cataract. As the signal to noise ratio (SNR) is too low, and the individual scans do not show clear peaks. In the composite scan (blue), the four individual scans are superimposed on each other, thus amplifying the real signals. This results in an improved signal to noise ratio and a clear peak representing the length of the eyes (adopted from [12]). **b** The longitudinal ssOCT based B-scan of the IOLMaster 700 produces an image with visible anatomical details instead of individual peaks. ssOCT based is the axial section (upper image), as well as the macular scan (far right) for fixation control. The keratometry, white-to-white measurement and the red-free image (for intra-operative alignment for toric artificial lenses) are not ssOCT based (from the ESCRS presentation in London 2014). **c** ssOCT based B-Scan of the Anterion with tomographic corneal image (top right) and signal intensity display for cornea, lens and axial length in mm (bottom)

(Fig. 3a). This amplifies real peaks because they occur in several scans and the other peaks (noise) cancel each other out. In a clinical evaluation of the composite scan, the rate of unsuccessful scans was reduced from 10% to less than 5% [12]. Later, another biometric device using the same method was launched on the market, the AL-Scan (Nidek Co., LTD, Japan) [13].

(c)

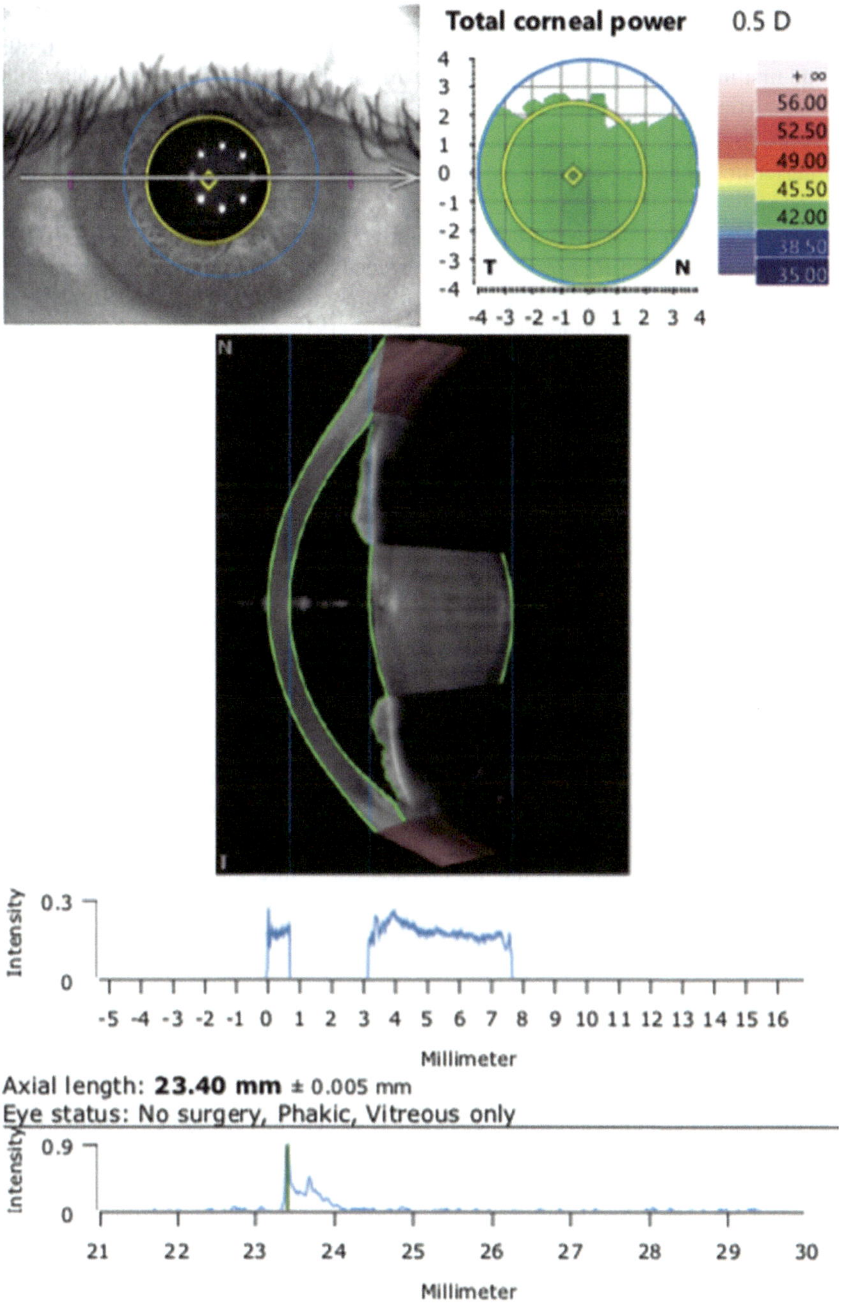

Fig. 3 (continued)

PCI-Like Procedures

The best-known A-scan alternative is optical low coherence reflectometry (OLCR). The first instrument on the market using this approach was the Lenstar (Haag-Streit Diagnostics, Switzerland) followed by the Aladdin (Topcon, Japan) [14]. Similar to the PCI method, an A-scan is used and the concept is also based on a Michelson interferometer but in contrast to the PCI method, a slightly longer wavelength is used (820 nm) [15].

In various comparative studies, the differences in axial length measurements between OLCR and PCI technology were not considered clinically relevant [15–17]. PCI and OLCR methods are also not different for the measurement of anterior chamber depth in any clinically relevant way [18].

Due to a software update, the number of successful scans could be increased from 94 to 98% [19]. However, the more modern generation of optical coherence tomography (OCT) technology appears to be even better than OLCR technology in terms of successful scans [20].

OCT Based Optical Biometry

Another development is the use of swept source OCT (ssOCT) for axial eye length. The principle is also based on the PCI method, but there are a few major differences. The first device on the market for longitudinal B-scans was the IOLMaster 700 [21] (Carl Zeiss Meditec AG, Germany), followed by Argos [22] (Movu, a Santec Company, USA) and Anterion [23] (Heidelberg Engineering, Germany). Spectral domain OCT-based methods have also made it to the market (B-OCT module for Revo OCT from Optopol, Poland) [24].

The comparison between ssOCT and PCI/OLCR technology showed a very good comparability between the two methods but with a better reproducibility for the ssOCT method [25]. The ssOCT technology also has some advantages over the PCI/OLCR method that should be considered. While the PCI/OLCR method is fundamentally based on A scans, ssOCT devices provide longitudinal B scans. In other words, instead of an amplitude (A scan) a brightness scan (B scan) is used, or more simply, instead of a one dimensional scan, a two-dimensional image is used (Fig. 3a–c). The image has the advantage that the anatomical structures can be clearly identified. Thus, the clinician can see with a glance whether, for example, the macula has been correctly recognized. We recently showed that this longitudinal B-scan can also be used directly for a rough macular screening [26].

A somewhat more futuristic approach is to use preoperative B-scans to make predictions for the postoperative lens position [27]. The most important advantage, however, is the longer wavelength (just over 1000 nm) of the ssOCT technology compared to the PCI/OLCR technology. This longer wavelength leads to a better penetration through dense media, such as a dense cataract. This even deeper penetration can increase the number of successful scans from about 95% [12] to over 99% [28], even in dense posterior subcapsular cataracts.

While it is not yet available, an even newer concept s to perform intra-operative ssOCT measurements [29] of the aphakic eye (Hienert et al., ESCRS 2019 in

Marrakesh). This could be a good alternative for a number of patient groups where preoperative biometry is particularly difficult. Paediatric patients with cataract and adult patients who cannot be successfully measured with optical biometry in a sitting position, whether due to compliance problems, physical limitations or a very dense cataract could benefit greatly from this approach.

Prediction of the Post-Operative IOL

The current greatest source of error in IOL calculation is the prediction of the IOL position, which currently accounts for more than 50% of the total error of the IOL power calculation [5, 30]. This uncertainty is also the reason why various IOL power calculation formulae have been developed in recent decades. While these formulae are discussed in detail elsewhere in this book, it is important to note that the prediction is difficult for two reasons: firstly, it is difficult to predict the post-operative IOL position [29, 31, 32] and secondly, in the weeks following implantation, there is an axial displacement of the IOL, which depends on the type of IOL and the degree of capsular fibrosis which varies greatly between patients [33–36].

Basically, there are three groups of IOL power calculations. Firstly, there is the optical approach which includes the simple vergence formulae ("thin" lens formulae) [2] all the way to complex ray tracing systems [37]. The calculation is subject to clear and established physical laws. Unfortunately, direct prediction of the IOL position is not possible with this model and either a fixed value must be assumed (very outdated model) or other non-ray tracing-based methods must be used.

Secondly, the empirical approach group, which is based on pre-existing data (biometric values, IOL power and measured post-operative refraction). These formulae are a sort of "black box" approach which always generates a constellation of a constants and various parameters that are taken into account for the prediction. By optimizing the constant, an IOL power calculation formula can then be used for different types of IOLs. This also underlines the importance of optimizing the constants for every new lens.

The third approach is artificial intelligence (AI). AI is an umbrella term for various concepts and a distinction is made between combination formulae [38] (basically not a "real" AI approach), big data [39] and chain algorithms [40].

References

1. Findl O, Drexler W, Menapace R, Heinzl H, Hitzenberger CK, Fercher AF. Improved prediction of intraocular lens power using partial coherence interferometry. J Cataract Refract Surg. 2001;27(6):861–7.
2. Olsen T. Calculation of intraocular lens power: a review. Acta Ophthalmol Scand. 2007;85 (5):472–85.
3. Drexler W, Findl O, Menapace R, Rainer G, Vass C, Hitzenberger CK, et al. Partial coherence interferometry: a novel approach to biometry in cataract surgery. At J Ophthalmol. 1998;126 (4):524–34.

4. Findl O, Kriechbaum K, Sacu S, Kiss B, Polak K, Nepp J, et al. Influence of operator experience on the performance of ultrasound biometry compared to optical biometry before cataract surgery. J Cataract Refract Surg. 2003;29(10):1950–5.
5. Norrby S. Sources of error in intraocular lens power calculation. J Cataract Refract Surg. 2008;34(3):368–76.
6. Hitzenberger CK. Adolf Friedrich Fercher: a pioneer of biomedical optics. J Biomed Opt. 2017;22(12):1–8.
7. Hitzenberger CK, Drexler W, Leitgeb RA, Findl O, Fercher AF. Key developments for partial coherence biometry and optical coherence tomography in the human eye made in Vienna. Invest Ophthalmol Vis Sci. 2016; 57(9):OCT460–74.
8. Hitzenberger C, Mengedoht K, Fercher AF. Laser optic measurements of the axial length of the eye. Progress Ophthalmol. 1989;86(2):159–61.
9. Findl O, Drexler W, Menapace R, Hitzenberger CK, Fercher AF. High precision biometry of pseudophakic eyes using partial coherence interferometry. J Cataract Refract Surg. 1998;24 (8):1087–93.
10. Drexler W, Baumgartner A, Findl O, Hitzenberger CK, Sattmann H, Fercher AF. Submicrometer precision biometry of the anterior segment of the human eye. Invest Ophthalmol Vis Sci. 1997;38(7):1304–13.
11. Kiss B, Findl O, Menapace R, Wirtitsch M, Drexler W, Hitzenberger CK, et al. Biometry of cataractous eyes using partial coherence interferometry: clinical feasibility study of a commercial prototype I. J Cataract Refract Surg. 2002;28(2):224–9.
12. Hirnschall N, Murphy S, Pimenides D, Maurino V, Findl O. Assessment of a new averaging algorithm to increase the sensitivity of axial eye length measurement with optical biometry in eyes with dense cataract. J Cataract Refract Surg. 2011;37(1):45–9.
13. Srivannaboon S, Chirapapaisan C, Chonpimai P, Koodkaew S. Comparison of ocular biometry and intraocular lens power using a new biometer and a standard biometer. J Cataract Refract Surg. 2014;40(5):709–15.
14. Mandal P, Berrow EJ, Naroo SA, Wolffsohn JS, Uthoff D, Holland D, et al. Validity and repeatability of the Aladdin ocular biometer. Br J Ophthalmol. 2014;98(2):256–8.
15. Hoffer KJ, Shammas HJ, Savini G. Comparison of 2 laser instruments for measuring axial length. J Cataract Refract Surg. 2010;36(4):644–8.
16. Chen YA, Hirnschall N, Findl O. Evaluation of 2 new optical biometry devices and comparison with the current gold standard biometer. J Cataract Refract Surg. 2011;37(3): 513–7.
17. Rabsilber TM, Jepsen C, Auffarth GU, Holzer MP. Intraocular lens power calculation: clinical comparison of 2 optical biometry devices. J Cataract Refract Surg. 2010;36(2):230–4.
18. Air N, brain sound N, Farrokhi S, Findl O. Comparability of anterior chamber depth measurements with partial coherence interferometry and optical low-coherence reflectometry in pseudophakic eyes. J Cataract Refract Surg. 2015; 41(8):1678–84.
19. Shammas HJ, Wetterwald N, Potvin R. New mode for measuring axial length with an optical low-coherence reflectometer in eyes with dense cataract. J Cataract Refract Surg. 2015;41 (7):1365–9.
20. Kurian M, Negalur N, Das S, Puttaiah NK, Haria D, J TS, et al. Biometry with a new swept-source optical coherence tomography biometer: Repeatability and agreement with an optical low-coherence reflectometry device. J Cataract Refract Surg. 2016; 42(4):577–81.
21. Srivannaboon S, Chirapapaisan C, Chonpimai P, Loket S. Clinical comparison of a new swept-source optical coherence tomography-based optical biometer and a time-domain optical coherence tomography-based optical biometer. J Cataract Refract Surg. 2015;41(10): 2224–32.
22. Shammas HJ, Ortiz S, Shammas MC, Kim SH, Chong C. Biometry measurements using a new large-coherence-length swept-source optical coherence tomographer. J Cataract Refract Surg. 2016;42(1):50–61.

23. Asam JS, Polzer M, Tafreshi A, Hirnschall N, Findl O. Anterior segment OCT. In: Bille JF, editor. High resolution imaging in microscopy and ophthalmology: new frontiers in biomedical optics. Cham (CH); 2019, pp. 285–99.
24. Kanclerz P, Hoffer KJ, Rozema JJ, Przewlocka K, Savini G. Repeatability and reproducibility of optical biometry implemented in a new optical coherence tomographer and comparison with an optical low-coherence reflectometer. J Cataract Refract Surg. 2019;45(11):1619–24.
25. Kunert KS, Peter M, Blum M, Haigis W, Sekundo W, Schutze J, et al. Repeatability and agreement in optical biometry of a new swept-source optical coherence tomography-based biometer versus partial coherence interferometry and optical low-coherence reflectometry. J Cataract Refract Surg. 2016;42(1):76–83.
26. Hirnschall N, Leisser C, Radda S, Maedel S, Findl O. Macular disease detection with a swept-source optical coherence tomography-based biometry device in patients scheduled for cataract surgery. J Cataract Refract Surg. 2016;42(4):530–6.
27. Brain sound N, Buehren T, Bajramovic F, Trost M, Teuber T, Findl O. Prediction of postoperative intraocular lens tilt using swept-source optical coherence tomography. J Cataract Refract Surg. 2017; 43(6):732–6.
28. Hirnschall N, Varsits R, Doeller B, Findl O. Enhanced penetration for axial length measurement of eyes with dense cataracts using swept source optical coherence tomography: a consecutive observational study. Ophthalmol Ther. 2018;7(1):119–24.
29. Hirnschall N, Farrokhi S, Amir-Asgari S, Hienert J, Findl O. Intraoperative optical coherence tomography measurements of aphakic eyes to predict postoperative position of 2 intraocular lens designs. J Cataract Refract Surg. 2018;44(11):1310–6.
30. Olsen T. Sources of error in intraocular lens power calculation. J Cataract Refract Surg. 1992;18(2):125–9.
31. Hirnschall N, Amir-Asgari S, Maedel S, Findl O. Predicting the postoperative intraocular lens position using continuous intraoperative optical coherence tomography measurements. Invest Ophthalmol Vis Sci. 2013;54(8):5196–203.
32. Shajari M, Sonntag R, Niermann T, Holland D, Kohnen T, Priglinger S, et al. Determining and comparing the effective lens position and refractive outcome of a novel rhexis-fixated lens to established lens designs. At J Ophthalmol. 2020.
33. Findl O, Hirnschall N, Nishi Y, Maurino V, Crnej A. Capsular bag performance of a hydrophobic acrylic 1-piece intraocular lens. J Cataract Refract Surg. 2015;41(1):90–7.
34. Findl O, Struhal W, Dorffner G, Drexler W. Analysis of nonlinear systems to estimate intraocular lens position after cataract surgery. J Cataract Refract Surg. 2004;30(4):863–6.
35. Kriechbaum K, Findl O, Preussner PR, Koppl C, Wahl J, Drexler W. Determining postoperative anterior chamber depth. J Cataract Refract Surg. 2003;29(11):2122–6.
36. Wirtitsch MG, Findl O, Menapace R, Kriechbaum K, Koeppl C, Buehl W, et al. Effect of haptic design on change in axial lens position after cataract surgery. J Cataract Refract Surg. 2004;30(1):45–51.
37. Hirnschall N, Buehren T, Trost M, Findl O. Pilot evaluation of refractive prediction errors associated with a new method for ray-tracing-based intraocular lens power calculation. J Cataract Refract Surg. 2019.
38. Ladas JG, Siddiqui AA, Devgan U, Jun AS. A 3-D "Super Surface" combining modern intraocular lens formulae to generate a "Super Formula" and maximize accuracy. JAMA Ophthalmol. 2015;133(12):1431–6.
39. Darcy K, Gunn D, Tavassoli S, Sparrow J, Kane JX. Assessment of the accuracy of new and updated intraocular lens power calculation formulae in 10 930 eyes from the UK National Health Service. J Cataract Refract Surg. 2020;46(1):2–7.
40. Siddiqui AA, Devgan U. Intraocular lens power calculations in atypical eyes. Indian J Ophthalmol. 2017;65(12):1289–93.

Scheimpflug Tomography and Measurement of Higher Order Aberrations

Jens Bühren

Scheimpflug Tomography

Scheimpflug photography of the eye lens is a method that has been in use in scientific ophthalmology for a long time. Originally this technique was practised as an analogue procedure with high-resolution films but with the advent of high-resolution digital cameras and powerful personal computers the introduction of fully digital units became possible. Scheimpflug tomographers have been used reliably to image the cornea for about 20 years. The first instrument with wide market distribution was the Pentacam® (Oculus Optikgeräte, Wetzlar, Germany). Scheimpflug tomographers use a camera rotating around a central axis to produce sectional images of the anterior eye segment, which are then assembled into a three-dimensional reconstruction. With the Pentacam HR®, for example, up to 50 sectional images are taken within one second. Other devices such as the Galilei® (Ziemer, Port, Switzerland) use two Scheimpflug cameras opposite each other and an additional Placido disc for precise measurement of the optically most relevant anterior corneal surface. In pure Placido topography and other methods based on the principle of reflection, the centre of the cornea has to be interpolated because of the position of the camera. In contrast, a rotating Scheimpflug camera represents the centre with a high density of measuring points (Fig. 1).

In addition to the interfaces of the cornea, the iris (anterior surface) and lens (but usually only the anterior surface) can also be represented and measured. This allows a full topography of the corneal anterior and posterior surface, but also further measurements such as corneal thickness and anterior chamber depth (Fig. 2). The representation of the lens strongly depends on pupil diameter. While the lenticular curvatures can also be measured, densitometry derived from the backscattered light is by far more important (see below).

J. Bühren (✉)
Praxis für Augenheilkunde Prof. Bühren, Frankfurt, Germany
e-mail: buehren@ophthalmologicum-ffm.de

M. Shajari et al. (eds.), *Cataract and Lens Surgery*,
https://doi.org/10.1007/978-3-031-05394-8_15

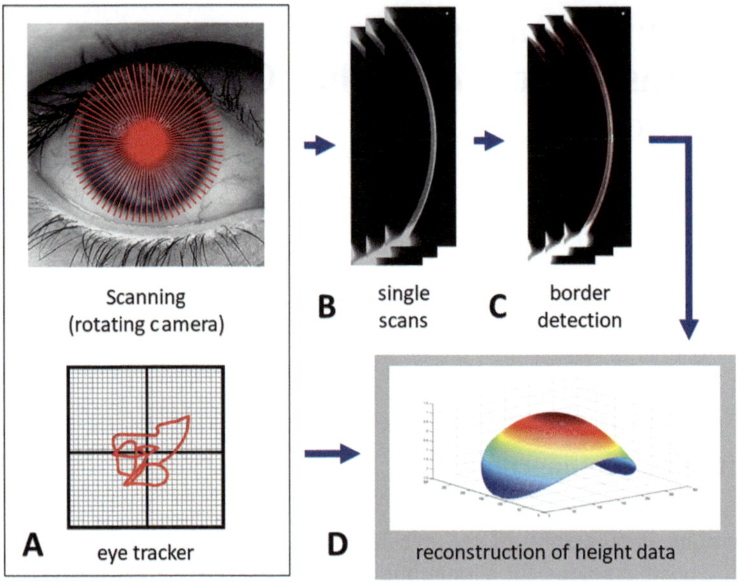

Fig. 1 Data collection by corneal Scheimpflug tomography. During the examination, optical sections are recorded in various corneal meridians and, at the same time, eye movements during the recording are measured (**A**). For each of the individual optical sections (**B**) an automatic interface recognition is performed (**C**). Finally, the sections are put together taking into account the eye movements and image distortion and from this the height data of the corneal interfaces are calculated by interpolation (**D**)

Author's recommendation

In modern lens surgery, tomography of the anterior segment of the eye is an indispensable examination method.

In the following section, the individual modalities and their significance for lens surgical procedures will be covered.

Corneal topography

Mathematical models can be applied to the raw data, tomographically determined, to represent the shape (curvature or reference body fitting such as "Best Fit Sphere") and the optical properties (Ray Tracing) [2]. The corneal topography of the anterior surface provides important information about the cornea prior to lens surgery. In addition to the height and axis of a corneal astigmatism, possible irregularities that would otherwise be overlooked or missed can be detected. For example, a long-standing non-progressive or undiagnosed keratoconus in cataract patients or other irregularities such as scars or a basement membrane dystrophy can lead to unpleasant postoperative surprises. This is especially true when considering the implantation of multifocal IOL. Therefore, the topography of the corneal anterior surface is one of the most essential preoperative examinations before implantation

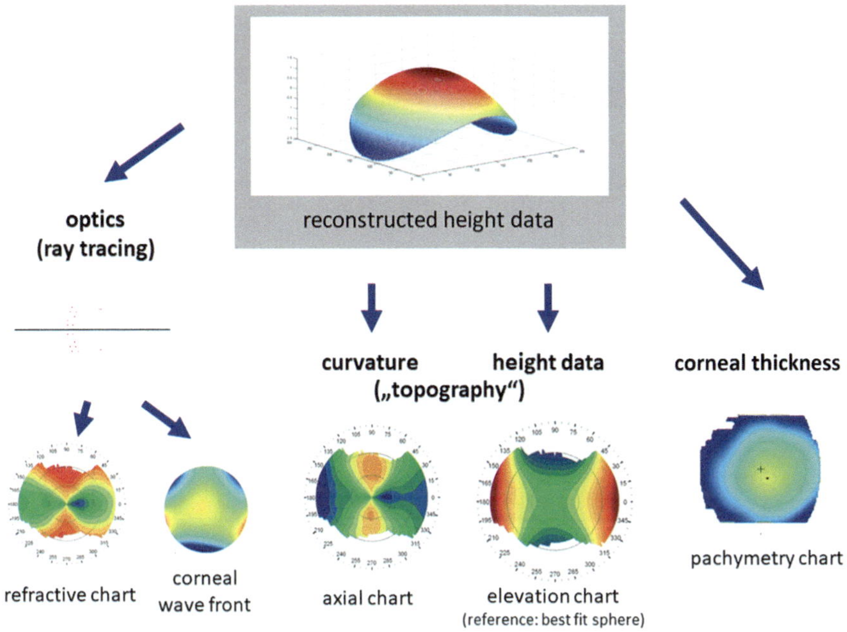

Fig. 2 Modalities of corneal Scheimpflug tomography derived from the raw data. The densitometry of the cornea is not included for the sake of clarity

of special lenses in cataract surgery, refractive lens exchange (RLA) and implantation of IOL into the phakic eye. The greatest advantage of Scheimpflug tomography over classical placido topography is the additional measurement of the posterior surface of the cornea.

Topographic maps show the corneal curvature as a function of location. The curvature is reconstructed by fitting circles of different radii to the raw data of the measurement over a defined area ("region of interest" or ROI). The topography map used in most cases is the axial or sagittal map (Fig. 3). Here, the centres of the circles lie on the optical axis. This does not apply to the tangential or meridional map. As a result, axial maps appear more regular and tangential maps more "noisy", because they emphasize local irregularities.

Author's recommendation

In practice, axial maps are sufficient to detect visually relevant irregularities.

It is important to note that these representations only show the **curvature** and not the **refractive power** of the cornea. Thus, the most important key figure of corneal topography, the simulated keratometry ("simK values", see also Fig. 3) is given in dioptres. The simK values correspond approximately to the values obtained with manual keratometry and characterise the curvature in the individual main sections of the cornea and consequently the corneal astigmatism.

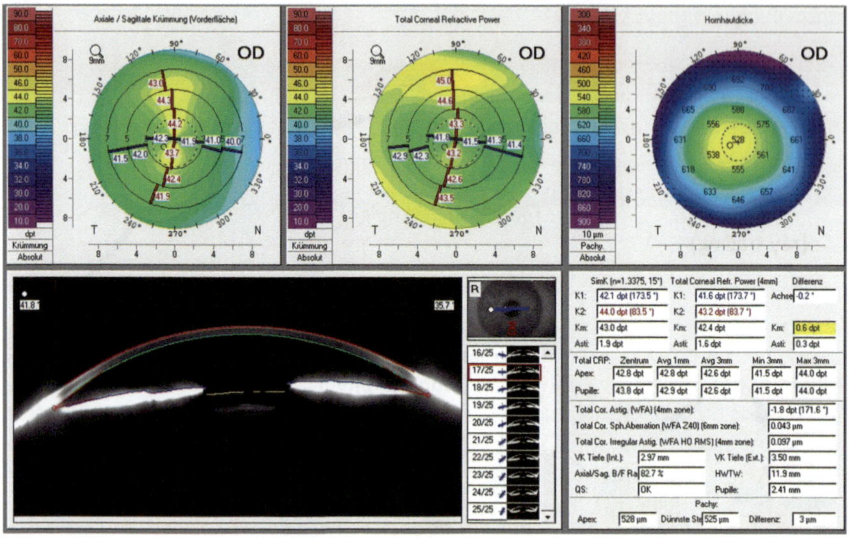

Fig. 3 "Cataract Preop" representation of the Pentacam® as an example of a special Scheimpflug tomography display. Note in particular the difference between the sagittal map (left) and the ray-tracing based refractive map in the middle ("Total Refractive Corneal Power"). Furthermore, there is a spatially resolved pachymetry map on the right. At the bottom right, various relevant key parameters such as astigmatism, anterior chamber depth and corneal spherical aberration (C_4^0) are shown

Scheimpflug tomographers can display the optical effect of the entire cornea by imaging the anterior and posterior corneal interface and by using ray tracing models. In contrast to the axial map, these representations take into account both the spherical aberration of the cornea and the effect of the posterior surface. Inclusion of the posterior surface is of particular advantage if the axial position of the posterior astigmatism deviates, since in these cases a sole measurement of the anterior surface can provide an imprecise axial position [8]. Modern tomographers output a ray tracing based total astigmatism of the cornea, analogous to the simK values of the simple topographers, (Fig. 3).

Corneal pachymetry

Corneal tomography methods also provide a spatially resolved image of the corneal thickness (pachymetry). Pachymetry maps and derived thickness profiles play an important role in the diagnosis of ectatic conditions like keratoconus. Pachymetry maps are occasionally required when a lens surgery procedure is combined with an incisional procedure (*e.g.,* limbal relaxation incisions). Most femtosecond laser units have an intraoperative OCT-controlled thickness measurement for planning the incisions.

Anterior chamber depth measurement

A Scheimpflug camera (but in a minimal form) can be found in optical biometers such as the first generation IOL-Master® (Carl Zeiss Meditec AG, Jena; Germany) and is used to determine anterior chamber depth. All devices currently on the market provide a spatially resolved measurement of the anterior chamber depth (Fig. 3). In most cases, a glance at the central anterior chamber depth value is sufficient to estimate the overall conditions. The anterior chamber depth plays a central role in planning the implantation of an intraocular lens (IOL) in the phakic eye. Therefore, many Scheimpflug tomographers have a module to simulate the postoperative position of the intraocular lens. This allows prediction of the post-operative distance between the IOL to the corneal endothelium to ensure that it does not fall below a critical value (Fig. 4). When evaluating the measurements, it is important to know whether the displayed value includes corneal thickness (measured from the epithelium) or is measured from endothelium and thus represents the "actual" anterior chamber depth. The former is the standard for ultrasound-based measurements and has also been adopted by optical biometers such as the IOL-Master®. The latter display method can be manually adjusted in modern

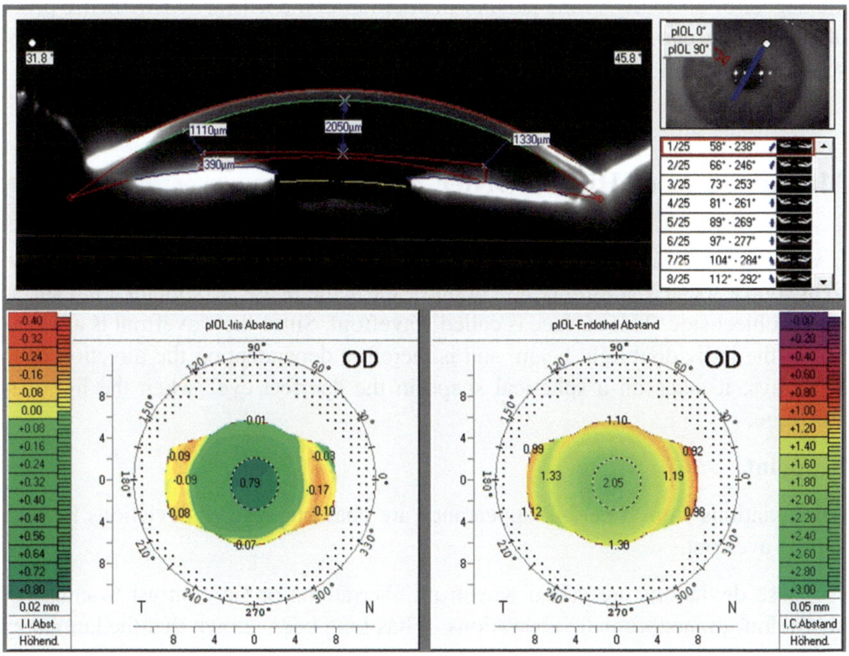

Fig. 4 Module of the Pentacam® for planning IOL implantations in the phakic eye (pIOL). The software predicts whether any critical distances between the implant and intraocular structures such as the endothelium may be undercut. The maps below show the distances between pIOL and iris (left) and pIOL and endothelium (right)

Scheimpflug tomographers. In daily practice, it is important to commit to one presentation in order to obtain the necessary practical routine in handling the measured values.

Lens densitometry

The light reflected by the lens represents the turbidity of the lens material, and can be quantified with a Scheimpflug image. This "density measurement" (lens densitometry) was the subject of the first analogue Scheimpflug cameras in ophthalmology. Since the semi-quantitative densitometry performed in the context of slit-lamp examination is sufficient in clinical routine, the automatic and objective quantification of lens opacity with Scheimpflug tomography is mainly reserved for scientific purposes though A future application could be the documentation of the preoperative lens status. A complete imaging of the lens with Scheimpflug cameras is only possible in mydriasis. Similarly, the posterior lens pole cannot be displayed in cases where the lenses are very thick. It is well-known that the opacity measured is often proportional to the degree of hardening of the lens material, or to the scattering. It should be mentioned, however, that it is the forward-scattered light and the optical aberrations induced by local changes in the lenticular refractive index that contribute to the deterioration of vision due to cataract formation [6]. As a result, the lens densitometry obtained by backscatter does not directly represent the degree of disability of the patient. In addition to the lens, a densitometric profile of the cornea can also be obtained. However, the practical value of these measurements has not yet been sufficiently evaluated.

Measurement of Higher Order Aberrations

If we consider light as electromagnetic waves and combine all waves emitted by a light source located at infinity at a point of the same phase, we obtain a flat surface on the object side. This surface is called wavefront. Since the wavefront is always at 90° to the individual light beam, and is therefore dependent on the direction of the light rays, it takes on a spherical shape in the "perfect eye" when the light rays converge.

Keypoint

All deviations from a perfect appearance are characterised by deviations from the ideal wavefront.

These deviations are called wavefront aberrations or (in contrast to chromatic aberration) monochromatic aberrations. It has long been known that the human eye is affected by optical aberrations that cannot be corrected with glasses. These are also known as higher order aberrations (HOA). The two main clinically relevant HOA are spherical aberration and coma [3]. If parallel rays of light from infinity fall on a spherical lens (e.g., the cornea), the peripherally incident light rays are

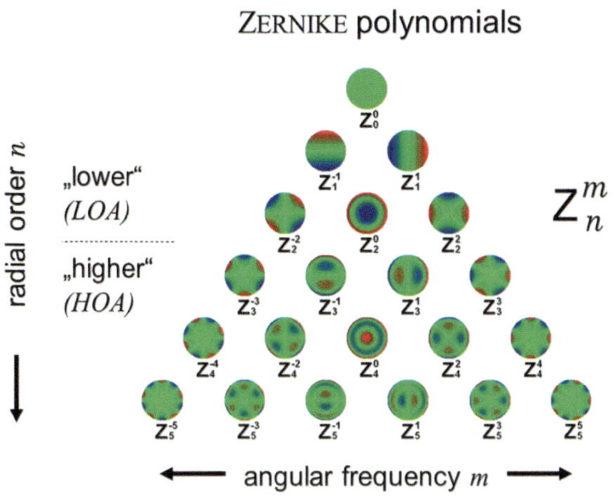

Fig. 5 Pyramid with Zernike polynomials (orders 1–5). Note the relationship between polynomials of the same order *n* and the same angular frequency *m*, but with opposite signs (*e.g.*, astigmatism Z_2^{2} and Z_2^{-2}). Similarity also exists between polynomials of the same angular frequency *m* but of different order *n* (e.g., Z_2^{0} and Z_4^{0})

deflected more strongly, and are not focused together with the centrally incident light rays (positive spherical aberration). This results in an overlay of the actual sharp image, which is perceived as a halo in the dark and as a weakened contrast under photopic conditions (Fig. 5). Spherical aberration is strongly dependent fon the pupil diameter. A negative asphericity of the cornea and a negative spherical aberration of the lens largely compensate for the inherent spherical aberrations of the cornea in the young human eye [1]. After refractive corneal surgery, spherical aberration of the cornea can increase significantly. Positive spherical aberration is observed after treatment for myopia and negative spherical aberration after treatment for hyperopia [7].

If a system with spherical aberration, e.g. a LASIK treatment or IOL, is decentred, the coma is formed (from gr. κώμη, tail). The result is the perception of a "comet" tail on point light sources or "shadows" and "ghost images" on letters (Fig. 6).

In addition to the most clinically relevant HOA, there are others like trefoil and other higher foiled astigmatism. In technical and physiological optics, the circular polynomials formulated by the Dutch mathematician Frits Zernike have long been used to quantify these irregularities [9]. Using these functions, a wavefront error can be reconstructed by mathematical approximation of the measured raw data and broken down into individual shape components (Zernike decomposition). A two-part index scheme (Z_n^m) allows a unique nomenclature of each polynomial, where *n* is the radial order (polynomial component) and *m* the angular frequency (sine or cosine component) (Fig. 7). Some of these functions represent long known imaging errors such as tilt, spherical defocusing, astigmatism, coma and spherical aberration. By fitting the Zernike polynomial functions to the raw data of the

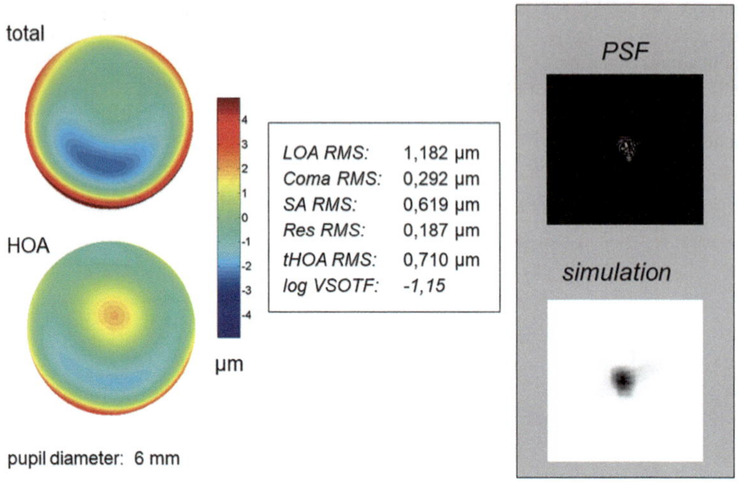

Fig. 6 Synopsis of the wavefront analysisWavefront analysis of an eye with high spherical aberrationSpherical aberration (Z.n. LASIK for −9.5 dpt). The wavefront map also shows an increased coma component. HOA: "higher-order aberrationsHigher-order aberrations", LOA: "lower-order aberrationsAberration", RMS: "root mean square", SA RMS: effective value of all spherical aberrationsSpherical aberration, Res RMS: RMS value of all HOA that are not coma or spherical aberrationSpherical aberration, tHOA RMS: RMS: RMS of all higher order aberrationsHigher order aberration, VSOTF: "Visual Strehl Ration based on the Optical Transfer Function", a optical qualityOptical quality metric, PSF: "Point Spread Function"

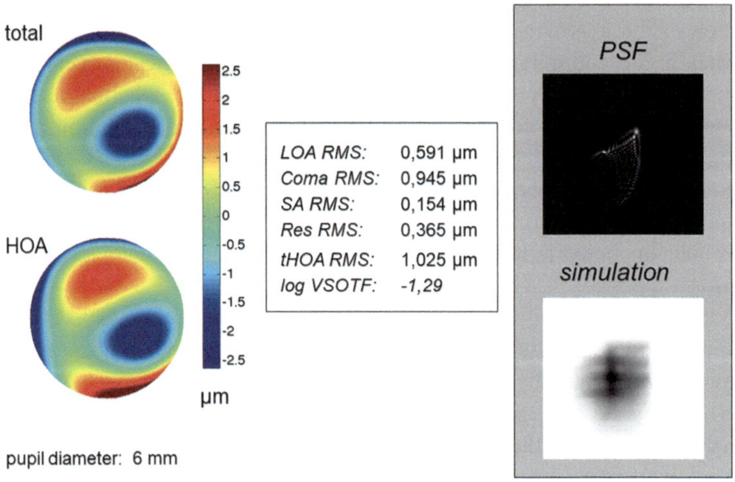

Fig. 7 Synopsis of the wavefront analysis of an eye with high coma (keratoconus). Compare the RMS values of the individual components with those in Fig. 5

aberrometer, coefficients (Zernike coefficients) which indicate the strength of the aberration represented by the single polynomial in the wavefront of the eye are obtained. The list of these coefficients is a quasi-representation of the code of the wavefront error. Thus, a wavefront map, the Point Spread Function (PSF) and simulations derived by convolution can be derived from them. It is also possible to calculate key figures that quantify the quality of the image (Figs. 5 and 6).

A number of systems have been developed to measure the wavefront error of the human eye. Either a pattern is projected onto the retina and the wavefront error is derived directly from the deformation of this pattern in the retinal image (*e.g.*, Ray-Tracing or Tscherning Aberrometer) or the light reflected back from the eye is divided by a lens matrix, and the resulting dot pattern is analysed (Hartmann-Shack-Sensor).

Zernike polynomials can be adapted not only to the raw data from the aberrometer, but also to corneal height data determined with Scheimpflug tomography. As mentioned above, it is also possible to simulate the optical properties of the entire cornea by means of ray tracing. The wavefront calculated in this way can also be described by a Zernike decomposition. This form of presentation is often referred to somewhat imprecisely as "corneal wavefront" though it is mathematically derived and should not be confused with aberrometrically obtained measurements. A module for Zernike analysis of the cornea is now part of most tomographers. Zernike analysis of the cornea is always of practical use when corneal shape characteristics and corneal optical properties are required. In surgical practice, this mainly concerns the exclusion of a keratoconus and other corneal irregularities (e.g., scars or basement membrane dystrophy). When planning the implantation of an intraocular lens (IOL) into the phakic eye or before phacoemulsification with the implantation of a multifocal or toric IOL, corneal irregularities that are masked as astigmatism in eyeglasses or autorefractometer measurements must be excluded. An overlooked keratoconus or visually significant basement membrane dystrophy, for example, are contraindications for the implantation of a multifocal IOL. The irregularities are sensibly quantified by stating the effective values of homologous Zernike coefficients ("root mean square" or RMS value) (Figs. 3, 6 and 7). One should familiarise oneself with the standard and limit values of these ratios for the most reliable interpretation of the measurement in practice.

The practical meaning of measured aberrations always depends on the clinical situation. While mild irregularities (corneal HOA RMS < 0.3 μm, measured over 4 mm) are very common in elderly people, higher values should be looked closer at. Values of coma RMS and primary spherical aberration beyond 0.5 μm point to pathological conditions. Particularly after early-generation laser refractive corrections with high attempted corrections and small optical zones excessive corneal HOA can be measured. Because of very high inter-individual differences in subjective perception of HOA, it is impossible to provide cut-off values for HOA if a patient desires the implantation of multifocal IOLs. A pragmatic approach can involve the patient's individual needs and expectations and his or her individual aberrations compared to a normative data base. In case of elevated HOA the patient should be at least informed thoroughly about the higher potential risk of postoperative visual disturbances.

Wavefront sensors provide the input data for wavefront-guided corneal surgery. In lens surgery they play a rather minor role, but can provide further information in case of unclear pre- and postoperative situations.

Author's recommendation

Combined units that provide both topography of the cornea and aberrometry of the entire eye are particularly helpful in everyday clinical practice.

The commercially available devices iTrace [Tracey Technologies, Inc.] and iDesign [Johnson & Johnson Vision, Albuquerque, NM, USA]) allow the measurement of "internal" aberrations (posterior corneal surface + lens); with the Pentacam AXL Wave (Oculus Optikgeräte, Wetzlar, Germany) even the posterior corneal surface and lens can be differentiated more precisely. The measurement of lenticular aberrations is particularly useful when deciding on surgery for early stages of cataract ("dysfunctional lens syndrome") [4]. In these cases, often only lenticular discontinuity zones are visible at the slit lamp, but patients already complain of significant visual deterioration, often as ghost images [5, 6]. In cases of postoperative IOL decentrations, the measurement of internal aberrations can assist clinical decision making. If in case of elevated coma the main source is from internal aberrations, a IOL decentration is likely.

References

1. Artal P, Berrio E, Guirao A, et al. Contribution of the cornea and internal surfaces to the change of ocular aberrations with age. J Opt Soc Am A Opt Image Sci Vis. 2002;19:137–43.
2. Bühren J. Corneal topography and keratoconus diagnostics using Scheimpflug photography. Ophthalmologist. 2014;111:920–6.
3. Bühren J, Kohnen T. Application of wavefront analysis in clinic and science. From irregular astigmatism to higher order aberrations - part I: fundamentals. Ophthalmologist. 2007;104:909–25.
4. Fernández J, Rodríguez-Vallejo M, Martínez J, et al. From presbyopia to cataracts: a critical review on dysfunctional lens syndromes. J Ophthalmol. 2018;2018:4318405. https://doi.org/10.1155/2018/4318405.
5. Fujikado T, Kuroda T, Maeda N, et al. Wavefront analysis of an eye with monocular triplopia and nuclear cataract. At J Ophthalmol. 2004;137:361–3.
6. Fujikado T, Kuroda T, Maeda N, et al. Light scattering and optical aberrations as objective parameters to predict visual deterioration in eyes with cataracts. J Cataract Refract Surg. 2004;30:1198–208.
7. Kohnen T, Mahmoud K, Bühren J. Comparison of corneal higher-order aberrations induced by myopic and hyperopic LASIK. Ophthalmology. 2005;112:1692.
8. Tonn B, Klaproth OK, Kohnen T. Anterior surface-based keratometry compared with Scheimpflug tomography-based total corneal astigmatism. Invest Ophthalmol Vis Sci. 2014;56:291–8.
9. Zernike F. Diffraction theory of the cutting method and its improved form, the phase contrast method. Physica. 1934;1:689–704.

OCT of the Anterior Segment

Nikolaus Luft

OCT-based corneal measurements

As an imaging modality with almost histological resolution ("optical biopsy"), optical coherence tomography (OCT) has a firm place in the examination of both the anterior and posterior segment of the eye prior to lens surgery.

OCT is a significant improvement over traditional keratometry methods, which only take into account the anterior corneal surface to calculate the total corneal refractive power. It is also becoming an increasingly popular alternative to Scheimpflug-based tomography techniques, the previous device of choice, for measuring both the anterior and posterior corneal surface. An extension of OCT-based tomography is the OCT-based ray-tracing principle, which is a purely physical method for IOL power calculation and, therefore, does not require empirical formula optimization. As a results, ray-tracing is a valuable option for IOL power calculation, particularly in cases of irregular corneas or corneas with previous keratorefractive procedures (Fig. 1).

In addition to thorough topographic measurements, OCT imaging can also be used for morphological preoperative examination of the cornea. For example, subtle ectatic corneal diseases (so-called form fruste keratoconus) can be easily missed by conventional Scheimpflug tomography but can be detected with high sensitivity with OCT-based epithelial thickness mapping [1]. Some devices can generate a color-coded map of the corneal epithelial thickness over a certain measurement area (typically between 6.0 mm and 9.0 mm of diameter). These epithelial maps can also be used to help differentiate between conditions that are difficult to distinguish clinically, such as between ectatic corneal disease and contact lens warpage syndrome [2].

N. Luft (✉)
Munich, Germany
e-mail: nikolaus.luft@med.uni-muenchen.de

M. Shajari et al. (eds.), *Cataract and Lens Surgery*,
https://doi.org/10.1007/978-3-031-05394-8_16

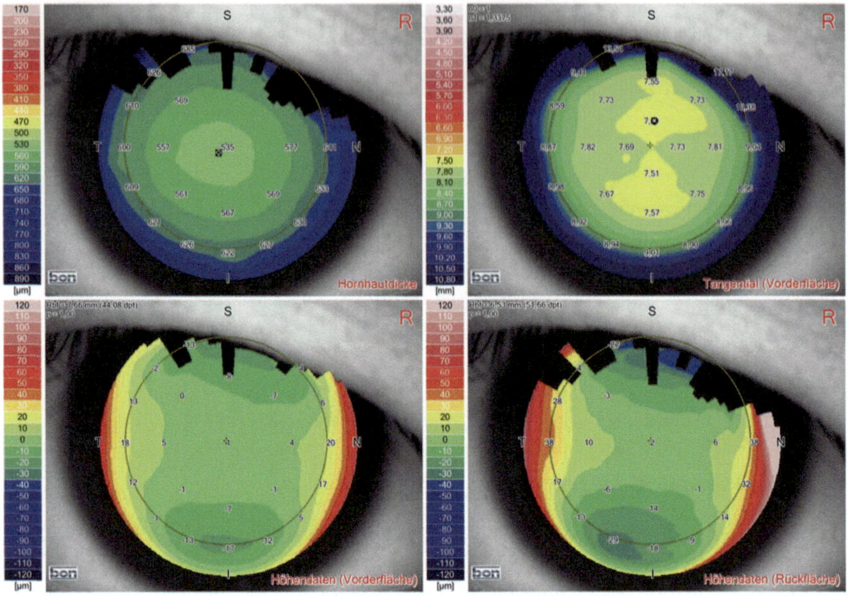

Fig. 1 Typical 4-field representation of an OCT-based pachymetry and tomography image before cataract surgery. The tangential view of the anterior surface shows regular with-the-rule astigmatism

In cases of endothelial disease (e.g. Fuchs' endothelial corneal dystrophy), OCT-based corneal layer pachymetry (epithelial mapping & stromal mapping) is also valuable as a basic examination before lens surgery to evaluate any abnormal increase in pachymetry. Finally, OCT can also be used as an objective parameter for non-invasive evaluation of the tear film prior to planned lens surgery.

OCT-based lens measurements

The commercialization of swept-source OCT technology (SS-OCT), with a higher wavelength (1050 nm) compared to traditional spectral-domain OCT (SD-OCT; ca 840 nm), has enabled significantly faster acquisition rates as well as a higher corneal penetration depth of OCT imaging. The deeper anterior segment measuring depth allows more comprehensive representations of the anatomy of the anterior eye segment including the entire anterior chamber and the back of the lens (Fig. 2). This improved anterior segment depth and resolution often comes at the cost of posterior segment OCT capabilities.

These technological improvements open up new potential to optimize IOL power calculation using previously unavailable SS-OCT based biometric parameters of the anterior segment (e.g. preoperative angle-to-angle distance) [3]. Likewise, the preoperative measurement of the crystalline lens by means of SS-OCT can allow improved predictability of the postoperative tilt of the intraocular lens (IOL), which might be of particular relevance for toric IOLs [4].

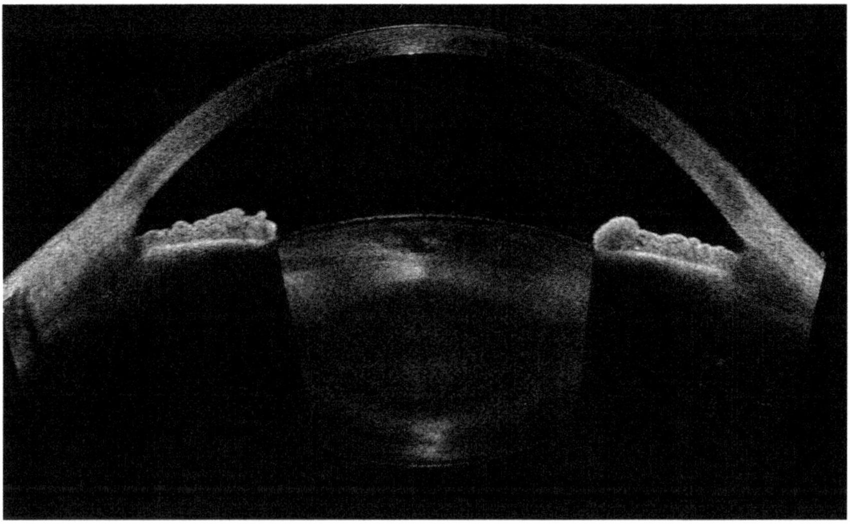

Fig. 2 SS-OCTSwept image of the anterior eye segment before cataract surgery

Pre-operative OCT of the crystalline lens also allows for the surgical approach to be individualized and optimized for each case. A preoperative measurement of the lens density by OCT is quantitatively possible and allows, for example, an adjustment of the femtosecond laser energy or the femtosecond laser fragmentation pattern of the nucleus according to the individual degree of lens opacity. A preoperative morphological evaluation of the cataract by OCT can be useful for the safety and efficiency of lens surgery in traumatic or polar cataracts. Moreover, in cases of mature lens opacity, subcapsular fluid accumulations can be visualized by OCT and aspirated with a curved 30-gauge cannula prior to capsulorhexis to prevent sudden uncontrolled expansion of the capsulorhexis, thus avoiding the dreaded "Argentinian flag sign" [5]. Similarly, by detecting the presence of a posterior polar cataract preoperatively by OCT, unpleasant intraoperative surprises such as a pre-existent posterior capsule defect can be anticipated [6]. This information in advance of the surgery enables the surgeon to tailor their technique, like performing a hydrodelineation instead of a hydrodissection tp avoid extending the posterior break. Similarly, in case of traumatic cataract where preoperative clinical evaluation of the posterior lens capsule may be insufficient, a pre-existing opening of the posterior capsule leaf can be detected by OCT thus allowing appropriate surgical precautions to be taken and preparations to be made [7].

As we have already seen in the posterior segment of the eye, a wider application of intraoperative OCT imaging in the anterior segment of the eye is expected be seen in the future. In addition to the improved IOL power calculation by intraoperative measurement of the capsule apparatus in the aphakic eye [8], an OCT analysis of the lens surgery could also be useful for improving the individual surgical technique. The incision architecture of different corneal incision techniques, for example, can be evaluated and adapted to the surgeon's needs [9]. In the future, OCT-based feedback could be applied to many aspects of intraocular surgery like notifying the surgeon in to lens pieces tumbling in the anterior chamber and making contact with the corneal endothelium [10]. This sort of feedback, and more, could provide objective goals for surgeons always seeking to improve their surgical techniques.

Author's recommendation

An SS-OCT system is recommended for routine pre-operative examination prior to lens surgery, which combines the functions of corneal tomography, corneal epithelial mapping and measurements of the anterior chamber and the crystalline lens in one device.

References

1. Temstet C, Sandali O, Bouheraoua N, Hamiche T, Galan A, El M, et al. Corneal epithelial thickness mapping using Fourier-domain optical coherence tomography for detection of form fruste keratoconus. J Cataract Refract Surg. 2015;41(4):812–20.
2. Schallhorn JM, Tang M, Li Y, Louie DJ, Chamberlain W, Huang D. Distinguishing between contact lens warpage and ectasia: usefulness of optical coherence tomography epithelial thickness mapping. J Cataract Refract Surg. 2017;43(1):60–6.
3. Goto S, Maeda N, Koh S, Ohnuma K, Hayashi K, Iehisa I, et al. Prediction of postoperative intraocular lens position with angle-to-angle depth using anterior segment optical coherence tomography. Ophthalmology. 2016;123(12):2474–80.
4. Hirnschall N, Buehren T, Bajramovic F, Trost M, Teuber T, Findl O. Prediction of postoperative intraocular lens tilt using swept-source optical coherence tomography. J Cataract Refract Surg. 2017;43(6):732–6.
5. Dhami A, Dhami AS, Singh H, Dhami GS. Role of anterior segment optical coherence tomography for safer management of mature white cataracts. J Cataract Refract Surg. 2019;45 (4):480–4.
6. Pavan G, Krishnamurthy P, Nath M, Baskaran P, Janani M, Venkatesh R. Can preoperative anterior segment optical coherence tomography predict posterior capsule rupture during phacoemulsification in patients with posterior polar cataract? J Cataract Refract Surg. 2018;44 (12):1441–5.
7. Tabatabaei SA, Soleimani M, Etesali H, Naderan M. Accuracy of swept source optical coherence tomography and ultrasound biomicroscopy for evaluation of posterior lens capsule in traumatic cataract. Am J Ophthalmol. 2020.
8. Hirnschall N, Farrokhi S, Amir- S, Hienert J, Findl O. Intraoperative optical coherence tomography measurements of aphakic eyes to predict postoperative position of 2 intraocular lens designs. J Cataract Refract Surg. 2018;44(11):1310–6.
9. Calladine D, Packard R. Clear corneal incision architecture in the immediate postoperative period evaluated using optical coherence tomography. J Cataract Refract Surg. 2007;33 (8):1429–35.
10. Amir- S, Hirnschall N, Findl O. Using continuous intraoperative optical coherence tomography to classify swirling lens fragments during cataract surgery and to predict their impact on corneal endothelial cell damage. J Cataract Refract Surg. 2016;42(7):1029–36.

OCT of the Posterior Segment

Jakob Siedlecki and Marcus Ang

Indication for preoperative posterior segment OCT

While preoperative posterior segment OCT is not an essential examination before every cataract procedure, it can be useful to supplement clinical fundoscopy for several reasons. First, the exclusion or diagnosis of a macular pathology can help to gauge postoperative outcomes after cataract surgery. Second, diseases that require therapy before cataract surgery itself (e.g. neovascular AMD) can be identified, and special precautions or therapeutic strategies for the postoperative period can be recommended (e.g., to prevent cystoid macular edema in diabetic patients). Finally, the exclusion of macular pathologies on OCT is absolutely essential prior to the implantation of "premium" IOLs (multifocal, EDOF) to exclude a macular pathology as any significant macular pathology is a contraindication to such implants [1].

Author's recommendation

For many patients, preoperative screening for maculopathy using OCT is very useful, particularly when considering a multifocal IOL.

Practical aspects of posterior segment OCT

While pharmacological mydriasis is not necessary for a good macular OCT image, the quality of the image may decrease in miosis as the crystalline lens becomes cloudier. OCT devices are offered by a variety of different manufacturers, and each comes with its own proprietary software. In all devices, macular scan patterns can

J. Siedlecki (✉)
Munich, Germany
e-mail: jakob.siedlecki@med.uni-muenchen.de

M. Ang
Singapore, Singapore
e-mail: marcus.ang@singhealth.com.sg

M. Shajari et al. (eds.), *Cataract and Lens Surgery*,
https://doi.org/10.1007/978-3-031-05394-8_17

be adjusted manually. A quick and practical line scan where only a horizontal section ("B-scan") is acquired through the fovea stands opposed to a full volume scan where additional macular sections are acquired above and below the line scan (e.g., a total of 49 sections (=B-scans) at a distance of 5.3 μm each over an area of 20° × 20 centered on the fovea). Although the line scan, often printed out or exported as a PDF into electronic health records is quick and easy to export, macular pathologies can easily be overlooked if they lie extrafoveally (but are likely to spread to the fovea in the next few years). Therefore, macular volume scans are suggested over single line scans.

Author's recommendation

Volume scans with several retinal sections across the entire macula are superior to line scans (a single section through the fovea) when screening for maculopathies.

Overview of the main pathologies

Age-related macular degeneration

Since both cataract and age-related macular degeneration (AMD) increase in incidence with age, preoperative OCT screening is an important part of the surgical planning. This is especially true when a patient has a positive family history or when the fundus is abnormal. AMD can manifest itself as an early form (drusen > 63 − 125 μm), intermediate form (drusen > 125 μm or pigment epithelial changes) or late form (neovascular AMD, geographic atrophy) [2].

Diagnosis may be obvious in the presence of classic foveal "soft" drusen which can also be seen on routine fundoscopy (Fig. 1 upper picture). However, the diagnosis is more complicated in patients with reticular pseudodrusen (Fig. 1 lower picture), which present as small, sharply defined lesions located in the subretinal layers. Reticular pseudodrusen are usually extrafoveal and can therefore be overlooked on a simple line scan. They are more conspicuous in the associated infrared or autofluorescence image, or in macular volume scans with multiple B-scans (Fig. 2). Despite their often-inconspicuous clinical appearance, reticular pseudodrusen represent a serious dysfunction of the choriocapillaris and a predisposing factor for retinal angiomatous proliferation (RAP), geographic atrophy and deposition of pseudovitelliform material (Fig. 2 lower picture). When considering patients for a multifocal IOL, reticular pseudodrusen in particular (and of course soft drusen) should therefore be carefully excluded. An assessment of the partner eye should never be omitted, especially with regard to possible signs of AMD.

Patients with neovascular AMD (Fig. 3) should first receive an intravitreal therapy with anti-vascular endothelial growth factor (VEGF) inhibitors prior to cataract surgery. The aim should be to establish a "dry" interval before reliable biometry and safe surgery can be performed. Patients with geographic atrophy should be informed about their reduced visual prognosis. A large number of studies however have shown that AMD patients of all stages (including late forms) benefit significantly from cataract surgery so it should not be considered a contraindication to surgery [3].

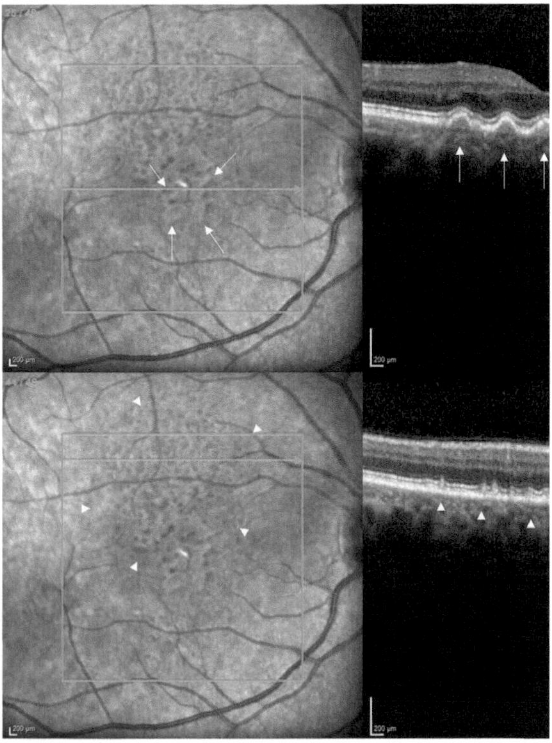

Fig. 1 Age-related macular degeneration (AMD). Drusen are the hallmark of AMD, which can present as soft drusen (upper picture, marked by arrows) or reticular pseudodrusen (lower picture, marked by arrowheads; also called: subretinal drusenoid deposits). The latter can often be overlooked on funduscopy and single-line scans of the fovea since they are often located extrafoveally. Near-infrared confocal scanning laser ophthalmoscopy will aid with detection

Author's recommendation

A normal foveal line scan does not rule out AMD - reticular pseudodrusen are often located extrafoveally and indicate a risk for more severe macular pathology in the future. a (GA, RAP).

Diabetic macular edema

Diabetic macular edema (DME) is seen as focal or diffuse thickening of the central retina, often with large intraretinal cystoid cavities (Fig. 4) and/or subretinal fluid. Hyperreflective foci (white intraretinal dots) indicate that the edema is more likely chronic. The treatment of DME with intravitreal anti-VEGF inhibitors or corticosteroids is recommended to achieve reliable biometry and perform safe surgery. In the case of anti-VEGF therapy, surgery can be performed between two injections (e.g., 2 weeks after the last injection), often augmented with an intraoperative application of steroids and postoperative prescription of NSAID eye drops, as the risk of DME relapse or Irvine-Gass syndrome is significantly increased [5]. Surgery under "steroid protection" has also proven to be a successful approach, where dexamethasone is administered as a three-month intravitreal implant and cataract

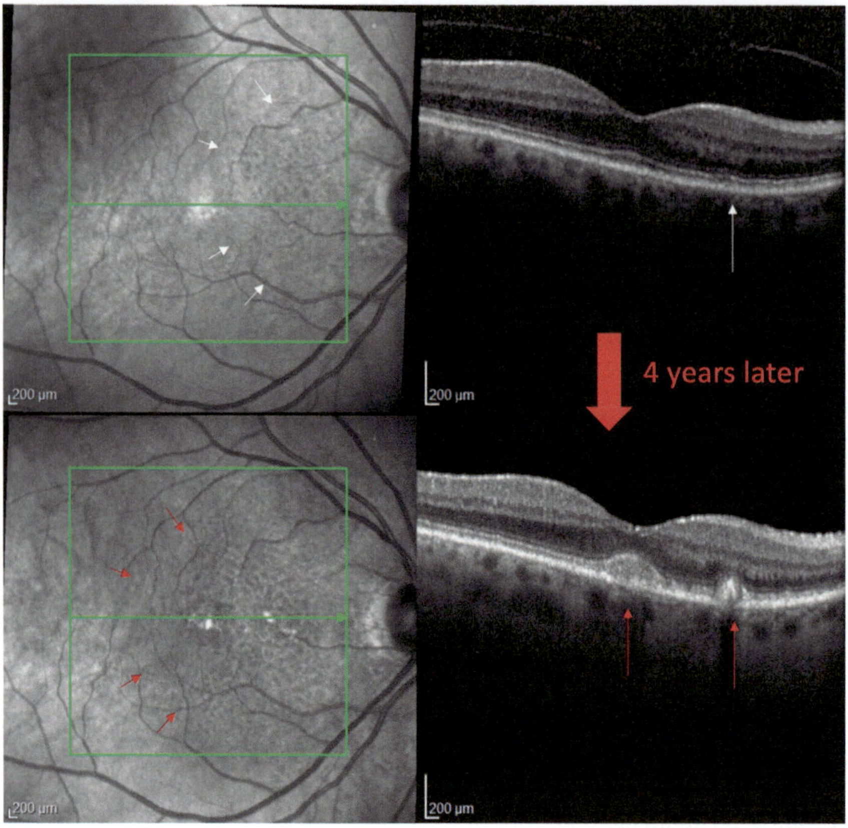

Fig. 2 Age-related macular degeneration (AMD) with reticular pseudodrusen. Reticular pseudodrusen can be easily overlooked on macular line scans (white arrow). Over time, subretinal pseudo-vitelliform material can develop (lower picture four years later). In such cases of maculopathy, the implantation of multifocal IOLs is not recommended

surgery is performed after 6 weeks, after which edema prophylaxis is provided for another 6 weeks by the steroid implant.

Retinal vein occlusion

Retinal vein occlusion can manifest as central retinal vein occlusion, hemi-central retinal vein occlusion or branch retinal vein occlusion. For the cataract surgeon they usually become problematic when associated with cystoid macular edema (Fig. 5). Intraretinal fluid may also be accompanied by subretinal exudation [6]. As with DME, anti-VEGF or steroid therapy is required intravitreally before cataract surgery can be performed. In these cases too, surgery during the interval between anti-VEGF injections or under steroid protection may be appropriate. The addition of intraoperative steroids can be beneficial in preventing a worsening of the CME postoperatively.

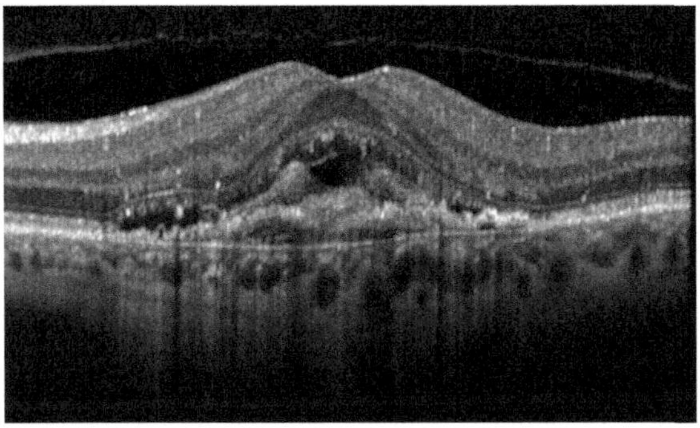

Fig. 3 Neovascular age-related macular degeneration. Pigment epithelium detachment and subretinal hyperreflective material (dense white matter subfoveally) are highly suggestive of choroidal neovascularization. Angiography (OCT or dynamic fluorescein) and subsequent timely anti-VEGF therapy is recommended before cataract surgery

Fig. 4 Diabetic macular edema with center involvement (giant cyst) and smaller intraretinal cysts. Note the hyperreflective dots in the nasal aspect of the macula

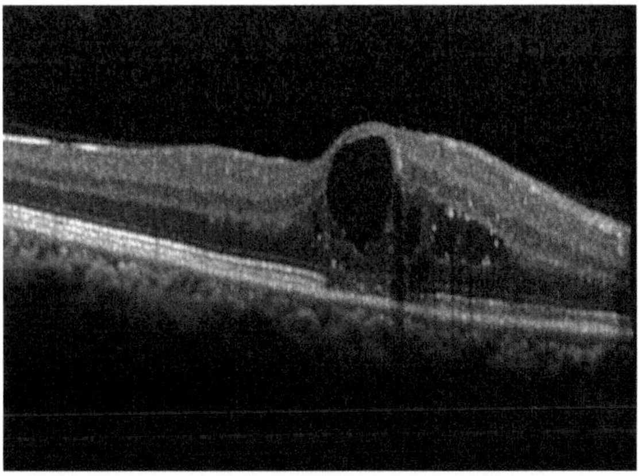

Fig. 5 Macular edema secondary to retinal vein occlusion. Note the intraretinal and subretinal fluid

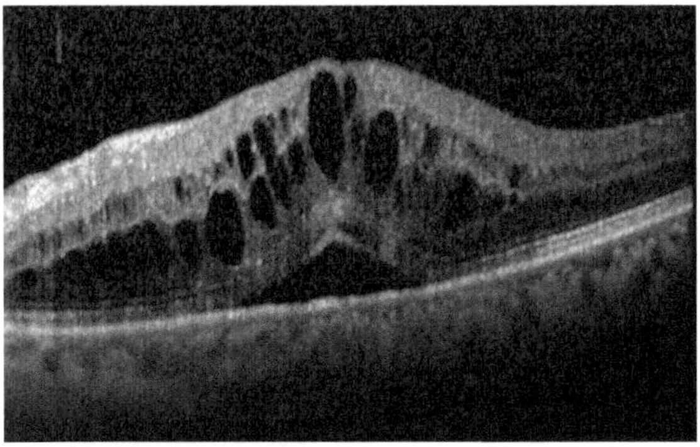

Pachychoroid maculopathies (including central serous chorioretinopathy).

Pachychoroid (pachy meaning thick) maculopathies are retinochoroidal pathologies characterized by a thickened, congested choroid. Central serous chorioretinopathy (CSC) is the most widely recognized representative of the pachychoroid spectrum and is defined by the presence of subretinal fluid (stage 2; Fig. 6; thickened choroid marked with a white arrow). Pachychoroid pigment epitheliopathy (PPE) is a preliminary stage, in which only RPE defects without subretinal fluid occur (stage 1). If choroidal neovascularisation (CNV) forms secondary to CSC (approx. 25–39%), this is called pachychoroid neovasculopathy (PNV; stage 3). If aneurysms form within the CNV, pachychoroid aneurysmal type 1 CNV (PAT1; former/also polypoidal choroidal vasculopathy (PCV), stage 4) occurs. In many patients, these stages progress over time though they can also regress under therapy. A classification system has recently been suggested to describe the various pachychoroid disease entities [7].

PPE without subretinal fluid does not pose a problem for cataract surgery but progress to CSC can be seen when steroids are given. In the case of CSC, PNV or PCV, pachychoroid maculopathy should be treated with anti-VEGF if CNV is present, micropulse or argon lasers and, in many cases, photodynamic therapy before cataract surgery is performed. In these cases, steroids should be used with care.

Pachychoroid disorders of the macula

Stage	
0	Uncomplicated pachychoroid (UCP)
I	Pachychoroid pigment epitheliopathy (PPE)
II	Central serous chorioretinopathy (CSC)
III	Pachchoroid neovasculopathy (PNV)
III a	with neurosensory detachment (overlap with CSC)
III b	without neurosensory detachment
IV	Pachychoroid aneurysmal type 1 CNV (PAT1) / Polypoidal Choroidal Vasculopathy (PCV)

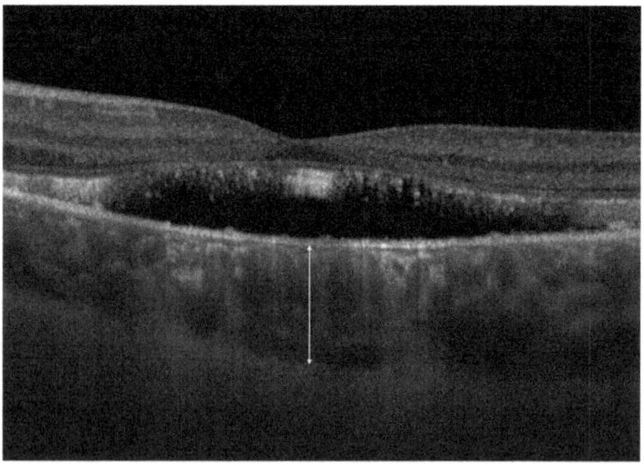

Fig. 6 Central serous chorioretinopathy with subretinal fluid. Central serous chorioretinopathy belongs to the Pachychoroid spectrum (stage II) which is defined by abnormal choroidal thickening (white arrow) and the presence of pachyvessels (thick vessels in the choroid >180 μm)

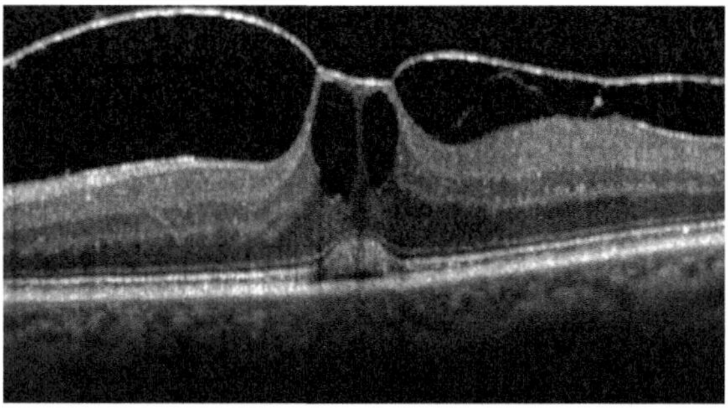

Fig. 7 Vitreomacular traction. Note the subretinal cleft ("subretinal fluid") which is indicating rather strong traction. Also note the epiretinal membrane nasally and temporally suggesting pars plana vitrectomy over intravitreal agents to release traction (ocriplasmin/gas)

Maculopathies of the vitreoretinal interface

The interaction of a pathological, detached vitreous body with the residual points of adhesion to the retina leads to maculopathies of the vitreoretinal interface [8]. These include vitreo-macular traction syndrome (VTMS), macular pucker and the macular holes. VMTS is characterized by a focal attachment of the partially detached vitreous body to the fovea, causing tractional deformation of the retina (Fig. 7). Intraretinal gaps are formed and in more pronounced pathology the photoreceptor layer may also be affected (delicate subretinal fluid accumulation in Fig. 7). In principle, marked VMTS, especially with concomitant pathologies like a macular pucker, should be treated by combined phaovitrectomy. In the case of moderate VMT, intravitreal orcriplasm or pneumatic vitreolysis (the latter with a relatively high risk of retinal detachment) can also be considered. In the case of mild VMT, primary cataract surgery can also be performed, as posterior vitreous detachment, which usually follows shortly after cataract surgery, is in many cases sufficient to resolve the VMT.

Where a macular pucker (Fig. 8) with strong traction is present with retinal thickening, marked metamorphopsia and visual impairment (Fig. 8, green reference arrow), a combined phacovitrectomy with ILM peeling should be performed. In case of a macular hole (Fig. 9), a combined phacovitrectomy is also recommended.

Rare maculopathies

In addition to the all of the common clinical entities mentioned above, a multitude of rare maculopathies can also be detected in patients scheduled for cataract surgery, e.g., myopia-related (myopic CNV), (vascular) degenerative (e.g., macular telangiectasia, angioid streaks) or hereditary (e.g., Stargardt's disease). In unclear cases, it is always advisable to consult a retina specialist.

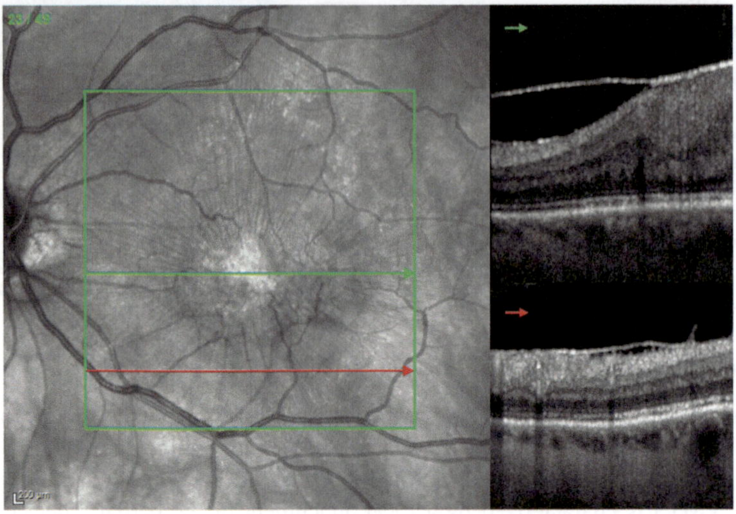

Fig. 8 Epiretinal membrane. Note that the vitreous is still attached in the foveal area (green arrow), while below the vitreous is already detached, leaving behind an epiretinal membrane

Fig. 9 Full-thickness macular hole, suggesting combined phacovitrectomy with ILM peeling

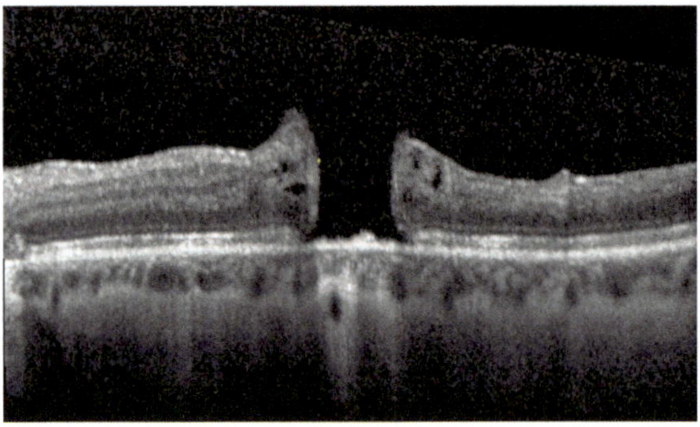

References

1. Alio JL, Plaza- AB, Fernandez- R, Pikkel J, Maldonado M. Multifocal intraocular lenses: an overview. Surv Ophthalmol. 2017;62(5):611–34.
2. Ferris FL 3rd, Wilkinson CP, Bird A, Chakravarthy U, Chew E, Csaky K, et al. Clinical classification of age-related macular degeneration. Ophthalmology. 2013;120(4):844–51.
3. Forooghian F, Agron E, Clemons TE, Ferris FL, 3rd, Chew EY. Visual acuity outcomes after cataract surgery in patients with age-related macular degeneration: age-related eye disease study report no. 27. Ophthalmology. 2009;116(11):2093–100.
4. Schmidt-Erfurth U, Garcia-Arumi J, Bandello F, Berg K, Chakravarthy U, Gerendas BS, et al. Guidelines for the management of diabetic macular edema by the European society of retina specialists (EURETINA). Ophthalmologica. 2017;237(4):185–222.

5. Wielders LHP, Schouten J, Winkens B, van den Biggelaar F, Veldhuizen CA, Findl O, et al. European multicenter trial of the prevention of cystoid macular edema after cataract surgery in nondiabetics. ESCRS PREMED study report 1st J Cataract Refract Surg. 2018;44(4):429–39.
6. Schmidt- U, Garcia- J, Gerendas BS, Midena E, Sivaprasad S, Tadayoni R, et al. Guidelines for the management of retinal vein occlusion by the European society of retina specialists (EURETINA). Ophthalmologica. 2019;242(3):123–62.
7. Siedlecki J, Schworm B, Priglinger SG. The pachychoroid disease spectrum-and the need for a uniform classification system. Ophthalmol Retin. 2019;3(12):1013–5.
8. DeCroos FC, Toth CA, Folgar FA, Pakola S, Stinnett SS, Heydary CS, et al. Characterization of vitreoretinal interface disorders using OCT in the interventional phase 3 trials of ocriplasmin. Invest Ophthalmol Vis Sci. 2012;53(10):6504–11.

Measurement of Endothelial Cells

Gernot Steinwender and Sheraz Daya

Endothelial cell analysis is an important evaluation for preparation and aftercare of all lens surgery procedures. The young and normal corneal endothelium represents a unicellular layer of delimited, semi-permeable, hexagonal cells of uniform size as the innermost layer of the cornea. In addition to their barrier function, endothelial cells also have a pump function, which allows aqueous humour to enter the cornea for nutritional purposes while at the same time ensuring transparency of the cornea by pumping out excess aqueous humour. Endothelial cells do not multiply to any significant degree and with increasing age, there is a gradual decrease in number of cells and regularity of cell size and shape. These changes can be measured and assessed by means of specular microscopy which can determine endothelial cell density (cells per mm^2), coefficient of variation (standard deviation of cell area/ average cell area) and percentage of hexagonality (percentage of hexagonal cells).

After the age of 40, endothelial cell density is typically between 2500 and 3000 cells/mm^2 [1]. Factors that influence endothelial cell density and morphology include trauma, contact lens use, refractive surgery, diabetes and corneal disease.

While endothelial cells can be seen using slit-lamp microscopy, the magnified image of the corneal endothelium obtained by a specular microscope allows a far better qualitative and quantitative assessment of endothelial diseases and possible dysfunction. The specular reflex resulting from the differing refractive indices of endothelial cells and aqueous humour can be recorded, allowing in most cases a clear distinction and good visibility of cell borders of the corneal endothelial layer.

In mild to moderate forms of Fuchs endothelial dystrophy, small endothelial excrescenses called guttae can be seen as dark spots between the bright cells on

G. Steinwender (✉)
Medical University of Graz, Graz, Austria
e-mail: steinwender.gernot@gmail.com

S. Daya
Centre for Sight, London, UK
e-mail: sdaya@centreforsight.com

M. Shajari et al. (eds.), *Cataract and Lens Surgery*,
https://doi.org/10.1007/978-3-031-05394-8_18

specular microscopy. Guttae typically first present in the centre of the cornea and over time increase in both size and density to the point that the can become confluent. As the disease evolves, the endothelial cells also lose their uniform hexagonal shape and cell loss and migration can occur. As cells die and shed, their neighbouring cells enlarge to repair the barrier function. This leads to both variations in size (polymegathism) and shape (pleomorphism). While most specular microscopy devices on the market offer automated cell density measurements, they can be fraught with error and false demarcation of cells which can include guttata and sometimes doubling of a large cell. The automated calculated results can thus vary considerably based on the location and size of the counting frame. The best counting results are achieved with a counting frame as large as possible together with the option of manually counting (Fig. 1).

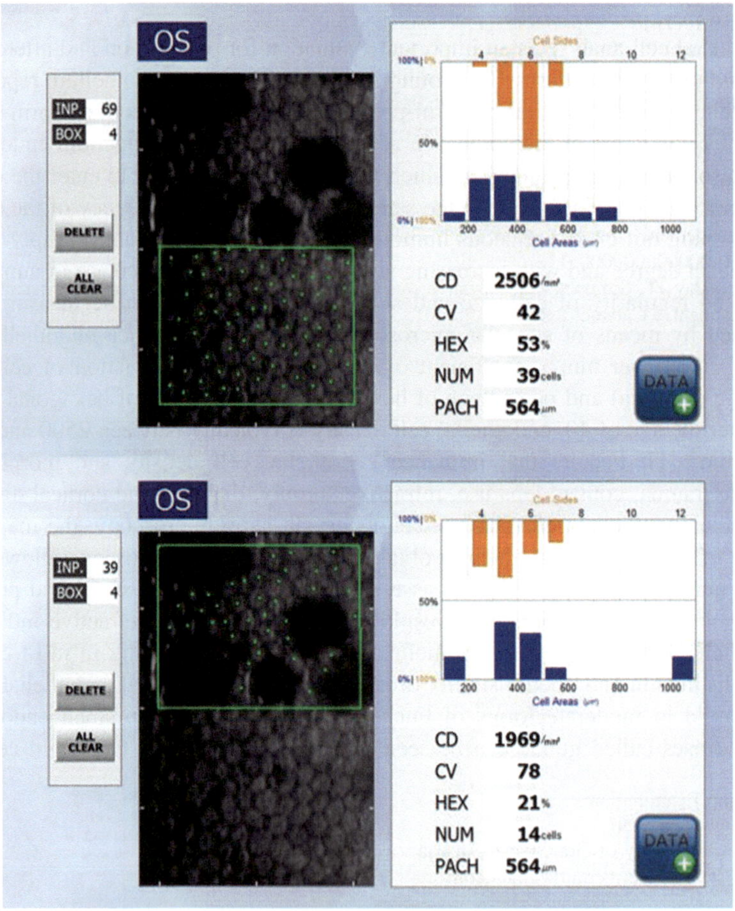

Fig. 1 When the endothelial cell density is determined by means of a specular microscope, the typical guttae in the presence of a Fuchs endothelial dystrophy becomes apparent. It should be noted that due to the guttae, the results vary considerably depending on the position of the counting frame

Scheimpflug tomography can also be a helpful tool to identify early Fuchs endothelial dystrophy. While it cannot provide estimates of endothelial cell density, eyes with subclinical corneal edema can be reliably distinguished from healthy eyes by features in tomographic pachymetry and elevation maps, like displacement of the thinnest point and focal posterior corneal surface depression [2].

Measurement of central corneal thickness alone, however, is of little help in understanding the extent of Fuchs endothelial dystrophy as there is a wide range of central corneal thickness in the healthy population. Sequential central corneal thickness measurements over time may be more useful in demonstrating an increase in corneal thickness from baseline.

When considering lens surgery, the analysis of corneal endothelium is relevant in several aspects. The initial diagnosis of a corneal pathology is often made during pre-operative examination before cataract surgery. Furthermore, a healthy endothelium is an important baseline criterion in patient selection for refractive lens surgery.

When a patient with Fuchs endothelial dystrophy presents for cataract surgery, the question arises what the sequence of surgeries should be or whether the cataract surgery should be combined with corneal endothelial keratoplasty. One reason why a two-stage approach favours prior phacoemulsification followed by Descemet membrane endothelial keratoplasty (DMEK) is that with DMEK in the phakic eye, the development of a visually relevant cataract is 76% due to intraocular manipulation and postoperative local steroid administration [3]. Additionally, phacoemulsification following endothelial transplantation can lead to endothelial cell loss on the transplant [4]. Another good argument for commencing with phacoemulsification is improved technical ease of performing the DMEK in pseudophakic eyes with deeper anterior chambers.

On the other hand, a reverse sequence with prior DMEK and subsequent phacoemulsification has the potential advantage of a more accurate IOL calculation, as the total corneal refractive power (anterior and posterior surface) can be significantly changed by DMEK [5].

A combined surgery, known as triple-DMEK, offers the patient advantage of a one-stage procedure. In triple-DMEK, the complexity of surgery is increased by pupil dilation and the need for complete removal of viscoelastic device. Although final visual outcomes do not differ between triple-DMEK and DMEK-alone [6], endothelial cell loss seems to be greater in the combined procedure [7].

In patient selection for **multifocal IOL** implantation, endothelial cell analysis is of particular importance. Even with only mild Fuchs endothelial dystrophy without corneal edema in slit-lamp examination, guttae may lead to light scattering and thus to visual disturbances [8]. The combination of guttata with the potentially reduced contrast sensitivity of multifocal IOLs, which can occur even in healthy eyes may result in significant impairment of visual quality [9]. In patients with Fuchs endothelial dystrophy highly motivated to have spectacle independence, the option of a "Duet implantation" with a multifocal add-on IOL in the ciliary sulcus may be consideration and has the benefit of facile removal of the add-on multifocal in the event vision is adversely affected. Good results have been reported for multifocal IOL implantation after DMEK [10].

Author's recommendation

Endothelial cell analysis is essential in preoperative diagnostics before refractive lens surgery.

When implanting **toric IOLs** in patients with endothelial dysfunction, possible changes in corneal astigmatism due to subsequent DMEK surgery must be taken into account for calculating cylindric power of the IOL [11]. However, good outcomes following use of toric IOLs in triple DMEK, has been reported in a case series [12].

A healthy corneal endothelium is important when considering implantation of **phakic IOLs**. Potential low grade endothelial cell loss after phakic IOL implantation has been reported [13], and can become problematic in young patients long term. Chronic endothelial cell loss 10 years after implantation of a rigid iris-fixated phakic IOL was 16.6% for the myopic and 21.5% for the toric IOL model [14], while it was about 10% 5 years after implantation of a foldable iris-fixated IOL [15]. Endothelial cell loss following implantation of sulcus-fixated phakic IOL was lower with a mean loss of 5.3% after 10 years, probably due to the greater distance between the IOL and the endothelium [16]. Nevertheless, annual endothelial cell analysis is recommended for all models of phakic IOLs to detect excessive endothelial cell loss at an early stage. When interpreting the measured values, it is important to consider normal physiological endothelial cell loss reported to be 0.6% per year [17].

Endothelial cells are responsible for maintenance of corneal clarity and loss can adversely influence both visual quality and corneal shape. It is therefore important to consider endothelial cell counts and morphology when indicated prior to intraocular surgery.

References

1. Mannis MJ, Holland EJ, directeurs. Cornea: fundamentals, diagnosis and management. Fourth ed. Edinburgh, N.Y: Elsevier; 2017.
2. Sun SY, Wacker K, Baratz KH, Patel SV. Determining subclinical edema in fuchs endothelial corneal dystrophy: revised classification using Scheimpflug tomography for preoperative assessment. Ophthalmology. Elsevier. 2019;126(2):195–204.
3. Burkhart ZN, Feng MT, Price FW, Price MO. One-year outcomes in eyes remaining phakic after Descemet membrane endothelial keratoplasty. J Cataract Refract Surg. 2014;40(3): 430–4.
4. Musa FU, Cabrerizo J, Quilendrino R, Dapena I, Ham L, Melles GRJ. Outcomes of phacoemulsification after Descemet membrane endothelial keratoplasty. J Cataract Refract Surg. 2013;39(6):836–40.
5. Alnawaiseh M, Rosentreter A, Eter N, Zumhagen L. Changes in corneal refractive power for patients with fuchs endothelial dystrophy after DMEK. Cornea. 2016;35(8):1073–7.

6. Chaurasia S, Price FW, Gunderson L, Price MO. Descemet's membrane endothelial keratoplasty: clinical results of single versus triple procedures (combined with cataract surgery). Ophthalmology. 2014;121(2):454–8.
7. Shahnazaryan D, Hajjar Sese A, Hollick EJ. Endothelial cell loss after Descemet's membrane endothelial keratoplasty for fuchs' endothelial dystrophy: DMEK compared to triple DMEK. Am J Ophthalmol. 2020;218:1–6.
8. Watanabe S, Oie Y, Fujimoto H, Soma T, Koh S, Tsujikawa M, et al. Relationship between corneal guttae and quality of vision in patients with mild fuchs' endothelial corneal dystrophy. Ophthalmology. 2015;122(10):2103–9.
9. de Vries NE, Webers CAB, Touwslager WRH, Bauer NJC, de Brabander J, Berendschot TT, et al. Dissatisfaction after implantation of multifocal intraocular lenses. J Cataract Refract Surg. 2011;37(5):859–65.
10. Price MO, Pinkus D, Price FW. Implantation of presbyopia-correcting intraocular lenses staged after Descemet membrane endothelial keratoplasty in patients with fuchs dystrophy. Cornea. 2020;39(6):732–5.
11. Shajari M, Kolb CM, Mayer WJ, Agha B, Steinwender G, Dirisamer M, et al. Characteristics of preoperative and postoperative astigmatism in patients having Descemet membrane endothelial keratoplasty. J Cataract Refract Surg. 2019;45(7):1001–6.
12. Yokogawa H, Sanchez PJ, Mayko ZM, Straiko MD, Terry MA. Astigmatism correction with toric intraocular lenses in Descemet membrane endothelial keratoplasty triple procedures. Cornea. 2017;36(3):269–74.
13. Kohnen T, Kook D, Morral M, Güell JL. Phakic intraocular lenses: part 2: results and complications. J Cataract Refract Surg. 2010;36(12):2168–94.
14. Jonker SMR, Berendschot TTJM, Ronden AE, Saelens IEY, Bauer NJC, Nuijts RMMA. Long-term endothelial cell loss in patients with artisan myopia and artisan toric phakic intraocular lenses: 5- and 10-year results. Ophthalmology. 2018;125(4):486–94.
15. Jonker SMR, Berendschot TTJM, Ronden AE, Saelens IEY, Bauer NJC, Nuijts RMMA. Five-year endothelial cell loss after implantation with artiflex myopia and artiflex toric phakic intraocular lenses. Am J Ophthalmol. 2018;194:110–9.
16. Nakamura T, Isogai N, Kojima T, Yoshida Y, Sugiyama Y. Posterior chamber phakic intraocular lens implantation for the correction of myopia and myopic astigmatism: a retrospective 10-year follow-up study. Am J Ophthalmol. 2019;206:1–10.
17. Bourne WM, Nelson LR, Hodge DO. Central corneal endothelial cell changes over a ten-year period. Invest Ophthalmol Vis Sci. 1997;38(3):779–82.

Tear Film Analysis

Anna Maria Schuh

Components and function

The three-layer model proposed by Wolff [1] (mucin layer - aqueous layer - lipid layer) is still frequently used to describe the tear film due to its simplicity. Today, however, we know that the precorneal tear film is a highly complex, dynamic functional unit consisting of different compartments [2], which also include cells of the immune system, cytokines, enzymes and antimicrobes that are necessary for its functionality [3].

In addition to the constant moistening of the ocular surface, the tear film has a key function in maintaining the refractive surface of the visual system.

Considerations before lens surgery

The presence of a dry eye has to be recognised before lens surgery in order to inform the patient about the possibility of postoperative worsening of the disease and to initiate appropriate therapeutic measures preoperatively. A detailed description of dry eye treatment in lens surgery can be found in Chapter "Postoperative Inflammation". It is also important to consider how the tear film plays an important role in the calculation of the intraocular lens. Light experiences its first strong refraction when passing from air to tear film [2]. Changes in the composition of the tear film and resulting instability can lead to aberrant keratometry readings and thus incorrect IOL calculations which can result in refractive surprises and ultimately functionally worse outcomes for the patient, which could have been avoided. Epitropoulus et al. show that a hyperosmolar tear film leads to a

A. M. Schuh (✉)
Department of Ophthalmology, Ludwig-Maximilians-University Munich, Munich, Germany
e-mail: anna.schuh@med.uni-muenchen.de

M. Shajari et al. (eds.), *Cataract and Lens Surgery*,
https://doi.org/10.1007/978-3-031-05394-8_19

higher variability of the mean K-value and anterior corneal astigmatism when measured repeatedly [4].

Author's recommendation

The tear film must be examined before IOL calculation and, if pathological, treated to avoid measurement errors in keratometry.

Evaluation of symptoms

In addition to taking the patient's history, there are different tests available to evaluate dry eye symptoms. The *OSDI* (*Ocular Surface Disease Index*) is the most widely used questionnaire measuring frequency of symptoms, environmental triggers and vision related quality of life [5]. It is recommended by the Dry Eye Workshop (DEWS) 2017 for clinical trials, as well as the *Dry Eye Questionnaire (DEQ-5)* [5]. Other current, but less validated, questionnaires include: *Impact of Dry Eye on Everyday Living (IDEEL), National Eye Institute's Visual Function Questionnaire (NEI VFQ-25), Dry Eye-Related Quality-of-Life Score (DEQS), Computer-vision symptom scale (CVSS17)* [5].

However, dry eye symptoms often do not correlate with the severity of tear film irregularities [6]. Patients might have an instable tear film without reporting any dry eye symptoms [4].

Author's recommendation

The absence of dry eye symptoms does not rule out tear film irregularities. Further tear film analysis is curial before lens surgery.

Methods of tear film analysis

Tear film stability

Tear film break-up time using fluorescent dye (Fluorescent Break-up time, FBUT).

The best way to apply the dye is via a fluorescent dye strip moistened with sodium chloride in the temporally inferior fornix (Figs. 1 and 2). The excess fluid should be shaken off the strip before application. After blinking several times to evenly distribute the stained tear film, the patient is then asked to look straight ahead and not to blink. Under cobalt blue light, the seconds from the last blink to the first break up of the tear film are counted. A normal BUT is >10 s [7]; if very little dye is used, values as low as 6 s may still be normal [8].

Author's recommendation

Moistening with sodium chloride avoids unnecessary irritation of the ocular surface. Local anaesthetics, however, reduce tear film stability. Local anaesthetics mixed with fluorescein (e.g., Thilorbin) lead to incorrect measurement results and should not be used.

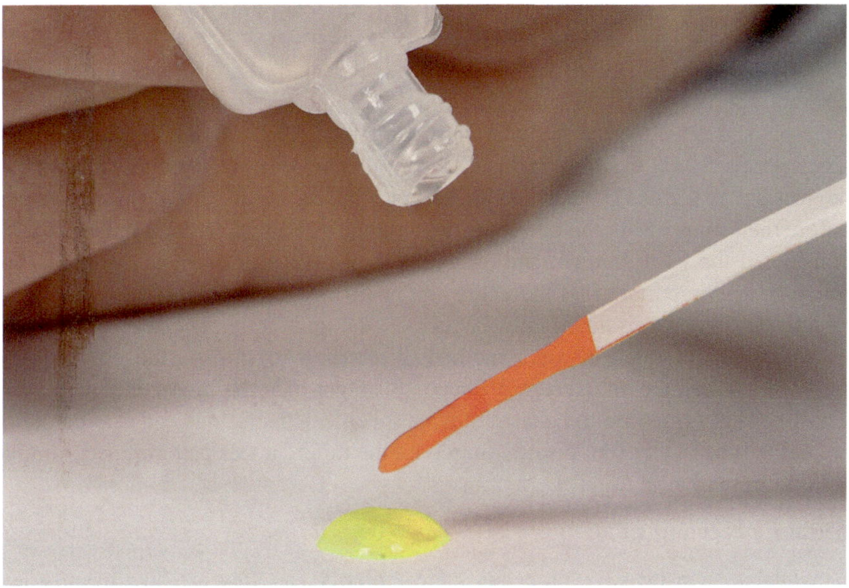

Fig. 1 Moistening of the fluorescent dye strip

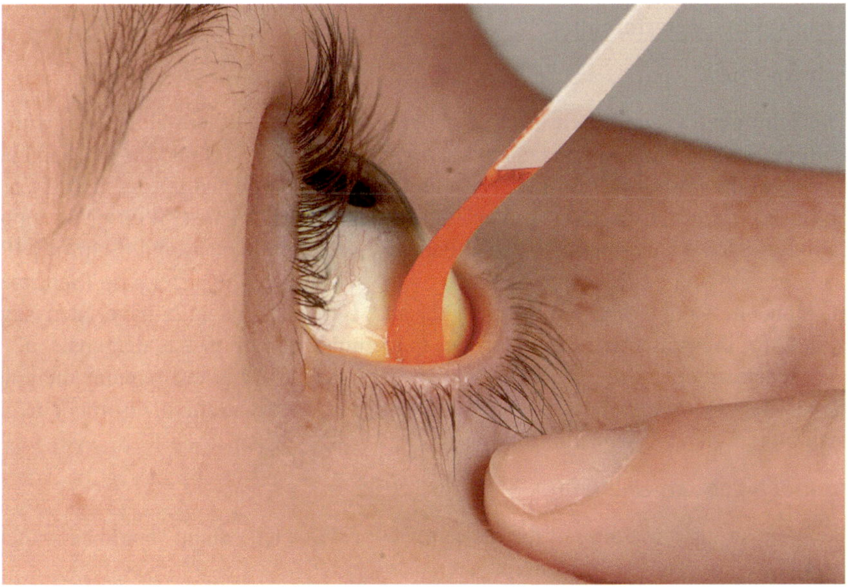

Fig. 2 Installation of fluorescent dye in the temporal inferior fornix

Non-invasive tear film break-up time (NIBUT)

Using NIBUT, an image of the eye surface is reflected as a grid pattern or placido disc and the rupture of the tear film, which leads to the interruption of the image pattern, is detected by a software program. This function is integrated in the Keratograph 5 M (Oculus, Wetzlar, Germany), as an example; though various other devices are available. The patient should first blink three times, in a relaxed manner, before then suppressing the blink for measurement. The first break in the tear film is considered the final moment and an average of three measurements is taken. For this test, it is important that the entire ocular surface is captured. Fluorescent dye, which also has a certain negative effect on the stability of the tear film, is not necessary for this non-invasive method. According to studies, the non-invasive measured values are on average 3.7 seconds longer than the invasive methods [9]. Thus, normal values are to be taken device specific. Conclusions can also be drawn about the type of tear film disorder based on the different tear patterns, according to a study by Yokoi et al. [10].

Author's recommendation

If available, non-invasive procedures are preferred, as they are significantly less dependent on the examiner. Invasive examinations that falsify the measurements (e.g. expression of the meibomian glands, dye application) should be carried out only after the break-up time is measured.

Tear volume determination

Schirmer test

The Schirmer test paper measuring strip consists of a thin piece of filter paper with a millimetre scale. This strip is bent at the upper end and hooked into the temporal lid margin of the lower eyelid. After five minutes, it is removed and the amount of tears produced up to that point is read off the moistened millimetres. With prior application of a local anaesthetic, the so-called base secretion is measured (Schirmer II); without it, the reflex tears are contained by the stimulus of the paper strip (Schirmer I). Standard values of 5 mm/5 min [11] and 10 mm/5 min [12] have been suggested for Schirmer II; for Schirmer I 15 mm/5 min. For the diagnosis of a hyposecretory deficit (e.g., Sjögren's syndrome) the Schirmer test remains the gold standard [13]; however, it is less suitable for hyperevaporative disorders (e.g., meibomian gland dysfunction).

Author's recommendation

To avoid strong variability of the measurement results, the patient should keep their eyes closed during the measurement.

Lacrimal meniscus determination

The height of the lacrimal meniscus above the lid margin of the lower eyelid can be determined under the slit lamp with the aid of fluorescent staining and cobalt blue light. Non-invasive meniscometry (volume and height) with anterior segment OCT

[5] is more complex but less examiner dependent. Measurements are taken just above the middle of the lid margin of the lower lid after blinking.

Corneal and conjunctival staining

In routine clinical practice, fluorescein dye is used. This is applied in the same manner as for the FBUT. Epithelial cell defects stain yellow and become clearly visible under cobalt blue light. An alternative stain, Rose Bengal stains dead cells, but also vital cells that are not protected by mucin or glycocalix. It is not frequently used as it has a strong irritant effect. Lissamine green exhibits less toxicity, and only stains non-vital cells with damaged cell walls.

Tear film osmolarity

Hyperosmolarity of the tear film, as often seen in dry eye, leads to a shift in the cytokine balance, which, by activating the JAK/STAT signalling pathway, leads to cell death of the epithelium. Tear film osmolarity tests have displayed a high correlation to the severity of the disease in dry eye [14]. A normal tear film typically has low osmolarity levels and little variability between different measurements. Values above 308 mOsm/L, or a difference of 8 mOsm/L between the two eyes, are good indicators of a tear film osmolarity disorder [15]. Osmolarity measuring devices are commercially available and one such device is the TearLabTM Osmolarity System (TearLab, CA, USA). The TearLab measurement is taken with the chin slightly raised in the tear meniscus above the lid margin of the lower eyelid, without touching the globe with the sensor.

Matrix Metalloproteinase-9 Test (MMP-9 Test)

MMPs destroy the tight junctions of the surface epithelium. MMP levels therefore reflect the loss of barrier function and the degree of inflammation. Normal MMP-9 levels range from 3 to 40 ng/mL [16]. Higher levels have been measured in patients with dry eye. One available device is InflammaDry (Rapid Pathogen Screening, Inc, Sarasota, FL, USA), which can detect MMP-9 levels within 10 min.

Both, osmolarity and MMP-9 test, are becoming increasingly relevant in routine clinical practice. The assessment of the tear film is especially important before refractive surgery as well as cataract surgery [17]. Preoperatively asymptomatic patients who already show changes in tear film, but in whom other clinical tests such as surface changes are not yet noticeable, can possibly be detected early with the help of these tests.

For subgroup determination of dry eye patients, other tests such as detailed inspection of the eyelid margins, meibomian glands and conjunctiva, and diagnostic tests such as meibography, lactoferrin test, Sjo test and interferometry tests may be helpful. A good overview can be found in the Diagnostic Methodology report of the DEWS of 2017 [5].

References

1. Wolff E. Mucocutaneous junction of lid-margin and distribution of tear fluid. Trans Ophthal Soc UK. 1946;66:291–308.
2. Willcox MDP, Argueso P, Georgiev GA, Holopainen JM, Laurie GW, Millar TJ, et al. TFOS DEWS II tear film report. Ocul Surf. 2017;15(3):366–403.
3. Albertsmeyer AC, Kakkassery V, Spurr-Michaud S, Beeks O, Gipson IK. Effect of pro-inflammatory mediators on membrane-associated mucins expressed by human ocular surface epithelial cells. Exp Eye Res. 2010;90(3):444–51.
4. Epitropoulos AT, Matossian C, Berdy GJ, Malhotra RP, Potvin R. Effect of tear osmolarity on repeatability of keratometry for cataract surgery planning. J Cataract Refract Surg. 2015;41 (8):1672–7.
5. Wolffsohn JS, Arita R, Chalmers R, Djalilian A, Dogru M, Dumbleton K, et al. TFOS DEWS II diagnostic methodology report. Ocul Surf. 2017;15(3):539–74.
6. Begley CG, Chalmers RL, Abetz L, Venkataraman K, Mertzanis P, Caffery BA, et al. The relationship between habitual patient-reported symptoms and clinical signs among patients with dry eye of varying severity. Invest Ophthalmol Vis Sci. 2003;44(11):4753–61.
7. Lemp MA, Hamill JR Jr. Factors affecting tear film breakup in normal eyes. Arch Ophthalmol. 1973;89(2):103–5.
8. Abelson MB, Ousler GW 3rd, Nally LA, Welch D, Krenzer K. Alternative reference values for tear film break up time in normal and dry eye populations. Adv Exp Med Biol. 2002;506 (Pt B):1121–5.
9. Nichols JJ, Nichols KK, Puent B, Saracino M, Mitchell GL. Evaluation of tear film interference patterns and measures of tear break-up time. Optom Vis Sci. 2002;79(6):363–9.
10. Yokoi N, Georgiev GA, Kato H, Komuro A, Sonomura Y, Sotozono C, et al. Classification of Fluorescein breakup patterns: a novel method of differential diagnosis for dry eye. Am J Ophthalmol. 2017;180:72–85.
11. The definition and classification of dry eye disease: report of the Definition and Classification Subcommittee of the International Dry Eye WorkShop. Ocul Surf. 2007;5(2):75-92.
12. Li N, Deng XG, He MF. Comparison of the Schirmer I test with and without topical anesthesia for diagnosing dry eye. Int J Ophthalmol. 2012;5(4):478–81.
13. Vitali C, Bombardieri S, Jonsson R, Moutsopoulos HM, Alexander EL, Carsons SE, et al. Classification criteria for Sjogren's syndrome: a revised version of the European criteria proposed by the American-European Consensus Group. Ann Rheum Dis. 2002;61(6):554–8.
14. Tomlinson A, Khanal S, Ramaesh K, Diaper C, McFadyen A. Tear film osmolarity: determination of a referent for dry eye diagnosis. Invest Ophthalmol Vis Sci. 2006;47 (10):4309–15.
15. Bron AJ, Tomlinson A, Foulks GN, Pepose JS, Baudouin C, Geerling G, et al. Rethinking dry eye disease: a perspective on clinical implications. Ocul Surf. 2014;12(2 Suppl):S1-31.
16. Sambursky R, O'Brien TP. MMP-9 and the perioperative management of LASIK surgery. Curr Opin Ophthalmol. 2011;22(4):294–303.
17. Gonzalez-Mesa A, Moreno-Arrones JP, Ferrari D, Teus MA. Role of tear osmolarity in dry eye symptoms after cataract surgery. Am J Ophthalmol. 2016;170:128–32.

Pupillometry

Helmut Wilhelm

In cataract surgery surgery pupil size plays a role before, during and after surgery. The pupil should be wide enough before surgery so that a proper and thorough examination can be performed. It also must be wide enough intraoperatively to allow a safe procedure. However, it should not be too large postoperatively as disturbing optical phenomena become more evident and reflections from the edge of the lens and haptics might become visible. The optical zone of the implanted lens must match the pupil. The pupil width can only be roughly estimated. If you want to know the exact pupil size, you have to measure it.

Pupillography or pupillometry devices are occasionally used before and after surgery [3, 5, 6]. Pupillometers measure the pupil width statically, while pupillographs can also record it and apply light stimuli. The measurement is performed using invisible near infrared light, so that pupil measurements are possible even in complete darkness, without the test itself influencing the pupil. Pupil size is determined by means of image processing from the acquired video images. The measurement resolution of devices varies, but is almost always better than 0.1 mm, which is sufficient for the purpose of pupil measurement before cataract surgery. Simultaneous binocular measurement devices are advantageous because the measurement conditions are more natural.

If no pupillography device is available, flash photography can be used. The duration of the camera flash is so short (a few milliseconds) that the pupil does not manage to contract before the camera sensor is exposed. It normally takes 200 ms before the pupil even begins to contract after a light stimulus. A scale can be photographed simultaneously and the pupil can be measured on the monitor and calculated using the rule of three. It makes sense to use the mean value of two perpendicular diameters, because the pupil is not perfectly round. Pupillography devices use a circular or elliptical fit, which still works even if the pupil is partially covered.

H. Wilhelm (✉)
Tübingen, Germany
e-mail: Helmut.Wilhelm@med.uni-tuebingen.de

M. Shajari et al. (eds.), *Cataract and Lens Surgery*,
https://doi.org/10.1007/978-3-031-05394-8_20

The pupil size depends on the brightness, the fixation distance, the emotional status of the patient and age. When assessing the risk of postoperative irritation caused by a pupil that is too large, measurements should be taken in the weakest light possible, either in complete darkness or deep mesopic conditions with corneal illumination below 1 lx. It should be noted that pupil dilation is slower than constricting to a light stimulus. The pupil must be allowed to dilate for at least 10 s until it reaches its approximate maximum width. The fixation should take place in at least 1 m distance, this is usually ensured in binocular devices by the optics. With monocular devices, one must ensure that the patient themselves does not accommodate. The difference between 1 and 5 m fixation distance is very small and can be neglected [1].

Stress, anxiety or annoyance cause the pupil to dilate, and in the case of fatigue, the pupil narrows and can fluctuate [2]. If this is the case, give the patient a task that challenges him or her, e.g. starting at 1000 and subtracting 13 again and again. This is usually very effective stabilizing pupil size. Due to feedback in the pupillomotor system, the pupil may oscillate with largest amplitudes at individually varying mesopic light conditions. This is also possible in complete darkness when the person being examined is sleepy. For the sake of safety, it is therefore advisable to measure several times to avoid underestimating pupil size. Pupillography devices have an advantage here, as they record pupil size over a certain time period and thus demonstrate pupil variability.

The most comprehensive data on the age-dependency of pupil size in darkness was collected by Irene Loewenfeld from 1969 to 1972 on 1263 randomly selected subjects [4]. Based on these data, humans have the widest pupils at about 15 years of age with a median value of about 7.2 mm and a maximum width of almost 9 mm. As we age, pupil size decreases by 0.4 mm every 10 years (Fig. 1). This value was confirmed in numerous other smaller collectives. In light conditions, the pupil width decreases with age, although somewhat less than in the dark [7].

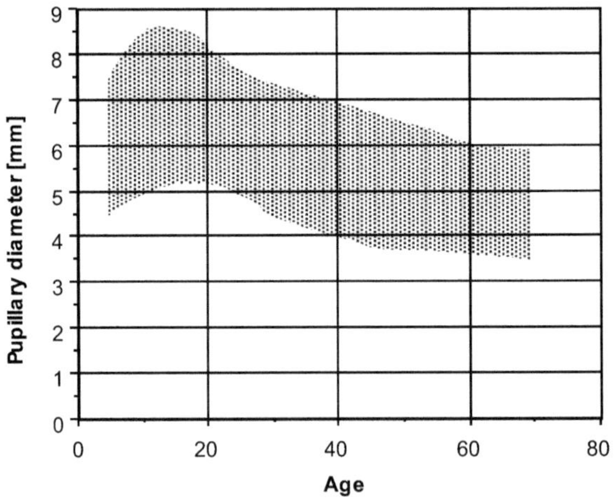

Fig. 1 The figure shows the range of pupil widths measured in this study based on data from Irene Löwenfeld. Beyond the age of 70 there were too few measured values. However, pupil widths over 6.5 mm no longer occurred at this age. A range of pupil sizes of 3 mm is also relatively constant in all age groups. It is therefore difficult to say where an abnormal pupil size begins

Conclusion

To avoid halos and glare, it is important to know the maximum pupil size that can be achieved. When measuring, ideally in the dark with infrared pupillography or photographically, disturbing influences must be controlled.

References

1. Heine C, Yazdani F, Wilhelm H. Pupil width in everyday situations. Klin Monbl Augenheilkd. 2013;230(11):1114–8.
2. Kelbsch C, Strasser T, Chen Y, Feigl B, Gamlin PD, Kardon R, Peters T, Roecklein KA, Steinhauer SR, Szabadi E, Zele AJ, Wilhelm H, Wilhelm BJ. Standards in pupillography. Frontal neurol. 2019;10:129.
3. Kohnen T, Terzi E, Kasper T, Kohnen EM, Buhren J. Correlation of infrared pupillometers and CCD-camera imaging from aberrometry and videokeratography for determining scotopic pupil size. J Cataract Refract Surg. 2004;30(10):2116–23.
4. Loewenfeld IE. The pupil. Anatomy, physiology and clinical applications. Boston, Oxford, Butterworth and Heineman;1999.
5. Rickmann A, Waizel M, Kazerounian S, Szurman P, Wilhelm H, Boden KT. Digital pupillometry in normal subjects. Neuroophthalmology. 2017;41(1):12–8.
6. Wickremasinghe SS, Smith GT, Stevens JD. Comparison of dynamic digital pupillometry and static measurements of pupil size in determining scotopic pupil size before refractive surgery. J Cataract Refract Surg. 2005;31(6):1171–6.
7. Winn B, Whitaker D, Elliott DB, Phillips NJ. Factors affecting light-adapted pupil size in normal human subjects. Invest Ophthalmol Vis Sci. 1994;35(3):1132–7.

Congenital and Childhood Cataract Examination and Indication for Newborns and Children

Günter Rudolph

Causes of congenital and childhood cataract

Congenital and childhood cataract is one of the most common causes of treatable amblyopia or blindness in newborns and children. Various forms of lens opacities can be described, based on phenotypic appearance. Considering the embryonic and foetal development of the lens, the morphology of congenital or infantile cataracts allows conclusions to be drawn about the pathogenesis, though a considerable proportion of congenital cataracts cannot be explained. For example, posterior polar cataract is due to an impaired regression of the tunica vasculosa lentis, while anterior polar cataract is due to insufficient separation of the lens from the surface ectoderm in early pregnancy.

In **bilateral congenital cataract**, various causes can be identified, in particular the hereditary, monogenic forms (autosomal dominant, autosomal recessive, x-linked), as well as cataracts in the context of chromosomal aberrations or syndromes (genetic counselling of parents is recommended due to risk of recurrence). Furthermore, there are metabolic cataracts or lens opacities of infectious origin, e.g. of the TORCH group (toxoplasmosis, rubella, syphilis, parvo B19, cytomegaly, herpes).

Unilateral cataract is associated with early intrauterine eye development and is not typically associated with systemic diseases. It is rather in the context with persistent hyperplastic primary vitreous (PHPV), a persistent hyaloid artery, an impaired regression of the tunica vasculosa of the lens, a microphthalmic or dysgenetic developmental disorder or anterior segment dysgenesis. The differential diagnosis is important when considering the strategy of the surgical procedure.

Another group of congenital and infantile cataracts are **polar cataracts**, which often do not require immediate surgical intervention. They occur unilaterally or bilaterally and have a very heterogeneous appearance. This ranges from minor

G. Rudolph (✉)
Munich, Germany
e-mail: guenther.rudolph@med.uni-muenchen.de

M. Shajari et al. (eds.), *Cataract and Lens Surgery*,
https://doi.org/10.1007/978-3-031-05394-8_21

central opacity with minimal central shading in retinoscopy, to pronounced central opacity, which, despite occlusion treatment of the unaffected or less affected eye, leads to deep amblyopia and is sometimes an indication for surgery even in early infancy.

Examination of the newborn or child

When examining the newborn, it is always advisable to place the baby on an examination pad and, after the application of a topical local anaesthetic, to insert an eyelid retractor to assess the fully opened eye. To do this, the infant is wrapped in a blanket to prevent grasping movements towards the eyelid retractor.The head is stabilised by an assistant using both hands. If desired, a parent can also be present and included in the examination. Firstly, a transillumination-test is carried out using a retinoscope/skiascope, where attention is paid to whether the fundus reflex is moving with or against the direction of light movement. The cataract can be evaluated further using an infrared camera device. This is first carried out in the undilated pupil, then in the dilated pupil followed by funduscopy. Next, the anterior segment of the eye should be inspected with a hand-held slit lamp to categorize the cataract, possible synechiae or other pathological changes (Fig. 1). The diameter of the cornea is then measured. An intraocular pressure measurement can be carried out with a rebound-tonometer by turning the child's head laterally or with Perkins- or Schiötz-tonometry. The dilation of the pupil is then induced with tropicamide eye drops and, if needed, additional phenylephrine hydrochloride 2.5% eye drops. The transillumination test is then repeated and, if there is sufficient fundus reflex, a

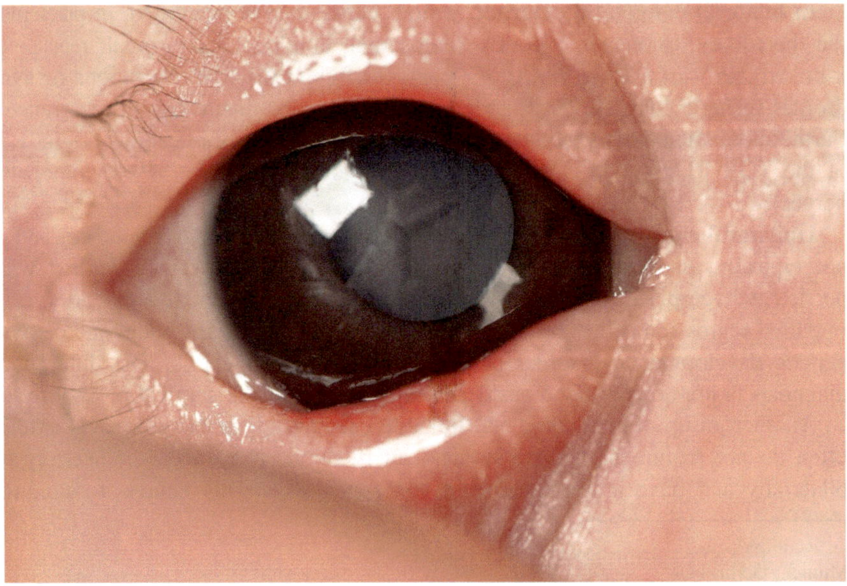

Fig. 1 Congenital dense cataract in Hallermann-Streiff syndrome

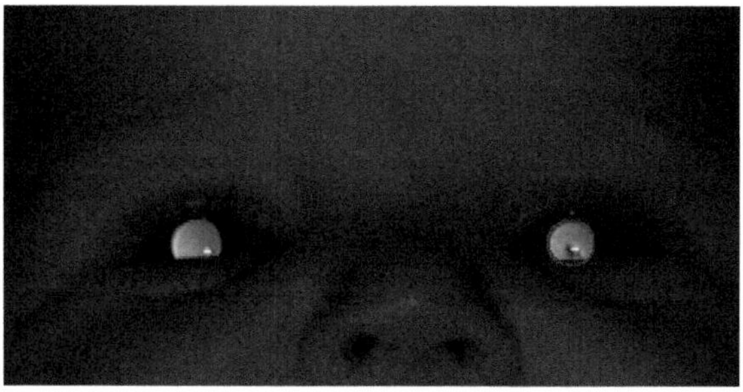

Fig. 2 Posterior polar cataract in the left eye in the infrared image

retinoscopy with refraction is performed. With a larger infant (from 6 months of age), the examination of the eye is preceded by an orthoptic assessment including Brückner's test.

If a dense cataract is present, an additional ultrasound examination is performed to assess the globe status. Preoperatively, keratometry is determined under general anaesthesia and the ultrasound examination is repeated with measurement of the axial length (ultrasound with water-immersion is preferred as it is more accurate). In the case of an implantation of an intraocular lens (IOL), these results are used to calculate the power of the IOL. The axial length also provides information about complications that may be expected later, including the possible occurrence of secondary glaucoma. In older children, IOL-calculation is performed in the same way as in adults (e.g. IOL-Master), but with the corresponding correction factor, taking into account the expected growth of the eye with age (myopic shift).

Author's recommendation

- Photo documentation of relevant anatomical changes
- Attempt to document lens opacities in infrared mode (Fig. 2)

Basis of decision for surgery

The basis for the decision to undergo cataract surgery is the assessment of the shading caused by the opacity of the lens in retinoscopy and the assessment of the lens by transillumination. In older children (from 6 months of age), functional parameters, e.g. the ability of fixation, following movements and fusion, are taken into account as far as possible. When assessing lens opacities with retinoscopy, it is crucial to estimate the reflex in miosis and in mydriasis. A sufficient light-reflex in mydriasis may otherwise lead to overestimation of the developmental potential of visual acuity, although the shading in miosis is too pronounced to allow for sufficient visual development.

Keypoint

The decision for surgery is determined by retinoscopy and transillumination of the lens, both in the undilatet and dilatet pupil.

Timing of surgery

Congenital cataract leads to immediate deprivation of the visual system and is therefore a significant risk factor for the development of deep amblyopia and even blindness. This deprivation can be expressed by the appearance of nystagmus (possible from 10–12 weeks of age) and secondary strabismus. This would suggest to opt for surgery as soon as possible [2, 4, 5]. However, it is also known, that with earlier operation there is higher risk of aphakic glaucoma. These risk factors must therefore always be weighed up against each other [1]. In unilateral cataract, which usually has a significantly lower visual prognosis than bilateral cataract (unilateral deprivation and often additional unfavourable anatomical conditions), the earliest possible time for surgery is usually around the 5th–6th week of life. In the case of bilateral cataract, there is no clear consensus on the optimal time for surgery. Studies have shown that children operated on in the 8th–10th week of life had a similar prevalence of amblyopia as those who had surgery between week 10–12 after birth. However, the children operated on earlier had a lower rate of secondary strabismus compared to the children having surgery later [3]. Surgery should definitely be performed before the manifestation of nystagmus, which will remain even after optical rehabilitation.

Author's recommendation

In unilateral cataract, surgery should be performed in the 5th–6th week of life and in the 8th–10th week of life in newborns with bilateral cataract.

Postoperative follow-up examination and care

The most frequent complications after cataract surgery in infants and children are the postoperative opacifications in the optical axis and secondary glaucoma. The former is usually caused by lens epithelial cells that proliferate along existing anatomical structures. This means that attention must be paid to prevent the retention of lens epithelial cells for proliferation. Visual axis obscuration is expected to occur with significant probability in the aphakic as well as pseudophakic eye. However, with IOL-implantation using an "optic capture" or bag-in-the-lens technique (BIL-IOL), this complication can be reduced according to the data currently available [6, 7].

Aphakic glaucoma requires regular follow-up examinations with slit-lamp examination, measurement of the intraocular pressure and during the first years of life measurements of the axial growth and length of the eye. The development of the axial length of the eye is an important diagnostic component, especially in infancy, and provides important information regarding the presence of raised intraocular pressure. The importance of the surgeon's expertise in avoiding secondary complications and with regard to the visual prognosis in infants and children with congenital or infantile cataracts cannot be emphasised enough. Essential components of post-operative care are, in addition to the recognition in time and treatment of secondary complications, refractive correction and treatment of amblyopia. In case of aphakia in newborns, the fitting of contact lenses for distant vision but also the correction for reading distance, using bifocal glasses, is important.

It requires many years of intensive cooperation between child, parents, pediatric ophthalmologist, optician and orthoptist to achieve the best possible visual result.

References

1. Beck AD, Freedman SF, Lynn MJ, Bothun E, Neely DE, Lambert SR. Glaucoma-related adverse events in the Infant Aphakia Treatment Study: 1-year results. Arch Ophthalmol. 2012;130(3):300–5. https://doi.org/10.1001/archophthalmol.2011.347.
2. Birch EE, Cheng C, Stager DR Jr, Weakley DR Jr, Stager DR Sr. The critical period for surgical treatment of dense congenital bilateral cataracts. J AAPOS. 2009;13(1):67–71. https://doi.org/10.1016/j.jaapos.2008.07.010.
3. Kuhli-Hattenbach C, Fronius M, Kohnen T. Impact of timing of surgery on outcome in children with bilateral congenital cataract. Ophthalmologe. 2017;114(3):252–8. https://doi.org/10.1007/s00347-016-0326-5.
4. Lagreze WA. The management of cataract in childhood. Klin Monbl Augenheilkd. 2009;226(1):15–21. https://doi.org/10.1055/s-2008-1027946.
5. Lambert SR. The timing of surgery for congenital cataracts: minimizing the risk of glaucoma following cataract surgery while optimizing the visual outcome. J AAPOS. 2016;20(3):191–2. https://doi.org/10.1016/j.jaapos.2016.04.003.
6. Plager DA, Lynn MJ, Buckley EG, Wilson ME, Lambert SR. Complications in the first 5 years following cataract surgery in infants with and without intraocular lens implantation in the Infant Aphakia Treatment Study. Am J Ophthalmol. 2014;158(5):892–8. https://doi.org/10.1016/j.ajo.2014.07.031.
7. Tassignon MJ, De Veuster I, Godts D, Kosec D, Van den Dooren K, Gobin L. Bag-in-the-lens intraocular lens implantation in the pediatric eye. J Cataract Refract Surg. 2007;33(4):611–7. https://doi.org/10.1016/j.jcrs.2006.12.016.

Anaesthesia for Cataract Surgery

Friedrich Lersch and Tom Eke

Introduction

For many types of surgery, the technique of anaesthesia could potentially influence the final outcome, and patient satisfaction. Cataract surgery is no exception. While the surgeon's preferences and cultural factors play an important role in the choice of anaesthesia, the greatest care should be given to customize the safest, anxiety-free —and pain-free surgical experience for the patient. This chapter stresses the need to consider a balance of safety (anaesthetic & surgical complications) and the team approach providing surgical safety and patient satisfaction. Nowadays it's not enough to have uncomplicated surgery but patients have rightly come to expect that they should have a good experience of the whole procedure.

Topics covered:

- Patient preparation & information
- Anxiolytic communication with the patient on surgery day
- Pharmacological sedation, analgesia & anxiolysis
- Topical and locoregional anaesthesia techniques
- Aims of general anaesthesia in cataract surgery.

Supplementary Information The online version contains supplementary material available at https://doi.org/10.1007/978-3-031-05394-8_22. The videos can be accessed individually by clicking the DOI link in the accompanying figure caption or by scanning this link with the SN More Media App.

F. Lersch (✉)
Bern, Switzerland
e-mail: friedrich.lersch@insel.ch

T. Eke
Norwich, United Kingdom
e-mail: tom.eke@nnuh.nhs.uk

M. Shajari et al. (eds.), *Cataract and Lens Surgery*,
https://doi.org/10.1007/978-3-031-05394-8_22

Table 1 Summary of the main anaesthetic agents used for topical and local ('block') anaesthesia in eye surgery

Topical	Ester/Amid	Pain on application	Duration	Corneal toxicity	Onset time
Tetracaine 0.5–1%	Ester	++	Intermediate	++	
Oxybuprocaine 0.4%	Ester	±	Short	±	2 min
Lidocaine	Amid	++	Intermediate	+	5 min
Proxymetacaine	Ester	±	15 min	+−	20-30 s
Proparacaine					
Local (=Block)	Ester/Amid	Onset	Duration	Myotoxicity	Potential cardiotoxicity
Lidocaine 2%	Amide	3 min	60–120 min	±	±
Bupivacaine 0.5%	Amide	5 min	>/=2 h	+++	++
Ropivacaine 0.5–1%	Amide		>/=2 h	±	±
Articaine 4%	Amide +Ester	3–4 min			
Mepicavaine 1–3%	Amide		1.5 h	+	
Levobupivacaine 0.75%	Amide		>5 h	+	++
Prilocaine					

A wide array of anaesthetic techniques may be needed for cataract patients. Options range from topical anaesthesia (TA) to locoregional anaesthesia (LA), sedation and general anaesthesia (GA) [1] (Table 1). These techniques can be combined with each other and with pharmacological techniques of anxiolysis, analgesia and sedation.

In the United Kingdom (UK), national guidelines have long recommended that either TA or LA should be the "default" technique for cataract surgery, and in 2017 NICE [2] stated that sharp-needle LA should only be used if less invasive techniques are contra-indicated. At the time of writing, needle LA is still in regular use in many countries.

Patient preparation & information

An important factor in patient anxiety and satisfaction is the information and guidance received during pre-operative counselling [2]. Research data is not unanimous whether better information really decreases anxiety [4], but it is felt that better pre-operative explanation and counselling will minimise the need for anxiolytic/analgesic interventions. As information provided in pre-surgery clinics is rarely absorbed to a sufficient extent, leaflets or online informational videos might be an effective way to familiarize patients with the surgery situation. The majority of eye clinics have little experience in putting electronic information at the patients disposal. Most publicly accessible videos on cataract surgery come with commercial bias [5] and have not been objectively evaluated.

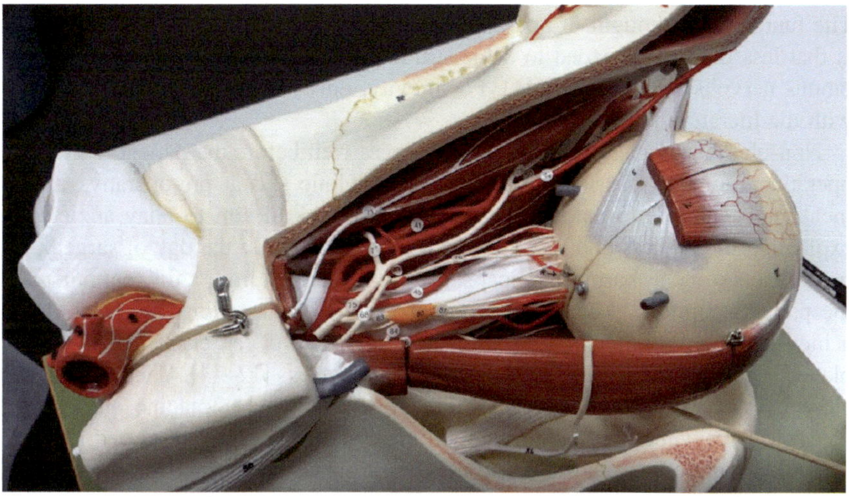

Video 1 Techniques for Anesthesia (▶ https://doi.org/10.1007/000-8d5)

While topical anaesthesia (TA) is sufficient for the vast majority of cataract patients, clinicians should be sensitive to increased needs in specific patients groups like chronic pain patients, or otherwise traumatized patients [6]. Some studies have suggested that (somewhat surprisingly), cataract surgery on the second eye is sometimes perceived to be more painful [7].

Fasting emerges as an unnecessary stressor in elderly patients. The UK national guideline [8] states that pre-operative fasting is unnecessary for patients who have LA without sedation. A 2019 French observational study showed that low-dose propofol sedation in non-fasted cataract surgery patients appeared to be safe [9]. Fluid restriction longer than 6 h constitutes an independent cause for postoperative delirium [10]. Systemic and ocular comorbidities have to be accounted for in a premedication clinic and patients should continue taking their regular medication-especially antihypertensive and anti-diabetic drugs.

Before discussing particular anaesthetic techniques individually, it needs to be pointed out that all components of the "anaesthetic toolbox"—ranging from handholding, topical and locoregional anaesthesia as well as sedation—can be combined by a well-informed surgical-anaesthetic team to provide "tailor-made" care for each patient. A certain degree of on-the-spot-improvisation based on ongoing communication can elevate rote procedure to a swift and elegant endeavour and epitomizes the qualities of "personal medicine". Including an "upgrade"-analgesia in very anxious patients, those with chronic pain or eyes likely to prove more problematic than anticipated often pays. It is important that a "safety net" strategy is defined in the team, should efforts at topical anaesthesia not be successful.

Non-pharmacological calming techniques

The fundamental thought of non-pharmacological interventions to counter anxiety is that less drugs are needed to achieve tranquillity, ensuing less stress on autonomous nervous system level [11]. For brevity, only sketchy information is given with the literature in question cited.

Non-pharmacological anxiolysis commences well before the patient reaches the operating room. Discussions in the outpatient clinic and at pre-operative assessment, and patient information leaflets/videos should all aim to allay anxiety, by explaining the process and risk-management strategies. On the day of surgery, the basic tenets of non-pharmacological sedation are derived from a diligent pursuit of the patients comfort: positioning avoiding discomfort, warming etc. Once this is achieved in a caring manner, distractive communication can ensue. Music can be played with the explained goal of soothing nervousness [12–14]. Cues are given to close eyes, keep a slow and steady breathing and maybe imagine oneself in a pleasant place while any monitoring and intravenous (iv)-line are placed [15, 16].

Children are offered music, small movies or games on a tablet held by a parent, especially to distract from iv-placement [17, 18]. Parents are left to remain with their child as soothing support until anaesthesia is successfully induced [19, 20]. Once the line is placed, the patient is given the choice to have iv-sedation, explaining that it can be administered at any time the need is felt. Handholding is offered and movement of the hand explained to be the means of communicating discomfort. Having a person to hold on to during surgery increases patient-satisfaction without reducing pain-ratings per se [21].

Pharmacological sedation in the anteroom

Most cataract patients will not need any sedative medication at all. For those who do need sedation or GA, it is preferable for the patient to be calm during surgery and also during emergence. In the majority of adult patients, topical anaesthesia together with non-pharmacological calming communication is sufficient. But upholding the offer of sedation being available at the patient's request is important. In very anxious patients a combination of several drugs in small boluses should reduce the risk of accumulating one particular drug beyond its therapeutic window. In this multimodal way, phases of apnea or delirious behaviour in disinhibited elderly patients can be avoided. Sedative drugs like propofol can provoke short bouts of disinhibition with incoherent speech or sudden movements. It is important to go through this phase in the anteroom, not when the patient is being draped. Different levels of sedation depth should be cautiously applied bearing in mind the food intake of the last hours [22].

Benzodiazepines

Given price and efficacy, Midazolam in sublingual form or in small boluses remains one of the pharmacological classes most often administrated. It provides fast-onset tranquillity with it's effects waning off reasonably fast. Many elderly patients use benzodiazepines chronically and are liable to react in unpredictable manner to sedation. Benzodiazepine use in children sometimes provoke paradoxical reactions and prolonged hang-over after GA. In elderly patients, there is increasing data reporting benzodiazepines as an agent provoking delirium in a sedative cocktail, so more scrutiny may be warranted [23]. Midazolam is currently marketed in the USA in sublingual troches together with ketamine and omeprazole to provide entirely oral sedation in cataract surgery and the claim to forego the necessity of iv-lines altogether [24]. These claims still have to stand up to unbiased trials.

Propofol

With it's swift and subjectively pleasant sedative action, low incidence of hang-over and anti-nausea effects, propofol is unparalleled as a bolus-drug. Combined with small boluses of iv lidocaine even the stinging on injection can be curbed and effect titrated by small boluses. Elderly patients often have a fast transition from claiming no subjective effect, to deep sedation with uncoordinated movements or speech. Finding out the deep-sedation threshold in the anaesthesia room before draping in operation theatre is wise. Propofol can easily be combined with dexmedethomidine, clonidine or opioids for deeper relaxation and analgesia, especially while a block is being administered. Paradoxical reactions have been reported, especially in heavy drinkers. Explaining to the patient that the drug's effect is pleasant but that ideal level of sedation is "not-anxious, cooperative, awake" helps to correct false expectations on the patients side and curbs the tendency to overdose. Long fasting does not seem to be required in light propofol sedation [9]. Increased incidence of sneezing during peri/retrobulbar blocks application has been observed under propofol sedation [25].

Opioids

Historically, opioids constitute the mainstay of analgesia and anxiolysis in monitored anaesthesia care (MAC) and they have an important role especially in the administration of regional anaesthesia alleviating "block-pain". While anaesthesia providers are intimately familiar with the immediate action of iv drugs like fentanyl, alfentanyl and remifentanil and often combine them successfully together with hypnotic drugs like benzodiazepines and propofol, a word of caution is needed. Repeated doses of opioids increase the risk of accumulation, and apnea-phases under surgical drapes due to closure of the airway or central opioid effect. Opioid-induced analgesia often comes at the price of nausea, vomiting, brain-fog and depressive moods after emergence from sedation and GA [26] Should longer need for analgesia be foreseen (i.e. in chronic pain patients, combined procedures) a long lasting locoregional anaesthesia should be considered as a valid substitute for more opioids.

Ketamine

A strong analgesia drug with dissociative and hallucinogenic properties, ketamine needs to be used with caution and in combination with GABAergic or alpha-agonistic drugs. The subjective patient situation ideally has to be tranquil before ketamine is administrated lest it provoke nightmares extending from the anxiety-inducing clinical situation. As an oral premedication drug it can be given to children with a small quantity of sweet-tasting syrup, ideally together with a benzodiazepine or an alpha-agonist like dexmedetomidine or clonidine. While ketamine use has seen a renaissance in "opioid-free" or "opioid-sparing anaesthesia" regimens, the anaesthesia team providing such care should be outspoken about the "deeper" character of sedation and the possibility of "colourful dreams". The need to secure the airway may arise from the sheer intensity of anaesthesia combinations like propofol-ketamine, even if spontaneous respiration can be upheld. Increased salivation is a frequently observed side-effect and can be countered by glycopyrrolate administration. Especially in combination with alpha-agonists and or propofol, ketamine does NOT increase intraocular pressure [27].

New combined oral lozenges of midazolam, ketamine and omeprazole ("MKO-troches") are currently being evaluated as sedation technique (as a replacement for intravenous cannulation) [24], but further research is needed on this topic.

Alpha-agonists

Both clonidine and dexmedetomidine have been successfully used in sedation for their sedative and co-analgesic properties. They produce a state considered physiologically most akin to NREM-sleep [28] and are proven to be a pharmacological component in anaesthesia-combinations safeguarding against emergence-delirium/post-operative delirium in children and elderly patients [29]. Both drugs can be administered intra-nasally as premedication in children. Although the same administration route has been shown to be effectively sedative in adults, significant hypotension complicated the use in elderly patients [30]. With iv use, one should aim for only light sedation, because deep sleep may produce startling to wakefulness. Patients arriving hypertensive should receive a propofol bolus before receiving 0.1–0.2 ug/kg as the initial effect of dexmedetomidine accentuates hypertension. Higher doses of dexmedetomidine (1 ug/kg bolus/10 min and continuous infusion resulted in higher patients satisfaction as midazolam, but higher rates of bradycardia, hypotension and delayed recovery room discharge [31].

Other sedation techniques:

Historically, **neuroleptic** drugs like droperidol were combined with opioids or locoregional anaesthesia to good sedative success. Given their anticholinergic potential of inducing cognitive side-effects, hallucinations and anxiety, these drugs are no longer used in elderly and Parkinson's patients.

Another new approach, maybe more in tune with cataract surgery's objective of cognitive improvement in the elderly, is the use of **melatonin** as premedication [32]. Sublingual or oral melatonin has a co-analgetic and anxiolytic effect and provides good surgical sedation in cataract surgery. In comparison to placebo, melatonin fared significantly better, while when compared to midazolam, comparable anxiolysis was achieved with significantly less cognitive side-effects [33]. Melatonin was also effective in another study compared with gabapentin and placebo [34]. Of note, doses used in the two cited studies differed widely and melatonin effectivity as anxiolytic in elderly patients is debated. The antiepileptic drugs **gabapentin** and **pregabalin** outline an interesting premedication perspective: apart from assuring anxiolysis and sedation without cognitive dysfunction like midazolam, both drugs consistently led to reduction of opioid-based postoperative analgesia being used. This trajectory may seem irrelevant for the uncomplicated phaco/IOL-patient, but may likewise be of consequence in combined surgery cases on patients suffering from chronic pain, substance abuse etc. [34, 35].

At surgical time-out, the caring anaesthesia person should be invited to voice concern over anxiety levels and the level of pharmacological sedation already administered to the patient during time-out. Switching to locoregional anaesthesia and deeper sedation or GA at this point needs to be a team decision.

General anaesthesia (GA)

GA is costly, and, and makes the presence of an anaesthesia team necessary during the whole case. Often induction and emergence in difficult cases take longer time than the surgical procedure itself, slowing progress of surgical lists. Nevertheless, it offers a nearly perfect surgical site for patients unable to cooperate while awake, even under sedation and regional anaesthesia. These are in most situations children, very anxious patients, patients with extreme claustrophobia or movement disorders and elderly patients with dementia prone to move and become agitated under sedation. The choice again is a team-responsibility [36].

GA should provide smooth induction and emergence and should aim at low nausea and delirium potential after surgery. Endotracheal intubation is a must where risk of aspiration is present but generally a laryngeal mask is the airway of choice for a cataract procedure. It allows to keep retching and coughing against the tube at a minimum. Endotracheal tubes demand "deeper" anaesthesia and the use of opioids to keep brainstem reflexes at bay. At least in part, such "deep" anaesthesia seems to be at the heart of post-operative delirium in the elderly [37]. Opting for an opioid-sparing anaesthesia regime along the lines of the Multimodal Anaesthesia concept might pay off in elderly patients [38]. With patients under GA, analgesia can safely be obtained by adding a topical/intracameral anesthesia, or sub-Tenon's block (STB) [39, 40]. This provides good postoperative analgesia, anti-nausea effects and safeguards against pain or opioid induced emergence delirium in children and elderly alike. This combination holds promise to reduce postoperative vomiting and cognitive dysfunction [41, 42]. It also helps to prevent oculo-cardiac reflex by interrupting the trigemino-parasympathetic reflex arc.

GA can be induced and maintained by either propofol or sevoflurane, while analgesia should be provided by adding topical drops, a locoregional block or systemically by opioids or ketamine. Adding dexmedetomidine as a slow low-dose bolus before induction provides an additional analgetic agent and smooth emergence. In elderly and children in case of bradycardia, atropine should be regarded as a delirogenic drug reserved for life-saving resuscitation. Glycopyrrolate can usually achieve the same hemodynamic effect without causing anticholinergic effects in the brain and tipping the balance toward postoperative delirium [43, 44]. Even atropine-eyedrops have been described as provoking delirium in the elderly [45] after cataract surgery.

Topical and locoregional anaesthesia

Local anaesthetic drugs can be chosen either from the ester or the amide group according to preferred characteristics for topical and injected locoregional anaesthesia. For detailed information on pharmacology please consult ophthalmic anaesthesia textbooks. Important characteristics of LA-drugs used topically and in blocks relate to structure, ionization and acidity, lipid solubility, protein-binding and metabolism. Only those aspects deemed most practically important are outlined here. Cocaine is not discussed as it is too fraught with pharmacological complications and regulative burden.

Especially in topical anaesthesia, irritation of the eye on application and toxicity to the and ocular corneal epithelium on repeated application are of concern. Corneal oedema will impair surgeon's view of intraocular structures, causing surgical difficulty, and can cause post-operative pain from epithelial erosions. Oxybuprocaine, an ester-local anaesthetic, gives little discomfort on application, has fast-onset and short duration, and can be used prior to sub-Tenon's block: by contrast, the amide tetracaine combines higher application discomfort with longer duration, but higher corneal toxicity. In locoregional anesthesia, onset and duration as well as myotoxicity matter [46, 47]. Not rarely, patient's allergies to a particular agent make changing to an alternative necessary, this applies mostly to ester local anaesthetics as these are metabolized by cholinesterase to PABA (p-amino-benzoic acid). Should sharp-needle blocks be applied, the rare but potentially grave systemic (cardiac, cerebral) toxicity on inadvertent vascular injection should be kept in mind [48]. Topical eye-drops preserve the eye in all its mobility, making this anaesthesia modality a choice for experienced surgeons. A newer trend in topical analgesia is the application of nonsteroidal anti-inflammatory drugs (NSAIDs) [49]. The reduction in nociception seems to correlate with diminished prostaglandin secretion.

As for needle and cannula based blocks, anatomical landmarks are being used for orientation by the vast majority of practitioners. The last decades saw more efforts of aligning especially sharp needle blocks with an ultrasound overview of the deep anatomy [50]. The basic two approaches are pre-screening of the eye for potentially problematic varieties (staphylomata, elongation) and informed but "blind" puncture or real-time ultrasound visualisation of anatomic structures and needles. Ultrasound research in some ways reiterated the importance of local anaesthetic to diffuse into the retrobulbar compartment to achieve satisfactory levels of the clinical endpoints analgesia and akinesia [51]. This is achieved by STB, peribulbar block (PBB) and retrobulbar block (RBB), and the functional precondition of supressing neuronal transmission in sensible and motor nerves to the eye [52]. Life-and sight-threatening complications, diplopia and retinal artery occlusion have been reported [53] for all methods. Injected volumes should always be adapted to systemic blood pressure (i.e. ocular perfusion pressure) [54].

Intracameral anaesthesia (see Fig. 1)

Topical analgesia can be improved in quality by injecting preservative free lidocaine. A commercially available combination of lidocaine 1% with low-dose tropicamide and phenylephrine (Mydrane®), can be used for mydriasis and analgesia. Combinations of viscoelastic and lidocaine are also available (e.g. Visthesia). Contrary to former concerns, intracameral lidocaine does not harm corneal endothelium [55].

Subconjunctival injection (see Fig. 1)

Sub-conjunctival anaesthetic injection will also anaesthetise the underlying sclera, making the technique useful for glaucoma surgery and scleral-tunnel phacoemulsification. Given sufficient time, the anaesthetic can reach the ciliary body, meaning that the technique can be useful for cyclodestructive procedures such as diode laser.

Retrobulbar block (RBB) (see Fig. 1)

After the shortlived initial success of injecting cocaine behind the eye [56], RBB became the standard locoregional anaesthesia in the 1930s due to Atkinson's work and a series of improved local anaesthetics being synthesized. In a time when

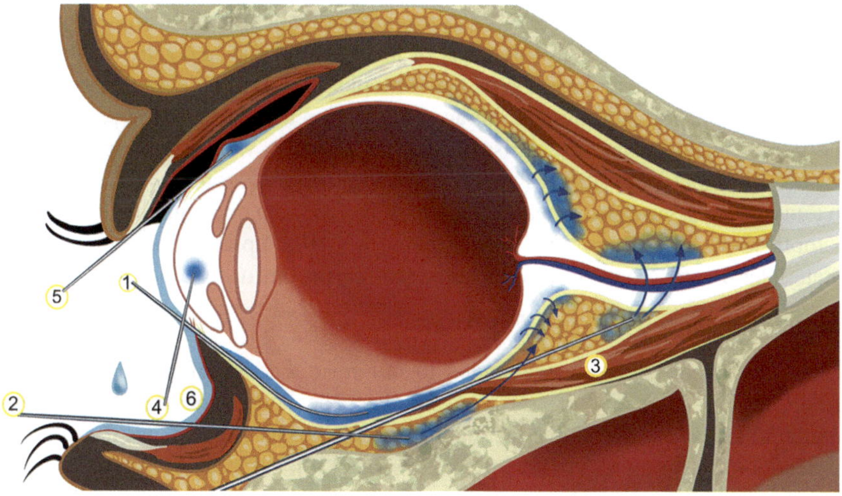

Fig. 1 Schematic representation of topical and locoregional ophthalmic anaesthesia techniques; The invasive techniques (STB, PBB, RBB) all lead to LA reaching the intra-conal area behind the globe, where sensory and motor nerves (not depicted) converge. Dense blood vessels behind the eye are not depicted. Blue color signifies topical and regional deposits of local anaesthetic. (1) sub-Tenon's block (STB); (2) peribulbar Block (PBB); (3) retro-bulbar block (RBB; note proximity of needle to globe and optic nerve); (4) intracameral LA-injection; (5) sub-conjunctival injection; (6) topical LA on cornea and conjunctiva. Arrows indicate dynamics of flow

cataract surgery was characterized by long hospital stays, anaesthesia mortality and complication, RBB was an elegant solution to a pervasive problem. Nowadays, with cataract surgery having undergone the revolutionary changes to minimal invasiveness, RBB's rare but potentially grave complications—bulbar perforation, intra-orbital bleeding, brainstem anaesthesia—make it appear more like a problem than a solution. This is reflected in the UK national guidelines [2] and also 2012 LA guideline [8], both of which advise against using RBB in cataract surgery. Because RBB is no longer recommended for cataract surgery, the technique will not be discussed in detail.

Historically, RBB was is effected by introducing a sharp or blunt straight needle through the lower eyelid or conjunctiva at the transition of the middle to the outer third of the orbital rim, aiming at the orbital floor. After having made contact with this bony structure, the needle's direction is changed upward and inward bringing the needle's tip behind the eye bulb and depositing 3–6 ml of local anaesthetic inside the conus being formed by the retroocular muscles. This brings LA into contact with sensory and motor nerves residing in the adipose body. This intraconal deposition was taken to be the hallmark of successful blockade [57] notwithstanding the fact that Ripart [58] had demonstrated-based on Koornneef's work [59]-that anatomical substrate for an intraconal compartment is non-existent. Going intraconal may be responsible for the excellent akinesia of RBBs given the deposition of LA close to the eye's motor nerves. But it may also be responsible for a less than perfect analgesia and often leaves the patient with an urge and motor capability to blink. Historically, facial nerve blocks were the answer to blepharospasm, leaving the eyelids paralyzed but the patient still feeling the urge to blink. Moreover, inadvertent injections of local anaesthetic into retro-orbital muscles leave them paralyzed and the patient diplopic, necessitating a second surgery in the worst case [60]. Adding risk, intraconal injection also has greatest proximity to the dense and tortuous vascularisation of the orbita as well as the optic nerve's sheath. Both these can serve as access ways for central nervous system anaesthetic toxicity causing seizures, apnea, hemiparesis, bradycardia or a combination of these complications [61]. Intraorbital bleeding and it's build-up of pressure may necessitate lateral canthotomy to provide sufficient perfusion for the eye [62].

Peribulbar block (PBB) (see Fig. 1)

This sharp-needle block was intended to minimise the risk of retrobulbar anaesthesia, though in reality the risks are similar. The effectiveness of PBB is also similar to RBB, illustrating the fact that no anatomical barrier impedes the diffusion of extraconal LA-deposits to the intraconal space [58]. PBB can be administrated in the classical 2-injection method, where the first injection is made at the RBB injection site and the second medially at the caruncle. Supero-nasal injections should be avoided (or more laterally), because of the risk of vascular injection and globe perforation. Modern PBB-application prefers to limit itself to one injection, trying to safeguard against perforating and injecting into the eyeball with the second bolus after the eye has been moved out of it's position by the first injection. Greater volumes of LA (8–10 ml) may be necessary and chemosis is not rare. All of the rare but significant complications of RBBs have been described for PBB and discussion about a lower frequency of them in PBB is ongoing [63].

It must be pointed out that both RBB and PBB are historically undertaken in the quadrant, which also has the highest probability of posterior staphylomata presence [64]. Thus the "traditional" infero-temporal injection is more likely to cause globe perforation, particularly in large myopic eyes. A single medial PBB injection appears to be less likely to cause sight-threatening complications [65].

Sub-Tenon's Block (STB) (see Fig. 1)

Sub-Tenon's block uses a blunt cannula to place the anaesthetic behind the globe. The intention is to have all of the benefits of sharp-needle LA (RBB,PBB) while minimising the risk of trauma to the globe, optic nerve or orbital structures [66]. It is performed by making a small incision in the double-layer of bulbar conjunctiva and Tenon's fascia in the intranasal quadrant. A blunt cannula is then slid backwards on the scleral surface into sub-Tenon's space and local anaesthetic slowly injected. Variations on the standard technique include using a pencil-point probe instead of scissors to open the conjunctiva/Tenon's, or the cannula can be passed directly to the sub-Tenon's space, using a "no-snip-technique". Various types of blunt-ended sub-Tenon cannulae (short plastic or longer metal cannula) exist. Some inject the sub-Tenon's using a needle, though this will of course increase the risk of a globe perforation. In recent surveys, STB has been the most commonly used anaesthesia modality for cataract surgery in the UK and several other countries. The technique recommends itself through an unparalleled analgesia combined to an outstanding safety profile in comparison to sharp-needle blocks [67]. STB is an intraconal block by way of transfusion, as testified by the "T-sign" visible on ultrasound examination after injection [52, 68] (see Figs. 1 & 2). Akinesia is usually achieved to a satisfactory degree, albeit with some minutes delay compared to RBB. This seeming disadvantage should be seen in balance with a much lower incidence of diplopia [60] and other sight-or life threatening complications.

Surgical factors

While akinesia of the eye is a factor often discussed in cataract surgery it needs to be seen in relation to skill and experience of the surgeon. Many trainee surgeons may prefer an akinetic local anaesthesia (sub-Tenon's, peribulbar), as this may be considered wise to facilitate surgical conditions and minimise the risk of surgical complications. However, this is a controversial area [69], as many trainers and trainees prefer topical/intracameral anaesthesia. Rarely, a patient may become unable to cope with the level of anaesthesia, so the team should be prepared to increase the level of anaesthesia if required: for example, topical/intracameral anaesthesia may need to be "topped up" to STB, or STB augmented with intravenous sedation.

Post-operative pain and management strategies

Postoperative pain afflicts a third of cataract surgery patients during the first hours after operation and relents over a short time period. Aching pain can usually be

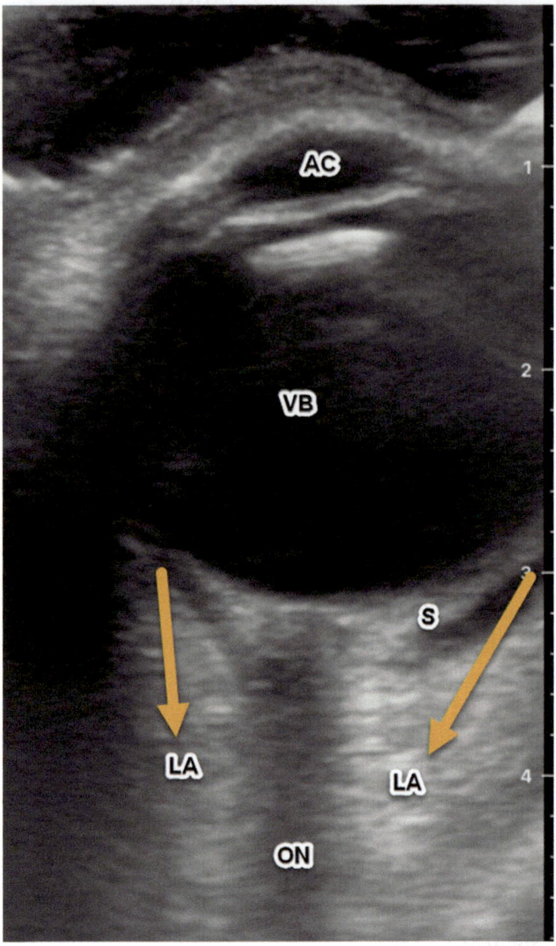

Fig. 2 T-sign after sub-Tenon's block; around 7 min after injection, LA-deposit (LA) diffuses from episcleral space (S) into the intraconal, retrobulbar space, increasing optic nerve (ON)-visibility forming a "T-sign"; VB = vitreous body; AC = anterior chamber

managed by simple analgesia using ibuprofen and paracetamol [70]. Persistent or worsening ache should trigger an urgent assessment to look for elevated intraocular pressure, inflammation or even endophthalmitis. These specific problems should be treated (e.g with anti-inflammatories, cycloplegics, ocular hypotensives and/or other medications), as appropriate. Quite often this discomfort presents as "foreign-body sensation" or dry eyes, therefore ocular lubricants (artificial tears or ointment) may be helpful. Myopia, operation on the second eye and dominance of the operated eye seem to predispose to postoperative pain [71]. Previous chronic, non-ocular pain also seems to increase the risk of dry-eye-like symptoms after cataract surgery [72].

Reduced vision and postoperative eye-patching constitute inherently hallucinogenic situations (Charles-Bonnet-syndrome) and these usually well tolerated hallucinations of the elderly can take on malign, delirious character [73]. Being in the company of loved ones and returning home as early as possible are important in cognitively frail patients [74].

Conclusion

Every cataract surgery patient needs to be treated as individual with individual anxiety and pain-thresholds. Furthermore, reducing anxiety starts with improved information and making sure that the content of pre-op discussions is retained and accessible beyond pre-op discussions. A safe, efficient and calm clinical environment, catering to the needs especially of pediatric and old patients needs to blend in with an anaesthesia strategy tailor-made to the patient at hand. A wide variety of anxiolytic, analgesic and sedative techniques along with topical or locoregional techniques are at the disposition of the anaesthetic/surgical team. A back-up anaesthesia plan should be agreed upon between the clinicians involved.

References

1. Hussain N, et al. Local anaesthetic-induced myotoxicity in regional anaesthesia: a systemic review and empirical analysis, BJA. 2018; 121(4):822–841. https://doi.org/10.1016/j.bja.2018.05.076
2. National Institute for Health and Care Excellence. Cataracts in adults: management NICE Guideline [NG77]. NICE Guid. 2017.
3. Elder MJ, Suter A. What patients want to know before they have cataract surgery. Br J Ophthalmol 2004.
4. Tipotsch-Maca SM, Varsits RM, Ginzel C, Vecsei-Marlovits P V. Effect of a multimedia-assisted informed consent procedure on the information gain, satisfaction, and anxiety of cataract surgery patients. J Cataract Refract Surg. 2016.
5. Bae SS, Baxter S. YouTube videos in the English language as a patient education resource for cataract surgery. Int Ophthalmol. 2018.
6. Rapoport Y, Wayman LL, Chomsky AS. The effect of post-traumatic-stress-disorder on intra-operative analgesia in a veteran population during cataract procedures carried out using retrobulbar or topical anesthesia: a retrospective study. BMC Ophthalmol. 2017; 17.
7. Ursea R, Feng MT, Zhou M, Lien V, Loeb R. Pain perception in sequential cataract surgery: Comparison of first and second procedures. J Cataract Refract Surg. 2011; 37.
8. Kumar CM, Eke T, Dodds C, et al. Local anaesthesia for ophthalmic surgery - new guidelines from the Royal College of Anaesthetists and the Royal College of Ophthalmologists. Eye. 2012.
9. Guerrier G, Rothschild PR, Bonnet C, Monnet D, Baillard C. Safety of low-dose propofol in non-fasted patients undergoing cataract surgery: a prospective cohort study. Br J Anaesth (Elsevier Ltd). 2019:e526–8.
10. Radtke FM, Franck M, MacGuill M, et al. Duration of fluid fasting and choice of analgesic are modifiable factors for early postoperative delirium. Eur J Anaesthesiol. 2010;27:411–6.
11. Bertelmann T, Strempel I. Self-relaxation techniques for glaucoma patients: significance of autogenic training, hypnosis and music therapy. Der Ophthalmol. 2016; 113.
12. Guerrier G, Abdoul H, Jilet L, et al. Musical intervention reduces anxiety-related hypertensive events during cataract surgery: a randomized controlled trial. Perioper Care Oper Room Manag. 2020; 20.
13. Cruise CJ, Chung F, Yogendran S, Little D. Music increases satisfaction in elderly outpatients undergoing cataract surgery. Can J Anaesth. 1997; 44.
14. Lunde SJ, et al. Music-induced analgesia: how does music relieve pain? Pain. 2019; 160(5); 989–93. https://doi.org/10.1097/j.pain.0000000000001452.

15. Agard E, Pernod C, El Chehab H, Russo A, Haxaire M, Dot C. A role for hypnosis in cataract surgery: report of 171 procedures. J Fr Ophtalmol. 2016; 39.
16. Chen X, Yuan R, Chen X, et al. Hypnosis intervention for the management of pain perception during cataract surgery. J Pain Res. 2018; 11.
17. De Queiroz Siqueira M, Tosseti S, Marechal C, Cogniat B, Berthilier J, Chassard D. Effect of Ipad tablet on children and parental anxiety during anesthesia. Anesth Analg. 2016; 123(3 Sup).
18. McQueen A, Cress C, Tothy A. Using a tablet computer during pediatric procedures. Pediatr Emerg Care. 2012; 28.
19. Chundamala J, Wright JG, Kemp SM. An evidence-based review of parental presence during anesthesia induction and parent/child anxiety. Can. J. Anesth. 2009.
20. Bailey KM, Bird SJ, McGrath PJ, Chorney JE. Preparing parents to be present for their child's anesthesia induction: a randomized controlled trial. Anesth Analg. 2015; 121.
21. Modi N, Shaw S, Allman K, Simcock P. Local anaesthetic cataract surgery: factors influencing perception of pain, anxiety and overall satisfaction. J Perioper Pract. 2008; 18.
22. M. L, S. L, K. K, et al. Sedation during surgery under regional anesthesia: which drug is best for my patient? Reg Anesth Pain Med. 2012; 37.
23. Kassie GM, et al. Preoperative medication use and postoperative delirium: a systematic review. BMC Geriatr. 2017; 17:298.
24. Dickson D, Padilla Conde T, Berdahl J, et al. Comparison of a new sublingual sedation troche with midazolam, ketamine, and ondansetron with intravenous sedation and the effects on vital signs. J Cataract Refract Surg. 2020.
25. Boezaart AP, Berry RA, Nell ML, Van Dyk AL. A comparison of propofol and remifentanil for sedation and limitation of movement during periretrobulbar block. J Clin Anesth. 2001; 13.
26. Stark N, Kerr S, Stevens J. Prevalence and predictors of persistent post-surgical opioid use: a prospective observational cohort study. Anaesth Intensive Care. 2017; 45(6):700–6. https://doi.org/10.1177/0310057X1704500609
27. Drayna PC, Estrada C, Wang W, Saville BR, Arnold DH. Ketamine sedation is not associated with clinically meaningful elevation of intraocular pressure. Am J Emerg Med (W.B. Saunders). 2012; 30:1215–8.
28. Akeju O, Hobbs LE, Gao L, et al. Dexmedetomidine promotes biomimetic non-rapid eye movement stage 3 sleep in humans: a pilot study. Clin Neurophysiol [Internet]. 2018; 129:69–78. https://linkinghub.elsevier.com/retrieve/pii/S1388245717310830.
29. Janssen TL, Alberts AR, Hooft L, Mattace-Raso FUS, Mosk CA, Van Der Laan L. Prevention of postoperative delirium in elderly patients planned for elective surgery: systematic review and meta-analysis. Clin Interv Aging. 2019.
30. Barends CRM, Driesens MK, Struys MMRF, Visser A, Absalom AR. Intranasal dexmedetomidine in elderly subjects with or without beta blockade: a randomised double-blind single-ascending-dose cohort study. Br J Anaesth Elsevier Ltd. 2020;124:411–9.
31. Alhashemi JA. Dexmedetomidine vs midazolam for monitored anaesthesia care during cataract surgery. Br J Anaesth. 2006; 96.
32. Chellappa S, Bromundt V, Frey S, et al. Impact of intraocular cataract lens replacement on circadian rhythms and sleep in older adults. J Sleep Res [Internet] (Blackwell Publishing Ltd). 2018; 27:87–8. https://rsm.idm.oclc.org/login?url=https://www.rsm.ac.uk?url=https://dialog.proquest.com/professional/docview/2112826815?accountid=138535.
33. Patel T, Kurdi MS. A comparative study between oral melatonin and oral midazolam on preoperative anxiety, cognitive, and psychomotor functions. J Anaesthesiol Clin Pharmacol. 2015.
34. Khezri MB, Oladi MR, Atlasbaf A. Effect of melatonin and gabapentin on anxiety and pain associated with retrobulbar eye block for cataract surgery: a randomized double-blind study. Indian J Pharmacol. 2013; 45.
35. Kong VKF, Irwin MG. Gabapentin: a multimodal perioperative drug? Br J Anaesth. 2007.

36. Jefferis JM, Clarke MP, Taylor JP, Brittain KR. Challenges for the cataract surgeon treating people with dementia: a qualitative study exploring anesthetic choices. Clin Ophthalmol. 2014; 8.
37. Fritz BA, Kalarickal PL, Maybrier HR, et al. Intraoperative electroencephalogram suppression predicts postoperative delirium. Anesth Analg [Internet]. 2016; 122:234. http://www.ncbi.nlm.nih.gov/pubmed/26418126.
38. Brown EN, Pavone KJ, Naranjo M. Special Article: Multimodal general anesthesia: theory and practice. Anesth Analg [Internet]. 2018; 127:1246. http://journals.lww.com/00000539-201811000-00023.
39. Chhabra A, Sinha R, Subramaniam R, Chandra P, Narang D, Garg SP. Comparison of sub-Tenon's block with i.v. fentanyl for paediatric vitreoretinal surgery. Br J Anaesth. 2009; 103.
40. Seo IS, Seong CR, Jung G, Park SJ, Kim SY, Kim MM. The effect of sub-Tenon lidocaine injection on emergence agitation after general anaesthesia in paediatric strabismus surgery. Eur J Anaesthesiol. 2011; 28.
41. Nordquist D, Halaszynski TM. Perioperative multimodal anesthesia using regional techniques in the aging surgical patient. Pain Res Treat. 2014.
42. Snir M, Bachar M, Katz J, Friling R, Weinberger D, Axer-Siegel R. Combined propofol sedation with sub-Tenon's lidocaine/mercaine infusion for strabismus surgery in adults. Eye. 2007; 21.
43. Longo VG. Behavioral and electroencephalographic effects of atropine and related compounds. Pharmacol Rev. 1966.
44. Dawson AH, Buckley NA. Pharmacological management of anticholinergic delirium - theory, evidence and practice. Br J Clin Pharmacol. 2016.
45. Maravi P, Mishra DK, Singh A, Niranjan V. Atropine eye-drop-induced acute delirium: a case report. Gen Psychiatry 2020; 33.
46. Gioia L, Prandi E, Codenotti M, et al. Peribulbar anesthesia with either 0.75% ropivacaine or a 2% lidocaine and 0.5% bupivacaine mixture for vitreoretinal surgery: a double-blinded study. Anesth Analg 1999; 89:739–42.
47. Oz Gergin O, Bayram A, Gergin S, et al. Comparison of myotoxic effects of levobupivacaine, bupivacaine and ropivacaine: apoptotic activity and acute effect on pro-inflammatory cytokines. Biotech Histochem (Taylor and Francis Ltd). 2019;94:252–60.
48. Eke T, Thompson JR. The national survey of local anaesthesia for ocular surgery. II. Safety profiles of local anaesthesia techniques. Eye 1999 132 [Internet]. 1999; 13:196–204. http://www.nature.com/articles/eye199950.
49. Hoffman RS, Braga-Mele R, Donaldson K, et al. Cataract surgery and nonsteroidal antiinflammatory drugs. J Cataract Refract Surg. 2016.
50. Luyet C, Eichenberger U, Moriggl B, Remonda L, Greif R. Real-time visualization of ultrasound-guided retrobulbar blockade: an imaging study. Br J Anaesth. 2008.
51. Luyet C, Eng KT, Kertes PJ, Avila A, Muni RH, McHardy P. Real-time evaluation of diffusion of the local anesthetic solution during peribulbar block using ultrasound imaging and clinical correlates of diffusion. Reg Anesth Pain Med. 2012; 37.
52. Gayer S, Palte HD. Ultrasound-guided ophthalmic regional anesthesia. Curr Opin Anaesthesiol [Internet]. 2016; 29:655–61. http://journals.lww.com/00001503-201612000-00004.
53. Tappeiner C, Garweg JG. Retinal vascular occlusion after vitrectomy with retrobulbar anesthesia-observational case series and survey of literature. Graefe's Arch. Clin Exp Ophthalmol. 2011:1831–5.
54. Kelly DJ, Farrell SM. Physiology and role of intraocular pressure in contemporary anesthesia. Anesth Analg [Internet] (Lippincott Williams and Wilkins). 2018 [cited 2021 May 6]; 126:1551–62 http://journals.lww.com/00000539-201805000-00024.
55. Minakaran N, Ezra DG, Allan BDS. Topical anaesthesia plus intracameral lidocaine versus topical anaesthesia alone for phacoemulsification cataract surgery in adults. Cochrane Database Syst Rev. 2020.

56. Knapp H. On cocaine and its use in ophthalmic and general surgery. Arch Ophthalmol. 1884; 13.
57. Luyet C, Eichenberger U, Moriggl B, Remonda L, Greif R. Real-time visualization of ultrasound-guided retrobulbar blockade: an imaging study. Br J Anaesth (Oxford University Press). 2008;101:855–9.
58. Ripart J, Lefrant JY, De La Coussaye JE, Prat-Pradal D, Vivien B, Eledjam JJ. Peribulbar versus retrobulbar anesthesia for ophthalmic surgery: an anatomical comparison of extraconal and intraconal injections. Anesthesiology. 2001.
59. Koornneef L. Details of the orbital connective tissue system in the adult. Acta Morphol Neerl Scand. 1977.
60. Guyton DL. Strabismus complications from local anesthetics [Internet]. 2009; 23:298–301. https://doi.org/10.1080/08820530802505914, http://www.tandfonline.com/doi/full/10.1080/08820530802505914.
61. Dettoraki M, Dimitropoulou C, Nomikarios N, Moschos MM, Brouzas D. Generalized seizures and transient contralateral hemiparesis following retrobulbar anesthesia: a case report. BMC Anesthesiol. 2015.
62. Roberto SA, Bayes J, Karner PE, Morley MG, Nanji KC. Patient harm in cataract surgery: a series of adverse events in Massachusetts. Anesth Analg (Lippincott Williams and Wilkins). 2018;126:1548–50.
63. Alhassan MB, Kyari F, Ejere HOD. Peribulbar versus retrobulbar anaesthesia for cataract surgery. Cochrane Database Syst Rev. 2015.
64. Ohno-Matsui K. Proposed classification of posterior staphylomas based on analyses of eye shape by three-dimensional magnetic resonance imaging and wide-field fundus imaging. Ophthalmology. 2014.
65. Ball JL, Woon WH, Smith S. Globe perforation by the second peribulbar injection [14]. Eye. 2002.
66. Chua MJ, Lersch F, Chua AWY, Kumar CM, Eke T. Sub-Tenon's anaesthesia for modern eye surgery—clinicians' perspective, 30 years after re-introduction. Eye (Springer Nature). 2021.
67. Eke T, Thompson JR. Serious complications of local anaesthesia for cataract surgery: a 1 year national survey in the United Kingdom. Br J Ophthalmol [Internet]. 2007; 91:470. http://www.ncbi.nlm.nih.gov/pubmed/17124243.
68. Winder S, Walker SB, Atta HR. Ultrasonic localization of anesthetic fluid in sub-Tenons, peribulbar, and retrobulbar techniques. J Cataract Refract Surg. 1999; 25.
69. Sivanesan O, Foot B, Eke T. Does local anaesthetic technique affect the incidence of posterior capsule rupture during phacoemulsification? An updated analysis of prospective randomized trials comparing "akinetic" (block) and "kinetic" (topical) anaesthesia. Clin Exp Ophthalmol. 2019.
70. Porela-Tiihonen S, Kaarniranta K, Kokki M, Kokki H. Recovery and patient satisfaction after cataract surgery. A one-year prospective follow-up study. Acta Ophthalmol. 2015.
71. Assam JH, Bernhisel A, Lin A. Intraoperative and postoperative pain in cataract surgery. Surv Ophthalmol. 2018.
72. Iglesias E, Sajnani R, Levitt RC, Sarantopoulos CD, Galor A. Epidemiology of persistent dry eye-like symptoms after cataract surgery. Cornea. 2018; 37.
73. Khadavi NM, Lew H, Goldberg RA, Mancini R. A case of acute reversible charles bonnet syndrome following postsurgical unilateral eye patch placement. Ophthal Plast Reconstr Surg. 2010; 26.
74. Lee RMH, Foot B, Eke T. Posterior capsule rupture rate with akinetic and kinetic block anesthetic techniques. J Cataract Refract Surg. 2013.

Choosing the Right Lens

Design and Material of Intraocular Lenses

Gerd U. Auffarth

Design of Intraocular lenses

The first implanted intraocular lens (Ridley lens) was a relatively thick one-piece implant, which was placed in the capsular bag after extracapsular cataract extraction [1] (Fig. 1).

The subsequent intraocular lenses were constructed from a central optic, which determined the imaging properties, and the so-called haptics, which serve to fix the artificial lens in the eye. Various anatomical intraocular structures, such as chamber angle, iris, and ciliary sulcus were explored as means of fixating the lens. Today, foldable intraocular lenses are usually implanted into the capsular bag. Foldable lenses are offered as one-piece or three-piece models. In the past, some three-piece IOL models were designed to meet the different material and design requirements of optics and haptics. However, the trend of most modern IOLs is towards manufacturing the lenses in one piece. For many years optics with soft edges were used but lens epithelial cells from the equatorial region of the capsular bag could migrate unhindered behind the IOL, so that a posterior capsule opacity would develop relatively early. The so-called posterior capsular opacification (PCO) is the most common cause of a postoperative reduction in visual acuity. The treatment consists of a capsulotomy with the neodymium:yttrium–aluminium-garnet (Nd:YAG) laser. Sharp optical edges can slow down or stop this epithelial migration. In early IOLs made of PMMA with rounded edges, Nd:YAG laser rates of around 30% were described but improvements in lens design and materials have significantly reduced the rate [2]. The 3-year incidence of Nd:YAG capsulotomy is reported to be 2.5–4.5% in hydrophobic and about 11% in hydrophilic acrylate lenses. The sharp trailing edge of the lens optics is mainly responsible for the reduction of the tendency to develop PCO (Fig. 2).

G. U. Auffarth (✉)
David J. Apple, MD Vision Research Center, Department of Ophthalmology,
University Clinic Heidelberg, Im Neuenheimer Feld 400, 69120 Heidelberg, Germany
e-mail: gerd.auffarth@med.uni-heidelberg.de

M. Shajari et al. (eds.), *Cataract and Lens Surgery*,
https://doi.org/10.1007/978-3-031-05394-8_23

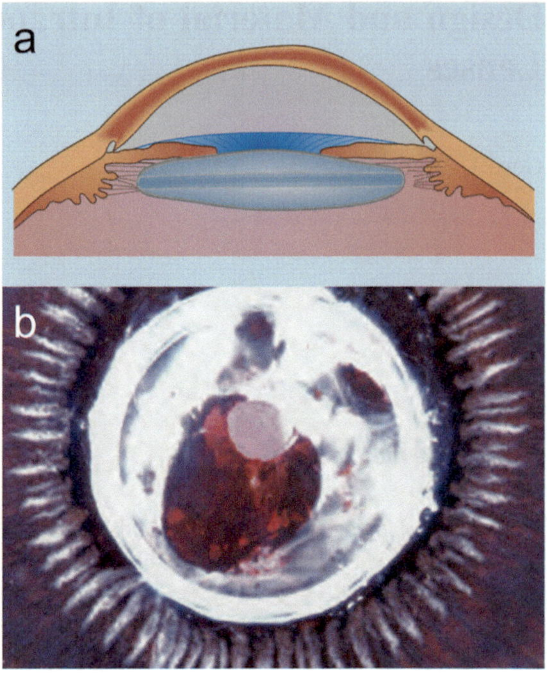

Fig. 1 Implanted Ridley lens. **a** schematic diagram, **b** photograph of an autopsy eye from the vitreous side onto the back surface of the lens and the ciliary body

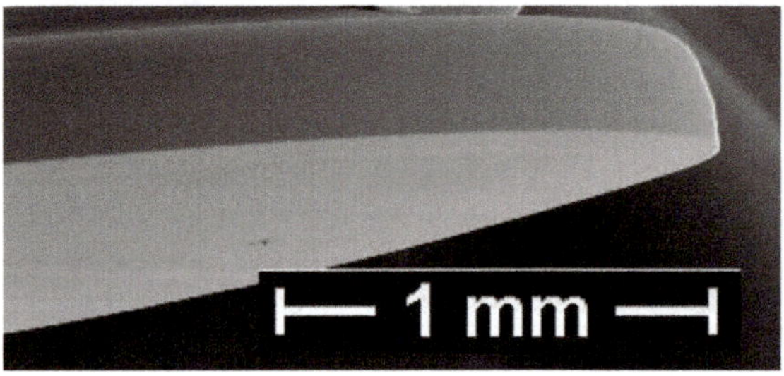

Fig. 2 Scanning electron microscope detail view. The front edge of the optic rim of the depicted hydrophobic folded acrylate lens is rounded, the optic rear edge is sharp

Unfortunately, sharp edges (especially anteriorly) also have disadvantages. Sometimes patients suffer from visual light phenomena (dysphotopsia). In rare cases, these photopic phenomena may even require lens removal. The optics of an IOL must be designed in such a way that the lens has the desired optical imaging properties [3]. The spherical aberration of the natural lens changes during life and becomes positive with age. The cornea, on the other hand, has a positive spherical aberration from the beginning, which remains largely constant throughout life and this knowledge has been applied by various lens manufacturers. Nowadays, IOLs are also available with appropriately modified surfaces. but the extent to which minimizing spherical aberration is beneficial is controversial. Since complete compensation of all spherical aberration leads to a reduction in depth of field, a certain amount of aberration could also be beneficial for the patient. The standard size for the optical diameter of an intraocular lens is 6 mm. However, some manufacturers also offer IOLs with a smaller (5.5 mm) or larger (7 mm) optic diameter.

Haptic design

Depending on the site of fixation (iris, ciliary sulcus, capsular bag, scleral sutured, etc.) there are certain requirements on the shape, size and stability of the artificial lens haptics. In the past, polypropylene was used for the production of haptics for three-piece IOLs. However, many manufacturers have switched to producing haptics from polymethylmetacrylate (PMMA) instead of polypropylene, since polypropylene can be degraded over years by oxidation in vascular tissue, among other things, and there is a certain UV sensitivity. The different materials used to produce artificial lenses are discussed separately in the next chapter. One of the most common reasons for posterior chamber lens explantation in the past has been IOL (sub)luxation [4]. To combat this, efforts have been made to optimize fixation methods. Based on the geometric shape, a distinction is made between C, J, Z or various panel haptic designs. The most popular designs nowadays are capsular bag-fixed IOLs which are one-piece and have a C or plate haptic design (Fig. 3).

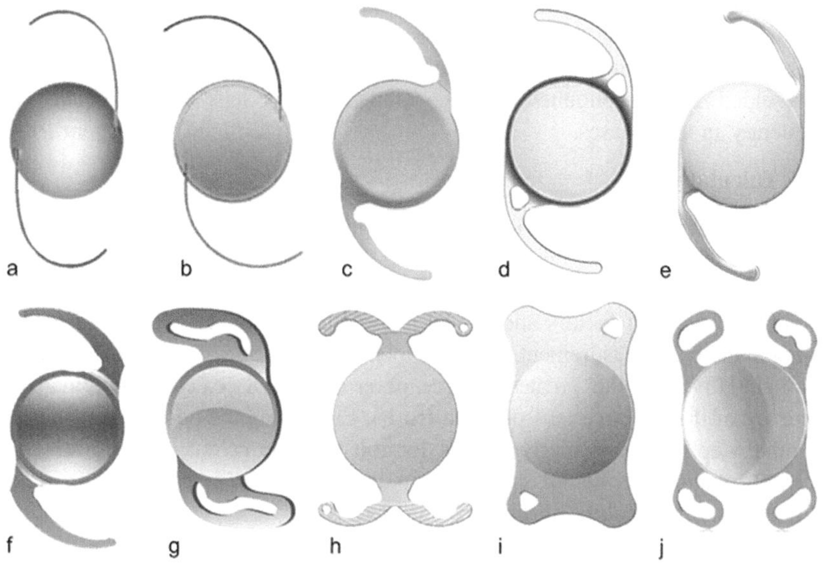

Fig. 3 Haptic designs of capsular bag-fixed posterior chamber lenses. a-b: Three-piece intraocular lenses (IOL) with a: J-Loop, b: C-Loop c-j: One-piece IOL with c-e: C-Loop, f: Z-Loop g: Plate loop, h: double C-loop i: plate haptic, j: multi-loop. The majority of routinely implanted monofocal IOLs today are one-piece C-loop IOLs with a sharp edge

Almost all classic plate haptic IOLs are made of hydrophilic acrylate. The main advantage is that they can be implanted through quite small incisions. However, in comparison to the one-piece C-Loop IOL with a sharp edge, these lenses are associated with higher rates of early PCO development. The idea behind the four-point fixation of the plate haptic IOL is to improve rotational stability, especially in the case of toric lenses. Early plate haptics, which consisted of an uninterrupted block, unfortunately showed rather poor rotational stability. As a result, some lens manufacturers implemented fenestrations in the lens haptics in subsequent generations of plate haptic IOLs. Lens epithelial cells can grow into these fenestrations, which leads to improved rotational stability in the long-term. With hydrophobic acrylic lenses, a multi-loop or double C-loop design is chosen for four-point fixation rather than a classic plate design.

Rotational stability

The first toric lens models were described in the early 1990s. These were often three-piece PMMA or silicone IOLs with an elaborate haptic design. The biggest challenge for all toric IOLs is the risk of IOL rotation, especially in the context of capsular bag shrinkage, since even an IOL rotation or deviation from the target axis by 15 degrees can cause a 50% reduction of the astigmatic effect of the toric IOL. Attempts have been made to minimize the rotational behavior by means of various haptic designs. Some lens haptics, for example, have a corrugated structure to confer more stability. This concept has been used particularly in sulcus-supported IOLs. For example, even high astigmatic refractive errors can be precisely compensated by means of additive sulcus-supported IOLs [5]. In the case of pseudoexfoliation, implantation of foldable intraocular lenses with plate haptics should be avoided, since pronounced fibrosis of the anterior lens capsule occurs more frequently in these cases.

Lens calculation

It is important to calculate the lens refractive power as accurately as possible for the individual adjustment of the lens power to compensate aphakia. Lens calculation formulae are an evolving field and have been developed with the aim of optimizing empirical correction factors and model assumptions. Sources of error in lens calculation include measurement errors in pre- and postoperative biometry and refraction. However, the greatest source of error in IOL calculation remains the accuracy of the effective lens position (ELP). Estimating the postoperative anterior chamber depth is particularly crucial for most of the calculation formulas used today. The haptics of the IOL contribute to determining the position of the IOL after surgery and after healing of the capsular bag.

Special fixation methods

A relatively new approach to fixing an IOL in the eye is to attach the lens to one or both leaves of the empty capsule bag. One of the benefits of these fixation methods is improved rotational stability by anchoring the IOL in the existing anatomical structure with a relatively fixed position. It may also lead to a better estimate of the

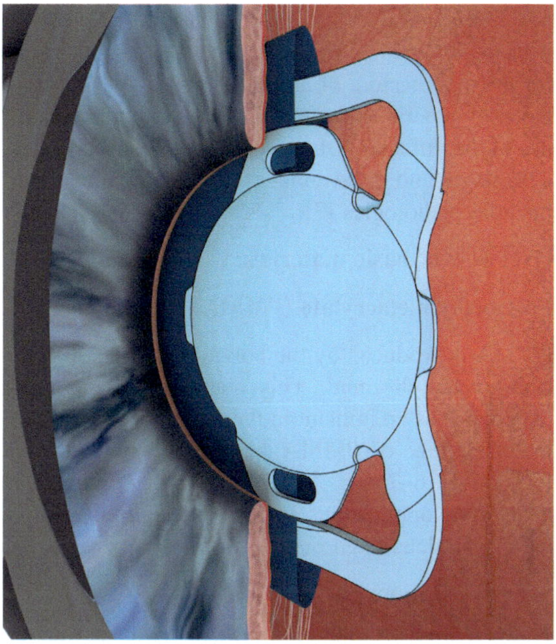

Fig. 4 Rhexis fixed posterior chamber lens. The rhexis-fixed intraocular lens is attached to the anterior leaf of the capsular bag

postoperative effective lens position. The results of the first study of an IOL which is attached to the anterior leaf of the capsule bag after femtosecond laser assisted cataract surgery are now available (Fig. 4).

The first results show an exceptionally high rotational stability. As all new lenses first have to be optimised for use in lens calculation formulae, it is not yet possible to make any conclusive statements regarding a better estimate of the effective lens position. However, the improvement seen with this approach seems to be plausible, because these IOL are independent of the lens posterior capsule and the postoperative position of the anterior capsule alone can be estimated better. With ever better predictability of the postoperative lens position, new possibilities for future examinations are emerging. It is still unclear which parameters should be used to optimally centre the IOL. Centering on the centre of the pupil—the centre of the visual axis—or on the centre of the vertex would be possible with this IOL approach.

Material of Intraocular lenses

The original material of the first intraocular lens was polymethylmetacrylate (PMMA). Sir Harold Ridley first became aware of the good biocompatibility of the material in the course of his medical work during the Second World War. When splinters from cockpit windows of fighter planes healed in the eyes of pilots without any foreign body reaction he realized the potential. He then implanted the first intraocular lens in 1949 [6]. Since then, many other materials have been developed for the manufacture of artificial lenses. Today, variousother polymers are used and have, in general, surpassed PMMA, though it is still used in certain implants. The use of the different IOL materials are determined, on the one hand by their different advantages and disadvantages, and on the other hand by the occurrence of different material pathologies [7].

Overview of basic materials:

Polymethylmetacrylate (PMMA)

PMMA is produced by the polymerisation of methyl metacrylate, which is derived from metacrylic acid. This material has the longest follow-up time and most experience as an implant in the eye because it has been in use since 1949. Implants made entirely of PMMA have to be implanted, as rigid lenses, through large incisions of 6–7 mm. As a result, PMMA lenses are hardly used nowadays, but do have some applications in more specialized areas, e.g. for the secondary implantation of sulcus-fixed or scleral-fixed lenses in aphakia.

Silicone elastomers

The first foldable silicone IOL was implanted by Mazzocco in 1984. Silicone is a particularly inert material and, together with acrylates, is a preferred material for foldable IOLs. Foldable silicone intraocular lenses paved the way for small incision cataract surgery in the 1980s and 1990s [8]. Even then they could be implanted through a small incision, only slightly larger than the phaco incision. Since then, however, silicone folded lenses have been almost completely replaced by foldable acrylate lenses and are hardly offered by the industry any more.

Foldable acrylates

Foldable acrylates found their way onto the intraocular lens market in the 1990s and have enjoyed increasing popularity ever since. The AcrySof intraocular lens from Alcon (Fort Worth, USA) was first implanted in 1994 by Richard Packard in England and the first commercial lens model, a three-part lens (MA60AL, Alcon) was launched in 1995 [9]. Folding acrylate lenses are divided into those with a high and a low water content. Although the terms hydrophilic and hydrophobic describe surface properties in the true sense of the word, they are commonly used to differentiate between the various classes of materials depending on their equilibrium water content (EWC). Today, the combination of different copolymers results in a variety of different acrylic lenses with different physical and chemical properties. Hydrophilic acrylates, or hydrogels, are a group of lenses made of copolymers that swell by more than 20% on contact with water, without dissolving in water. Examples of monomers that are processed in various mixing and polymerisation processes by lens (material) manufacturers are polyurethane and methacrylates, phenylethyl acrylate (PEA), phenylethyl methacrylate (PEMA), hydroxyethyl methacrylate (HEMA) although there are many more. These are mixed in a certain

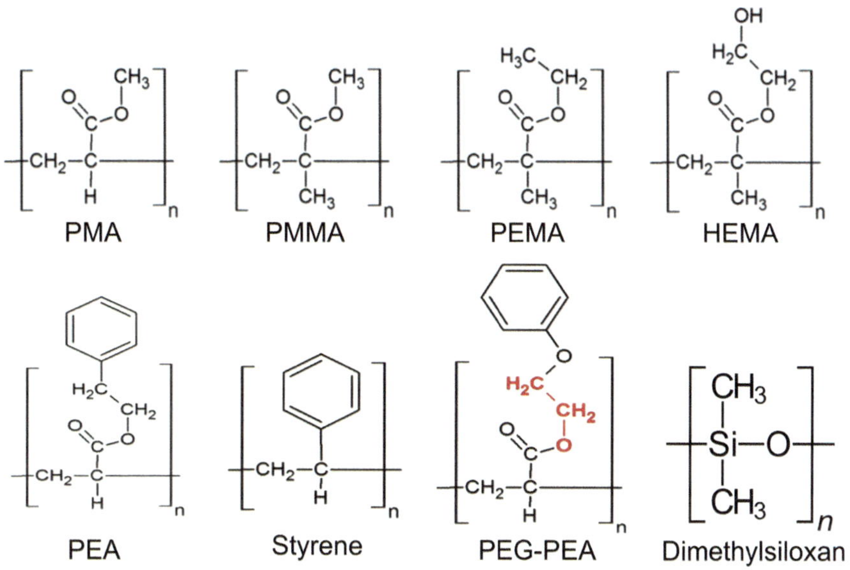

Fig. 5 Basic components of today's materials for intraocular lenses. Polymethyl acrylate (PMA), polymethyl metacrylate (PMMA), phenylethyl methacrylate (PEMA), hydroxyethyl methacrylate (HEMA), phenylethyl acrylate (PEA), polyethylene glycol (PEG)

ratio and bonded together with cross-linkers, e.g. butanediol diacrylate (BDDA), to give the desired properties (Fig. 5).

Depending on the polymer composition, materials have a different refractive index, which is important for the thickness and geometry of the lens (Table 1).

RI refractive index, Equilibrium water content (EWC)

The various materials have different advantages and disadvantages. For example, hydrophilic IOLs have a better uveal tolerance and as a result all phakic sulcus-supported intraocular lenses available today are made of hydrophilic acrylates. On the other hand, hydrophobic IOLs have a lower rate of PCO.

Equilibrium water content and surface Coating

By coating the lens surface, manufacturers try to combine the advantages of different materials. In some lenses made of hydrophobic acrylate, for example, attempts are being made to create a more hydrophilic surface by surface modification with heparin, which should reduce IOL-induced inflammation. This should also reduce injuries to cell membranes caused by the generation of electrostatic forces. On the other hand, hydrophobic surface coatings of hydrophilic IOLs are used to counteract a complication observed in hydrophilic IOLs - the incorporation and deposition of calcium phosphates.

Table 1 Examples of refractive indices and equilibrium water content of different lens materials. Material designation (company) RI EWC (%)

Material designation (company)	Refractive Index (RI)	EWC (%)
PMMA	1.49	0
Hydrophobic silicone	1.41–1.46	<0.03
Aaris (Zeiss)	1.49	0.3
AcrySof (Alcon)	1.55	<0.4
Sensar/Tecnis (Johnson & Johnson)	1.47	0.7
AF-1 (Hoya)	1.50	0.8
Clareon (Alcon)	1.55	1.5
Zaraccom and Delight	1.51	2.5
Envista MX60T (Carl Zeiss)	1.54	4.5
Akreos (Bausch & Lomb), Pod F (PhysIOL), Asphina (Zeiss), C-Flex (Rayner)	1.46	25–28
Hydrohpil Staar hydrophilic (Staar)	1.44	34

PCO treatment and IOL material

Different IOL materials differ with regards to the treatment of PCO. If the lens is accidently hit during Nd:YAG laser capsulotomy, different typical defect shapes can be seen depending on the IOL material. The defects resulting from photodisruption within a PMMA IOL are impressive and appear as radially running material cracks. In silicone IOLs, small whitish stars are formed after laser exposure, whereas in poly-HEMA IOLs display very small, localised, easily distinguishable brightenings are formed in the material. In the PMMA IOL, the melted and raised edge after Nd:YAG laser photodisruption indicates a heat effect, which causes less damage to the hydrous IOL when, applying the same high energy.

Individual material selection

In modern cataract surgery today, we have a large number of high-quality intraocular lens materials that are suitable for a wide range of patients. Nowadays, the standard, typical intraocular lens is a monofocal lens made of a material that is highly resistant to material changes. In the case of patients at who may need retinal or corneal surgery in future, choosing a hydrophobic IOL can avoid the complication of IOL calcification. On the other hand, hydrophilic acrylates are said to have a better biocompatibility in case of increased inflammatory tendencies, e.g. in patients with diabetes mellitus. Overall, none of the lens materials has become dominant as the single best treatment of all patient groups. As a result is important to know the differences between the various materials in the clinical context in order to be able to advise and treat patients adequately.

New materials

In addition to the established basic materials, new substances are being investigated for their suitability for production of intraocular lenses, which may confer better biocompatibility and material stability. Cross-linked polyisobutylene, for example, theoretically should have a better inflammatory reaction profile and should not be prone to glistening. Initial stress tests in the laboratory showed good results. However, many investigations still have to be carried out before clinical application and it remains to be seen which new biomaterials will prevail in the future production of IOLs.

Author's recommendation

Starting with PMMA (polymethylmetacrylate = Plexiglas), various foldable acrylates have been developed which have either a low (hydrophobic) or higher (hydrophilic) equilibrium water content. Other foldable materials (e.g. silicone elastomers) are hardly used today.

References

1. Auffarth GU, Apple DJ. The history of the development of intraocular lenses. The ophthalmologist. 2001;98:1017–31.
2. Apple DJ, Peng Q, Visessook N, Werner L, Pandey SK, Escobar-Gomez M, et al. Eradication of posterior capsule opacification: documentation of a marked decrease in Nd:YAG laser posterior capsulotomy rates noted in an analysis of 5416 pseudophakic human eyes obtained postmortem. Ophthalmology. 2020;127(4S):S29–42.
3. Thomas BC, Khoramnia R, Auffarth GU, Holzer MP. Clinical outcomes after implantation of a toric intraocular lens with a transitional conic toric surface. Br J Ophthalmol. 2018;102(3): 313–6.
4. Auffarth GU, Wesendahl TA, Brown SJ, Apple DJ. Reasons for the explantation of posterior chamber lenses. Ophthalmologist. 1994;91(4):507–11.
5. Thomas BC, Auffarth GU, Rider J, Holzer MP, Rabsilber TM. Implantation of three-piece silicone toric additive IOLs in challenging clinical cases with high astigmatism. Journal of refractive surgery (Thorofare, NJ : 1995). 2013;29(3):187–93.
6. Auffarth GU, Apple DJ. History of the development of intraocular lenses. Ophthalmologist. 2001;98(11):1017–28.
7. Yildirim TM, Auffarth GU, Łabuz G, Bopp S, Son H-S, Khoramnia R. Material analysis and optical quality assessment of opacified hydrophilic acrylic intraocular lenses after pars plana vitrectomy. Am J Ophthalmol. 2018;193:10–9.
8. Auffarth GU, Wilcox M, Sims JC, McCabe C, Wesendahl TA, Apple DJ. Analysis of 100 explanted one-piece and three-piece silicone intraocular lenses. Ophthalmology. 1995;102 (8):1144–50.
9. Mehdorn E, Hunold W, Auffarth G. First experiences with a new foldable acrylic lens (Acrysof™). In: 6 Congress of the German-speaking Society for intraocular lens implantation. Berlin, Heidelberg: Springer; 1993. p. 115–20.

New materials

In addition to the established basic materials, new substances are being investigated for their suitability for production of intraocular lenses, which may confer better

General Introduction to IOL Calculation

Peter Hoffmann and Tyll Jandewerth

Models

The law of refraction was defined in 1618 by Willebrord van Roijen Snell:

$$n_1 \cdot \sin \delta_1 = n_2 \cdot \sin \delta_2$$

where refractive indices = n_i and angle of incidence/reflection = δ_i. The application of Snell's law to the refractive surfaces enables, in principle, the calculation of any optical system (ray tracing). Unfortunately, this was not practical at the time, because the resulting equations could not be solved analytically without powerful computers due to the enormous computational power required. Carl Friedrich Gauss simplified this for paraxial space (cases of very small angular incidence) by replacing the sinusoidal functions with the angle itself. This made it much easier to calculate and introduces the familiar terms such as focal length, principal focal point, principal plane etc.

A further simplification is the approximation of real lenses by modelling them as infinitely thin lenses with a fictitious refractive index.

The Gullstrand Eye

The Gullstrand eye model was developed by the Swedish ophthalmologist and Nobel Prize winner Allvar Gullstrand and is a simplified eye model with standardized optical data (refractive indices, refractive values, spherical refractive surfaces, etc.) with which calculations can be made for optical systems/aids such as contact lenses and intraocular lenses [1]. All "classical" IOL formulas are based on the Gullstrand model.

P. Hoffmann (✉) · T. Jandewerth
Castrop-Rauxel, Germany
e-mail: ph@augenklinik-castrop-rauxel.de

M. Shajari et al. (eds.), *Cataract and Lens Surgery*,
https://doi.org/10.1007/978-3-031-05394-8_24

Liou and Brennan eye model

In contrast to the Gullstrand eye model, this newer model uses four aspherical surfaces and a gradient refractive index of the lens [2]. It offers a considerably more precise modelling ability but cannot be handled in its entirety with Gaussian optics. Computer-aided ray tracing is required for this purpose.

Historical development

With the advent of acoustic length measurement for the eye, formulae were developed to predict the refraction of the pseudophakic eye, before surgery. The first-generation formulae [3–6] were similar in that they all worked with Gaussian optics where lenses were assumed to be infinitely thin and the axial position of the IOL was assumed to be constant. These formulae were improved over several generations, but two input parameters, namely axial length and radius of curvature of the corneal anterior surface, must be taken into account in all formulae.

Sources of error

Axis length

The first generation of axial length measurements were made using ultrasound. Acoustic measurement with A-scan sonography, mostly used in the 10 MHz band and in the applanation mode, has an average tolerance of $\approx$ 0.2 mm. This corresponds to 0.5 dpt at eyeglass level for a normal eye. Significantly better results could be achieved by immersion A-scan because the indentation of the cornea as a source of error is eliminated. In small eyes (and in children in particular) the effect of measurement error is significantly bigger.
For most cases, acoustic axial length measurement has been surpassed by devices that use optical axial length measurement, such as the Zeiss IOL-Master introduced in 1999/2000. The measurement tolerance is reduced to 0.03–0.05 mm which corresponds to 0.15–0.2 dpt at eyeglass level. Newer methods such as OLCR (optical low coherence reflectometry) and ssOCT (swept source OCT) reduce the tolerances even further to $\approx$ 0.01 mm, increase the measurability on very turbid media and provide measurement data for all sections of the optical path, which is advantageous when newer algorithms are used.

Cornea

Normally, the corneal refractive power is estimated from paraxially measured local radii of the anterior surface. Some assumptions are hidden here, namely those of a sphere or minimal prolate asphere and a constant ratio of anterior and posterior surface radii. Measurement errors, asphericity and anterior or posterior surface ratio can all cause an error of $\approx$ 1/8 dpt [7]. The moisture of the patient's eye and fixation can also have dan effect on measurement accuracy. In device comparisons, corneal measurement accounts for more than 75% of the total refractive difference between the devices.

IOL position

The prediction of the axial position of the lens is the largest single source of error in IOL calculation [7]. Considerable improvements can be achieved by providing information on the partial distances of the optical path [8, 9]. In the near future, algorithms using ssOCT image data to determine the lens equator can be expected to provide further improvements, especially for short eyes.

Refraction

The postoperative refraction determination is a subjective procedure in which human factors of the examinee and examiner have an impact on the results. In addition, refraction can only be measured in discrete intervals. Distance, ambient light and other factors can also influence the results. Higher-order aberrations cause device dependence and overall less precisive values. The actual tolerance of refraction of pseudophakic patients ranges from 0.18 to 0.39 dpt, depending on the source and there is a strong dependence on visual acuity and type of IOL [9].

Formula error

The approximations of the Gaussian space and the infinitely thin lens are inaccurate for the human eye, because not all optical surfaces are rotationally symmetrical, large aperture angles and curvatures exist, and the lens thickness is not negligible. A major source of error is the corneal model. Using the Gullstrand model, the refractive power of the cornea is overestimated by $\approx$ 0.5 dpt, using the American keratometry indices, it is overestimated by more than 1.2 dpt. The estimation of the "effective lens position" (ELP, a fictitious value which should not be confused with the measured postoperative anterior chamber depth) is done by using the preoperatively measured parameters; axial length and keratometry values (Holladay, Hoffer Q, SRK/T) or axial length and anterior chamber depth (Haigis).

The ELP is usually significantly deeper than the actual IOL position. Its implicitly includes factors that have nothing to do with the geometric position of the IOL, such as refractive indices (corneal model), pupil size, decentration and tilting of the IOL, pseudoacocommodation, asphericity of cornea and lens, atypical ratio of anterior to posterior eye segment, surgical technique, etc. This compensates for systematic errors in the ELP by taking different quantities into consideration, which is correct on average but can be occasionally incorrect when evaluated on an individual basis. If ray tracing is used instead of Gaussian optics, these adjustments become less important, but here too, the calculation accuracy is affected by the modelling of the individual optical surfaces and by measurement errors, centration, and tilt.

Formulae

First generation

The first-generation formulae mentioned above shared the problem that the effective position of the lens was assumed to be constant. This meant that the refractive power was calculated as much too high for short eyes and too low for long eyes. Therefore, these formulae are obsolete.

Second generation

The unsatisfactory results of the early formulae led to the development of a purely empirical formula that established a relationship between IOL power, axial length and corneal power ("k readings") via a bivariate linear regression [10]. To adjust the prediction error, an offset "A" was used, which can still be found today on almost every lens package and is supposed to describe specific properties of the lens. The formula is:

$$P_{IOL} = A - 2.5 \cdot AL - 0.9 \cdot K$$

This formula can only achieve good results if the eye is statistically similar to the "standard eye". Myopic and hyperopic eyes as well as deviating anterior segments in particular can result in extremely large errors.

Third generation

The first published formula of the so-called third generation was the Holladay formula [11]. For the first time, a formula was presented that provided useful results for almost all eyes except for very long axial lengths, depending on the correct input data. The systematic errors are small for axial lengths less than 25 mm and are almost negligible when no other anomalies are present, especially for steep and flat corneal radii. Adjustment is done by a "surgeon factor" (SF), which is supposed to describe the axial position of the IOL in relation to the cornea. The SRK authors followed suit and developed a similar formula: SRK/T [12]. At the same time, the authors declared their earlier statistical formulae obsolete. In 1993 the Hoffer Q-formula was introduced though they all have a common weakness in very high myopic eyes (see model error above). Another common feature is the adjustment via a single offset (sf, A, pACD), which requires at least 50 refractions per lens model in order to be optimized.

Haigis [13] pursued a somewhat different approach with a modification of the Gernet formula. He used axial length and anterior chamber depth as predictors for ELP estimation. Thereby certain systematic errors were avoided. The adjustment is done by three variables a_0, a_1, a_2 (offset, coefficients for axis length and anterior chamber depth), but requires at least 200 data sets per IOL type. The Haigis formula is somewhat more robust than its American counterparts and for axial lengths over 26 mm it is superior to the American formulas.

Newer approaches

Multivariate formulas

Based on our clinical experience, the Holladay 2 formula, with its numerous coefficients, has no advantages over the classical ones, even if the optically measured lens thickness and corneal diameter are additionally included.

Very good results for most eyes except high hyperopic ones (see Sect. 27.1) are obtained with the Barrett Universal II formula [14]. Although the lens thickness is processed, it has, as with Holladay 2, almost no effect on the result.

The Kane formula [15] is also said to be superior to the classical ones, but the data published so far is so sparse that, apart from statistical significance, there is no clinical relevance. However, preliminary results of our own research indicate that the Kane formula could consistently deliver very good results even with hyperopic eyes and is close to the ray tracing results. In particular, the optically measured lens thickness is processed appropriately. Unfortunately, this formula is not published either.

Thick Lens formulas

Gaussian optics with "thick lenses", i.e. those in which the cornea and lens are not approximated by a single infinitely thin surface, have advantages, especially in the case of abnormal corneas or those whose front-to-back surface ratio deviates from what is typical. In addition, well-known modelling errors are avoided. The best-known representative in this group is the Olsen formula which is either pre-installed in Gaussian optics on biometric devices or available "stand-alone" in the PhacoOptics software.

Of course, this approach requires an exact measurement of both curvatures of the cornea.

The general lens formula can be adapted easily "do it yourself" to a "thick cornea", for that see Sect. 27.1. The simplified variant of the Haigis formula provides results that are at least equivalent to the Kane or Olsen formula, but the re-parameterization of the constants is quite complex.

Ray tracing

Ray tracing or beam tracing is nothing more than the application of Snell's law at all optical boundaries. In the optical industry such calculations have been standard for decades. The angles and refractive indices must be known for each interface, which also includes internal information from IOL manufacturers. Different devices can be used as data source, e.g. Okulix can import topography/tomography from devices of different manufacturers. This is important for abnormal corneas, for example after refractive surgery, and provides valuable additional information, e.g. for the selection of the individual best IOL asphericity. The quality of the imported data is absolutely crucial for the quality of the calculation. In comparison to the classical formulae, a greater amount of data and more complex data are included in the calculation (Fig. 1).

"Artificial intelligence"

A new approach is to calculate the refractive power without any formula at all based on pattern recognition by a software that has been trained with large amounts of data from past results. This can be realized with the "Hill Radial Basis Function". Unfortunately, only axial length, corneal radii and anterior chamber depth are included in the calculation. Other inputs such as lens thickness and corneal diameter

Patient: 860234 OS 2019/11/22

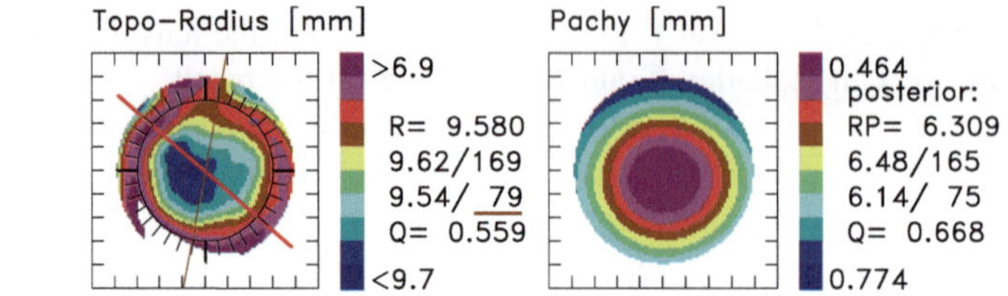

OS 22/11/19

R1= 9.62mm

R2= 9.54mm 0.06D/139.9°

RP= 6.31mm

AL=26.98mm ->26.96mm

ACDP=3.08mm, LT=3.58mm

Tomey OA-2000

HOYA: Vivinex iSert XY1/XC1
ACD=4.29mm

	[parax]	bf pup 2.5	
22.00 ->	[1.03]	0.98	(1.01/ -0.06/ 50)
22.50 ->	[0.65]	0.60	(0.63/ -0.06/ 50)
23.00 ->	[0.31]	0.26	(0.29/ -0.06/ 50)
23.50 ->	**[-0.07]**	**-0.12**	(-0.09/ -0.06/ 50)
24.00 ->	[-0.45]	-0.50	(-0.47/ -0.06/ 50)
24.50 ->	[-0.83]	-0.87	(-0.85/ -0.06/ 50)
25.00 ->	[-1.22]	-1.26	(-1.23/ -0.06/ 50)
25.50 ->	[-1.56]	-1.60	(-1.57/ -0.06/ 50)

Bausch&Lomb: enVista MX60
ACD=4.47mm

	[parax]	bf pup 2.5	
22.00 ->	[1.35]	1.17	(1.20/ -0.06/ 50)
22.50 ->	[0.86]	0.70	(0.72/ -0.06/ 50)
23.00 ->	[0.50]	0.34	(0.37/ -0.06/ 50)
23.50 ->	**[0.14]**	**-0.03**	(0.00/ -0.06/ 50)
24.00 ->	[-0.22]	-0.39	(-0.36/ -0.06/ 50)
24.50 ->	[-0.58]	-0.76	(-0.73/ -0.06/ 50)
25.00 ->	[-1.00]	-1.18	(-1.15/ -0.06/ 50)
25.50 ->	[-1.36]	-1.54	(-1.52/ -0.06/ 50)

J&J: Sensar AAB00
ACD=4.24mm

	[parax]	bf pup 2.5	
21.50 ->	[1.32]	1.11	(1.14/ -0.06/ 50)
22.00 ->	[0.94]	0.73	(0.76/ -0.06/ 50)
22.50 ->	[0.55]	0.34	(0.37/ -0.06/ 50)
23.00 ->	**[0.17]**	**-0.05**	(-0.02/ -0.06/ 50)
23.50 ->	[-0.20]	-0.42	(-0.39/ -0.06/ 50)
24.00 ->	[-0.59]	-0.81	(-0.78/ -0.06/ 50)
24.50 ->	[-0.99]	-1.22	(-1.19/ -0.06/ 50)
25.00 ->	[-1.37]	-1.60	(-1.58/ -0.06/ 50)

J&J: Tecnis ZCB00/ZMB00
ACD=4.51mm

	[parax]	bf pup 2.5	
22.00 ->	[1.26]	1.28	(1.30/ -0.06/ 50)
22.50 ->	[0.89]	0.91	(0.93/ -0.06/ 50)
23.00 ->	[0.51]	0.53	(0.56/ -0.06/ 50)
23.50 ->	**[0.14]**	**0.16**	(0.18/ -0.06/ 50)
24.00 ->	[-0.25]	-0.22	(-0.20/ -0.06/ 50)
24.50 ->	[-0.65]	-0.62	(-0.60/ -0.06/ 50)
25.00 ->	[-1.02]	-1.00	(-0.97/ -0.06/ 50)
25.50 ->	[-1.41]	-1.39	(-1.36/ -0.06/ 50)

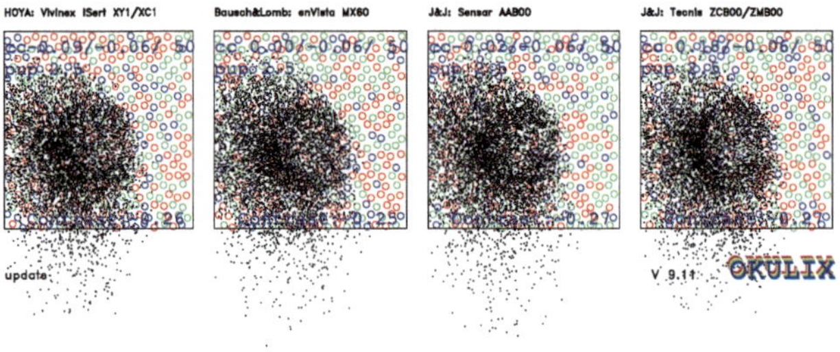

Fig. 1 Printout of the raytracing software Okulix 9.11 with a data set of the Heidelberg Anterion ssOCT. The eye has undergone myopic LASIK of approx. -8 dpt. The central flattening is clearly visible, the ratio of the anterior to posterior radii is only 0.66 and the anterior surface is an oblate asphere. In addition to the calculation of refractive power, the retinal image is also simulated with a measure. This allows an estimation which IOL would probably achieve the highest local contrast on the retina

seem to serve primarily to collect data for the operator, but do not influence the result.

Practically achievable accuracy

Firstly, on the basis of postoperative refractions, the "constants" must be adjusted such that either the mean or median error become zero. The appropriate measure of the accuracy of the method is the standard deviation or variance of the prediction error. With the classical formulae, standard deviations of the prediction error of 0.4–0.5 dpt. can be achieved (corresponds to MAE ≈ 0.3–38 dpt., ≈ 80% within 0.5 dpt.), provided that the basis conditions are well designed. With aspherical lenses and high visual acuity, the accuracy will be better, because spherical aberration is reduced and refraction precision is improved (Fig. 2).

In statistically abnormal eyes (long axis, steep or flat radii, anterior segment not corresponding to the axial length), the error of the classical formulae is considerably greater, but not in raytracing, Olsen or Kane.

If the optically measured lens thickness is included and the problems of Gaussian optics are avoided, improvements of 6–20% can be achieved depending on the algorithm, visual acuity level and lens type [9]. In the best case (high visual acuity, aspherical lens) the standard deviation is 0.29 dpt and the MAE 0.21 dpt, more than 90% of eyes are within 0.5 dpt [9].

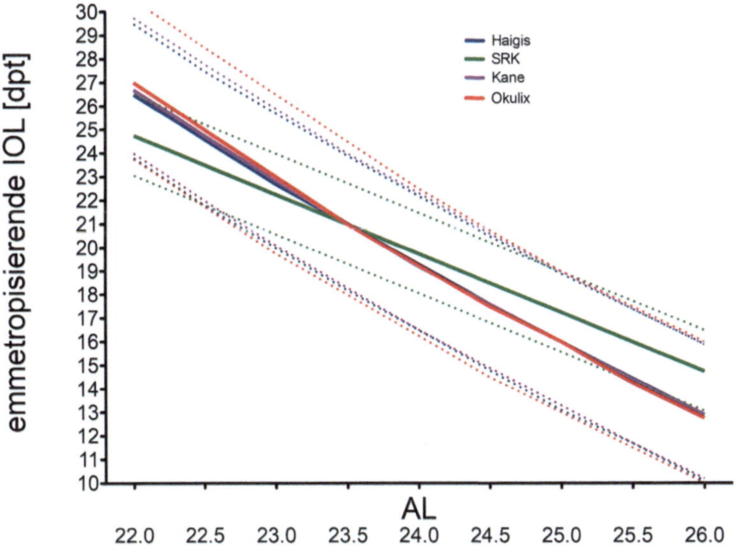

Fig. 2 Calculation of emmetropizing IOL power for axial lengths 22 - 26 mm ("normal" eyes). Solid line: Corneal radii and anterior chamber depth on the 50th percentile, dashed lines: 10th and 90th percentile. It is clear to see that the old SRK formula differs greatly, while the classical formula (Haigis), the latest formula (Kane) and raytracing (Okulix) differ only very slightly and are not clinically relevant. The biggest differences are shown in hyperopic eyes with a large anterior segment. For reasons of clarity, only one method per category has been listed

Second eye

Since the refractive prediction error of both eyes is positively correlated with r $\approx$ 0.5, the result of the first eye can be used to improve the calculation of the second one [16–18]. In practice, 50% of the error of the first eye is removed. If, for example, a prediction error of + 0.6 dpt occurred, the target refraction in the 2nd eye would be -0.3 dpt instead of 0.0 dpt.

In ray tracing programs, the anatomical IOL position of the 1st eye can also be used directly for the 2nd eye [8]. The optically measured anterior chamber depth is entered directly into the pACD field for the 2nd eye. The potential for improvement of both methods is $\approx$10% on average and significantly more for short eyes.

Author's recommendation

Optimal biometry is essential for good refractive results. Without precise input data, no IOL calculation can yield good results. ssOCT is currently the most precise and reliable method for measuring axial length and other sections of the optical path. The measurement of corneal radii or calculation of corneal refractive power remains the main source of error in diagnostics of "normal" eyes. The choice of formula is of secondary importance in the vast majority of eyes, provided that the adjustment is correct for the individual types of IOL. Larger deviations can occur with statistically abnormal combinations of values. If raytracing (our preference) is not available, the Kane formula currently seems to process the data generated by modern biometers in the most meaningful way and may have the smallest deviations at the edges of the distribution.

References

1. Gullstrand A. The dioptrics of the eye. 3rd ed. Helmholtz by H, editor. Hamburg/Leipzig: Voss; 1909. 307p.
2. Liou HL, Brennan NA. Anatomically accurate, finite model eye for optical modeling. J Opt Soc Am A Opt Image Sci Vis. 1997;14(8):1684–95.
3. Gernet H, Ostholt H, Werner H. The preoperative calculation of intraocular Binkhorst lenses. 122 Meeting of the Association of Rheinisch-Westfälischer Ophthalmologists. Carpenter. Balve; 1970. p. 54–5.
4. Fyodorov SN, Kolinko AI. Estimation of optical power of the intraocular lens. VestnOftalmol. 1967;4:27–37.
5. Colenbrander MC. Calculation of the power of an iris clip lens for distant vision. Br J Ophthalmol. 1973;57:735–40.
6. Binkhorst RD. Intraocular lens power calculation. IntOphthalmolClin. 1979;19(4):237–52.
7. Norrby S. Sources of error in intraocular lens power calculation. J Cataract Refract Surg. 2008;34(3):368–76.
8. Olsen T, Hoffmann PC. C constant: New concept for ray tracing-assisted intraocular lens power calculation. J Cataract Refract Surg. 2014;40(5):764–73.
9. Hoffmann PC, Wahl J, Prussian P-R. Accuracy of intraocular lens calculation with ray tracing. J Refract Surg. 201;28(9):650–5.

10. Sanders DR, Retzlaff J, Kraff MC. Comparison of the accuracy of the Binkhorst, Colenbrander and SRK implant power prediction. J Am Intraocul Implant Soc. 1981;7:337–40.
11. Holladay JT, Prague TC, Chandler TY, Musgrove KH, Lewis JW, Ruiz RS. A three-part system for refining intraocular lens power calculations. J Cataract Refract Surg. 1988;14 (1):17–24.
12. Retzlaff JA, Sanders DR, Kraff MC. Development of the SRK/T intraocular lens implant power calculation formula. J Cataract Refract Surg. 1990;16(3):333–40; erratum1990; 16:528.
13. Haigis W. IOL calculation according to Haigis [Internet]. 1996 [cited 08.05.2020]. Available from: http://www.augenklinik.uni-wuerzburg.de/uslab/ioltxt/haie.htm
14. Melles RB, Holladay JT, Chang WJ. Accuracy of intraocular lens calculation formulas. Ophthalmology. 2018;125(2):169–78.
15. Darcy K, Gunn D, Tavassoli S, Sparrow J, Kane JX. Assessment of the accuracy of new and updated intraocular lens power calculation formulas in 10 930 eyes from the UK National Health Service. J Cataract Refract Surg. 2020;46(1):2–7.
16. Olsen T. Prediction of the effective postoperative (intraocular lens) anterior chamber depth. J Cataract Refract Surg. 2006;32(3):419–24.
17. Olsen T. Use of fellow eye data in the calculation of intraocular lens power for the second eye. Ophthalmology. 2011;118(9):1710–5.
18. Covert DJ, Henry CR, Koenig SB. Intraocular lens power selection in the second eye of patients undergoing bilateral, sequential cataract extraction. Ophthalmology. 2010;117 (1):49–54.

Formula Optimisation and Use of the IOL WEB Platform IOLCon

Achim Langenbucher

The majority of cataract lenses today are calculated with lens power calculation formulae. In addition to the lens formulae, procedures are used today that work with numerical ('full-aperture') ray tracing, which projects a bundle of rays onto the eye and optimises the retinal image quality. With the lens formulae, a distinction is made between empirical approaches that work without an anatomical-physiological eye model and theoretical optical formulae that are based on a pseudophakic eye model. Not all available calculation strategies are disclosed, so that the underlying algorithm cannot always be understood.

Lens calculation formulae are generalised calculation concepts that can be adapted to the special situations and conditions of a lens type. They can also be adapted to the surgical technique, the characteristics of the patients or the calibration of the biometer or the refraction measurement technique. To allow for this adaptation, the formulae include formula constants or lens constants, which can be used, for example, to minimise or eliminate average deviations between achieved and intended refraction after cataract surgery. However, the characteristics of the formulae are not lost in the process. This means, for example, that if a formula incorrectly estimates the refraction result in long eyes in the direction of postoperative myopia, the characteristics will be retained even if the formula constant is optimised.

Keypoint

The optimisation of formula constants has a very high value in modern cataract surgery and is of fundamental importance for achieving the target refraction and thus patient satisfaction.

A. Langenbucher (✉)
Homburg, Germany
e-mail: achim.langenbucher@uks.eu

M. Shajari et al. (eds.), *Cataract and Lens Surgery*,
https://doi.org/10.1007/978-3-031-05394-8_25

In general, formulae with more than one constant, such as the Haigis formula or Castrop formula, can be adapted more individually to boundary conditions, but in return can induce a more significant error when boundary conditions change. As a rule of thumb, at least 80–100 clinical data sets are required for the optimisation of formula constants, and in the case of more than one formula constant, a correspondingly higher number of data sets is required.

The minimum requirements for optimisation from preoperative biometry are eye length, corneal radii (and for some formulae other variables such as the phakic external anterior chamber depth in the Haigis formula, the horizontal corneal diameter in the Holladay2 or Barrett formula or the axial lens thickness in the Olsen or Castrop formula), in addition to the refractive power and type of the implanted lens and the manually measured refraction at least 4–6 weeks after the procedure. In the case of intraocular lenses with pseudo accommodation (especially EDOF lenses with a plateau in the defocus curve), not only should the refraction be determined, but a check should be made by defocusing with plus lenses to ensure that the determined refraction actually corresponds to the distant refraction and that visual acuity is reduced if additional plus lenses are added.

The strategy for optimising the formula constant depends on whether the lens calculation formula requires one or more formula constants. If a constant is required, by changing the calculation formula and resolving according to the formula constant, the constant can be determined directly for each clinical data set. This constant is used to calculate the achieved refraction on the basis of preoperative biometry and the implanted lens. The 'optimal' constant can then be determined using statistical measures such as the arithmetic or geometric mean or the median using the individual formula constants of all clinical cases.

For formulae that require more than one formula constant, however, linear or non-linear optimisation procedures are required for constant optimisation. Currently, the formula constants for the Haigis formula (a0/a1/a2 or a0 with default values for a1/a2), the SRK/T formula (A), Hoffer-Q formula (pACD) as well as Holladay1 formula (SF) and Castrop formula (C/H/R), for the SRK2 formula the A constant is available on request. For the Holladay2 formula (ACD) and Barrett U2 formula (LF and DF) no optimisations have been carried out due to the non-disclosure of the formula algorithm via IOLCon, but the lens manufacturer can make these constants available via IOLCon (Fig. 1) in the print or file output.

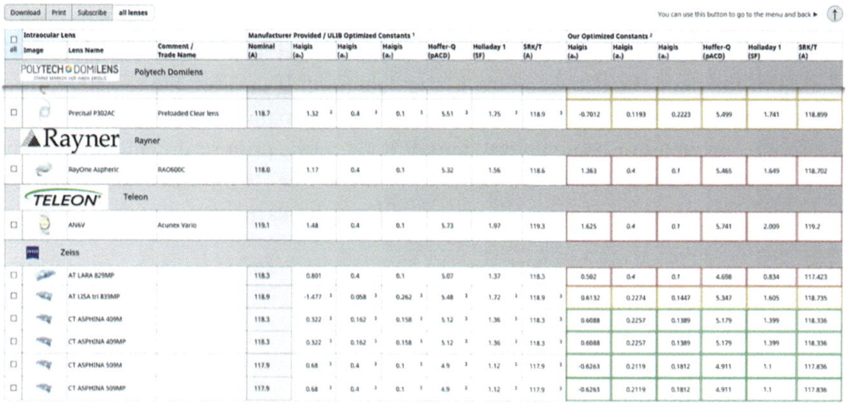

Fig. 1 Detail of the standard view in IOLCon (567 lens types and 31 manufacturerm 12.09.2022). The lenses are sorted by manufacturer. Next to the icon and the lens name the nominal formula constant, a block with the constants recommended by the manufacturer and on the right side another block with the constants optimised by IOLCon are shown. The technical specifications and delivery ranges can be displayed by selecting the 'Visible columns' option

Keypoint

The internet platform IOLCon (www.iolcon.org) serves as an almanac not only for technical data and specifications of all intraocular lenses currently on the market, but also displays the available delivery ranges and gradations of the lenses as well as the formula constants.

With the option 'Show all lenses' all lenses of the manufacturers are listed alphabetically and with the option 'Visible columns' the display is further specified by the user. The 'Search for lenses' option provides a selection of lenses that can be limited by manufacturer or criteria, and several selections can be activated by holding the 'CTRL' key. For both options the selection can be further specified by activating the checkbox to the left of the lens icon. The technical data, delivery ranges and formula constants can optionally be output to the standard printer via 'Print' or saved in a standardised.xml database format for further processing in the biometer. Via 'Constants to download' it is specified which data sets are to be used for the optimisation. Here, for example, the biometer used or the ethnicity of the patients can be chosen as selection criteria. However, care must be taken that the number of data sets is not reduced by the selection to the extent that the formula constants can no longer be loaded.

The constants recommended by the manufacturer are always included in the print or file output, even if no or too little clinical data for optimisation is stored in the IOLCon platform. The 'Add clinical results' option allows clinical data to be added to the data pool for optimisation of formula constants. To ensure the traceability of the data a user ID is required (email to admin@iolcon.org). After registration, a template in.csv format (for Office Excel applications) or in.xml format can be generated, which can then be uploaded via 'Upload results file' after being filled with anonymised clinical data. After an automated and a subsequent manual verification of the data, the data is added to the data pool. If desired, the registered user who uploaded the data receives the corresponding personalised formula constants as a report via email or can convert them directly into a print or download template via the options 'Show all lenses' or 'Search for lenses' 'Constants for download' 'Surgeon' (here you can optionally select 'all' or the user themselves).

Surgically Induced Corneal Astigmatism

Nino Hirnschall

Due to the constant development of cataract surgery, post-operative manifest refraction has become increasingly important. This post-operative refraction depends on many parameters, including the changes of the cornea due to the cataract operation itself. Surgically induced corneal astigmatism (SICA) is the change in the radius and thus the refractive power of the cornea because of the operation. Only the astigmatism of the cornea is taken into account, but not other sources of astigmatism, such as the lens or the (minor) influence of the posterior pole. Morphologically speaking, the incision reduces tissue tension by cutting through corneal lamellae and fibres. However, it is not only the incision width determined by the keratome itself that has an influence on the SICA, but also the manipulations within the incision during surgery.

The SICA is interesting for any form of cataract surgery, but it is particularly relevant when using toric intraocular lenses (IOLs) and when calculating any possibility of intra-operative astigmatism reduction [1] In a recent study it was shown that SICA accounts for 7–8% of the total error in a 2.2 mm temporal incision and correction of 3.0D corneal astigmatism [2, 3].

In the following section, we will discuss the most relevant parameters that influence SICA, such as the type of incision, incision size, position of the incision and the biomechanical properties of the cornea.

Type of incision

In the classic extracapsular cataract extraction, which is very rarely performed nowadays, the approach is usually scleral. Scleral incisions have a lower SICA (per mm) than the clear corneal incisions described below. In a scleral incision, a preliminary incision is made at a distance from the limbus and then a scleral tunnel is created, which ends in a corneal "lip". This technique is still used today with a

N. Hirnschall (✉)
Department of Ophthalmology and Optometry, Johannes Kepler University, Linz, Austria
e-mail: nino.hirnschall@kepleruniklinikum.at

M. Shajari et al. (eds.), *Cataract and Lens Surgery*,
https://doi.org/10.1007/978-3-031-05394-8_26

smaller incision (approx. 7.5 mm) in manual small incision surgery. Manual small incision cataract surgery is a procedure that does not require phacoemulsification and is used in several countries, such as parts of India. With this technique, the type of pre-cut plays a role and there are three types: an incision parallel to the limbus has the highest induced astigmatism, a straight incision has lower induced astigmatism and a so-called “frown” incision has the lowest induced astigmatism. In this last type of incision, the preliminary incision is made antiparallel to the limbus [4].

In the clear corneal incision, which is the most frequently performed in Europe today, the incision area (length x width of the incision) is important [5]. This is particularly evident for the historical larger incisions and concerns especially incision sizes over 4.0 mm (see below) [6].

In some centers, this clear corneal incision is performed with a femtosecond laser but the laser method does not seem to be significantly different from the manual method with regard to SICA [7–10].

Presumably, the speed of IOL implantation also has an influence on the wound architecture. Ouchi has shown in a case series that the cartridge diameter temporary increases the wound size significantly during the implantation process. Furthermore, in the same publication it was shown that a very slow IOL implantation leads to added stretching of the wound [11]. How relevant this is for the type of incision, however, has yet to be verified in further studies and an overly hasty implantation of an IOL also carries risks.

Incision size

The incision size has a significant influence on the SICA. Strictly speaking, the incision area should be taken into account, but since the length of the tunnel varies from surgeon to surgeon and from case to case, the literature usually only refers to the incision size. In a Cochrane review of 26 included trials, 4 different incision sizes were compared (up to 1.5 mm, 1.8 mm, 2.2 mm and 3.0 mm). This review showed that although a small incision induces less astigmatism, the variation between patients is still large [12].

Although a smaller incision correlates with a lower SICA, very small incisions have been shown to cause more wound stress, which in turn results in a higher SICA. The question is if there is a cut-off value concerning incision size and induced astigmatism. Although there is no general agreement, there are good references in the literature. For larger incisions (5 mm vs 4 mm vs 3.5 mm) [13] there are clear and significant differences. Incisions between 2.5 mm and 3.0 mm should also have a significant influence on SICA. Masket et al. [14] (2.2 mm vs. 3.0 mm), Luo et al. [15] (2.2 mm vs. 3.0 mm), Wang et al. [16] (2.6 mm vs. 3.0 mm) and Wilczynski et al. [17] (1.8 mm vs. 2.75 mm) all measured lower SICA values for the smaller incision size. No significant difference was observed for incision size comparisons of 2.2 mm versus 2.6 mm [16] and 2.2 mm versus 2.8 mm [18]. Because the SICA depends on many factors, this discrepancy between the studies can be easily explained.

For an incision size up to 2.0 mm there are no significant differences and therefore an incision size of less than 2.0 mm is probably not relevant for SICA at present [15, 19].

In summary, an incision size of less than 3.0 mm is recommended, and there is a current trend in the field to aim for incisions below 2.5 mm. No good evidence is available, however, for a smaller incision size.

Position of the incision

The cornea is approximately ellipsoid, with the horizontal diameter being larger than the vertical. In addition, the refractive power of the cornea decreases from the centre to the periphery and the thickness increases. An incision made superior, therefore, is closer to the centre of the cornea and the cornea is thinner than in a temporal incision. This is why superior incisions result in a higher SICA than temporal incisions. Marek et al. showed that temporal incisions not only generally induce less astigmatism (0.6 vs. 1.0 D), but also have a lower spread of SICA (0.3 D vs. 0.5 D) [20]. Nikose et al. have confirmed this difference with an overall higher SICA (0.8 vs 1.3 D) [21].

In theory, there should be no relevant difference between nasal and temporal, as Ermis et al. observed no relevant difference in SICA between superotemporal and superonasal access [22]. However, any nasal access increases difficulty of the surgery significantly.

With the "on axis" incision, the incision is made according to the steepest astigmatic axis during corneal measurement (for example, keratometry). The aim is to reduce corneal astigmatism as effectively as possible through the flattening effect of the incision. This concept is still used in many clinics, though some surgeons have left this concept because the predictability of temporal incisions seems to be better compared to on axis incisions. However, the data available on this topic is not yet sufficiently evident to make a conclusive statement.

Biomechanical properties of the cornea

The biomechanical properties of the cornea are viscosity and elasticity. Since these two parameters are not easily measurable in vivo, most studies use the viscoelastic properties. The viscoelastic properties are mainly determined by corneal hysteresis and the corneal response factor (CCF). The relationship between biomechanical corneal properties and viscoelastic properties is difficult to elucidate. Glass, Roberts et al. [23] showed in a model that the relation of hysteresis and elasticity is complex. Low hysteresis can mean either high or low elasticity, depending on the viscosity. In addition, there is a significant negative correlation between age and hysteresis, and hypermetropic eyes have less elasticity than myopic eyes [24] Since all these parameters have an influence and the viscoelastic properties are a surrogate parameter for the biomechanical properties, the measured influence of hysteresis and CCF is still debated. Denoyer et al. have shown that the pre-operatively measured hysteresis has an influence on SICA [25].

The SICA also exhibits a certain "fading" effect, which can also be explained by its viscoelastic properties. This effect occurs mainly in the first 4 months, but can continue to a lesser extent up to one year after the operation [26].

Measurement and calculation of SICA

The measurement of SICA is device-dependent and it should be taken into account that the measured SICA always includes a certain measurement error. In principle, however, different measurement methods provide similar SICA average values [27].

As mentioned at the beginning of the chapter, SICA is calculated as a vector. It is therefore wrong to simply subtract astigmatism values from each other; instead, a vector calculation should be performed. To understand this concept, one should take a short look at the concept of astigmatism representation. A vector can always be represented in two ways, either by means of Cartesian coordinates, or as polar coordinates. In ophthalmology, polar coordinates are more commonly used. The two properties of each vector are a certain length (mode) and an orientation. To calculate the difference between two vectors, both properties of both vectors should be considered. With this vector calculation the total effect of the incision on the cornea can be shown. But sometimes it is also interesting to calculate the direct effect of the incision at the incision site. This is the so-called "flattening" effect. Detailed instructions for calculating this flattening effect were published by Naeser in 2008 [28].

Author's recommendation

On the ASCRS homepage there is a much simpler method to calculate and display corneal astigmatism (Fig. 1): https://ascrs.org/tools/corneal-sia-tool

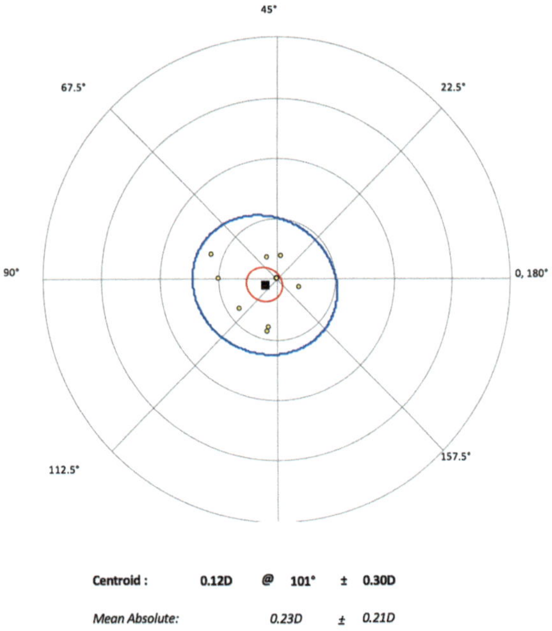

Fig. 1 Representation of the induced astigmatism in a so-called "double angle" plot. "Double" angle refers to the fact that the circle is divided into 180° instead of the usual 360°, thus corresponding to astigmatism. Each ring represents 1.0 D astigmatism. Each small empty circle represents a difference vector (keratometry), the black square is the centroid, the red circle the 95% confidence interval of the centroid and the blue circle the 95% confidence interval of the data. In this case the SICA would be 0.12 D at 101° with a dispersion of 0.30 D and the mean absolute induced astigmatism would be 0.23 D with a dispersion of 0.21 D

For this purpose, the preoperative and postoperative values are entered by the keratometry and all relevant parameters are calculated automatically.

References

1. Kohnen T, Cook DD. Methods to control astigmatism in cataract surgery. Curr Opin Ophthalmol. 1996;7(1):75–80.
2. Brain ultrasound NF, O. Bayer N., Leisser, C. Norrby, S. Zimper, E. Hoffmann, P. Sources of error in toric intraocular lens power calculation. J Refract Surg. Submitted 2020.
3. Hirnschall N, Hoffmann PC, Draschl P, Maedel S, Findl O. Evaluation of factors influencing the remaining astigmatism after toric intraocular lens implantation. J Refract Surg. 2014;30 (6):394–400.
4. Singer JA. Frown incision for minimizing induced astigmatism after small incision cataract surgery with rigid optic intraocular lens implantation. J Cataract Refract Surg. 1991;17 (Suppl):677–88.
5. Armeniades CD, Boriek A, Tuber GE. Effect of incision length, location, and shape on local corneoscleral deformation during cataract surgery. J Cataract Refract Surg. 1990;16(1):83–7.
6. Leen MM, Ho CC, Yanoff M. Association between surgically-induced astigmatism and cataract incision size in the early postoperative period. Ophthalmic Surg. 1993;24(9):586–92.
7. Fernandez J, Rodriguez-Vallejo M, Martinez J, Tauste A, Pinero DP. Prediction of surgically induced astigmatism in manual and femtosecond laser-assisted clear corneal incisions. Eur J Ophthalmol. 2018;28(4):398–405.
8. Pereira A, Somani S, Tam ES, Chiu H, Maini R. Comparison of surgically induced astigmatism and corneal morphological features between femtosecond laser and manual clear corneal incisions. J Refract Surg. 2019;35(12):796–802.
9. Diakonis VF, Yesilirmak N, Cabot F, Kankariya VP, Kounis GA, Warren D, et al. Comparison of surgically induced astigmatism between femtosecond laser and manual clear corneal incisions for cataract surgery. J Cataract Refract Surg. 2015;41(10):2075–80.
10. Ferreira TB, Ribeiro FJ, Pinheiro J, Ribeiro P, O'Neill JG. Comparison of surgically induced astigmatism and morphologic features resulting from femtosecond laser and manual clear corneal incisions for cataract surgery. J Refract Surg. 2018;34(5):322–9.
11. Ouchi M. Effect of intraocular lens insertion speed on surgical wound structure. J Cataract Refract Surg. 2012;38(10):1771–6.
12. Jin C, Chen X, Law A, Kang Y, Wang X, Xu W, et al. Different-sized incisions for phacoemulsification in age-related cataract. Cochrane Database Syst Rev. 2017;9:CD010510.
13. Kohnen T, Dick B, Jacobi KW. Comparison of the induced astigmatism after temporal clear corneal tunnel incisions of different sizes. J Cataract Refract Surg. 1995;21(4):417–24.
14. Masket S, Wang L, Belani S. Induced astigmatism with 2.2- and 3.0-mm coaxial phacoemulsification incisions. J Refract Surg. 2009;25(1):21–4.
15. Luo L, Lin H, He M, Congdon N, Yang Y, Liu Y. Clinical evaluation of three incision size-dependent phacoemulsification systems. On J Ophthalmol. 2012;153(5):831–9 e2.
16. Wang J, Zhang EK, Fan WY, Ma JX, Zhao PF. The effect of micro-incision and small-incision coaxial phaco-emulsification on corneal astigmatism. Clin Exp Ophthalmol. 2009;37(7):664–9.
17. Wilczynski M, Supady E, Loba P, Synder A, Palenga-Pydyn D, Omulecki W. Evaluation of surgically induced astigmatism after coaxial phacoemulsification through 1.8 mm microincision and standard phacoemulsification through 2.75 mm incision. Clin Oczna 2011;113(10–12):314–20.
18. Sethi HS, Saluja K, Naik MP. Comparative analysis of coaxial phacoemulsification with 2.2- and 2.8-mm clear corneal incisions. Int Ophthalmol. 2018;38(1):215–22.

19. Yu YB, Zhu YN, Wang W, Zhang YD, Yu YH, Yao K. A comparable study of clinical and optical outcomes after 1.8, 2.0 mm microcoaxial and 3.0 mm coaxial cataract surgery. Int J Ophthalmol. 2016;9(3):399–405.
20. Marek R, Klus A, Pawlik R. Comparison of surgically induced astigmatism of temporal versus superior clear corneal incisions. Clin Oczna. 2006;108(10–12):392–6.
21. Nikose AS, Saha D, Laddha PM, Patil M. Surgically induced astigmatism after phacoemulsification by temporal clear corneal and superior clear corneal approach: a comparison. Clin Ophthalmol. 2018;12:65–70.
22. Ermis SS, Inan UU, Ozturk F. Surgically induced astigmatism after superotemporal and superonasal clear corneal incisions in phacoemulsification. J Cataract Refract Surg. 2004;30(6):1316–9.
23. Glass DH, Roberts CJ, Litsky AS, Weber PA. A viscoelastic biomechanical model of the cornea describing the effect of viscosity and elasticity on hysteresis. Invest Ophthalmol Vis Sci. 2008;49(9):3919–26.
24. Roberts CJ, Reinstein DZ, Archer TJ, Mahmoud AM, Gobbe M, Lee L. Comparison of ocular biomechanical response parameters in myopic and hyperopic eyes using dynamic bidirectional applanation analysis. J Cataract Refract Surg. 2014;40(6):929–36.
25. Denoyer A, Ricaud X, Van Went C, Labbe A, Baudouin C. Influence of corneal biomechanical properties on surgically induced astigmatism in cataract surgery. J Cataract Refract Surg. 2013;39(8):1204–10.
26. Hirnschall N, Wiesinger J, Draschl P, Findl O. Factors influencing efficacy of peripheral corneal relaxing incisions during cataract surgery. J Ophthalmol. 2015;2015:706508.
27. Ofir S, Abulafia A, Kleinmann G, Reitblat O, Assia EI. Surgically induced astigmatism assessment: comparison between three corneal measuring devices. J Refract Surg. 2015;31(4):244–7.
28. Naeser K. Assessment and statistics of surgically induced astigmatism. Acta Ophthalmol. 2008;86(Suppl 1):5–28.

Lens Calculation in Short and Long Eyes

Peter Hoffmann and Tyll Jandewerth

Calculation problems with long eyes

All "classical" formulae tend to underestimate the IOL refractive power in high myopic eyes, which leads to undesirable hyperopic outcomes. The source of the underlying problem is mainly the cornea model and, in particular, the concept of refractive power calculation. In most formulae, the cornea is treated as an infinitely thin lens and this requires some assumptions. The most important assumptions are the refractive index of the cornea (usually 1.376), a spherical shape and a constant ratio of front and back surface radii (usually 1:0.9). Under these assumptions, a fictitious refractive index of the cornea as a thin lens of 1.3315, 1.3320 or 1.3375 results, depending on whether one refers to the main plane on the object side, the front or rear vertex.

Unfortunately, especially the last two assumptions do not apply, which leads to both systematic and individual deviations. Most significant is the systematic overestimation of the refractive power, which, depending on the fictitious index used, leads to a deviation of 0.45, 0.52 or 1.23 dpt. for an average cornea.

With the classical formulae this deviation is compensated by the previously mentioned "effective lens position", and the IOL is virtually "lowered". This is no longer the case in high myopic eyes because of the low refractive power of the implant.

Various approaches for solving this problem have been described.

Statistical corrections of existing models

The Haigis formula has less systematic error in high myopic eyes than Hoffer Q, Holladay I, Holladay II and SRK/T. Haigis recommends eliminating the systematic error completely by adjusting the "constants" for lenses of low refractive power [1].

P. Hoffmann (✉) · T. Jandewerth
Castrop-Rauxel, Germany
e-mail: ph@augenklinik-castrop-rauxel.de

M. Shajari et al. (eds.), *Cataract and Lens Surgery*,
https://doi.org/10.1007/978-3-031-05394-8_27

The result is that the effective main plane is located far behind the eye for lenses with positive refractive power and far in front of the eye for lenses with negative refractive power. Furthermore, this constant adjustment can only be performed on an empirical basis for a single IOL model on the market (Alcon MA60MA). Despite a mean error of zero in a given data set, an error still exists because a lens of +5.0 dpt. needs a completely different "constant" than one of +1.0 dpt. In addition, calculations of aphakic eyes could not be correct either. Therefore, this approach has to be scrutinized [2].

An alternative approach is the transformation of the axial length, which can be designed in such a way that the refractive result is correct and independent of the type of lens. This approach has also been criticized as it does not address the underlying cause of the error.

Finally, another very simple method to avoid any errors is to use the known systematic error of the formula (by analysis of previous refraction results) in a certain IOL refractive power range with reversed sign as target refraction. If it is known, for example, that the Haigis formula produces about +0.75 dpt. hyperopia with a certain IOL type in the refractive power range of −5 dpt. To +5 dpt., it is very easy to use −0.75 dpt. as the target refraction in the calculation to arrive at zero.

Improved models

In our view, it is better to address the underlying cause of the error. As explained above, the overestimation of corneal refractive power can no longer be compensated by virtually lowering the IOL.

Ray tracing avoids this error in principle, and special corrections are not necessary as "refractive power" does not occur at all and systematic errors do not occur, provided that the input variables are correct.

In Gaussian optics, the problem can be minimized if a refractive index of ≈ 1.328 is used for the cornea when modelled as a thin lens. Another possibility is to modify the basic lens formula to avoid the problem with the fictitious refractive index by including both corneal curvatures (mod. according to Langenbucher):

from

$$P_{IOL} = \frac{n_{GK}}{AL - ELP} - \frac{1}{\frac{1}{\frac{1}{\frac{1}{P_{Brille}} - d_{HSA}} + P_{HH}} - \frac{ELP}{n_{KW}}}$$

will then be

$$P_{IOL} = \frac{n_{GK}}{AL - ELP} - \frac{1}{\frac{1}{\frac{1}{\frac{1}{\frac{1}{\frac{1}{P_{Brille}} - d_{HSA}} + P_{HH\alpha}} - \frac{d_{HH}}{n_{HH}}} - P_{HHp}} - \frac{ELP}{n_{KW}}}$$

Axial length that is determined as being "too long" plays a smaller role because a PCI-based optical biometer uses an average refractive index (1.35491 for the

IOL-Master) for the entire eye. For high myopia, however, the posterior segment is longer than the anterior segment relative to a model of a normal eye, so the resulting average refractive index is smaller than assumed. In a case of pathological myopia, for example, where an axial length of 36.00 mm is measured by the biometer, the actual axial length would then be 35.84 mm (effect on spectacle plane $\approx$ 0.17 dpt.). Newer devices, which can measure sections of the optical path, could represent the axial length directly as a segment sum, but this has only been used experimentally so far.

The uncertainty of the refractive index of the cataract lens remains a problem regardless, so an optical axial length measurement can never be completely free of assumptions and thus free of potential error.

In addition, optical biometers were calibrated against acoustic biometers before the IOLMaster was introduced in 1999. This also generated systematic errors in long and short eyes. This can be counteracted at least approximately by transforming the output value for the axis length [3].

Formulas like the Olsen or Barrett (neither are published but are available in many biometers) compensate the abovementioned problems to a large extent. Whether this happens on the basis of another model or by statistical corrections is unclear. In any case, both mentioned formulae are free of systematic errors in high myopic eyes.

In this context, little can be said about the Hill RBF methodology, because the function is mainly based on IOL refractive powers between 6 and 30 dpt. and therefore may not sufficiently cover the very highly myopic problem cases.

In our own clinical routine, we use ray tracing software for high myopic eyes. If this is not possible, the target refraction is modified as described above.

Author's recommendation

Model errors lead to deviations towards hyperopia in long eyes. Use formulae or software that avoids this problem (Okulix, Olsen, Barrett) or use the known prediction error of your favorite formula with the reversed sign as target refraction to target emmetropia (Fig. 1).

Calculation problems with short eyes

High hyperopic eyes are also a particularly difficult problem for IOL calculation. There are several reasons for this. The allowed tolerances of the IOL refractive power are higher, and the form factor of the lenses (thickness, radii ratios) can vary and change the ELP Errors in the measurements have a greater impact than in normal eyes as large angles κ or α lead to aberrations which show in the refraction. Last but not least, the prediction of the final IOL position is extremely critical. An axial change in position of 0.1 mm has a 2.5 times greater effect with a +35 dpt. lens compared to a +20 dpt. lens.

Since many of the variables cannot be influenced mathematically, the prediction of the IOL position is the decisive factor when the measuring technique is used

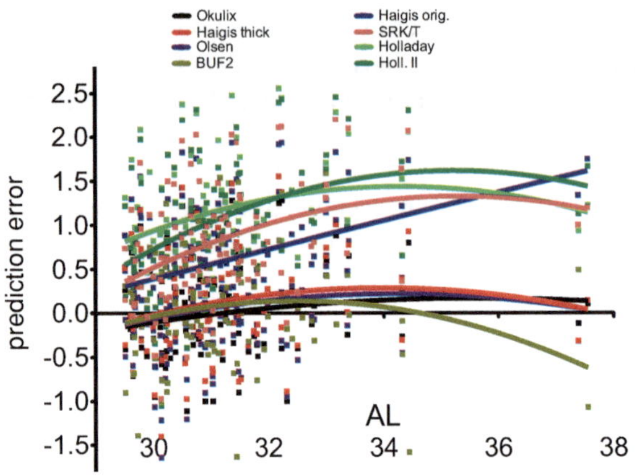

Fig. 1 Prediction error of different formulae and calculation methods for very long eyes over 30 mm. It can be clearly seen that the classical formulae produce deviations in hyperopia due to the abovementioned model errors, whereas Okulix, Olsen formula, Barrett formula and the modified Haigis formula according to Langenbucher show hardly any systematic deviations. The classical formulae used constants that produce a mean error of zero for all eyes

carefully. To make matters worse, in very long and short eyes the anatomy of the anterior segment does not often correlate with the overall size of the eye [4].

Statistical approaches

Some IOL formulae attempt to improve the reliability in high hyperopic eyes by using special terms and case distinctions. In essence, the aim is to detect an "exotic" or "outlying" anterior segment. Hoffer and Holladay use the corneal radii for this purpose, while Holladay II also considers refraction, lens thickness, corneal diameter, etc. But these final variables only have a slight influence on the result. Barrett also uses the lens thickness, but again this appears to have little influence on the result. Hill RBF is mainly designed for "pattern recognition" of axial length and radius combinations, but currently (2019) works no better than standard formulae for high hyperopic eyes and high IOL refractive powers (Fig. 2).

In our own separate study on 100 high hyperopic eyes (mean axial length 21.05 ± 0.64 mm) we could not find any significant differences between the formulae mentioned except for small systematic offsets, whereas the SRK-family performs significantly worse here. This has also shown in other studies [5].

Anatomical approaches

The standard formulae summarize the refractive power in an infinitely thin plane called the ELP. This plane is typically much deeper than the actual principal plane of the IOL due to the abovementioned modelling errors and is not measurable postoperatively due to its fictitious character. For the estimation of ELP, axial length and anterior chamber depth (Haigis), axial length and corneal radii (SRK/T,

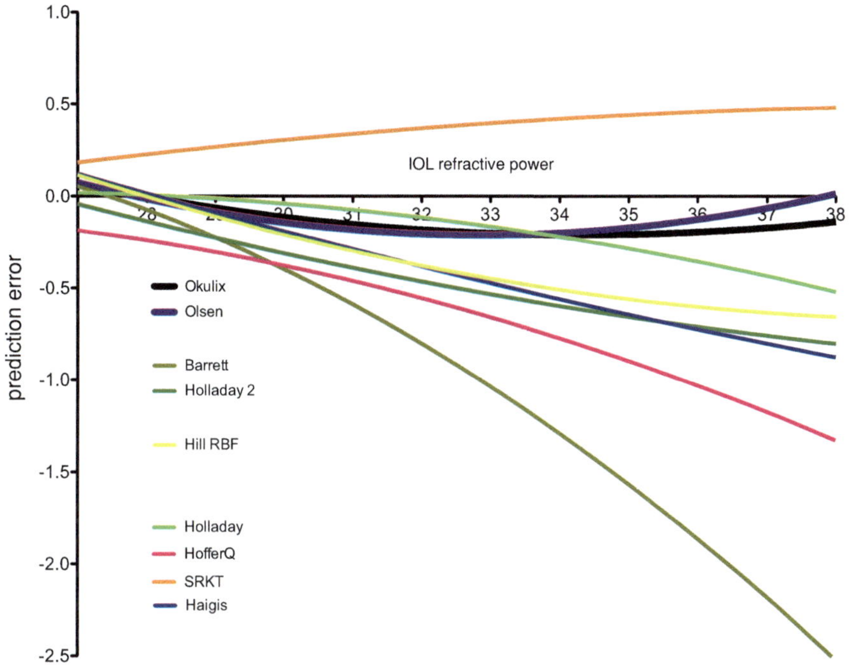

Fig. 2 Prediction error as a function of IOL refractive power in high hyperopic eyes. Ray tracing with Okulix or PhacoOptics/Olsen provides significantly better results than the classical formulae. Especially the "new" unpublished formulae like Holladay 2 and Barrett Universal 2, which do not perform better than the classical ones

Holladay, Hoffer Q, Barrett, Hill RBF) or anterior chamber depth and lens thickness (Olsen) are used.

It is obvious that the implanted lens is in the capsular bag and that the haptics are spread out in the plane of the equator/zonula. Laser interferometric measurement series confirm that the IOL is, on average, about 1/3 of the thickness of the former natural lens [6]. If the thickness of the IOL and the position of the posterior corneal surface and the anterior and posterior capsule are known, the expected position of the IOL can be predicted quite well [2, 7]. Haptic angulations seem to play only a minor role in the long run, whereas steps, as seen in the Tecnis 1-piece, lead to a systematically deeper lens position than planar haptics.

As postoperative anterior chamber depth is a also defined anatomical size which can be verified, and the algorithms can be adapted accordingly.

The refractive results of ray tracing programs, which use the aforementioned anatomical parameters, are in any case very accurate and clearly superior to conventional formulae, provided that optical measurement data for the partial distances are available (Fig. 2). If only a conventional data set with axial length and corneal radii is available then, ray tracing has little or no advantage over the standard formulae because the main error is remains the axial IOL position.

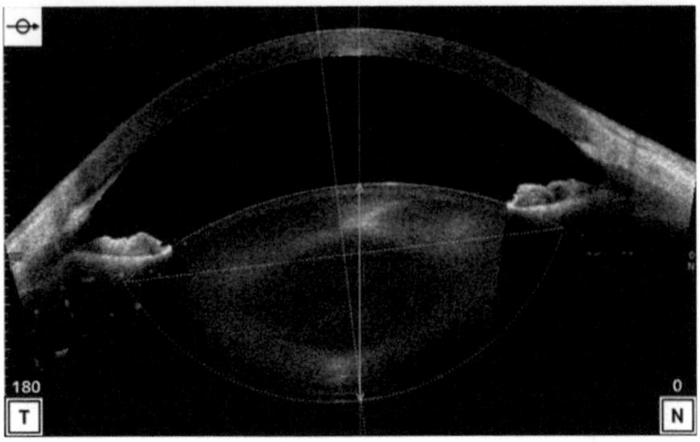

Fig. 3 Geometric analysis of the cataract lens. Both the radii of the lens surface and the position of the equator as the later plane of the haptic end piece as well as decentration and tilting of the lens relative to the line of sight are clearly visible

An extremely interesting approach for the near future is the intraoperative OCT-supported measurement of the empty capsular bag [8].

Swept source OCTs now also allow the cataract lens to be modelled in terms of curvatures and the equator (Fig. 3). Our own investigations have shown that this allows for even better predictions of the later IOL position than with algorithms using anterior chamber depth and lens thickness. Newer and better approaches are to be expected in this field in the near future.

Author's recommendation

For hyperopic eyes, tolerances in diagnostics, IOL and surgery have a much greater impact on IOL prediction. The largest single factor is the axial position of the IOL. All classical formulae have weaknesses in this aspect, the Holladay formula from 1988 is the most likely to provide consistent results. Using the Olsen formula or Okulix Raytracing is by far the most accurate method, provided that precise and complete input data is available.

References

1. Haigis W. Intraocular lens calculation in extreme myopia. J Cataract Refract Surg. 2009;35 (5):906–11.
2. Preußner P-R, Olsen T, Hoffmann PC, Findl O. Intraocular lens calculation accuracy limits in normal eyes. J Cataract Refract Surg. 2008;34(5):802–8.
3. Wang L, Shirayama M, Ma XJ, Kohnen T, Koch DD. Optimizing intraocular lens power calculations in eyes with axial lengths above 25.0 mm. J Cataract Refract Surg. 2011;37 (11):2018–27.
4. Hoffmann PC, Hütz WW. Analysis of biometry and prevalence data for corneal astigmatism in 23,239 eyes. J Cataract Refract Surg. 2010;36(9):1479–85.
5. Aristodemou P, Knox Cartwright NE, Sparrow JM, Johnston RL. Formula choice: Hoffer Q, Holladay 1, or SRK/T and refractive outcomes in 8108 eyes after cataract surgery with biometry by partial coherence interferometry. J Cataract Refract Surg. 2011;37(1):63–71.

6. Preußner P-R. Intraocular lens calculation in extreme myopia. J Cataract Refract Surg. 2010;36 (3):531–2; authorreply532–4.
7. Olsen T, Hoffmann PC. C constant: New concept for ray tracing-assisted intraocular lens power calculation. J Cataract Refract Surg. 2014;40(5):764–73.
8. Hirnschall N, Amir- S, Maedel S, Findl O. Predicting the postoperative intraocular lens position using continuous intraoperative optical coherence tomography measurements. Invest Ophthalmol Vis Sci. 2013;54(8):5196–203.

IOL Calculation for Particularly Dense Lenses

Efstathios Vounotrypidis

The thickness of the human crystalline lens increases with age, which has been confirmed by many large studies [1–3]. The increase in thickness is usually associated with a change in the refractive index of the lens, and the formation of cataract. In some cases, usually depending on the severity of the cataract, standard axial length measurement with partial coherence interferometry (PCI) is not possible. In cases of mature or posterior subcapsular cataract especially, optical biometry is usually not even possible [4–6], but even a less severe change of the lens thickness can lead to inaccurate measurements of the axis length (AL), because of the change of the refractive index of the crystalline lens [7].

These limitations in optical biometry have been partially remedied by new technological developments [8–10]. The newer "Swept-Source" OCT-based biometry (OA-2000, IOLMaster700) and "Optical-Low Coherence Reflectometry" show significantly better penetration through highly opaque lenses when compared to previous PCI generation. In recent studies, both the IOLMaster 700 and the OA-2000 have successfully measured the AL in almost all patients where PCI biometry was not possible [11–14]. In addition, the latest OLCR has shown a higher penetration rate in patients with posterior subcapsular cataract, where PCI measurements of AL were not possible [13].

Nevertheless, biometry is not always possible and AL must still be determined by ultrasound from time to time. It has been shown that accurate axial length measurement is the most important parameter for determining the correct IOL Power [15]. The refractive result using optical biometry is therefore proven to be significantly more accurate compared with applanation ultrasound (US) biometry [16]. However, it did not show a higher accuracy when compared to measurement using an optimized immersion US technique making it a very acceptable backup option in cases where optical biometry cannot be performed [17].

E. Vounotrypidis (✉)
Department of Ophthalmology, University Clinic Ulm, Ulm, Germany
e-mail: efstathios.vounotrypidis@uni-ulm.de

M. Shajari et al. (eds.), *Cataract and Lens Surgery*,
https://doi.org/10.1007/978-3-031-05394-8_28

Author's recommendation

The newest biometric devices are highly effective in achieving precise and accurate results, even in cases of severely opacified lenses and posterior subcapsular cataract. If biometry is not possible even with newest biometric devices, axial length should be determined using immersion US technique.

Measurement of anterior segment parameters is usually possible using different devices such as the PCI biometer, the OLCR, "Swept-Source" OCT-assisted biometers, or the Pentacam. If this is not possible, other anterior segment-OCT devices can be used to ensure precise measurement of the anterior segment of the eye [18]. These devices are preferred for obtaining anterior segment biometric parameters and only in the event that this is not possible, should it be substituted with immersion US.

While AL measured with ultrasound extends from the anterior corneal vertex to the inner limiting membrane (ILM), in optical biometry the distance between the corneal epithelium and the retinal pigment epithelium is defined as AL [19]. Therefore, optical and acoustic axial lengths, as well as the measured axis (optical vs. anatomical) are different [20]. For this reason, AL measured with the US is usually shorter than measured with optical biometry.

Nowadays, due to the technological evolution, a wide range of biometric devices with increased penetration in severely opacified lenses is available to the surgeon. In rare cases where optical biometry is not possible, AL should be determined with the immersion US technique. Since the AL measured with US is shorter, the surgeon should bear that in mind when choosing the correct lens power in order to avoid any postoperative hyperopic shift.

References

1. Shammas HJ, Shammas MC. Measuring the cataractous lens. J Cataract Refract Surg. 2015;41(9):1875–9.
2. Jivrajka R, Shammas MC, Boenzi T, Swearingen M, Shammas HJ. Variability of axial length, anterior chamber depth, and lens thickness in the cataractous eye. J Cataract Refract Surg. 2008;34(2):289–94.
3. 3rd Hoffer KJ. Axial dimension of the human cataractous lens. Arch Ophthalmol (Chicago, Ill: 1960). 1993;111(7):914–8.
4. Freeman G, Pesudovs K. The impact of cataract severity on measurement acquisition with the IOLMaster. Acta Ophthalmol Scand. 2005;83(4):439–42.
5. 5th Lege BA, Haigis W. Laser interference biometry versus ultrasound biometry in certain clinical conditions. Graefes Arch Clin Exp Ophthalmol. 2004;242(1):8–12.
6. Tehrani M, Krummenauer F, Blom E, Dick HB. Evaluation of the practicality of optical biometry and applanation ultrasound in 253 eyes. J Cataract Refract Surg. 2003;29(4):741–6.
7. 7th Prince A, Neumayer T, Buehl W, Kiss B, Sacu S, Drexler W, et al. influence of severity of nuclear cataract on optical biometry. J Cataract Refract Surg. 2006;32(7):1161–5.
8. Moshirfar M, Buckner B, Ronquillo YC, Hofstedt D. Biometry in cataract surgery: a review of the current literature. Curr Opin Ophthalmol. 2019;30(1):9–12.

9. Shammas HJ, Wetterwald N, Potvin R. New mode for measuring axial length with an optical low-coherence reflectometer in eyes with dense cataract. J Cataract Refract Surg. 2015;41 (7):1365–9.
10. 10th Brainwave N, Murphy S, Pimenides D, Maurino V, Findl O. Assessment of a new averaging algorithm to increase the sensitivity of axial eye length measurement with optical biometry in eyes with dense cataract. J Cataract Refract Surg. 2011;37(1):45–9.
11. Reitblat O, Levy A, Kleinmann G, Assia EI. Accuracy of intraocular lens power calculation using three optical biometry measurement devices: the OA-2000, Lenstar-LS900 and IOLMaster-500. 2018;32(7):1244–52.
12. 12th Hirnschall N, Varsits R, Doeller B, Findl O. Enhanced penetration for axial length measurement of eyes with dense cataracts using swept source optical coherence tomography: a consecutive observational study. Ophthalmol Ther. 2018;7(1):119–24.
13. Einan-Lifshitz A, Rozenberg A, Wang L, Koch DD, Shoshany N, Zadok D, et al. Accuracy and feasibility of axial length measurements by a new optical low-coherence reflectometry-based device in eyes with posterior subcapsular cataract. J Cataract Refract Surg. 2017;43(7):898–901.
14. Akman A, Asena L, Gungor SG. Evaluation and comparison of the new swept source OCT-based IOLMaster 700 with the IOLMaster 500. Br J Ophthalmol. 2016;100(9):1201–5.
15. Olsen T. Sources of error in intraocular lens power calculation. J Cataract Refract Surg. 1992;18(2):125–9.
16. Drexler W, Findl O, Menapace R, Rainer G, Vass C, Hitzenberger CK, et al. Partial coherence interferometry: a novel approach to biometry in cataract surgery. At J Ophthalmol. 1998;126 (4):524–34.
17. Kiss B, Findl O, Menapace R, Wirtitsch M, Petternel V, Drexler W, et al. Refractive outcome of cataract surgery using partial coherence interferometry and ultrasound biometry: clinical feasibility study of a commercial prototype II. J Cataract Refract Surg. 2002;28(2):230–4.
18. Fukuda S, Ueno Y, Fujita A, Mori H, Tasaki K, Murakami T, et al. Comparison of anterior segment and lens biometric measurements in patients with cataract. Graefes Arch Clin Exp Ophthalmol. 2020;258(1):137–46.
19. 19th Hitzenberger CK. Optical measurement of the axial eye length by laser Doppler interferometry. Invest Ophthalmol Vis Sci. 1991;32(3):616–24.
20. Nemeth J, Fekete O, Pesztenlehrer N. Optical and ultrasound measurement of axial length and anterior chamber depth for intraocular lens power calculation. J Cataract Refract Surg. 2003;29(1):85–8.

Intraocular Lens Calculation: Toric and Multifocal Intraocular Lenses

Nino Hirnschall and Oliver Findl

Introduction

The use of toric IOLs for corneal astigmatism has become the gold standard [1, 2]. Hoffmann et al. have shown that corneal astigmatism of 1.5 D and 2.0 D occurs in approximately 17% and 8% in the cataract population [3]. For the calculation of toric IOLs, the accurate measurement of the cornea plays a decisive role [4–6]. Therefore, it is strongly recommended to rely on different corneal measurement techniques.

Posterior Surface of the Cornea

The methods of measuring the cornea can be divided into two groups. Either only the front surface of the cornea is measured and the influence of the back surface of the cornea is estimated. This method includes, for example, keratometry (either from one ring, 2 rings or a telecentric figure [7]) and Placido disc-based procedures. In the second group, the back surface of the cornea (and the corneal thickness) is measured as well as the front surface. This measurement is quite susceptible to interference, however, so eye drops prior to the measurement should be avoided (except for artificial tears) [8]. Both methods have their advantages and disadvantages and the current recommendations from the literature are contradictory [9–11].

N. Hirnschall (✉)
Department of Ophthalmology and Optometry, Johannes Kepler University, Linz, Austria
e-mail: nino.hirnschall@kepleruniklinikum.at

O. Findl
VIROS-Vienna Institute for Research in Ocular Surgery, Hanusch Hospital, Vienna, Austria

M. Shajari et al. (eds.), *Cataract and Lens Surgery*,
https://doi.org/10.1007/978-3-031-05394-8_29

Estimation of the astigmatism of the posterior surface of the cornea is possible, because it shows an astigmatism with the rule in approximately 85% of all cases [12–14]. This results in the following important characteristic: if only the front surface of the cornea is measured and astigmatism with the rule is found, then the total astigmatism of the cornea is less than that measured on the front surface. This is because astigmatism with the rule on the front surface and negative astigmatism with the rule on the back surface of the cornea cancel [15]. Consequently, if the astigmatism is against the rule on the anterior surface of the cornea, the total astigmatism of the cornea is larger than measured purely from the anterior surface. It is important to note, however, that in the studies, a corneal posterior astigmatism was defined relatively generously (60°–120°) with the rule, but about 15% of the patients did not follow this pattern [13, 16].

Due to the different measurement methods, there are also different terms for how the refractive power of the cornea is represented. These terms include conventional keratometry (=simulated keratometry, or simK), true net power, total corneal refractive power and total keratometry (TK). Conventional keratometry (simK) is based on measuring the anterior corneal surface and the posterior corneal surface is calculated using a fixed ratio. The other terms measure the total cornea and indicate the refractive power in different ways. For example, true net power is a measurement of the corneal front and back surface and the refractive power is then calculated using Gaussian optics. Total corneal refractive power uses ray tracing using Snell's law to determine the total refractive power of the cornea. The TK value is a modified keratometry parameter that is used specifically for a biometric device and also describes the total corneal refractive power. The special feature of the TK value is that it can be directly transferred to any IOL formula without transversion [9].

All calculation models for toric IOLs, where the back surface of the cornea is estimated, could be replaced in the future as better measurement methods become available. For example, high-resolution OCT allow significantly better measurements compared to more conventional measurement techniques [5]. In the meantime, there are various OCT devices that can produce high-resolution corneal images (Anterion (Heidelberg Engineering, Germany) [17], Casia ss-1000 [5, 18] (Tomey, Japan), MS-39 (CSO, Italy)).

It is essential to always use at least 2, better 3, different measurement methods for the calculation of toric IOLs. There is no gold standard for the fusion of the different measurements. It is important to repeat the measurements in case of deviations and to choose undercorrection rather than overcorrection in case of doubt and, above all, to inform the patient if the different measurement methods differ. As already mentioned above, tomography also measures the back of the cornea and therefore a deviation from topographic methods should be expected. It should also be remembered that differences between different measurement methods often have a relevant impact on the quality of measurements, such as tear film problems, an irregular cornea or other problems.

Formulae for Toric IOLs

Toric IOL power calculation formulae vary depending on the method of measurement used for corneal measurement. Abulafia et al. [16] clearly showed that a pure measurement of the corneal anterior surface without estimating or measuring the posterior surface performs significantly worse. In the same study it was shown that the Abulafia-Koch formula (AK correction) can be used directly for most toric online calculators to achieve better post-operative toric refraction results (Fig. 1).

An important point is that it would be a mistake to measure and additionally estimate the posterior corneal surface, as otherwise the posterior corneal surface would be included twice in the formula. This has to be taken into account, especially with the companies' online calculators.

Most companies that offer toric IOLs have recently adapted their online calculators and offer a correction method for the posterior surface of the cornea. In most cases the AK (Abulafia, Koch [16]) correction (formerly Baylor Nomogram) is applied to estimate the influence of the posterior surface of the cornea.

Alternatively, the Barrett Toric Calculator on the APACRS website or on the ASCRS website can be used (Fig. 2). This calculator uses a very similar concept, is not a correction option for existing other formulae, but rather an independent formula. In the meantime, the Barrett calculator has also integrated the function of using the measured corneal back surface.

Another alternative is the EVO calculator, which also offers a calculation of toric IOLs. One advantage of this calculator is that it also offers a calculation of toric IOLs after myopic LASIK/PRK.

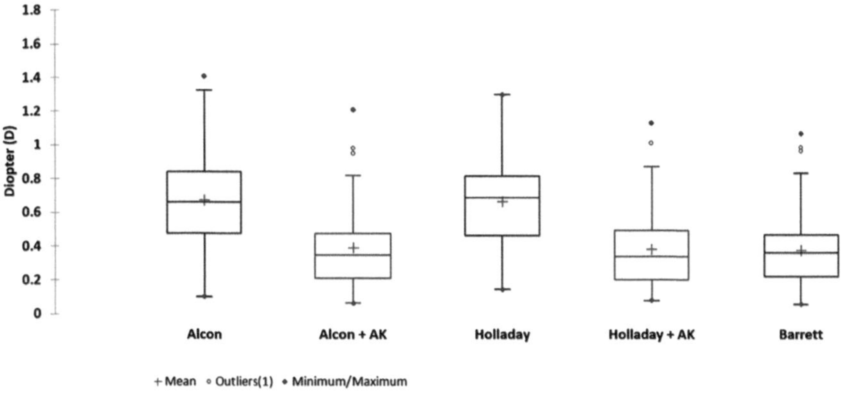

Fig. 1 Abulafia et al. [16] have developed the Abulafia-Koch formula (AK correction). The aim of this correction is to estimate the influence of the posterior corneal surface and to correct the resulting error

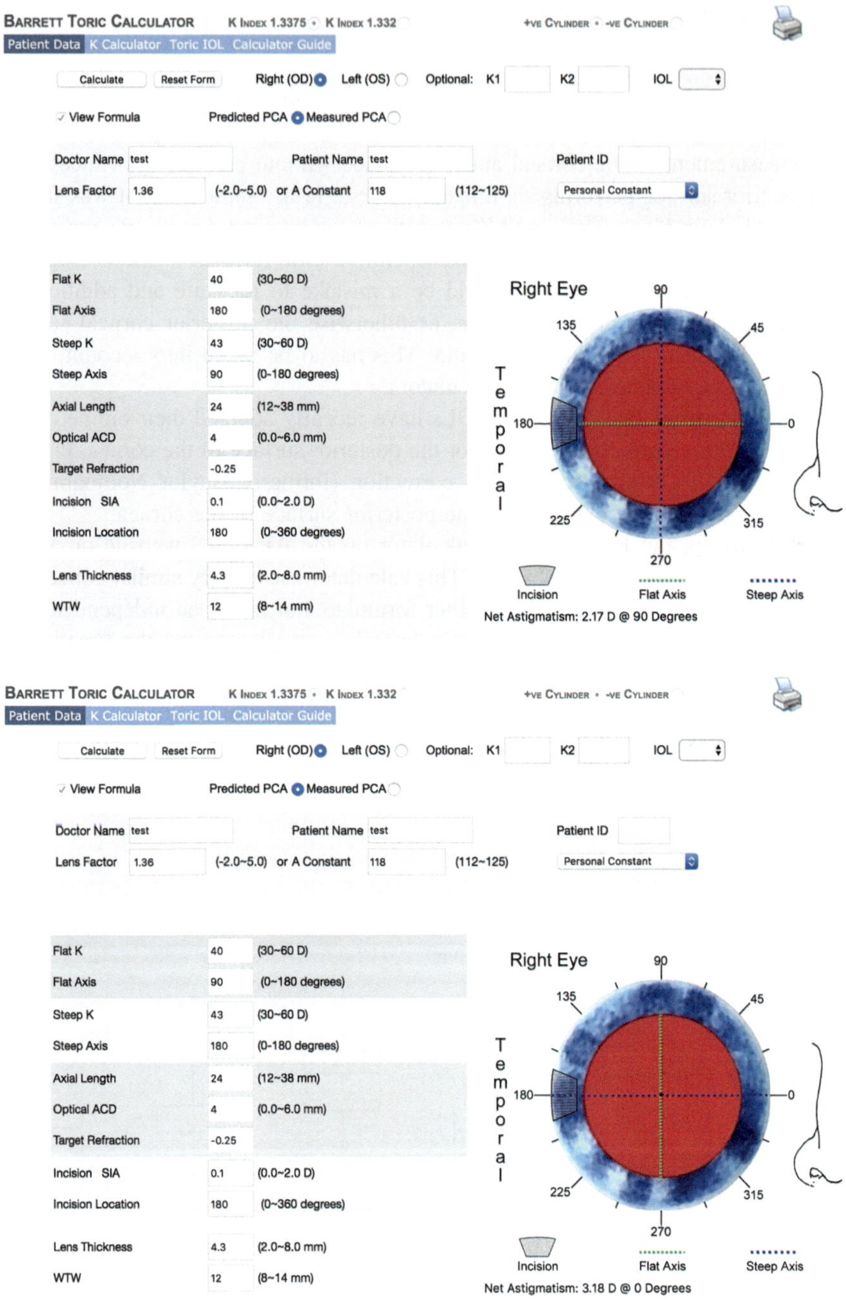

Fig. 2 Barrett Toric calculator. **a** shows a 3 D astigmatism of the corneal anterior surface with the rule (90°). However, due to the influence of the posterior corneal surface, the total corneal astigmatism is only 2.17 D (bottom left in the figure). In **b** the same data are used, only the astigmatism of the anterior surface is now against the rule (180° instead of 90°). The total corneal astigmatism has increased to 3.18 D

Finally, ray tracing concepts are also useful to calculate toric IOLs [19–21]. Ray tracing concepts are especially relevant for cases after refractive surgery, or if IOL tilt should be included in the calculation [22]. Another important advantage of ray tracing is that irregular astigmatism can be better calculated and corrected.

Author's recommendation

From our point of view, it is essential to measure the back surface of the cornea with a modern measurement technique, such as OCT. On the one hand, this is to exclude anticipated corneal ectasia, and on the other hand, to determine the orientation and extent of astigmatism of the corneal surface. In cases where the posterior corneal surface has a classical orientation with the rule, estimation methods (AK correction, Barrett toric calculator) can be used, in all other cases it is better to use the measured value and choose a formula where the measured posterior corneal surface can also be used.

References

1. Visser N, Beckers HJ, Bauer NJ, Gast ST, Zijlmans BL, Berenschot TT, et al. Toric vs aspherical control intraocular lenses in patients with cataract and corneal astigmatism: a randomised clinical trial. JAMA Ophthalmol. 2014;132(12):1462–8.
2. Cohen T, Klaproth OK. Correction of astigmatism during cataract surgery. Klin Monbl Ophthalmol. 2009;226(8):596–604.
3. Hoffmann PC, Hutz WW. Analysis of biometry and prevalence data for corneal astigmatism in 23,239 eyes. J Cataract Refract Surg. 2010;36(9):1479–85.
4. Brain Sound N, Hoffmann PC, Draschl P, Maedel S, Findl O. Evaluation of factors influencing the remaining astigmatism after toric intraocular lens implantation. J Refract Surg. 2014;30(6):394–400.
5. Hoffmann PC, Abraham M, Hirnschall N, Findl O. Prediction of residual astigmatism after cataract surgery using swept source Fourier domain optical coherence tomography. Curr Eye Res. 2014;39(12):1178–86.
6. Norrby S, Hirnschall N, Nishi Y, Findl O. Fluctuations in corneal curvature limit predictability of intraocular lens power calculations. J Cataract Refract Surg. 2013;39(2):174–9.
7. Shajari M, Cremonese C, Petermann K, Singh P, Muller M, Kohnen T. Comparison of axial length, corneal curvature, and anterior chamber depth measurements of 2 recently introduced devices to a known biometer. At J Ophthalmol. 2017;178:58–64.
8. Brain sound N, Crnej A, Gangwani V, Findl O. Effect of fluorescein dye staining of the tear film on Scheimpflug measurements of central corneal thickness. Cornea. 2012;31(1):18–20.
9. Fabian E, Wehner W. Prediction accuracy of total keratometry compared to standard keratometry using different intraocular lens power formulae. J Refract Surg. 2019;35(6):362–8.
10. Ferreira TB, Ribeiro P, Ribeiro FJ, O'Neill JG. Comparison of methodologies using estimated or measured values of total corneal astigmatism for toric intraocular lens power calculation. J Refract Surg. 2017;33(12):794–800.
11. Fityo S, Buhren J, Shajari M, Kohnen T. Keratometry versus total corneal refractive power: analysis of measurement repeatability with 5 different devices in normal eyes with low astigmatism. J Cataract Refract Surg. 2016;42(4):569–76.
12. Koch DD, Ali SF, Weikert MP, Shirayama M, Jenkins R, Wang L. Contribution of posterior corneal astigmatism to total corneal astigmatism. J Cataract Refract Surg. 2012;38(12):2080–7.

13. Koch DD, Jenkins RB, Weikert MP, Yeu E, Wang L. Correcting astigmatism with toric intraocular lenses: effect of posterior corneal astigmatism. J Cataract Refract Surg. 2013;39 (12):1803–9.
14. Core C, Cortum K, Muller M, Kampik A, Priglinger S, Mayer WJ. Comparison of two toric IOL calculation methods. J Ophthalmol. 2018;2018:2840246.
15. Abulafia A, Barrett GD, Kleinmann G, Ofir S, Levy A, Marcovich AL, et al. Prediction of refractive outcomes with toric intraocular lens implantation. J Cataract Refract Surg. 2015;41 (5):936–44.
16. Abulafia A, Koch DD, Wang L, Hill WE, Assia EI, Franchina M, et al. New regression formula for toric intraocular lens calculations. J Cataract Refract Surg. 2016;42(5):663–71.
17. Asam JS, Polzer M, Tafreshi A, Hirnschall N, Findl O. Anterior segment OCT. In: Bille JF, editor. High resolution imaging in microscopy and ophthalmology: new frontiers in biomedical optics. Cham (CH);2019. pp. 285–99.
18. Fukuda S, Ueno Y, Fujita A, Mori H, Tasaki K, Murakami T, et al. Comparison of anterior segment and lens biometric measurements in patients with cataract. Graefes Arch Clin Exp Ophthalmol. 2020;258(1):137–46.
19. de Sanctis U, Donna P, Penna RR, Calastri MI, Eandi CM. Corneal astigmatism measurement by ray tracing versus anterior surface-based keratometry in candidates for toric intraocular lens implantation. At J Ophthalmol. 2017;177:1–8.
20. Hoffmann PC, election J, Hutz WW, Preussner PR. A ray tracing approach to calculate toric intraocular lenses. J Refract Surg. 2013;29(6):402–8.
21. Hirnschall N, Buehren T, Trost M, Findl O. Pilot evaluation of refractive prediction errors associated with a new method for ray-tracing-based intraocular lens power calculation. J Cataract Refract Surg. 2019;45(6):738–44.
22. Brain sound N, Buehren T, Bajramovic F, Trost M, Teuber T, Findl O. Prediction of postoperative intraocular lens tilt using swept-source optical coherence tomography. J Cataract Refract Surg. 2017;43(6):732–6.

Multifocal Intraocular Lens

Annika Müller-Kassner and Kleopatra Varna-Tigka

The selection of a suitable formula for the calculation of multifocal intraocular lenses (IOLs) is of great importance in achieving the desired spectacle independence. Due to high visual demands on the postoperative result, residual refractive errors should be avoided as far as possible as this is the most common cause of dissatisfaction after multifocal lens implantation. The postoperative refraction should generally be targeted to the lowest positive refraction value.

Our working group retrospectively compared nine formulae of the 3rd and 4th generation to calculate a multifocal IOL. A significant difference in the formulas regarding absolute predictive errors could be shown ($p < 0.001$). The Barrett Universal II-, the Hill RBF- and the Olsen formula showed the smallest refractive prediction errors [1]. In a study by Raufi et al., the Barrett Universal II- and Hill RBF-formulas similarly showed the smallest absolute errors. 84%, respectively 83% of the patients were within ±0.5 D of the predicted spherical equivalent [2]. The Barrett Universal II-formula belongs to the vergence-based formulas and takes 5 variables into account for calculation. The Olsen-formula is based on a theoretical physical concept called "ray tracing". The Hill RBF-formula belongs to a newer generation of formulas based on large databases, artificial intelligence and complex statistical models [3].

Secondly, in addition to the selection of the IOL, the corneal topography should be analysed preoperatively to plan astigmatism reducing incisions. Incisions made orthogonally to the steep meridian of the cornea lead to a so-called "coupling effect", where the steep meridian is flattened, and the flat meridian is raised. In a prospective, randomized study, Ren et al. investigated the influence of "single clear corneal incisions (SCCI) and "opposite clear corneal incisions" (OCCI) of different

A. Müller-Kassner · K. Varna-Tigka (✉)
Department of Ophthalmology, Goethe-Universität, Frankfurt, Germany
e-mail: kleopatra.varna-tigka@kgu.de

A. Müller-Kassner
e-mail: annikamaria.mueller-kassner@kgu.de

M. Shajari et al. (eds.), *Cataract and Lens Surgery*,
https://doi.org/10.1007/978-3-031-05394-8_30

sizes on preoperatively existing astigmatisms ≥ 0.75 D. The largest reduction was achieved with 3.0 mm OCCIs [4].

Lastly, a preoperative examination of the angle kappa is recommended to avoid optical phenomena. If this angle is increased, light rays of an object are pictured parafoveally, and thus cause glare and halos. In a prospective study by Prakash et al., a relationship between a high angle kappa and increased optical phenomena after implantation of multifocal IOLs could be shown [5]. In 2015, Karhanová et al. showed the dependence of the angle kappa on the effective lens position and the refractive power of the cornea using a theoretical model and defined a combination of a flat anterior chamber and a higher angle kappa to be a risk combination for optical phenomena [6].

Conclusion

For the calculation of multifocal IOLs, the Barrett Universal II-, the Hill RBF- and the Olsen-formula formula show good results in terms of low refractive prediction errors. In general, a comparison of results of different formulas is recommended, also with regard to a continuous new development and advancement of formulas. Accurate preoperative measurement, planning of astigmatism reducing incisions based on corneal topography and the observation of the angle kappa are essential for satisfactory postoperative results.

References

1. Shajari M, Kolb CM, Petermann K, Böhm M, Herzog M, de'Lorenzo N, Schönbrunn S, Kohnen T. Comparison of 9 modern intraocular lens power calculation formulas for a quadrifocal intraocular lens. J Cataract Refract Surg. 2018; 44:942–8.
2. Raufi N, James C, Kuo A, Vann R. Intraoperative aberrometry vs modern preoperative formulas in predicting intraocular lens power. J Cataract Refract Surg. 2020;46:857–61.
3. Koch DD, Hill W, Abulafia A, Wang L. Pursuing perfection in intraocular lens calculations: I. logical approach for classifying IOL calculation formulas. J Cataract Refract Surg. 2017;43:717–8.
4. Ren Y, Fang X, Fang A, Wang L, Jhanji V, Gong X. Phacoemulsification with 3.0 and 2.0 mm opposite clear corneal incisions for correction of corneal astigmatism. Cornea. 2019;38:1105–10.
5. Prakash G, Prakash DR, Agarwal A, Kumar DA, Agarwal A, Jacob S. Predictive factor and kappa angle analysis for visual satisfactions in patients with multifocal IOL implantation. Eye (Lond). 2011;25:1187–93.
6. Karhanova M, Pluhacek F, Mlcak P, Vlacil O, Sin M, Maresova K. The importance of angle kappa evaluation for implantation of diffractive multifocal intra-ocular lenses using pseudophakic eye model. Acta Ophthalmol. 2015;93:e123-128.

IOL Power Calculation for Secondary IOL Implantation

Vincent Qin

Alternative strategies for IOL implantation can be required in several different situations. Typical situations that require secondary lens implantation techniques include complicated cataract surgery with posterior capsular rupture (with or without remaining capsular support), post-trauma with loss of the lens, in congenital cataract surgery in children or infants, or during the course of an IOL exchange. IOL exchange, in turn, can occur for a number of reasons; incorrect IOL power/refractive surprise, IOL luxation, IOL opacification, dissatisfied patients with multifocal IOLs, IOL-induced endothelial decompensation, or any other cause of IOL-induced inflammatory response.

In these circumstances, the IOL often needs to be implanted somewhere other than in the capsular bag, as the capsular bag can be partially or completely absent or otherwise unreliable or unavailable. In these situations, there are 4 classical alternative lens implantation choices: sulcus-fixated IOLs, iris-fixated IOLs, scleral-fixated IOLs, and anterior chamber angle supported IOLs. In all four cases, the lens position of the IOL is not in the capsular bag anymore and this is a significant parameter change to the IOL calculation process, as the estimated lens position (ELP) is a crucial part of the equation. In all three cases, the IOL usually comes to lie more anteriorly when compared to a classic in-the-bag implant. As such, a lower IOL power, than that for the capsular bag is needed. The most frequent indication for alternative lens placement is the scenario of a capsular bag tear, where an in-the-bag implantation is not possible, but there is sufficient anterior capsular support. In these cases, a sulcus-fixated IOL is a simple solution and can

V. Qin (✉)
Université Catholique de Louvain, Ottignies-Louvain-la-Neuve, Belgium
e-mail: vincent.qin@live.be

M. Shajari et al. (eds.), *Cataract and Lens Surgery*,
https://doi.org/10.1007/978-3-031-05394-8_31

be used. If on the other hand, the capsular bag is completely absent or there is insufficient anterior capsular support, the IOL can either be fixated on the iris, on the sclera, or very rarely, put in the anterior chamber, supported by the angle.

Sulcus-Fixated IOLs

Sulcus implantation involves the placement of a 3-piece IOL directly into the space between the posterior iris and anterior capsule, the ciliary sulcus. This may or may not be augmented by a technique known as optic capture, where the optic of the lens is pushed through the anterior capsulorhexis and lies behind it, while the haptics remain in the sulcus. Optic capture usually confers an increased stability and a better centration of the IOL, while reducing the risk of postoperative vitreous prolapse. It also leads to a lower myopic shift, when compared to standard sulcus placement. Other variants of the optic capture exist, including placing the haptics in the sulcus and the optic behind the posterior rhexis (assuming there is one), placing the haptics in the bag and the optic behind the posterior rhexis, and "reverse optic capture" where the haptics are sited in the capsular bag and the optic is located in the sulcus (captured by the anterior capsulorhexis).

Every standard biometric IOL calculation formula can be used for secondary implantation in the sulcus. However, an important adaptation needs to be made: Standard biometric IOL calculation formulas calculate the lens power for in-the-bag implantation, so if a classic sulcus-fixated implantation is needed, the formulas cannot be used without adjustment. Rather, a reduction of the IOL power by 0.5D to 1D is needed to take into account the anterior shift of the IOL position (ELP). Not doing this and using the same IOL power proposed for in-the-bag placement will lead to probable postoperative myopia, as the lens position in the sulcus is anterior to the plane of the capsular bag. This has to be nuanced however: if one does a classic optic capture, with the IOL optic in the bag, then no lens power adjustment is needed and the original in-the-bag IOL power can be used, as the IOL plane is the same as a normal in-the-bag IOL.

It has also been shown that, depending on the axial length of the eye, the value of the adjustment can change. In hyperopic eyes with short axial lengths, and IOL powers >25D, the IOL power reduction needed is larger, and should be rather around 1-2D instead of 0.5-1D. It is also worth noting that, although every IOL calculation formula can be used for the IOL calculation, a modified Haigis formula has been shown in some studies to be the most accurate [1].

Iris-Fixated IOLs

In cases of insufficient capsular support, sulcus-fixated IOLs cannot be used and iris-fixated IOLs may be used for secondary implantation. Iris-claw IOLs (e.g. Artisan, Artiflex), can be placed on either the anterior or posterior surface of the iris, depending on the choice of the surgeon. The artisan is entirely composed of PMMA material and while it requires a larger incision, has a longer history of aphakia correction than the Artiflex model.

Fixation of the IOL posterior to the iris (retropupillary fixation) appears to result in less endothelial cell loss than pre-iris fixation, and thus could have less risk of corneal decompensation in the long term. As in the case of sulcus-fixated IOLs, iris-fixated IOLs are implanted in a plane anterior to the capsular bag, and there is an anterior shift of the IOL position and anterior iris attachment is even more anteriorly sited than retropupillary fixation. As such, the IOL power should be reduced compared to an in-the-bag implantation, otherwise a postoperative myopic shift could result. Most commercial biometers contain adapted IOL calculations for iris claw lenses for both anterior and posterior iris placement, deciding at the moment of surgery prone to error and is not advisable. It is safe to consider that the IOL power reduction should be around 1–1.5D. Formulas that have been specifically assessed in this regard are: Haigis, Holladay 1, SRK/T, although classic formula could achieve similar results. A mix-and-average approach is always safer than basing a decision on one formula alone.

Scleral-Fixated IOLs

As in the case of iris-fixated IOLs, insufficient capsular support can also orient the surgeon towards the use of a scleral-fixated IOL for secondary implantation. One reasonable approach is to consider scleral fixation as the preferred option when neither sufficient capsular bag support nor iris tissue can be used, as in cases of iris atrophy, trauma or uveitis. Scleral-fixated IOLs are also the implant of choice, should there be a high risk of corneal decompensation or a very shallow anterior chamber, which might preclude the use of an iris-fixated IOL as well. Scleral-fixated IOLs have achieved good visual outcome with relatively low complication rates.

Scleral IOLs may be fixated to the sclera either by sutureless or sutured techniques [2–7] . Different materials have been used for sutures, including: 10-0 or 9-0 polypropylene, 7-0 Gore-tex (CV-8) or 6-0 Prolene [8]. Sindal et al. Sutureless or sutured techniques do not appear to differ in terms of postoperative outcomes, visual results or complications. They are not without problems, however, and Hayashi et al. have shown that scleral-fixated IOLs exhibit more tilt and decentration than standard in-the-bag implantation. Matsuki et al. have shown that 4-haptic IOLs display more intraocular stability when compared to 2-haptic C loop IOLs.

In sutureless scleral-fixated IOLs, the scleral tunnel is prepared 1.5–2 mm behind the limbus (Scharioth technique) or a tunnel is created directly in the sclera using a needle (Yamane technique). For sutured scleral-fixated IOLs, the sclerotomy sites are placed either 2 or 3 mm posterior to the limbus. It has been shown that in IOL calculation, the postoperative myopia shift is greater when the sclerotomy sites are placed 2 mm posterior to the limbus than when the sclerotomy is performed 3 mm posterior to the limbus [9].

Regarding IOL calculation for scleral-fixated IOLs, few studies have been conducted. Botsford et al. have shown that classic IOL calculation formulas were relatively equivalent, with no significant difference between Barrett, HofferQ, SRK/T and Holladay2. Haigis showed a statistically higher error rate. Similarly, McMillin and colleagues found that Refractive outcomes of the Yamane technique were less predictable than those of standard cataract surgery with all formulae (Barrett Universal II, Holladay 1, Hoffer Q, SRK/T) leading to a hyperopic arithmetic refractive prediction error in average [10].

References

1. Eom Y, Song JS, Kim HM. Modified Haigis formula effective lens position equation for ciliary sulcus-implanted intraocular lenses. Am J Ophthalmol. 2016;161(142–49):e1-2. https://doi.org/10.1016/j.ajo.2015.09.040.
2. Barca F, Caporossi T, de Angelis L, Giansanti F, Savastano A, Di Leo L, et al. Sutureless scleral fixation using Carlevale lens: surgical and refractive outcomes. J Cataract Refract Surg. 2020. https://doi.org/10.1097/j.jcrs.0000000000000135.
3. Barca F, Caporossi T, de Angelis L, Giansanti F, Savastano A, Di Leo L, et al. Trans-scleral plugs fixated IOL: a new paradigm for sutureless scleral fixation. J Cataract Refract Surg. 2020;46(5):716–20. https://doi.org/10.1097/j.jcrs.0000000000000135.
4. Boral SK, Agarwal D. A simple modified way of glueless sutureless scleral fixation of IOL—a retrospective case series. Am J Ophthalmol. 2020. https://doi.org/10.1016/j.ajo.2020.03.021.
5. Dimopoulos S, Dimopoulos V, Blumenstock G, Trevino-Rodriguez H, Bartz-Schmidt KU, Spitzer MS, et al. Long-term outcome of scleral-fixated posterior chamber intraocular lens implantation with the knotless Z-suture technique. J Cataract Refract Surg. 2018;44(2):182–5. https://doi.org/10.1016/j.jcrs.2017.11.009.
6. Veritti D, Grego L, Samassa F, Sarao V, Lanzetta P. Scleral fixation of a single-piece foldable acrylic IOL through a 1.80 mm corneal incision. J Cataract Refract Surg 2020; 46(5):662–666. https://doi.org/10.1097/j.jcrs.0000000000000138.
7. Yamane S, Inoue M, Arakawa A, Kadonosono K. Sutureless 27-gauge needle-guided intrascleral intraocular lens implantation with lamellar scleral dissection. Ophthalmology. 2014;121(1):61–6. https://doi.org/10.1016/j.ophtha.2013.08.043.
8. Stem MS, Todorich B, Woodward MA, Hsu J, Wolfe JD. Scleral-fixated intraocular lenses: past and present. J Vitreoretin Dis. 2017;1(2):144–52. https://doi.org/10.1177/2474126417690650.
9. Su D, Stephens JD, Obeid A, Borkar D, Storey PP, Khan MA, et al. Refractive outcomes after pars plana vitrectomy and scleral fixated intraocular lens with Gore-Tex suture. Ophthalmol Retina. 2019;3(7):548–52. https://doi.org/10.1016/j.oret.2019.02.012.
10. McMillin J, Wang L, Wang MY, Al-Mohtaseb Z, Khandelwal S, Weikert M, Hamill MB. Accuracy of intraocular lens calculation formulas for flanged intrascleral intraocular lens fixation with double-needle technique. J Cataract Refract Surg. 2021;47(7):855–8. https://doi.org/10.1097/j.jcrs.0000000000000540 PMID: 33315743.

IOL Power Calculation After Refractive Surgery

Giacomo Savini and Kenneth J. Hoffer

The calculation of intraocular lens (IOL) power in eyes with prior corneal refractive surgery has remarkably improved over the last decade and is now approaching the accuracy of unoperated eyes, with about 70% of eyes showing a prediction error (PE) within ±0.50 diopters (D) [1–8]. These results can be obtained using a combination of the latest generation technologies and the best formulas. Moreover, historical clinical data—such as the pre-refractive surgery keratometry and the laser-induced refractive change—can still provide an advantage, on the condition they are reliable.

To select the most appropriate methods and achieve the best outcomes it is recommended to understand the reasons why "standard" IOL power calculation fails after corneal refractive surgery. Knowing the sources of error helps, in fact, to find the solution.

Why Does "Standard" IOL Power Calculation Fail After Corneal Refractive Surgery?

Excimer laser surgery

There are three sources of error [9, 10]:

G. Savini (✉)
Studio Oculistico D'azeglio, Bologna, Italy
e-mail: dr.giacomo.savini@gmail.com

G. Savini
G.B. Bietti Foundation I.R.C.C.S, Rome, Italy

K. J. Hoffer
Stein Eye Institute, University of California, Los Angeles, CA, USA
e-mail: khoffermd@startmail.com

St. Mary's Eye Center, Santa Monica, CA, USA

M. Shajari et al. (eds.), *Cataract and Lens Surgery*,
https://doi.org/10.1007/978-3-031-05394-8_32

(1) **The Keratometric Index Error**. Keratometers and corneal topographers adopt a fictitious keratometric irefractive index (in most cases 1.3375) to calculate the total corneal power from the measured radius of the anterior corneal surface. The corneal power is obtained by means of the following formula:

$$P = (n - 1)/r$$

where P is the corneal power (in D), n is the keratometric index of refraction and r is the anterior corneal radius (in meters). The 1.3375 index is not the "real" corneal refractive index, but is rather an arbitrary value enabling a conversion a corneal radius of 7.5 mm into a corneal power of 45 D [11]. It relies on the assumption that the ratio between the anterior and posterior corneal surfaces is constant. Since corneal refractive surgery fundamentally disrpupts this ratio, the keratometric refractive index becomes invalid and leads to corneal power overestimation and subsequent IOL power underestimation in previously myopic eyes [12–16]. The opposite occurs in eyes with a previous hyperopic correction [17].

(2) **The Radius Error**. All instruments extrapolate the central corneal curvature from paracentral measurements. In cases of small or decentered optical zones, it is likely that the curvature of the paracentral and central areas are different, so that keratometers and corneal topographers measure a value that is steeper, with respect to the central corneal region. We previously reported that this error is negligible when the optical zone is equal to or larger than 6 mm [18].

(3) **The Formula Error**. Traditional thin-lens formulas (Hoffer Q, Holladay 1 and SRK/T) [19–21] as well as more recent formulas (e.g. Barrett Universal II) use the corneal power to estimate the effective lens position (ELP). Since myopic excimer laser flattens the cornea, the ELP is artificially underestimated, which further contributes to IOL power underestimation. Again, the opposite occurs after hyperopic surgery. The formula error can be solved by the Aramberri Double-K method, which uses two K-values: the pre-refractive surgery K to calculate the ELP and the post-refractive surgery K for the vergence formula [22]. The Haigis formula, [23] which uses the anterior chamber depth (ACD, measured from corneal epithelium to lens) instead of the corneal power to estimate the ELP, is an alternative solution.

Incisional surgery

Radial keratotomy (RK) induces a stronger flattening effect on the posterior surface than the anterior corneal surface, so that RK eyes are also significantly affected by the keratometric index error [24]. In addition, eyes with previous RK typically have small optical zones and are very likely to suffer from the radius error as well. As a consequence, corneal power can be overestimated and IOL power underestimated, with subsequent postoperative hyperopia [25–27]. The unpredictability of IOL power calculation after RK is further worsened due to the mechanical instability of the cornea immediately following the cataract surgery.

How Can We Calculate IOL Power After Lasik And PRK?

(A) NO-HISTORY METHODS

The pre-LASIK/PRK keratometry and the surgically induced refractive change are often not available, so No-History methods often represent the only solution for many eyes.

Barrett True-K No History formula

The "basic" version of Barrett's True-K formula works without historical data and is available on most optical biometers as well as on the website of the Asia–Pacific Association of Cataract and Refractive Surgeons (www.apacrs.org). The results are quite good (56 to 63% of eyes with a PE within ± 0.50 D, [8, 28, 29] and can be improved by adding the posterior corneal curvature (up to 70% of eyes with a PE within ± 0.50 D) [8, 28, 30] Compared to other No-History formulas, it is the most accurate solution when the axial length (AL) is shorter than 28 mm [31].

Haigis-L formula

This formula is based on the regular Haigis formula [10, 23] and adopts a correlation to compensate for the radius and keratometric index errors. The results reported have been satisfactory (34 to 61% of eyes with a PE within ± 0.50 D), with a trend towards myopic outcomes [10, 28–32]. It is available on the IOLMaster 500 and 700 (Carl Zeiss Meditec, Jena, Germany) and on the ASCRS website (https://ascrs.org/tools/post-refractive-iol-calculator).

Haigis formula + Total Keratometry

Total Keratometry (TK) is a new calculation method of total corneal power developed by Zeiss using the swept-source OCT measurements of the anterior and posterior corneal curvature provided by the IOLMaster 700. It has two advantages: (1) it does not suffer from the keratometric index error and (2) it can be entered into standard IOL power formulas without changing the constants, because its values are adjusted to match, on average, those by standard keratometry in unoperated eyes [33, 34]. After myopic LASIK or PRK, TK is lower than standard keratometry [34]. When entered into the Haigis formula, TK can lead to results (58 to 64% of eyes with a PE within ± 0.50 D) that are equal to or better than those obtained by the Haigis-L and Barrett True-K No-History formulas [30, 31].

Intraoperative Aberrometry

Based on the concept of the aphakic refraction technique, [35] intraoperative aberrometry (Ora System, Alcon, Fort Worth, TX) is a technology that can calculate the IOL power in the operating room once the crystalline lens has been extracted. It measures the intraoperative wavefront aberrometry and enables real-time IOL power calculations. Satisfactory results have been reported, though with no pronounced advantages, however, compared to other formulae [36, 37].

Ray-Tracing

With respect to most IOL formulas, ray-tracing is a thick-lens approach that calculates the refraction of rays at each optical surface from the tear film to the retina, based on Snell's law. It does not suffer from the keratometric index error, the radius error and the formula error; in addition, ray-tracing does not need any historical data and can include corneal aberrations in IOL power calculation [38]. Many studies have reported good outcomes in eyes with previous excimer laser surgery [6, 39–41]. Those commercially available include Okulix and Phaco-Optics, [42, 43] which support exact ray-tracing and can be applied to many instruments, and the internal software of the Sirius Scheimpflug camera and the MS-39 anterior segment OCT. More than 70% of eyes can obtain a PE within ±0.50 D with solution.

Shammas-PL and PHL formulas (for previously myopic and hyperopic eyes)

These formulae adjust the corneal power by means of a published equation: Corneal power = 1.14 x Kpost −6.8, where Kpost is the post-refractive surgery average keratometry [44]. The adjusted corneal power value is entered into the Shammas formula, which does not require the Double-K solution as it does not estimate the ELP from keratometry [45]. Relatively good results (PE within ± 0.50 D in 46 to 60% of eyes) have been reported [5, 29, 46–48]. Compared to other No-History methods, the Shammas PL-formula achieved the highest accuracy in eyes longer than 30 mm [31]. A specific version (Shammas-PHL formula) can be used for eyes with previous hyperopic LASIK [49].

Triple-S Method (Seitz/Speicher/Savini) and Maloney's Method

The Triple-S adjusts the keratometric power by subtracting a mean value of 4.98 D from the anterior corneal power. Originally described as "separate consideration of anterior and posterior corneal curvature", [50] it has been reported as Seitz/Speicher/Savini for many years and has finally been abbreviated into Triple-S [7]. It does not require pre-LASIK/PRK keratometry, but the calculated corneal power has to be entered into either a Double-K formula or the Haigis formula. The results have been good, as the PE was within ± 0.50 D in 53 to 70% of eyes [5, 7, 31]. It has also been reported to be the best No-History formula in eyes with AL between 28 and 30 mm (compared to Barrett True-K, Haigis-L and Shammas PL) [31].

A similar option is Maloney's method. The main difference lies in the choice of the topographic value, which in Maloney's method is the single power at the center of the axial map and the mean posterior power (−4.90 D rather than -4.98D) [51].

(B) Methods Requiring Pre-Excimer Laser Data

Barrett True-K formula

The "history" version of the Barrett True-K formula requires the surgically induced refractive change and is more accurate for IOL power calculation with respect to the No-History version, as the PE is within ± 0.50 D in 64 to 67% of eyes [8, 28, 29]. Its results are further improved by adding the posterior corneal curvature data [8].

Masket Formula

In this formula (available at https://ascrs.org/tools/post-refractive-iol-calculator) the IOL power is calculated, as if the eye had not undergone previous excimer laser surgery, by means of the SRK/T (in the case of myopia) or the Hoffer Q formula (in the case of hyperopia). The values obtained are then adjusted according to the equation: IOL power adjustment = surgically induced refractive change x (−0.326) + 0.101. This value is added to the standard IOL power calculation in patients with previous myopic laser correction and subtracted in patients with previous hyperopic laser correction [52]. Accurate results have been reported by several studies, with up to more than 70% of eyes with a PE within ± 0.50 D [5, 28, 29, 46–48].

Savini's Method

With this method, the keratometric index of 1.3375 is decreased proportionally to the amount of myopic correction increases, according to the formula: Post-refractive surgery index of refraction = 1.338 + 0.0009856 x SIRC (surgically induced refractive change). With the adjusted keratometric index, the corneal power is recalculated [53]. This method provides accurate results when combined with the Double-K SRK/T formula, as the percentage of eyes with a PE within ± 0.50 D ranges between 64 and 73% [5–8, 47].

Methods Developed To Calculate IOL Power After RK

Fewer methods are available to calculate the IOL power in eyes that previously underwent RK. Using standard keratometric values leads to corneal power underestimation (and consequent myopic error after IOL implantation) because the keratometric index (1.3375) is altered in the opposite direction compared to myopic PRK and LASIK [24]. The corneal power underestimation may be compensated by the radius error caused by the small optical zone. However, in order to reduce the radius error, we recommended discarding SimK values and consider more central measurements of the corneal power [54–57]. These values should be entered into Double-K formulas. Alternative options that have been tested with similar results are Barrett True-K, Haigis formula with Total Keratometry, and intraoperative aberrometry [32, 58–60].

In conclusion, theoretically, ray-tracing is the best option for eyes with such irregular corneas, but so far there are is insufficient evidence to confirm this hypothesis.

References

1. Kane JX, Van Heerden A, Atik A, Petsoglou C. Intraocular lens power formula accuracy: comparison of 7 formulas. J Cataract Refract Surg. 2016;42:1490–500.
2. Liu J, Wang L, Chai F, Han Y, Qian S, Koch DD, Weikert MP. Comparison of intraocular lens power calculation formulas in Chinese eyes with axial myopia. J Cataract Refract Surg. 2019;45:725–31.

3. Rong X, He W, Zhu Q, Qian D, Lu Y, Zhu X. Intraocular lens power calculation in eyes with extreme myopia: comparison of Barrett Universal II, Haigis, and Olsen formulas. J Cataract Refract Surg. 2019;45:732–7.
4. Wang L, Cao D, Weikert MP, Koch DD. Calculation of axial length using a single group refractive index versus using different refractive indices for each ocular segment: theoretical study and refractive outcomes. Ophthalmology. 2019;126:663–70.
5. Savini G, Barboni P, Carbonelli M, Ducoli P, Hoffer KJ. Intraocular lens power calculation after myopic excimer laser surgery: selecting the best method using available clinical data. J Cataract Refract Surg. 2015;41:1880–8.
6. Savini G, Hoffer KJ, Schiano-Lomoriello D, Barboni P. Intraocular lens power calculation using a Placido disk-Scheimpflug tomographer in eyes that had previous myopic corneal excimer laser surgery. J Cataract Refract Surg. 2018;44:935–41.
7. Savini G, Hoffer KJ, Barboni P, Balducci N, Schiano-Lomoriello D. Validation of the SToP formula for calculating intraocular lens power in eyes with previous myopic excimer laser surgery. J Cataract Refract Surg. 2019;45:1562–7.
8. Savini G, Hoffer KJ, Barrett GD. Results of the Barrett True-K formula for IOL power calculation based on Scheimpflug camera measurements in eyes with previous myopic excimer laser surgery. J Cataract Refract Surg. 2020;46:1016–9.
9. Hoffer KJ. Intraocular lens power calculation after previous laser refractive surgery. J Cataract Refract Surg. 2009;35:759–65.
10. Haigis W. Intraocular lens calculation after refractive surgery for myopia: Haigis-L formula. J Cataract Refract Surg. 2008;34:1658–63.
11. Speicher L. Intra-ocular lens calculation status after corneal refractive surgery. Curr Opin Ophthalmol. 2001;12:17–29.
12. Odenthal MT, Eggink CA, Melles G, Pameyer JH, Geerards AJ, Beekhuis WH. Clinical and theoretical results of intraocular lens power calculation for cataract surgery after photorefractive keratectomy for myopia. Arch Ophthalmol. 2002;120:431–8.
13. Seitz B, Langenbucher A, Nguyen NX, Kus MM, Küchle M. Underestimation of intraocular lens power for cataract surgery after myopic photorefractive keratectomy. Ophthalmology. 1999;106:693–702.
14. Ladas JG, Boxer Wachler BL, Hunkeler JD, Durrie DS. Intraocular lens power calculations using corneal topography after photorefractive keratectomy. Am J Ophthalmol. 2001;132:254–5.
15. Feiz V, Mannis MJ, Garcia-Ferrer F, Kandavel G, Darlington JK, Kim E, et al. Intraocular lens power calculation after laser in situ keratomileusis for myopia and hyperopia: a standardized approach. Cornea. 2001;20:792–7.
16. Latkany RA, Chokshi AR, Speaker MG, Abramson J, Soloway BD, Yu G. Intraocular lens calculations after refractive surgery. J Cataract Refract Surg. 2005;31:562–70.
17. Wang L, Jackson DW, Koch DD. Methods of estimating corneal refractive power after hyperopic laser in situ keratomileusis. J Cataract Refract Surg. 2002;28:954–61.
18. Savini G, Carbonelli M, Barboni P, Hoffer KJ. Clinical relevance of radius of curvature error in corneal power measurements after excimer laser surgery. J Cataract Refract Surg. 2010;36:82–6.
19. Hoffer KJ. The Hoffer Q formula: a comparison of theoretic and regression formulas. J Cataract Refract Surg. 1993;19: 700:712. Errata: J Cataract Refract Surg. 1994:20: 677. J Cataract Refract Surg. 2007;33: 2–3.
20. Holladay JT, Prager TC, Chandler TY, Musgrove KH, Lewis JW, Ruiz RS. A three-part system for refining intraocular lens power calculations. J Cataract Refract Surg. 1988;14:17–24.
21. Retzlaff JA, Sanders DR, Kraff MC. Development of the SRK/T intraocular lens power calculation formula. J Cataract Refract Surg. 1990; 16: 333–340. Erratum: J Cataract Refract Surg. 1990);16: 528.
22. Aramberri J. Intraocular lens power calculation after corneal refractive surgery: double-K method. J Cataract Refr Surg. 2003;29:2063–8.

23. Haigis W, Lege B, Miller N, Schneider B. Comparison of immersion ultrasound biometry and partial coherence interferometry for intraocular lens calculation according to Haigis. Graefe's Arch Clin Exp Ophthalmol. 2000;238:765–73.
24. Camellin M, Savini G, Hoffer KJ, Carbonelli M, Barboni P. Scheimpflug camera measurement of anterior and posterior corneal curvature in eyes with previous radial keratotomy. J Refract Surg. 2012;28:275–9.
25. Chen L, Mannis MJ, Salz JJ, Garcia-Ferrer FJ, Ge J. Analysis of intraocular lens power calculation in post-radial keratotomy eyes. J Cataract Refract Surg. 2003;29:65–70.
26. Cellikol L, Pavlopoulos G, Weinstein B, Cellikol G, Feldman ST. Calculation of intraocular lens power after radial keratotomy with computerized videokeratography. Am J Ophthalmol. 1995;120:739–50.
27. Koch DD, Liu JF, Hyde LL, Rock RL, Emery JM. Refractive complications of cataract surgery after radial keratotomy. Am J Ophthalmol. 1989;108:676–82.
28. Abulafia A, Hill WE, Koch DD, Wang L, Barrett GD. Accuracy of the Barrett True-K formula for intraocular lens power prediction after laser in situ keratomileusis or photorefractive keratectomy for myopia. J Cataract Refract Surg. 2016;42:363–9.
29. Wang L, Tang M, Huang D, Weikert MP, Koch DD. Comparison of newer intraocular lens power calculation methods for eyes after corneal refractive surgery. Ophthalmology. 2015;122:2443–9.
30. Yeo K, Heng WJ, Pek D, Wong J, Fam HB. Accuracy of intraocular lens formulas using total keratometry in eyes with previous myopic laser refractive surgery. Eye (in press)
31. Whang WJ, Hoffer KJ, Kim SJ, Chung SSH, Savini G. Comparison of intraocular lens power formulas according to axial length after myopic corneal laser refractive surgery. J Cataract Refract Surg (in press)
32. Wang L, Spektor T, de Souza RG, Koch DD. Evaluation of total keratometry and its accuracy for intraocular lens power calculation in eyes after corneal refractive surgery. J Cataract Refract Surg. 2019;45:1416–21.
33. Srivannaboon S, Chirapapaisan C. Comparison of refractive outcomes using conventional keratometry or total keratometry for IOL power calculation in cataract surgery. Graefes Arch Clin Exp Ophthalmol. 2019;257:2677–82.
34. Savini G, Taroni L, Schiano-Lomoriello D, Hoffer KJ. Repeatability of total keratometry and standard keratometry by the IOLMaster 700 and comparison to total corneal astigmatism by Scheimfplug imaging. Eye. 2021;35:307–15.
35. Ianchulev T, Salz J, Hoffer K, et al. Intraoperative optical refractive biometry for intraocular lens power estimation without axial length and keratometry measurements. J Cataract Refract Surg. 2005;31:1530–6.
36. Ianchulev T, Hoffer KJ, Yoo SH, Chang DF, Breen M, Padrick T, Tran DB. Intraoperative refractive biometry for predicting intraocular lens power calculation after prior myopic refractive surgery. Ophthalmology. 2014;121:56–60.
37. Fram NR, Masket S, Wang L. Comparison of intraoperative aberrometry, OCT-based IOL formula, Haigis-L, and Masket formulae for IOL power calculation after laser vision correction. Ophthalmology. 2015;122:1096–101.
38. Canovas C, Abenza S, Alcon E, et al. Effect of corneal aberrations on intraocular lens power calculation. J Cataract Refract Surg. 2012;38:1325–32.
39. Rabsilber TM, Reuland AJ, Holzer MP, Auffarth GU. Intraocular lens power calculation using ray tracing following excimer laser surgery. Eye. 2007;21:697–701.
40. Jin H, Rabsilber T, Ehmer A, et al. Comparison of ray-tracing method and thin-lens formula in intraocular lens power calculations. J Cataract Refract Surg. 2009;35:650–62.
41. Savini G, Bedei A, Barboni P, Ducoli P, Hoffer KJ. Intraocular lens power calculation by ray-tracing after myopic excimer laser surgery. Am J Ophthalmol. 2014;157:150–3.
42. Preussner PR, Wahl J, Lahdo H, Dick B, Findl O. Ray tracing for intraocular lens calculation. J Cataract Refract Surg. 2002;28:1412–9.
43. Olsen T, Hoffmann P. C constant: new concept for ray tracing-assisted intraocular lens power calculation. J Cataract Refract Surg. 2014;40:764–73.

44. Shammas HJ, Shammas MC, Garabet A, Kim JH, Shammas A, LaBree L. Correcting the corneal power measurements for intraocular lens power calculations after myopic laser in situ keratomileusis. Am J Ophthalmol. 2003;136:426–32.
45. Shammas HJ, Shammas MC. No-history method of intraocular lens power calculation for cataract surgery after myopic laser in situ keratomileusis. J Cataract Refract Surg. 2007;33 (31):6.
46. McCarthy M, Gavanski GM, Paton KE, Holland SP. Intraocular lens power calculations after myopic laser refractive surgery: a comparison of methods in 173 eyes. Ophthalmology. 2011;118:940–4.
47. Savini G, Hoffer KJ, Carbonelli M, Barboni P. Intraocular lens power calculation after myopic excimer laser surgery: clinical comparison of published methods. J Cataract Refract Surg. 2010;36:1455–65.
48. Wang L, Hill WE, Koch DD. Evaluation of intraocular lens power prediction methods using the American society of cataract and refractive surgeons Post-Keratorefractive Intraocular lens power calculator. J Cataract Refract Surg. 2010;36:1466–73.
49. Shammas HJ, Shammas MC, Hill WE. Intraocular lens power calculation in eyes with previous hyperopic laser in situ keratomileusis. J Cataract Refract Surg. 2013;39:739–44.
50. Savini G, Barboni P, Zanini M. Intraocular lens power calculation after myopic refractive surgery: theoretical comparison of different methods. Ophthalmology. 2006;113:1271–82.
51. Wang L, Booth MA, Koch DD. Comparison of intraocular lens power calculation methods in eyes that have undergone LASIK. Ophthalmology. 2004;111:1825–31.
52. Masket S, Masket SE. Simple regression formula for intraocular lens power adjustment in eyes requiring cataract surgery after excimer laser photoablation. J Cataract Refract Surg. 2006;32:430–4.
53. Savini G, Barboni P, Zanini M. Correlation between attempted correction and keratometric refractive index after myopic excimer laser surgery. J Refract Surg. 2007;23:461–6.
54. Kim SH, Lee JH. Videokeratography to calculate intraocular lens power after radial keratotomy. J Refract Surg. 2004;20:284–6.
55. Packer M, Brown LK, Hoffman RS, Fine IH. Intraocular lens power calculation after incisional and thermal keratorefractive surgery. J Cataract Refract Surg. 2004;30:1430–4.
56. Maeda N, Klyce SD, Smolek MK, McDonald MB. Disparity between keratometry-style readings and corneal power within the pupil after refractive surgery for myopia. Cornea. 1997;16:517–24.
57. Awwad ST, Dwarakanathan S, Bowman W, et al. Intraocular lens power calculation after radial keratotomy: estimating the corneal power. J Cataract Refract Surg. 2007;33:1045–50.
58. Geggel HS. Intraocular lens power selection after radial keratotomy: topography, manual, and IOLMaster keratometry results using Haigis formulas. Ophthalmology. 2015;122:897–202.
59. Curado SX, Hida WT, Vilar CMC, Ordones VL, Chaves MAP, Tzelikis PF. Intraoperative aberrometry versus preoperative biometry for IOL power selection after radial keratotomy: a prospective study. J Refract Surg. 2019;35:656–61.
60. Dawson VJ, Patnaik JL, Ifantides C, Miller DC, Lynch AM, Christofer KL. Comparison of refractive prediction for intraoperative aberrometry and Barrett True K no history formula in cataract surgery patients with prior radial keratotomy. Acta Ophthalmol (in press).

IOL Calculation in Patients with Fuchs' Endothelial Dystrophy

Carolin Kolb-Wetterau and Mehdi Shajari

In eyes with Fuchs' endothelial dystrophy (FED), phacoemulsification with lens implantation can be performed before or after an endothelial keratoplasty or as a combined technique in an approach known as a triple-DMEK. The ratio of anterior to posterior corneal surface in these patients is typically very different to healthy eyes. Hence, ideally, the preoperative measurements for the IOL power calculation should include the posterior surface. It should be noted that calculations with TCRP instead of SimK values result in a myopic shift.

In FED, corneal edema leads to flattening of the back surface, resulting in a myopic shift. In addition, the refractive indices change due to the disordered arrangement of the corneal collagen fibrils. As a result, the accurate measurement of eyes is more difficult. In order to minimise error, it is reasonable to perform the measurements as late as possible during the course of the day and to apply hyperosmolar eye drops previously. Triple-DMEK is not recommended in the case of a pronounced cornea guttata, as central guttae lead to unreliable values.

An exact prediction of refractive changes by endothelial keratoplasty is not currently possible. The refractive power of the anterior corneal surface only decreases slightly, whereas the absolute value of the refractive power of the posterior surface increases and thus the TCRP decreases. Due to the corneal detumescence after endothelial keratoplasty there is usually a hyperopic shift. This is even more pronounced the thicker, i.e. more oedematous and decompensated, the cornea is prior to corneal transplantation, the greater is the ratio of the radius of the back to the front surface, and the higher is the posterior asphericity quotient (Q value), i.e. the flatter is the back surface. The sole consideration of corneal thickness or posterior corneal radius is not suitable for assessing the risk of a hyperopic shift [1].

C. Kolb-Wetterau (✉) · M. Shajari
Goethe University Frankfurt, Frankfurt, Germany
e-mail: carolin.kolb-wetterau@outlook.de

M. Shajari et al. (eds.), *Cataract and Lens Surgery*,
https://doi.org/10.1007/978-3-031-05394-8_33

In comparison to the Hoffer Q, Holladay I, and Haigis, calculations with the SRK/T and the use of K-values of the IOLMaster, i.e. without considering the posterior corneal surface, show the smallest deviations from ray-tracing based calculations (of the OKULIX software) which includes the corneal front and back surface [2]. However, there are currently no recommendations as to which formula leads to the best results.

Toric lenses can be implanted in selected cases of severe astigmatism. The unpredictable change in astigmatism caused by endothelial keratoplasty, especially in its orientation, should be taken into account [3].

Due to the rather poor predictability of the refractive outcome in patients with FED, the surgeon must choose individually whether first the lens should be exchanged, a DMEK or DSAEK should be done, or a triple-DMEK procedure would be the best choice. For example, in a patient with advanced corneal decompensation but only a mild cataract it is a reasonable approach to first perform DMEK and, after the corneal situation is stable, exchange the lens, as in a mild cataract the required ultrasound energy to remove the lens will be minimal and probably will not reduce the endothelial cell density significantly. On the other hand, if a patient has a very dense cataract but only mild corneal decompensation it is a better approach to first remove the lens and afterwards perform an endothelial keratoplasty to prevent corneal damage. A triple procedure is probably the best choice when the cataract and corneal decompensation is advanced and the patient is rather old or has a generally bad health condition and the number of surgeries should be reduced to the lowest number possible.

Author's recommendation

The following recommendations are suitable for reducing hyperopic errors during cataract surgery after or combined with DMEK:

- Due to the hyperopic shift after endothelial keratoplasty, a myopic outcome of -0.5 to -1.0 dpt should be targeted. The higher the preoperative posterior Q-value, the higher the risk of a hyperopic shift and the more myopic the target refraction should be chosen. It should be set slightly less if hyperosmolar eye drops were applied before the measurement.
- If surgery is indicated on both eyes, the calculation of the second eye can be based on the refractive results of the contralateral eye.
- Due to the overall poor predictability it is recommended to decide individually whether the DMEK or the lens exchange should be performed first or a triple-DMEK is the best choice.

References

1. Fritz M, Grewing V, Böhringer D, Lapp T, Maier P, Reinhard T, u. a. Avoiding hyperopic surprises after descemet membrane endothelial keratoplasty in Fuchs dystrophy eyes by assessing corneal shape. Am J Ophthalmol. 2019;197:1–6.
2. Alnawaiseh M, Zumhagen L, Rosentreter A, Eter N. Intraocular lens power calculation using standard formulas and ray tracing after DMEK in patients with Fuchs endothelial dystrophy. BMC Ophthalmol. 23. August 2017;17(1):152.
3. Shajari M, Kolb CM, Mayer WJ, Agha B, Steinwender G, Dirisamer M, u. a. Characteristics of preoperative and postoperative astigmatism in patients having Descemet membrane endothelial keratoplasty. J Cataract Refract Surg. Juli 2019;45(7):1001–6.

IOL Calculation in Patients with Keratectasia

Carolin Kolb-Wetterau and John Kanellopoulos

Idiopathic keratectasia is a commonly seen problem in refractive practices and refers most frequently to keratoconus (KC). Typical findings of keratoconus are progressive myopia and/or irregular astigmatism. Residual refractive errors and even refractive "surprises" after cataract surgery are common, as the cornea is irregular and conventional keratometry may not provide reliable values. In addition, the measured keratometry (K)-values and axial length (AL) often do not correspond to those at the effective optical axis, since the corneal apex is usually located inferiorly to the centre of the cornea.

The reliability of corneal measurements decreases further in cases of advanced KC. Stability in KC is therefore pivotal to obtain accurate IOL calculations. In some cases, preoperative crosslinking may be required to stabilize the disease prior to lens surgery. Scheimpflug-based corneal tomography devices, like the Pentacam, tend to measure lower K-values than optical biometry devices like the IOLMaster or Lenstar LS 900, that usually assess the central 2.8–3.2 mm of the cornea around the vertex [1]. Devices considering the anterior and posterior corneal surface curvature and thus keratometric power, like the Pentacam, are advised in order to better determine the total refractive power. An IOL calculation using the TCRP (total corneal refractive power) of the central 3 mm zone instead of the simulated K-values (SimK) may lead to a myopic shift. SimK-values that are only based on anterior surface measurements commonly overestimate the corneal refractive power. This is one reason for unpleasant "surprise" of hyperopic outcomes. For severe KC, a standard K-value of 43.25 dpt can be used for IOL power calculation instead of actual K-values.

The selection of a suitable calculation formula is also of importance. The HICSOAP software offers a Holladay II version especially for KC. However, it was shown to be inferior to the standard Holladay II formula. In addition, there is

C. Kolb-Wetterau (✉) · J. Kanellopoulos
Goethe University Frankfurt, Frankfurt, Germany
e-mail: carolin.kolb-wetterau@outlook.de

M. Shajari et al. (eds.), *Cataract and Lens Surgery*,
https://doi.org/10.1007/978-3-031-05394-8_34

also a version of the Kane formula modified for KC (Kane-KC) that also includes calculations of toric IOL (http://iolformula.com). The Kane-KC achieves better results in all stages of KC than the Hoffer Q, SRK/T, Holladay I and II, Haigis, Barrett Universal II, and Standard-Kane [2]. Alternatively, good results can also be obtained with the Barrett Universal II [1]. For long eyes in particular, the SRK/T is another option as it leads to a myopic shift at high K-values and AL. To a certain extent, this can compensate for the rather hyperopic outcome of KC patients [3]. Using the SRK/T, the following adjustments of the target refraction are recommended to correct errors in the prediction of the effective lens position: -0.75 to -1.5 dpt in stage II and -2.0 to -3.0 dpt in stage III of KC [2].

Another alternative in pursuit of an accurate refractive outcome may be an intraoperative refraction measurement, with the option of immediate lens exchange if warranted.

The lens design should also be chosen with care. Toric intraocular lenses have proven to be a good option for correcting regular astigmatism. In KC, however, astigmatism is often irregular and more difficult to correct. Difficulties arise both in IOL power calculation and in the axis positioning. Toric IOL are not recommended in situations where the patient intends to wear rigid contact lenses postoperatively, or when a keratoplasty might be necessary in the future. Higher order aberrations (HOA) can also be amplified, especially with multifocal lenses so they should be avoided in KC cases. The pinhole lens IC-8 may be another alternative especially in advanced cases and if an adjunct corneal transplant is not a realistic additional option for the specific patient, as it is suitable in order to reduce HOA and can improve central visual acuity [4].

Author's recommendation

The predictability of IOL power calculation in eyes with keratoconus is challenging. There is no consensus or distinct guidelines for the optimal preoperative measurement and calculation. Hyperopic errors, commonly encountered post-operatively, can be reduced by the following recommendations:

- The posterior corneal surface should be included in the measurement of the K-values. Central values within the optical axis should be used for IOL calculation.
- A myopic outcome should be targeted.
- The Kane-KC or Barrett Universal II currently appear to be the most accurate formulas.
- Toric lenses are only suitable in selected cases when the cornea is assessed as stable, the KC is mild to moderate and the measured astigmatism is rather regular with a similar corneal curvature in the upper and lower hemisphere within the central 3 mm zone.
- In very irregular corneas the pinhole lens may be another alternative especially if a corneal transplant is not a realistic additional option.

References

1. Wang KM, Jun AS, Ladas JG, Siddiqui AA, Woreta F, Srikumaran D. Accuracy of intraocular lens formulas in eyes with Keratoconus. Am J Ophthalmol. 2020;212:26–33.
2. Kane JX, Connell B, Yip H, McAlister JC, Beckingsale P, Snibson GR, u. a. Accuracy of intraocular lens power formulas modified for patients with Keratoconus. Ophthalmology. 9. April 2020;127(8):1037–42.
3. Savini G, Abbate R, Hoffer KJ, Mularoni A, Imburgia A, Avoni L, u. a. Intraocular lens power calculation in eyes with keratoconus. J Cataract Refract Surg. 2019;45(5):576–81.
4. Shajari M, Mackert MJ, Langer J, Kreutzer T, Wolf A, Kohnen T, u. a. Safety and efficacy of a small-aperture capsular bag-fixated intraocular lens in eyes with severe corneal irregularities. J Cataract Refract Surg. Februar 2020;46(2):188–92.

Planning Lens Calculation in Pediatric Cataract

Luc Van Os, Sorcha Ní Dhubhghaill, and Marie-José Tassignon

When performing cataract surgery in children, implanting an IOL is the silent wish of all pediatric cataract surgeons. A child provided with an IOL will be easier to manage during the postoperative visual rehabilitation than a child who is left aphakic. The reduced need for contact lens correction, improved comfort and image quality (even when some additional supplementary spectacle correction is required) will help to the goals of visual rehabilitation, provided the child does not develop posterior capsule opacification (PCO) during the follow-up. The largest group of children presenting with congenital cataract are newborns, requiring cataract surgery as soon as 2 to 3 months of age. Studies such as IATS and IOLunder2 have recently advised against IOL implantation in these very young children because of a higher risk of secondary surgery in pseudophakic children of a young age using a classic lens-in-the bag (LIB) IOL technique [1, 2].

When using classical LIB implants, these recommendations should be strictly followed because a classical LIBhas a diameter of 12 to 13 mm, which is extremely large for those small eyes. The authors have worked extensively on a novel technique since the late 1999s/early 2000s. This technique, called the Bag-In-the-Lens (BIL) technique (Fig. 1) uses an IOL of 7.5 mm in total width [3]. The IOL is not implanted in the capsular bag but rather is supported two matching diameter anterior and posterior capsulorhexes in the capsular bag. Recently, an entire book dedicated to this implantation technique has been published [4]. Motivated by the the very encouraging results in eyes of adults, the BIL implantation technique was then applied to younger patients with cataract; first in teenagers and toddlers and later in babies [5, 6].

The results of the clinical outcomes using this lens [7], as well as those published by Swedish [8, 9], German [10, 11], French [12] and Norwegian [13] pediatric cataract surgeons have demonstrated that, if the BIL is correctly implanted,, there is

L. Van Os · S. N. Dhubhghaill · M.-J. Tassignon (✉)
Antwerp University Hospital, Edegem, Belgium
e-mail: marie-jose.tassignon@uza.be

M. Shajari et al. (eds.), *Cataract and Lens Surgery*,
https://doi.org/10.1007/978-3-031-05394-8_35

Fig. 1 Bag-in-the-lens implant 8 years postoperative, surgery at 6 months of age

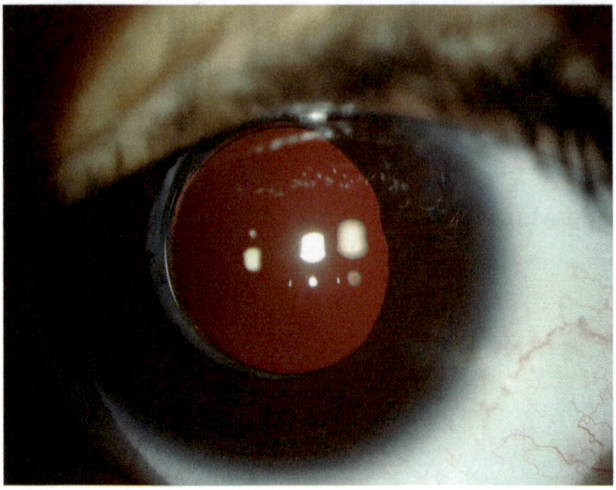

a very low rate of complications and need for secondary interventions. Pediatric cataract is a rare disease with a high potential for visual disability if not corrected on time. It is therefore particularly important to know and use the most suitable technique that allows immediate visual rehabilitation and reduces the need for repeated examinations under anaesthesia. Being the inventors of this technique, our surgical experience in pediatric cataract is primarily based on the use of the BIL. This chapter will therefore focus on our strategy in calculating the IOL power when using the BIL IOL device in childhood cataract.

In addition to the more complex the technical aspects of implanting an IOL in children, particular care should be taken to define the biometrical parameters of the child eye on which the calculation of the power of the IOL will be based. Firstly, it is not easy to obtain reliable measurements of the biometrical parameters of the eyes in young patients. The younger the child, the lesser the reliability. In contrast with adults or older children, in whom optical biometers can be used, small babies or children with an intellectual disability do not have the capacity to fixate long enough to allow capture of measurements. Biometry in these patients must therefore be performed under anaesthesia, using an A-scan for axial measurement and a hand-held keratometry device. For the A-scan, it is not always possible to measure along the exact optical axis of the eye and, when using the contact method (if an immersion-based device is not available) care should be taken not to push on the cornea. Contact measurements depend on the expertise of the surgeon/ nurse/ technician performing them. When using an immersion probe, contact with the eye is avoided but orientation of the measurement can be even more difficult to define. In the authors opinion, the axis of measurement is extremely important, we prefer to use the contact A-scan. In small eyes, the A-scan is frequently unable to automatically recognize the anatomical landmarks. The manual mode, therefore, should be used in these eyes, which might result in a lower degree of measurement accuracy.

When performing keratometry, care should be taken to perform the measurement as well centered as possible and to avoid parallax measurements. In addition, care should be taken that the eye speculum is not exerting any pressure on the eye while measuring. It is also important not to forget about the potential impact of the surgery on these biometrical parameters. A good example is the centripetal forces exerted by retrolental fibrovascular membranes in primary fetal vitreous accounting for the very curved corneas measured preoperatively, which after dissection and cutting will gradually flatten. The degree of flattening can only be generally estimated preoperatively and included in the calculation strategy when choosing the IOL power. Secondly, a child's eye will continue to grow postoperatively, so the target of the IOL-calculation will have to take this expected growth into account. Some data on eye growth progression are available in the literature though they are not conclusive.

The SRK/T formula, which was considered in the IATS to be one of the more accurate formulas in children [14], is also our preferred formula to calculate the BIL power. We will discuss the different factors that are considered in this formula:

The effective lens position, reflected by the a-constant of the IOL is, in our experience, not extremely different from that of adult eyes, provided there is a normal anatomical development of the eye but as mentioned previously, abnormal anatomical variations are very prevalent in children presenting with cataract. For example, in anterior vitreolenticular interface dysgenesis (AVLID) [15] there might be a clearly defined and intact posterior capsule but a dysgenic anterior hyaloid (or vice versa). Both membranes may also show significant dysgenesis. When these structures that are so crucial in determining the lens position in the eye are abnormal, it is evident that the estimation of the final lens position will be extremely unpredictable and adds to the unpredictability of the balance of the relationship between corneal curvature and axial length growth.

The corneal curvature is steeper in babies. It will flatten in harmony with the elongation of the eye to obtain emmetropia by ageing. If both parameters evolve differently however, it will result in ametropia. As previously mentioned, normal eye growth will cause an increase of *the axial length*. However, postoperative intraocular hypertension adds to the natural and relatively rapid growth of the eye during the first year of age, which might result in quite important long term postoperative ametropia. It is thus important to differentiate the cause for the eye growth, especially in children younger than 1 year. The growth of the eye also slows down somewhat in the second year of life but will continue to progressively increase until the age of 7 to 10 years, at which normally emmetropia is reached.

It is not yet known whether the growth of pseudophakic eyes follows the same curves as normal eyes. To answer this question and evaluate the degree of evolution in eye growth in the phakic and pseudophakic eyes of children, a registry has been developed under the auspices of the ESCRS-EUREQUO platform. This registry, called the European Registry of Childhood Cataract (EuReCCa) is ready to be launched shortly and the authors of this chapter are actively involved in the development of this EuReCCa registry as such data will be essential in improving outcomes for children after cataract surgery. It is therefore evident that the selection of the IOL power is clearly much more complicated in children than in adults. The choice of the IOL power must be guided by the specific eye characteristics considering the underlying type of cataract as well as the specific age of the child at the time of surgery. Furthermore, in unilateral cases, care should be taken to avoid the induction of large anisometropia to help mitigate the inherent high risk for amblyopia.

The BIL has the enormous advantage over standard lenses in that while it not only prevents PCO (or visual axis re-opacification, VAR, in cases where a posterior capsulorhexis has been performed) it can also be easily explanted and exchanged, even may years after explantation [16]. This major advantage has allowed us to challenge the current paradigm on IOL calculation. However, in our series, BIL exchange has only rarely been required in children so far. When the biometric calculation results in an IOL power of over 30 diopters, we opt to implant a 30D IOL and to correct the remaining refraction error with a contact lens, or spectacles if the refraction error is reasonable, and the child's nose is sufficiently developed. We have adopted this rule for three reasons: firstly, the thickness of the IOL makes it more difficult to implant in these small eyes, secondly, to avoid myopic overcorrection with time, and thirdly to avoid spherical aberrations that are extremely prominent in high power IOLs and in addition may turn to coma aberrations in case of IOL decentration or tilt. For unilateral cataract in children under 6 years of age, we aim for a light hyperopia, depending on the refraction of the opposite eye. We strive to stay within a 2D difference between both eyes to minimize the amblyogenic anisometropia. For bilateral cataract in children under 6 years of age, we aim for hyperopia, decreasing with age. Over 6 years of age we aim for emmetropia, unless in cases of unilateral cataract with high ametropia where we aim for an aniseikonia of less than 5% between both eyes.

Case illustration

This case is one of a 10-month-old girl who underwent surgery for a unilateral cataract due to posterior lenticonus on the left eye. The axial length was 20.36 mm on the right eye and 19.57 mm on the left eye. The values for keratometry were as follows: right eye K1: 43.00 @ 13° - K2: 45.75 @ 103°, left eye K1: 41.12 @ 168° - K2: 43.12 @ 78°. Refraction of the right eye was + 2.25 (-1.25 @ 16°).

Because of the difference is axial length, a slightly more hyperopic target refraction was chosen for the left eye: + 4.5. Using the SRK/T formula, this resulted in the implantation of a Morcher 89A IOL of + 29.0 Diopters. The remaining refractive error (+4.5D) for the left eye was then corrected with a contact lens and occlusion therapy was started. Three months after the surgery, a switch was made to spectacle correction because the contact lens had to be replaced frequently due to spontaneous loss of the contact lens. Refraction of the left eye at that time was + 4.5 (-2.25 @ 175°). Over time, the hyperopia gradually decreased. At the most recent follow-up, the child was 5 years old and the refraction was + 0.75 (-0.50 @ 179°) on the right eye and + 0.25 (-2.75 @ 171°) on the operated left eye. Corrected distance acuity was 0.63 in both eyes using the Tumbling E-chart. The axial length was 22.25 mm on the right eye and 21.81 mm on the left eye. The values for keratometry were as follows: right eye K1: 42.27 @ 176° - K2: 43.22 @ 186°, left eye K1: 40.92 @ 174° - K2: 43.52 @ 84°.

Author's recommendation

For a detailed overview of the bag-in-the-lens IOL we recommend the book: "Innovative Implantation Technique: Bag-in-the-lens Cataract Surgery" (Springer).

References

1. Plager DA, Lynn MJ, Buckley EG, Wilson ME, Lambert SR. Infant Aphakia treatment study. Complications in the first 5 years following cataract surgery in infants with and without intraocular lens implantation in the Infant Aphakia Treatment Study. Am J Ophthalmol. 2014;(58):892–8.
2. Solebo AL, Cumberland P, Rahi JS. British Isles congenital cataract interest group. 5-year outcomes after primary intraocular lens implantation in children aged 2 years or younger with congenital or infantile cataract: findings from the IoLunder2 prospective inception cohort study. Lancet Child Adolesc Health. 2018 Dec;2(12):863–71. https://doi.org/10.1016/S2352-4642(18)30317-1. Epub 2018 Oct 31.
3. Tassignon MJ, De Groot V, Vrensen GF. Bag-in-the-lens implantation of intraocular lenses. J Cataract Refract Surg. 2002;28(7):1182–8.
4. Tassignon MJ, Ní Dhubhghaill S, Van Os L, eds. Innovative implantation technique—Bag-in-the-lens Cataract Surgery. 1st ed. Springer Nature Switzerland: 2019, ISBN 978-3-030-03085-8.
5. Tassignon MJ, De Veuster I, Godts D, Kosec D, Van den Dooren K, Gobin L. Bag-in-the-lens intraocular lens implantation in the pediatric eye. J Cataract Refract Surg. 2007;33(4):611–7.
6. Tassignon MJ, Gobin L, De Veuster I, Godts D. Advantages of the bag-in-the-lens intraocular lens in pediatric cataract surgery. J Fr Ophtalmol. 2009 Sep;32(7):481–7.
7. Van Looveren J, Ní Dhubhghaill S, Godts D, Bakker E, De Veuster I, Mathysen DG, Tassignon MJ. Pediatric bag-in-the-lens intraocular lens implantation: long-term follow-up. J Cataract Refract Surg. 2015;41(8):1685–92.
8. Nyström A, Almarzouki N, Magnusson G, Zetterberg M. Phacoemulsification and primary implantation with bag-in-the lens intraocular lens in children with unilateral and bilateral cataract. Acta Ophthalmol. 2018;96(4):364–70.
9. Nyström A, Magnusson G, Zetterberg M. Secondary glaucoma and visual outcome after paediatric cataract surgery with primary bag-in-the-lens intraocular lens. Acta Ophthalmol. 2020 May;98(3):296–304.
10. Lytvynchuk LM, Thiele MV, Schmidt W, Lorenz B. Precision of bag-in-the-lens intraocular lens power calculation in different age groups of pediatric cataract patients: report of the giessen pediatric cataract study group. J Cataract Refract Surg. 2019;45(10):1372–9.
11. Lytvynchuk LM, Thiele MV, Lorenz B. Analysis and management of intraoperative and early postoperative complications of bag-in-the-lens intraocular lens implantation in different age groups of paediatric cataract patients: report of the Giessen Paediatric Cataract Study Group. Acta Ophthalmol. 2020;98(2):e144–54.
12. Bailleul H. Rate of re-intervention in paediatric cataract surgery with the bag-in-the-lens fixation: ten years of experience. Poster at the 38th Meeting of ESCRS; 2020.

13. Nils-Erik Boonstra, Olav H Haugen; Bag-in-the-lens intraocular lens in paediatric cataract surgery: intraoperative and postoperative outcomes. Acta Ophthalmol. 2021 May https://doi.org/10.1111/aos.14878 (online ahead of print).
14. Vanderveen DK, Trivedi RH, Nizam A, Lynn MJ, Lambert SR; Infant Aphakia Treatment Study Group. Predictability of intraocular lens power calculation formulae in infantile eyes with unilateral congenital cataract: results from the Infant Aphakia Treatment Study. *Am J Ophthalmol.* 2013 Dec;156(6):1252–60.
15. Van Looveren J, Vael A, Ideler N, Sillen H, Mathysen D, Tassignon MJ. Influence of the vitreolenticular interface in pediatric cataract surgery. J Cataract Refract Surg. 2018 Oct;44(10):1203–10.
16. Ní Dhubhghaill S, Van Os L, De Keizer RJ, Taal M, Zakaria N, Tassignon MJ. Intraocular lens exchange technique for an opacified bag-in-the-lens. J Cataract Refract Surg. 2015 May;41(5):924–8.

IOL Calculation in Patients with Retinal Diseases

Efstathios Vounotrypidis

The correct calculation of intraocular lens (IOL) power in cataract surgery is essential for achieving a successful postoperative refractive and visual outcome. Cataract surgery is being increasingly performed combined with vitrectomy in the presence of retinal pathology. Both the high precision of lens power calculation using partial coherence interferometry (PCI) [1, 2] and the wide spectrum of biometric formulas lead to highly satisfying outcomes [3, 4]. Furthermore, implementing new biometric technologies offers even more precise calculation even in severely opacified lenses [5, 6].

There are many reasons to combine cataract surgery together with pars plana vitrectomy, especially in macular pathologies such as epiretinal membranes (ERM), macular holes (MF), or vitreomacular traction syndrome (VMTS), because a preexisting cataract may lead to increased difficulties during surgery by reduced retinal visualization [7]. Furthermore, the majority of eyes undergoing vitrectomy suffer from cataract formation in the first postoperative years [8]. It has also been proposed that cataract surgery is more complex in vitrectomized eyes because the capsular bag is significantly more mobile due to the lack of vitreous support. As a result, vitrectomized eyes have been shown to have a higher rate of complications, such as a dropped nucleus or retinal detachment [9]. Combining the two surgeries is also more time and cost effective [10] and avoiding a second surgical procedure (with its own risks) has led to the increasing popularity of the combined procedure approach. Overall, combined phacovitrectomy for cataract and retinal diseases offers numerous advantages. Recent technological advances such as microincision cataract surgery and small-gauge vitrectomy have further established phacovitrectomy as a safe and efficient surgical procedure [11, 12].

The calculation of IOL power in cataract surgery is very precise but may still be challenging in combined phacovitrectomy [13]. The vitreous removal affects the

E. Vounotrypidis (✉)
Department of Ophthalmology, University Clinic Ulm, Ulm, Germany
e-mail: efstathios.vounotrypidis@uni-ulm.de

M. Shajari et al. (eds.), *Cataract and Lens Surgery*,
https://doi.org/10.1007/978-3-031-05394-8_36

axial length (AL) and the expected postoperative position of the IOL. The reliability of biometric measurements is also decreased in maculopathies such as in advanced epiretinal gliosis [14]. Because of the clinical diversity of these cases, studies on the precision of IOL power calculation for phacovitrectomy have shown variable results so far [13, 15–19]. However, the use of new biometric devices, such as "swept-source" OCT-based biometry, has continued to increase the accuracy of IOL-power calculation in such surgeries and has shown better results compared to PCI biometry [17].

Despite the variable results published in the literature, this procedure offers high precision, especially in vitreomacular pathologies but there are cases where optical biometry may not be possible. This can occur in cases of vitreous hemorrhage or retinal detachment, for example. In the case of vitreous hemorrhage, measurement of the axial length is hardly possible due to the hemorrhage (opacity), whereas in the case of retinal detachment, the detached retina deceives the device and often reports a falsified shorter axial length [20–22]. In these cases, measurement of the axial length by means of ultrasound (preferably using an immersion technique) remains the most reliable option [23]. However, recent studies have shown that AL can be measured with latest biometric devices even in cases with dense vitreous hemorrhage [24].

In the case of retinal detachment with macular involvement, there are a number of options available to the surgeon, in addition to the use of ultrasound biometry. One is to manually adjust the AL determined by the PCI biometer, [25] or to use the measurements of the partner eye [26]. Nevertheless, the precision of AL measurement with US remains limited compared to PCI biometry or latest biometer used in a normal eye (swept-source OCT; OLCR) [27].

Regarding the refractive outcome after combined phacovitrectomy, numerous studies have been published and have shown a wide range of refractive results [7, 11, 13, 15, 16, 18, 19, 28–30]. Overall, it can be concluded that most studies have shown a tendency toward a postoperative myopic "shift." This occurs mainly in cases of retinal detachment, where the source of error is most often the incorrect (and inaccurate) measurement of AL performed with ultrasound [15]. However, recent studies have shown that the reproducibility of axial length two years after phacovitrectomy for retinal detachment is very high, and changes in anterior chamber depth or effective lens position also contribute in the residual refractive error [31].

It has been shown recently that gas tamponade in phacovitrectomy leads to anterior displacement of the IOL, whereas phacovitrectomy without gas tamponade does not lead to any IOL displacement, when compared with cataract surgery alone [32, 33]. Conversely, the use of a gas tamponade in phacovitrectomy did not lead to increased tilt or decentration of the IOL, [34] which would lead to higher refractive error. There was no significant difference in postoperative complication rate found between one- and three-piece intraocular lenses [35]. On the contrary, in another study, the haptics and the angulation of the IOL did seem to play a role on its anterior displacement after combined phacovitrectomy with gas tamponade [36].

The choice of the IOL model and its power is up to the surgeon, but we recommend a realistic discussion with the patient preoperatively, regarding expectations and rare complications like IOL opacification or calcification after phacovitrectomy or vitrectomy [37, 38]. Similarly, the choice of biometric formula is also individual. Most studies have published results based on SRK-T, Haigis, Holladay 1, or Holladay 2 formulae. Recently, eight formulas, including the newest formulae, such as Barrett, Kane, Hill-RBF were compared in the context of phacovitrectomy for ERM and cataract. All formulae showed equally good results, with the Kane formula being more accurate. Furthermore, it was shown that constant optimization for phacovitrectomy may be beneficial, particularly for patients undergoing combined procedures [39]. In cases of combined procedures with silicon oil removal and cataract surgery, the newest biometric formulas should be employed in order to achieve satisfactory refractive results [40]. Another large study showed comparable performance of the newest biometric formulas after cataract surgery in vitrectomized eyes, with no apparent effect of silicone oil tamponade on the prediction accuracy of the evaluated formulae, when using the IOLMaster 700 [41]. If the silicone oil fill cannot be removed, the surgeon should consider the implantation of a convex-plano monofocal polymethyl methacrylate or foldable hydrophobic acrylic IOL, with large optic diameter, to minimize possible long-term complications [42].

References

1. Drexler W, Findl O, Menapace R, Rainer G, Vass C, Hitzenberger CK, et al. Partial coherence interferometry: a novel approach to biometry in cataract surgery. At J Ophthalmol. 1998;126 (4):524–34.
2. Connors R 3rd, Boseman P 3rd, Olson RJ. Accuracy and reproducibility of biometry using partial coherence interferometry. J Cataract Refract Surg. 2002;28(2):235–8.
3. Narvaez J, Zimmerman G, Stulting RD, Chang DH. Accuracy of intraocular lens power prediction using the Hoffer Q, Holladay 1, Holladay 2, and SRK/T formulas. J Cataract Refract Surg. 2006;32(12):2050–3.
4. Melles RB, Holladay JT, Chang WJ. Accuracy of intraocular lens calculation formulas. Ophthalmology. 2018;125(2):169–78.
5. Brain Sound N, Varsits R, Doeller B, Findl O. Enhanced penetration for axial length measurement of eyes with dense cataracts using swept source optical coherence tomography: a consecutive observational study. Ophthalmol Ther. 2018;7(1):119–24.
6. Einan-Lifshitz A, Rozenberg A, Wang L, Koch DD, Shoshany N, Zadok D, et al. Accuracy and feasibility of axial length measurements by a new optical low-coherence reflectometry-based device in eyes with posterior subcapsular cataract. J Cataract Refract Surg. 2017;43(7):898–901.
7. Hamoudi H, La Cour M. Refractive changes after vitrectomy and phacovitrectomy for macular hole and epiretinal membrane. J Cataract Refract Surg. 2013;39(6):942–7.
8. Cherfan GM, Michels RG, de Bustros S, Enger C, Glaser BM. Nuclear sclerotic cataract after vitrectomy for idiopathic epiretinal membranes causing macular pucker. At J Ophthalmol. 1991;111(4):434–8.
9. Cole CJ, Charteris DG. Cataract extraction after retinal detachment repair by vitrectomy: visual outcome and complications. Eye (Lond). 2009;23(6):1377–81.

10. Seider MI, Michael Lahey J, Fellenbaum PS. Cost of phacovitrectomy versus vitrectomy and sequential phacoemulsification. Retina. 2014;34(6):1112–5.
11. Steel DH. Phacovitrectomy: expanding indications. J Cataract Refract Surg. 2007;33(6):933–6.
12. Oshima Y, Wakabayashi T, Sato T, Ohji M, Tano Y. A 27-gauge instrument system for transconjunctival sutureless microincision vitrectomy surgery. Ophthalmology. 2010;117 (1):93–102 e2.
13. van der Geest LJ, Siemerink MJ, Mura M, Mourits MP, Lapid-Gortzak R. Refractive outcomes after phacovitrectomy surgery. J Cataract Refract Surg. 2016;42(6):840–5.
14. Kojima T, Tamaoki A, Yoshida N, Kaga T, Suto C, Ichikawa K. Evaluation of axial length measurement of the eye using partial coherence interferometry and ultrasound in cases of macular disease. Ophthalmology. 2010;117(9):1750–4.
15. Shiraki N, Wakabayashi T, Sakaguchi H, Nishida K. Optical biometry-based intraocular lens calculation and refractive outcomes after Phacovitrectomy for rhegmatogenous retinal detachment and Epiretinal membrane. Sci Rep. 2018;8(1):11319.
16. Hamoudi H, Correll Christensen U, La Cour M. Epiretinal membrane surgery: an analysis of 2-step sequential- or combined phacovitrectomy surgery on refraction and macular anatomy in a prospective trial. Acta Ophthalmol. 2018;96(3):243–50.
17. Vounotrypidis E, Haralanova V, Muth DR, Wertheimer C, Shajari M, Wolf A, et al. Accuracy of SS-OCT biometry compared with partial coherence interferometry biometry for combined phacovitrectomy with internal limiting membrane peeling. J Cataract Refract Surg. 2019;45 (1):48–53.
18. Hotte GJ, de Bruyn DP, de Hoog J. Post-operative refractive prediction error after Phacovitrectomy: a retrospective study. Ophthalmol Ther. 2018;7(1):83–94.
19. Shi L, Chang JS, Suh LH, Chang S. Differences in Refractive Outcomes between Phacoemulsification for Cataract Alone and Combined Phacoemulsification and Vitrectomy for Epiretinal Membrane Retina. 2019;39(7):1410-5.
20. Pongsachareonnont P, Tangjanyatam S. Accuracy of axial length measurements obtained by optical biometry and acoustic biometry in rhegmatogenous retinal detachment: a prospective study. Clin Ophthalmol. 2018;12:973–80.
21. Abou-Shousha M, Helaly HA, Osman IM. The accuracy of axial length measurements in cases of macula-off retinal detachment. Can J Ophthalmol. 2016;51(2):108–12.
22. Lege BA, Haigis W. Laser interference biometry versus ultrasound biometry in certain clinical conditions. Graefes Arch Clin Exp Ophthalmol. 2004;242(1):8–12.
23. Olsen T, Nielsen PJ. Immersion versus contact technique in the measurement of axial length by ultrasound. Acta Ophthalmol (Copenh). 1989;67(1):101–2.
24. Wang Q, Huang Y, Gao R, Chen H, Song B, Tu R, et al. Axial length measurement and detection rates using a swept-source optical coherence tomography-based biometer in the presence of a dense vitreous hemorrhage. J Cataract Refract Surg. 2020;46(3):360–4.
25. Rahman R, Kolb S, Bong CX, Stephenson J. Accuracy of user-adjusted axial length measurements with optical biometry in eyes having combined phacovitrectomy for macular-off rhegmatogenous retinal detachment. J Cataract Refract Surg. 2016;42(7):1009–14.
26. El-Khayat AR, Brent AJ, Peart SAM, Chaudhuri PR. Accuracy of intraocular lens calculations based on fellow-eye biometry for phacovitrectomy for macula-off rhegmatogenous retinal detachments. Eye (Lond). 2019;33(11):1756–61.
27. Kang EC, Lee KH, Koh HJ. Comparison of refractive error in phacovitrectomy for epiretinal membrane using ultrasound and partial coherence interferometry. Eur J Ophthalmol. 2016;26 (4):356–60. https://doi.org/10.5301/ejo.5000732.
28. Tranos PG, Allan B, Balidis M, Vakalis A, Asteriades S, Anogeianakis G, et al. Comparison of postoperative refractive outcome in eyes undergoing combined phacovitrectomy vs cataract surgery following vitrectomy. Graefes Arch Clin Exp Ophthalmol. 2020;258(5):987–93.
29. Sakamoto M, Yoshida I, Sodeno T, Sakai A, Masahara H, Maeno T. Postoperative Refractive Prediction Error Measured by Optical and Acoustic Biometry after Phacovitrectomy for

Rhegmatogenous Retinal Detachment without Macular Involvement J Ophthalmol. 2019;2019:5964127.
30. Ercan ZE, Akkoyun I, Yaman Pinarci E, Yilmaz G, Topcu H. Refractive outcome comparison between vitreomacular interface disorders after phacovitrectomy. J Cataract Refract Surg. 2017;43(8):1068–71.
31. Kang TS, Park HJ, Jo YJ, Kim JY. Long-term reproducibility of axial length after combined phacovitrectomy in macula-sparing rhegmatogenous retinal detachment. Sci Rep. 2018;8 (1):15856.
32. Shiraki N, Wakabayashi T, Sakaguchi H, Nishida K. Effect of gas tamponade on the intraocular lens position and refractive error after phacovitrectomy: a swept-source anterior segment OCT analysis. Ophthalmology. 2020;127(4):511–5.
33. Sato T, Korehisa H, Shibata S, Hayashi K. Prospective comparison of intraocular lens dynamics and refractive error between phacovitrectomy and phacoemulsification alone. Ophthalmol Retina. 2020.
34. Leisser C, Hirnschall N, Findl O. Effect of air tamponade on tilt of the intraocular lens after phacovitrectomy. Ophthalmologica. 2019;242(2):118–22.
35. Leiderman YI, Andreoli MT, Sun B, Dawood S. PARS Plana vitrectomy combined with cataract extraction: a comparison of surgical outcomes using single-piece and multipiece foldable intraocular lenses. Retina. 2015;35(6):1059–64.
36. Hwang HS, Jee D. Effects of the intraocular lens type on refractive error following phacovitrectomy with gas tamponade. Curr Eye Res. 2011;36(12):1148–52.
37. Marcovich AL, Tandogan T, Bareket M, Eting E, Kaplan-Ashiri I, Bukelman A, et al. Opacification of hydrophilic intraocular lenses associated with vitrectomy and injection of intraocular gas. BMJ Open Ophthalmol. 2018;3(1): e000157.
38. Yildirim TM, Auffarth GU, Labuz G, Bopp S, Son HS, Khoramnia R. Material analysis and optical quality assessment of opacified hydrophilic acrylic intraocular lenses after pars plana vitrectomy. On J Ophthalmol. 2018;193:10–9.
39. Vounotrypidis E, Shajari M, Muth DR, Hirnschall N, Findl O, Priglinger S, et al. Refractive outcomes of 8 biometric formulas in combined phacovitrectomy with internal limiting membrane peeling for epiretinal membrane. J Cataract Refract Surg. 2020;46(4):591–7.
40. Zhang J, Wang W, Liu Z, Yang G, Qiu X, Xu J, Jin G, Li Y, Zhang S, Tan X, Luo L, Liu Y. Accuracy of new generation intraocular lens calculation formulas in eyes undergoing combined silicone oil removal and cataract surgery. J Cataract Refract Surg. 2020 Nov 30. https://doi.org/10.1097/j.jcrs.0000000000000509. Epub ahead of print. PMID: 33278232.
41. Tan X, Zhang J, Zhu Y, Xu J, Qiu X, Yang G, Liu Z, Luo L, Liu Y. Accuracy of new generation intraocular lens calculation formulas in vitrectomized eyes. Am J Ophthalmol. 2020;217:81–90.
https://doi.org/10.1016/j.ajo.2020.04.035 Epub 2020 May 6 PMID: 32387430.
42. Kanclerz P, Grzybowski A. Accuracy of intraocular lens power calculation in eyes filled with silicone oil. Semin Ophthalmol. 2019;34(5):392–7.
https://doi.org/10.1080/08820538.2019.1636097 Epub 2019 Jul 1 PMID: 31257972.

Aspheric Intraocular Lens: Indications

Carlos Lisa, Luis Fernández-Vega Cueto, Belén Alfonso, David Madrid-Costa, and Jose F. Alfonso

The main aim of cataract surgery or refractive lens exchange is to satisfy the patient's visual requests for visual correction as well as providing the best possible quality of vision. The design of the intraocular lens (IOL) to be implanted is, a crucial factor in meeting this aim. Currently, several IOL designs are commercially available with various degrees of sphericity or asphericity. There are spherical designs with positive spherical aberration (SA) and aspheric designs which can be further differentiated into IOLs without SA or offering different degrees of negative SA. In order to make the challenging decision regarding the best IOL for each patient it is important to consider several aspects of the patient's ocular anatomy and the IOL, which could conditionate the postoperative visual performance. Preoperatively, all patients should undergo an exhaustive ocular exploration, which, in addition to the routine biometric tests for IOL power calculations, should include the following: Anterior Segment Optical Coherence Tomography (AS-OCT); Pupil Size; Macular OCT, corneal topography, and aberrometry.

AS-OCT provides excellent insights into the anterior segment anatomy and the potential future behavior of the IOL inside the capsular bag, but it is important to choose the best platform in relation to the angle-to-angle measurement and the anterior chamber depth. It is also very important for predicting the effective lens position. For example, a large IOL diameter in a short capsular bag could provide an axial displacement and consequently a refractive instability. On the other hand, a short IOL diameter in a large capsular bag could lead to IOL tilting or decentration.

C. Lisa (✉) · L. Fernández-Vega Cueto · B. Alfonso · J. F. Alfonso
Fernández-Vega Ophthalmological Institute, Oviedo, Spain
e-mail: carloslisa@fernandez-vega.com

D. Madrid-Costa
Complutense University of Madrid, Madrid, Spain

M. Shajari et al. (eds.), *Cataract and Lens Surgery*,
https://doi.org/10.1007/978-3-031-05394-8_37

Tilt and decentration of the IOLs have an impact on visual quality, and aspheric IOLs have a greater effect than the spherical ones [1].

Larger pupils are associated with a higher risk of dysphotopsias secondary to increased Higher Order Aberrations (HOAs) [2]. An analysis of studies reporting on the implantation of IOLs found a reduction of HOAs in eyes with an aspheric IOL for pupil sizes of 5.0 mm and 6.0 mm. However, there was no statistically significant difference with a pupil size of 4.0 mm [3, 4]. Hence, we need to measure pupil size under photopic and mesopic conditions to better predict the outcome of the chosen IOL and its influence on HOAs in every eye.

A good balance between the IOL design and optical characteristics of the cornea is therefore crucial to reach an optimal visual function after cataract surgery. Since the introduction of wavefront technology in ophthalmology, a primary area of interest for cataract and refractive surgery has been the role of HOAs, and mainly SA, in relation to the quality of vision. An increase in the total amount of SA of the eye results in an increase in the total amount of HOAs, thereby decreasing the patient's visual function [5]. However, SA increases depth of focus and the implications of this have been debated. Cataract surgery with some residual SA may be helpful in achieving an acceptable compromise between depth of focus and visual quality. The residual SA after cataract surgery relies mainly on two sources: SA of the cornea and SA of the IOL which can be corrected by a range of spheric or aspheric lens options. Ophthalmologists will also encounter a range of untreated healthy corneas as well as post-refractive corneas that induce a varying degrees of SA that the surgeons should be prepared to deal with.

The aspheric IOLs are designed to totally or partially compensate for the averaged SA of the cornea in the normal population, which, although varying between individuals, is estimated to be about +0.135 μm, at 5.0 mm [7]. Therefore, considering the collaborative effect of the corneal SA and SA of the IOL, it would seem that an aspheric IOL should be the choice to provide the best visual quality. However, the IOL design is not the only factor for achieving a good postoperative visual quality after cataract surgery. There are other issues, such as centration or tilt of the IOL, that also have an important impact on visual performance [1]. As previously mentioned, IOL misalignments have a greater negative effect on the aspheric IOLs [1] hence, the preoperative angle-to-angle measurement for choosing the best platform is crucial to ensure a correct alignment. For patients with untreated corneas, the criteria to select the optical design of presbyopic-correcting IOLs (EDOF, bifocal, trifocal) should be based on the visual demands, age, refractive error...., rather than the corneal SA. Nevertheless, it is well known that a reduction in total HOAs can improve contrast sensitivity and visual quality. This is the main reason why aspheric IOLs are de usual chosen lenses despite of complete HOA correction decreases the depth of field.

There are two types of aspheric IOLs: Aberration-neutral, or aberration-free, that have the same refractive power over their entire surface. They are meant to have a neutral effect on the SA of the eye and thus prevent the induction of new aberrations rather than correcting existing aberrations. They are therefore well suited for patients who have little to no HOA preoperatively and want a particularly sharp focal point with the best contrast vision postoperatively.

Aberration-correcting IOLs, on the other hand, have negative sphericity. They were developed to correct positive corneal SA as thoroughly as possible. The radius of curvature of these lenses is highest in the centre and decreases steadily in a radial form towards the periphery. They are recommended for patients with high SA preoperatively in order to neutralize them and to provide a higher imaging quality, as well as to improve contrast sensitivity and vision under mesopic conditions.

An important factor when considering the implantation of an aspheric IOL is the patients age and the pupillary diameter. Patients with larger pupils can obtain a greater benefit from aspheric IOLs than people with smaller pupils. In untreated corneas, the patient′s wishes (better contrast sensitivity/visual acuity vs depth of field) and the pupillary diameter are the main criteria which need to be considered when planning the implantation of an aspheric IOL.

The balance between the IOL design (both asphericity and optical design) and optical characteristics of the cornea takes on particular importance for those patients who have previously undergone refractive corneal surgery. The corneal shape and, consequently, its optical properties are significantly modified after corneal refractive surgery. Notedly, millions of patients have undergone corneal refractive surgeries worldwide. In general, if these patients were looking for spectacle independence for far distance, they will prefer to have spectacle independence in near tasks. Consequently, surgeons should choose an IOL that meets two needs: to provide the best visual quality as well as the highest level of spectacle independence. A decade ago, we carried out a research project in which we concluded that for patients with previous myopic corneal ablation, the bifocal aspheric IOL works better than the spherical ones [8–11]. In contrast, for post-hyperopic corneal ablations, the bifocal spherical IOL performed better. Since then, the optical design of the presbyopic-correcting IOL has experimented a revolution. To make the challenging decision of choosing the best IOL for each case it is essential to pay attention to several aspects. Firstly, the impact of residual SA on the visual quality and depth of focus [6] and secondly, the coupling effect of SA changes induced by corneal refractive surgery and optical design of the IOL itself.

A theoretical study suggests that a SA value of +0.2 or –0.2 μm is the limit from which the visual acuity decreases by more than 1 line [12]. In contrast, for these SA values, the depth of focus increase by 0.5D. Based on this finding, we prefer to select an IOL where the postoperative SA (coupling from cornea + IOL) does not exceed +0.2 or –0.2 μm. Taking this into account, we have come up with the following guideline (see Tables 1 and 2).

Table 1 Strategy with aspheric IOLs in eyes with previous myopic ablation

Corrected myopia	Mean K post excimer laser	Induced spherical aberration	IOL selection	Postop target refraction
–1,00/ – 4,00 D	39–42 D	+0.1 μ	Trifocal diffractive	0,00 D
–5,00/– 6,00 D	37–38 D	+0.2 μ	Bifocal diffractive or EDoF	0,00 or +0,50 D
–7,00/– 10.00 D	33–36 D	+0.3 μ	Intermediate enhanced	–0,50 D

Table 2 Strategy with IOLs in eyes with previous hyperopic ablation

Corrected hyperopia	Mean K post excimer laser	Induced spherical aberration	IOL selection	Postop target refraction
+1,00/ +2,50 D	42–44,5 D	–0.1 μ	Trifocal/EDOF	0,00/ –0,50 D
+3,00/ +5,00 D	44,5–48 D	–0.2 μ	Monofocal (aberration–free)	–0,50/ –1.00 D

Author's recommendation

1. The corneal SA for a patient who underwent corneal refractive surgery for low myopia (between –1 and –4 D), is around 0.2 μm for a pupil of 4.5 mm coming from 0.1 μm of the virgin cornea (pre-corneal refractive surgery) plus +0.1 μm which is the amount of SA induced to correct this magnitude of myopia). We recommend implanting an aspheric diffractive trifocal lens with SA of –0.1 μm to compensate for induced-corneal refractive surgery SA in these cases. In this way, we obtain a standard distance vision and preserve the trifocal performance of the lens.
2. For moderate myopia (between –5 and –6 D), the induced SA is around +0.2 m, and therefore, the SA of the cornea reaches high values (around +0.3 μm). We recommend implanting one of the following three aspheric lenses: bifocal classic diffractive with a 65:35 light distribution (i.e. AcriLISA 809; Zeiss) or non-diffractive EDOF (i.e. Vivity; Alcon), both with a SA of –0.1 μm, to partially compensate the laser induced SA. Finally, a diffractive EDOF lens (Tecnis Synfony; Johnson&Johnson Vision) could be another option due to its spherical aberration of –0.27 μm. With this technology, we can get the best possible distance vision, and two more advantages: far defocus tolerance and near functional vision, as a consequence of combining the performance of the lens and the residual positive SA of the cornea.

3. In cases of higher myopia (between –7 and –10 D) previously corrected the induced SA is approximately +0.3 μm. Hence, the corneal SA reaches values higher than 0.4 μm. In these cases, we opt for a monofocal lens with intermediate enhanced vision (Tecnis Eyhance; Johnson&Johnson Vision) and SA of –0.27 μm. With this lens, we are aiming at improving distance visual acuity by compensating the corneal SA. Furthermore, providing a functional intermediate vision secondary to the IOL performance, residual SA (lower than –0.20 μm), and intentional residual myopic refraction. We consider these cases as a relative contraindication for trifocal lenses. In addition to the corneal SA, we found that 50% of myopic eyes with an axial length greater than 25 mm had a posterior staphyloma. If the macular inclination in these cases forms an angle greater than 30 degrees, lines of vision can be lost after trifocal IOL implantation, even when there is no evident maculopathy [13].
4. For patients whose cornea asphericity has been modified by a hyperopic corneal ablation, we could apply a similar approach, but considering that the cornea becomes more prolate and its SA values become more negative [14]. In this scenario, considering the magnitude of SA induced by hyperopic correction, our preference for low hyperopia is a trifocal IOL or non-diffractive EDOF, with an SA value not higher than –0.10 μm. If the hyperopic correction was greater, the corneal SA will likely be higher than –0.10 μm. As a result, the implantation of an aspheric IOL would lead to a residual postoperative SA, which will exceed the limit of –0.2 μm. Currently, there are no available presbyopic-correcting IOLs with neutral or positive SA. For these cases, we recommend monofocal IOLs without SA (aberration-free IOL) and with a slightly myopic postoperative refractive target (around –0.50/–1D).

References

1. Madrid-Costa D, Ruiz-Alcocer J, Pérez-Vives C, et al. Visual simulation through different intraocular lenses using adaptive optics: effect of tilt and decentration. J Cataract Refract Surg. 2012;38:947–58.
2. De Vries NE, Webers CA, Touwslager WR, et al. Dissatisfaction after implantation of multifocal intraocular lenses. J Cataract Refract Surg. 2011;37:859–65.
3. Zeng M, Liu Y, Liu X, et al. Aberration and contrast sensitivity comparison of aspherical and monofocal and multifocal intraocular lens eyes. Clin Exp Ophthalmol. 2007;35:355–60.
4. Lin IC, Wang IJ, Lei MS, Lin LL, Hu FR. Improvements in vision-related quality of life with AcrySof IQ SN60WF aspherical intraocular lenses. J Cataract Refract Surg. 2008;34:1312–7.
5. Li J, Xiong Y, Wang N, et al. Effects of spherical aberration on visual acuity at different contrasts. J Cataract Refract Surg. 2009;35:1389–95.
6. Ruiz-Alcocer J, Pérez-Vives C, Madrid-Costa D, García-Lázaro S, Montés-Micó R. Depth of focus through different intraocular lenses in patients with different corneal profiles using adaptive optics visual simulation. J Refract Surg. 2012;28:406–12.

7. Wang L, Dai E, Koch DD, Nathoo A. Optical aberrations of the human anterior cornea. J Cataract Refract Surg. 2003;29:1514–21.
8. Alfonso JF, Fernández-Vega L, Baamonde B, Madrid-Costa D, Montés-Micó R. Visual quality after diffractive intraocular lens implantation in eyes with previous hyperopic laser in situ keratomileusis. J Cataract Refract Surg. 2011;37:1090–6.
9. Alfonso JF, Fernández-Vega L, Baamonde B, Madrid-Costa D, Montés-Micó R. Refractive lens exchange with spherical diffractive intraocular lens implantation after hyperopic laser in situ keratomileusis. J Cataract Refract Surg. 2009;35:1744–50.
10. Alfonso JF, Madrid-Costa D, Poo-López A, Montés-Micó R. Visual quality after diffractive intraocular lens implantation in eyes with previous myopic laser in situ keratomileusis. J Cataract Refract Surg. 2008;34:1848–54.
11. Fernández-Vega L, Madrid-Costa D, Alfonso JF, Montés-Micó R, Poo-López A. Optical and visual performance of diffractive intraocular lens implantation after myopic laser in situ keratomileusis. J Cataract Refract Surg. 2009;35:825–32.
12. Yi F, Iskander DR, Collins M. Depth of focus and visual acuity with primary and secondary spherical aberration. Vision Res. 2011;51:1648–58.
13. Alfonso-Bartolozzi B, Villota E, Fernández-Vega-González Á, et al. Implantation of a trifocal intraocular lens in high myopic eyes with nasal-inferior staphyloma. Clin Ophthalmol. 2020;14:721–7.
14. Llorente L, Barbero S, Merayo J, et al. Total and corneal optical aberrations induced by laser in situ keratomileusis for hyperopia. J Refract Surg 2004; 20: 203e16.

Indications for Toric Intraocular Lenses

Myriam Böhm, Li Wang, and Douglas D. Koch

Background

Astigmatism is the most common refractive error after hyperopia and myopia [1]. Approximately 41% of patients undergoing age-related cataract surgery have a preoperative astigmatism of more than 0.75 diopters (D), meaning about 1/3 of patients would benefit from astigmatism correction during a lens surgery procedure [2]. Surgical treatment options for astigmatism include implantation of toric intraocular lenses, limbal relaxing incisions, or alteration of the corneal curvature using corneal ablative procedures. The following chapter provides an overview of the indications for toric intraocular lenses in surgical astigmatism correction.

Astigmatism Correction

Most ophthalmic surgeons plan a surgical correction of preoperative astigmatism to target postoperative refractive astigmatism of less than 0.5 D. Lower values often do not show any effect of the correction as perceived by the patient, and the predictability of the procedure does not yet allow for a more accurate correction [3]. If the measurement of manifest refraction shows a cylinder, keratometry and corneal topography are the next steps and can determine whether it is a corneal or lenticular astigmatism. If corneal astigmatism is present, it can be decided, depending on the magnitude and type of astigmatism, whether the patient can be

M. Böhm (✉)
Goethe University Frankfurt, Frankfurt, Germany
e-mail: myriam.boehm@kgu.de

L. Wang · D. D. Koch
Baylor College of Medicine, Houston, Texas, USA
e-mail: dkoch@bcm.edu

M. Shajari et al. (eds.), *Cataract and Lens Surgery*,
https://doi.org/10.1007/978-3-031-05394-8_38

offered a correction of their astigmatism using a toric intraocular lens or limbal relaxing incisions.

Table 1 shows a systematic overview to provide the indication for astigmatism correction. Patients with varying degrees of corneal astigmatism are divided into different dioptric categories based on corneal measurements.

A precise estimation of the total corneal refractive power and the anterior and posterior surface astigmatism measurements can be obtained using ray tracing, Scheimpflug imaging, optical coherence tomography (OCT), and direct measurement of the second Purkinje image. A recent study has shown that corneal astigmatism measured by ray tracing has a higher measurement repeatability when compared to two autokeratometers and two placido topographers, and therefore shows promise for the accurate determination of total corneal power and corneal astigmatism (e.g. for calculating toric IOLs) [4].

Memo record

Neglecting astigmatism from posterior corneal surface may lead to incorrect estimation of total corneal astigmatism [5, 6].

End of memo

The selection of a toric intraocular lens based on anterior astigmatism, for example, can lead to overcorrection in eyes with "with-the-rule" astigmatism and undercorrection in eyes with "against-the-rule" astigmatism. In order to counteract this over- or undercorrection, we recommend using a toric IOL calculator that takes into account the posterior surface astigmatism. Several are available, including the Baylor nomogram, Barrett, Abulafia-Koch, and Holladay. Each incorporates estimated posterior corneal astigmatism, calculating lower power toric IOLs for corneas that have WTR astigmatism and higher power toric IOLs for corneas that have ATR astigmatism [7].

Table 1 Systematic overview of indications for corneal astigmatism correction during lens surgery

Magnitude of anterior corneal astigmatism steep along the vertical meridian	**Treatment approach**
≤ 1.00 D	- No correction needed
1.0 – 1.50 D	- Limbal relaxing incisions
> 1.50 D	- Toric intraocular lens or - Relaxing incisions if toric IOL not feasible
Magnitude of anterior corneal astigmatism steep along the horizontal meridian	**Treatment approach**
≤ 0.25 D 0.26 - 0.49 D	- Temporal incision - Relaxing incisions
≥ 0.5 D	- Toric IOL - Limbal relaxing incisions with maximal length of 45 degrees

Indications for Toric Monofocal Intraocular Lenses

To determine the surgical indication, the surgeon must consider the type of astigmatism. Corneal astigmatism is divided into regular, "with-the-rule" (WTR)(rectus), "against-the-rule" (ATR)(inversus), "oblique" (obliquus), and irregular.

Author's recommendation

Three factors determine the threshold for and planned magnitude of the surgical correction of astigmatism: (1) site of the steep meridian due to the effect of posterior corneal astigmatism, [5, 7] (2) known long-term ATR drift that occurs naturally, [8] and (3) IOL tilt, which can add ATR refractive astigmatism [9, 10]. Incorporating these, toric IOLs are recommended only when WTR astigmatism is 1.5 D or more but are implanted when ATR astigmatism is $\geq$ 0.5 D (Table 1). For oblique astigmatism, the astigmatism is targeted based on the anterior corneal magnitude and meridian.

Keypoint

Overcorrection of WTR astigmatism should be avoided due to the long-term ATR shift, whereas a small amount of overcorrection of ATR astigmatism may provide the patient with greater long-term benefit.

When calculating toric intraocular lenses, the surgically induced astigmatism (SIA) of the respective surgeon should always be considered. As a rule, it is usually between 0.1 D and 0.2 D with clear-corneal temporal incisions. Larger amounts of SIA will occur in longer temporal incisions and when incisions are made superiorly.

Keypoint

The SIA should be taken into account when determining the indication for a toric IOL, as it may increase corneal astigmatism to such an extent that the implantation of a toric IOL becomes reasonable.

Furthermore, the patient's eyelid position should be considered preoperatively as the presence of blepharochalasis or ptosis can also affect astigmatism [11]. If an eyelid correction is performed after implantation of a toric lens, this can lead to a postoperative change in astigmatism and thus generate residual astigmatism.

For an optimal refractive result, an eyelid correction should preferably be performed 3 to 6 months before corneal astigmatism is measured, using topography to calculate a toric IOL. However, there are also arguments for first performing lens surgery and then eyelid surgery (see Chap. "Eyelids").

The ideal conditions for the implantation of a toric monofocal lens include some basic criteria that should be considered, specifically for astigmatism correction. The patient should generally have regular astigmatism and it is important to have at least 2 measurements that show consistent values. This can be from 2 different devices or from the same device measuring the corneas on separate days.

Keypoint

There must be excellent capsular and zonular integrity for the implantation of the toric lens to ensure stable IOL positioning and minimize the risk of postoperative rotation.

Indications for Toric Multifocal Intraocular Lenses

There are extensive preoperative tests to ensure that a patient meets the criteria for implantation of a multifocal lens. Astigmatism of > 0.5 D after the implantation of multifocal IOLs leads to impairment of intermediate and distance vision, a reduction in optical quality and increase in halos [12]. Toric multifocal lenses allow the correction of astigmatism and therefore can often provide freedom from glasses at nearly all distances.

Author's recommendation

The implantation of toric multifocal lens shows several advantages when compared to the implantation of a non-toric multifocal lens in combination with LRIs. Both procedures can treat astigmatism, but toric multifocal lenses show a more successful astigmatism correction with better predictability, good rotational stability, and no regression effect, making them preferable to non-toric multifocal lenses combined with LRIs [13].

In cases of regular astigmatism, correction can be made with predictable and satisfactory results. However, patients with irregular astigmatism are often not good candidates for implantation of multifocal IOLs, as correction is challenging, and the visual results are often questionable and disappointing for the patient.

Indications for Limbal Relaxing Incisions

Limbal Relaxing Incisions (LRI) are incisions made on the steep meridian of the cornea with the effect of inducing flattening of the cornea, thereby reducing corneal astigmatism. The size and effect of the incisions depend on their depth, length, and position. LRIs are placed at the edge of the cornea, near the limbus, at both ends of the steep meridian at a pre-set depth to prevent accidental perforation of the cornea. The length of the incisions can be determined by a nomogram, and depends on how much astigmatism is to be corrected, the patient's age, and the axial position of the steep meridian. Nowadays, the use of a femtosecond laser allows incisions to be made with very high precision. Caution, however, is needed in incisions made along the horizontal meridian, as incisions over 45 degrees in length can induce irregular astigmatism.

Both LRIs and toric IOLs can successfully reduce low to moderate regular corneal astigmatism of 0.75–2.50 D (maximum 3.0 D). However, toric IOLs have some additional advantages in astigmatism correction over LRIs.

Keypoint

Advantages of toric IOLs over LRIs are:

1. A higher probability of achieving a postoperative astigmatism of < 0.5 D if the induced astigmatism is known and the axis positioning is accurate.
2. An unaltered corneal curvature so no regression of the corrected cylinder can develop.
3. Much higher limits for the treatable diopters are available.
4. It is a reversible technique [14].

A disadvantage of toric IOLs is the occasional need for secondary intervention to correct the axial position or even exchange the IOL if there is an unacceptably large postoperative refractive error [15].

Author's recommendation

LRIs are a good alternative to toric IOLs 1) if there is inadequate capsular support for a toric IOL, e.g., severe zonulopathy in case of a pseudoexfoliation syndrome, and therefore the implantation of a toric IOL would not be possible, or 2) for small amounts of astigmatism, eg, < 1 D. However, toric IOLs can still be used in the presence of zonulopathy if one can augment the capsular support with capsular tension rings and sutured capsular support devices.

LRIs are associated with limitations such as reduced predictability, dry eye, and wound healing disorders, in addition to the disadvantage of additional surgery. The economic factors of the individual patient should also be taken into account when deciding to choose one of the two techniques. If additional surgical costs are an issue for the patient, LRIs are a more cost-effective alternative for low to moderate astigmatism. When cost is not an issue, toric lenses are more accurate, particularly for addressing astigmatism of over 1 D.

Treatment Options of Irregular Astigmatism

In cases of irregular astigmatism, generally, the implantation of toric IOL is often contraindicated, as the postoperative results are not predictable. However, certain types of irregular astigmatism can be effectively reduced with toric IOLs, for example, after penetrating keratoplasty or Descemet membrane endothelial keratoplasty (DMEK), with some types of corneal scars, or in selected patients with keratoconus. For these types of cases, it is important to remember that the prediction of the refractive outcome of cataract surgery is already difficult with non-toric IOLs. The surgeon should be aware of the various sources of biometric errors and the possible consequences [16, 17].

In eyes with irregular corneal astigmatism, the goal is to correct the regular component of the astigmatism. Patient selection and accurate measurement including the IOL calculation would increase successful treatment of corneal irregular astigmatism [18].

In general, we consider toric IOLs in eyes with irregular astigmatism if (1) there are fairly consistent measurements of astigmatism magnitude and meridian using a biometer and topographer, (2) compared to the corneal readings, the spectacle correction for the patient is within ~1 D for magnitude and ~20 degrees for axis, (3) the central 3-mm of the topography displays the astigmatic pattern, (4) the corneal condition is stable, and (5) postoperative contact lens wear is not planned or possible.

Another patient group that can have irregular astigmatism and certainly challenging toric IOL calculations is those who have undergone corneal refractive surgery. In eyes with previous LASIK or PRK, Cao and colleagues reported that, in those who met 3 criteria, 80 to 84% of eyes had postoperative residual astigmatism $\leq$0.50 D and 95 to 100% had residual astigmatism 1.00 D following toric IOL implantation [19] The 3 inclusion criteria were:

- Regular bow-tie astigmatism within central 3-mm zone,
- Difference in corneal astigmatism magnitude between 2 devices (the IOLMaster and Lenstar in our study) was $\leq$ 0.75 D, and
- Difference in corneal astigmatism meridian between 2 devices was $\leq$ 15°.

Likewise, in eyes with previous RK who met the above criteria, Canedo et al. found that 73 and 88% of eyes had postoperative refractive astigmatism 0.5 D and 1.0 D following toric IOL implantation, respectively [20].

Advanced corneal irregularities cause higher-order aberrations and therefore severely impair quality of vision but a pinhole system is known to improve this condition. Recently, two small-aperture intraocular lenses have been introduced: One for capsular fixation as the sole IOL (IC 8, AcuFocus, Irvine, CA, USA) and the other as an add-on lens implanted in the sulcus in front of a standard capsular-fixated IOL (Trindade XtraFocus, MORCHER® GmbH, Stuttgart, Germany). Both provide an extended depth of focus and improved quality of vision in eyes with irregular corneal astigmatism. Adequate patient selection for pinhole IOL implantation involves several critical success factors: (1) Check whether the cornea is really irregular, (2) Check whether there is no central scarring, (3) Check the benefit of a small-aperture intraocular lens by testing pinhole visual acuity, (4) Check the pupillary diameter: if too small or atonic, no pinhole IOL indicated; if mesopic pupillary diameter > 5 mm, there is a risk of unwanted optical phenomena from IOL aperture, and (5) target the postoperative refraction to -0.5 D to -0.75 D. The small-aperture IOL is a useful tool to treat eyes with severe corneal astigmatism with a high safety index, providing high patient satisfaction and leading to better visual quality [21].

Measurement of Corneal Astigmatism

As noted above, several technologies are available to measure total corneal astigmatism. Prior studies have shown that anterior corneal astigmatism measurements obtained by automated (eg, IOL Master 500, Lenstar, SMI Reference Unit 3), manual (eg, Javal), corneal topography (eg KR-1 W) and Scheimpflug imaging (Pentacam) provide comparable results. The repeatability of astigmatism magnitudes of these devices is acceptable; however, the repeatability of astigmatism meridians is moderate. This might be clinically relevant when calculating the toric IOL [22].

Theoretically, patients needing astigmatism correction should benefit from direct measurement of posterior corneal astigmatism using available technologies such as Scheimpflug, OCT, and direct measurement of the second Purkinje image [23]. Unfortunately, studies to date have not demonstrated superior outcomes for toric IOLs using direct measurement of posterior corneal curvature compared to toric calculators based on mathematical models in conjunction with anterior corneal measurements [24].

Conclusion

Toric IOLs are superior to non-toric IOLs, even in combination with LRIs, in that they have lower postoperative residual astigmatism and no regression effect, allow a wider range of astigmatism correction, and offer better predictability. Therefore, we primarily recommend the implantation of toric IOLs for astigmatism correction to provide postoperative refractive astigmatism of 0.5 D or less. We recommend treatment with LRIs in cases of astigmatism > 0.75–2.0 D, if implantation of a toric IOL is not possible due to a defective capsular support or economic reasons.

References

1. Hassan H, Akbar F, Abbasali Y, Reza P, Hadi O, Mehdi K. Global and regional estimates of prevalence of refractive errors: Systematic review and meta-analysis. J Curr Ophthal [Internet]. 2018; 30(1):3–22.
2. Ferrer-Blasco T, Montés-Micó R, Peixoto-de-Matos SC, González-Méijome JM, Cerviño A. Prevalence of corneal astigmatism before cataract surgery. J Cataract Refract Surg. 2009;35 (1):70–5.

3. Kohnen T, Klaproth OK. Correction of astigmatism during cataract surgery. Klin Monatsbl Augenheilkd. 2009;226(8):596–604.
4. Fityo S, Buhren J, Shajari M, Kohnen T. Keratometry versus total corneal refractive power: analysis of measurement repeatability with 5 different devices in normal eyes with low astigmatism. J Cataract Refract Surg. 2016;42(4):569–76.
5. Koch DD, Ali SF, Weikert MP, Shirayama M, Jenkins R, Wang L. Contribution of posterior corneal astigmatism to total corneal astigmatism. J Cataract Refract Surg. 2012;38 (12):2080–7.
6. Tonn B, Klaproth OK, Kohnen T. Anterior surface-based keratometry compared with Scheimpflug tomography-based total corneal astigmatism. Invest Ophthalmol Vis Sci. 2014;56(1):291–8.
7. Koch DD, Jenkins RB, Weikert MP, Yeu E, Wang L. Correcting astigmatism with toric intraocular lenses: effect of posterior corneal astigmatism. J Cataract Refract Surg. 2013;39 (12):1803–9.
8. Hayashi K, Hirata A, Manabe S, Hayashi H. Long-term change in corneal astigmatism after sutureless cataract surgery. Am J Ophthalmol. 2011;151(5):858–65.
9. Weikert MP, Golla A, Wang L. Astigmatism induced by intraocular lens tilt evaluated via ray tracing. J Cataract Refract Surg. 2018;44(6):745–9.
10. Wang L, Guimaraes de Souza R, Weikert MP, Koch DD. Evaluation of crystalline lens and intraocular lens tilt using a swept-source optical coherence tomography biometer. J Cataract Refract Surg. 2019;45(1):35–40.
11. Brown MS, Siegel IM, Lisman RD. Prospective analysis of changes in corneal topography after upper eyelid surgery. Ophthalmic Plast Reconstr Surg. 1999;15(6):378–83.
12. Hayashi K, Manabe S, Yoshida M, Hayashi H. Effect of astigmatism on visual acuity in eyes with a diffractive multifocal intraocular lens. J Cataract Refract Surg. 2010;36(8):1323–9.
13. Gangwani V, Hirnschall N, Findl O, Maurino V. Multifocal toric intraocular lenses versus multifocal intraocular lenses combined with peripheral corneal relaxing incisions to correct moderate astigmatism. J Cataract Refract Surg. 2014;40(10):1625–32.
14. Lake JC, Victor G, Clare G, Porfirio GJ, Kernohan A, Evans JR. Toric intraocular lens versus limbal relaxing incisions for corneal astigmatism after phacoemulsification. The Cochrane database of systematic reviews. 2019;12:Cd012801.
15. Kessel L, Andresen J, Tendal B, Erngaard D, Flesner P, Hjortdal J. Toric intraocular lenses in the correction of astigmatism during cataract surgery: a systematic review and meta-analysis. Ophthalmology. 2016;123(2):275–86.
16. Allard K, Zetterberg M. Toric IOL implantation in a patient with keratoconus and previous penetrating keratoplasty: a case report and review of literature. BMC ophthalmology. 2018;18 (1):215-.
17. Yokogawa H, Sanchez PJ, Mayko ZM, Straiko MD, Terry MA. Astigmatism correction with toric intraocular lenses in descemet membrane endothelial keratoplasty triple procedures. Cornea. 2017;36(3):269–74.
18. Gao Y, Ye Z, Chen W, Li J, Yan X, Li Z. Management of cataract in patients with irregular astigmatism with regular central component by phacoemulsification combined with toric intraocular lens implantation. J Ophthalmol. 2020;30(2020):3520856. https://doi.org/10.1155/2020/3520856.
19. Cao D, Wang L, Koch DD. Outcome of toric intraocular lenses implanted in eyes with previous corneal refractive surgery. J Cataract Refract Surg. 2020;46(4):534–9.
20. Canedo ALC, Wang L, Koch DD, Al Mohtaseb Z. Accuracy of Astigmatism Correction with toric Intraocular Lens Implantation in Eyes with Prior Radial Keratotomy. J Cataract Refract Surg. Submitted.
21. Shajari M*, Mackert MJ*, Langer J, Kreutzer T, Wolf A, Kohnen T, Priglinger S, Mayer WJ. Safety and efficacy of a small-aperture capsular bag-fixated intraocular lens in eyes with severe corneal irregularities. J Cataract Refract Surg. 2020 Feb;46(2):188–92. https://doi.org/10.1097/j.jcrs.0000000000000045.

22. Visser N, Berendschot T, Verbakel F, Brabander J, Nuijts R. Comparability and repeatability of corneal astigmatism measurements using different measurement technologies. J Cataract Refract Surg. 2012;38(10):1764–70.
23. Shajari M, Cremonese C, Petermann K, Singh P, Mueller M, Kohnen T. Comparison of axial length, corneal curvature, and anterior chamber depth measurements of 2 recently introduced devices to a known biometer. Am J Ophthalmol. 2017;178:58–64.
24. Abulafia A, Hill WE, Franchina M, Barrett GD. Comparison of Methods to Predict Residual Astigmatism After Intraocular Lens Implantation. J Refract Surg. 2015.

Indications for Multifocal and Extended Depth of Focus Intraocular Lenses

Mehdi Shajari and Jorge L. Alio

Introduction

For the majority of our daily tasks, we need good visual acuity in the near distance (approx. 40 cm, e.g. when reading a book), in the intermediary range (approx. 60 - 80 cm, e.g. when working at the laptop and monitor) and at the far distance [1]. When replacing the natural lens with a monofocal intraocular lens, the patient must decide what distance he or she wants to see sharply, without additional visual aids. To reduce spectacle dependance for near vision spectacles, one of the most frequently used options is Monovision, in which the dominant eye is usually corrected to plano and the non-dominant eye to a target refraction of -0.75 to -2.5D. The larger the targeted myopia in the non-dominant eye, the better the patient can see in the near distance, but the more difficult it is to achieve stereopsis. As a result, the patient might develop symptoms such as dizziness or headache.

An alternative way to reduce dependence on visual aids is to use multifocal lenses (today mainly trifocal IOLs) or the so-called extended depth of focus (EDOF) IOLs. In multifocal lenses, multiple foci are created, either by means of diffractive or refractive technologies. EDOF IOLs, on the other hand, create a single elongated focal point to enhance depth of focus [2]. Diffraction, refraction and/or aberration, multifocal and EDOF lenses distribute the incoming beam of light into several distances, by various technologies. Both types of lenses may lead to a decrease in contrast sensitivity, increased glare and an increase in undesirable optical phenomena such as halos and glare. Since the lens used should, ideally, remain in the eye for a lifetime, the inclusion and exclusion criteria must be strictly adhered to.

M. Shajari (✉) · J. L. Alio
Goethe University, Frankfurt, Germany
e-mail: gms400@gmail.com

J. L. Alio
e-mail: jlalio@vissum.com

M. Shajari et al. (eds.), *Cataract and Lens Surgery*,
https://doi.org/10.1007/978-3-031-05394-8_39

The most important points to consider when planning the implantation of a multifocal lens are explained in this chapter.

The patient-doctor interview and preoperative ophthalmic evaluation:

Firstly, the patient´s lifestyle and demands of spectacle independence should be considered. There are many patients who have worn glasses all their live and have become so accustomed to them that they would not feel comfortable without them. On the other hand, there are patients who are already annoyed by light reading glasses and therefore wish to have their clear lenses replaced at the relatively young age of 50 years in order to be spectacle independent. A clear discussion of the patient's wishes should clarify the therapeutic goal in terms of expectations of the cataract/refractive lens exchange surgery and can avoid unnecessary diagnostics. The conversation should also include a discussion of how the patient spends his or her daily life and what profession and hobbies they have, in order to better assess which of the options for reducing dependency on visual aids would be most suitable for the patient. We must be aware that most patients do not want to give up the capability to be spectacle independent for near in spite of the common and more frequent use that today is necessary for intermediate vision tasks. Statements that can help lead the discussion to the most appropriate option could be:

- "I would like to be spectacle independent and above all I would like to see well in the near distance" -> Most probably trifocal IOL or combination of sectorial refractive mf IOLs with the power + 1.5 in the dominant and + 3 in the non-dominant eye
- "I work a lot at the monitor and I do not care at all for near vision" -> Low power + 1.5 sector refractive IOLs or low power multifocal/ EDOF hybrid IOLs
- "I drive a lot at night" -> monovision with aspheric IOL or low power refractive sectorial Mf IOLs
- "I already feel very disturbed by optical phenomena (e.g. halos) and cannot cope with them" -> Monovision with aspherical or aberration-correcting IOL or the modern "monofocal-plus" IOLs
- "I want the best possible optical quality, but also a certain freedom from glasses at a distance" -> Micro monovision with aberration-correcting IOL
- "I would like to achieve the greatest possible freedom from glasses and am prepared to make compromises in terms of optical quality" -> trifocal IOL or EDOF Mini Monovision
- "I want to see perfect in near, intermediate and far distance" -> currently no option available

Remember

It is important that the patient understands that there is no perfect option for achieving spectacle independence, but that each option has advantages and disadvantages, which may be more or less relevant depending on the patient's wishes. A clear informed consent should be offered to the patient in this regard.

It is critical to educate the patient about the phenomenon of neuro-adaptation before the surgical procedure. The neural system needs some time to "get used" to the new visual impression. This process usually takes about three to six months. During this period, patients usually get accustomed to optical phenomena and the perception of them will reduce in time. Therefore, if no optical cause for an unsatisfactory result is found during the follow-up examination, such as a residual refractive error or decentration of the IOL optic, the patient should be advised to wait for the process of neuro-adaptation and the ophthalmologist should not intervene too early. The possibility of neuroadaptation failure should be discussed in the informed consent the potential of an IOL exchange in the worst-case scenario should be discussed.

Author's recommendation

Before the use of multifocal lenses, it is essential to educate the patient about the phenomenon of neuroadaptation. The justification for delaying an intervention by the surgeon in case of dissatisfaction is much easier for the patient to understand if it was discussed beforehand.

Clinical examination

At the slit lamp, special attention should be paid to the following points during the anterior segment examination, as they have a high prevalence and can severely affect the result:

- Changes in the tear film? Reduced "break-up time"? Is there any level of punctate keratopathy?
- Signs of epithelial dystrophy (especially map-dot-fingerprint dystrophy)?
- Is there a Fuchs endothelial dystrophy?
- Signs of pseudoexfoliation syndrome (PEX)? Loosening of the capsule apparatus?
- Risk factors for complications during cataract surgery
- Pupil size in mesopic conditions and photopic reactivity

An insufficient tear film can easily be overlooked so it is extremely important to ask the patient about symptoms of keratoconjunctivitis sicca in detail (possibly with a standardized questionnaire). Keraconjunctivitis sicca can lead to incorrect measurements and associated postoperative refractive errors, which considerably reduce the optical quality of multifocal lenses (MIOL). Accordingly, keratoconjunctivitis sicca is one of the most common causes of dissatisfaction after implantation of multifocal lenses. Therefore, dry eyes must be intensely treated in advance and, if severe symptoms exist, multifocal lenses should not be used.

Author's recommendation

If the patient has clinically relevant dry eyes, the measurements should be repeated until reliable values are obtained. In case of high fluctuations in the data, the topical dry eye therapy should be intensified. If there is no high repeatability of the measurements despite intensive therapy, multifocal lenses should not be used.

During the posterior segment examination, pathological changes to the optic nerve, maculopathies and the presence of retinal pathology requiring laser coagulation should be excluded. It is well known that the patient has an increased risk of developing a retinal detachment due to lens replacement—particularly patients who suffer from high myopia or where the vitreous is still attached. It is also important to note that progressive diseases (particularly retinal diseases) should be detected at an early stage because the use of a multifocal lens in these cases should be evaluated very critically. Cellophane maculopathy, for example, does not usually affect the patient's vision and in milder cases would not have a negative effect on the final result when a MIOL is used. In many cases, however, the disease does progress and a pronounced epiretinal gliosis, which both reduces contrast sensitivity and can cause aberrations, leads to significant visual impairment, especially in the case of a MIOL.

Author's recommendation

Under certain circumstances, the use of sulcus-supported multifocal add-on lenses may make sense in patients where progression of an ocular pathology is possible, but who currently have no symptoms. These can be removed if the disease is progressive without posing too much of a risk of damaging the capsule or the zonula fibres. However, before an explantation is performed, it is important to exclude other potential reasons for a decrease in contrast sensitivity like age or other ocular comorbidities.

The correct centration of the lens plays a crucial role, especially in a multifocal IOL and even a large angle alpha can have a negative effect. Similarly, although it is still widely debated, it is generally accepted that if the visual axis deviates >0.5 mm from the optical axis, the visual result is worse and disturbing optical phenomena such as halos increase (large angle k). Fu et al. showed, by means of a regression analysis, that even if the visual axis deviates from the optical axis by <0.5 mm, there is a negative influence on the visual result and accordingly, a low angle k should ideally be present when using a multifocal lens [3]. This emphasizes how important it is that the lens is positioned centrally, when using multifocal optics but this can be a challenge, especially for myopic patients. Zhu et al. found that myopic patients often experience downward decentration postoperatively, resulting in a corresponding decrease in vision and satisfaction [4]. Tandogan et al. were also able to demonstrate that, in comparison to monofocal IOLs, multifocal IOLs show a stronger decrease in optical quality due to decentration of the lens [5].

Considering the corneal astigmatism is another decisive factor that should be addressed in order to achieve the best possible postoperative refractive result [6, 7]. Although the measurement repeatability of the magnitude of astigmatism is high with the currently available devices, there may still be cases of wide deviations when determining the axis of the astigmatism [8]. It should be noted that most devices only measure the corneal front surface and simulate the total refractive power. In a study by Tonn et al. of almost 4000 eyes measured using a Scheimpflug device, it was shown that large discrepancies to the actual total corneal refractive power can result from this [9]. In patients with astigmatism against the rule in particular, there can be large deviations and an actual measurement of the total corneal refractive power are useful here. Especially when using multifocal lenses, it is of utmost importance that there is no residual astigmatism postoperatively. If the postoperative astigmatism is between 0.3D and 1D, taking into account the surgically induced astigmatism, the use of limbal relaxing incisions is recommended. Due to the higher reproducibility, it is recommended these incisions be performed with a femtosecond laser. Toric lenses should be used in cases where residual astigmatism is expected to be above 1D. Furthermore, strong irregularities of the cornea are an important contraindication to the use of a MIOL. Most surgeons consider a value over 0.3 or 0.5 μm in total HOA RMS for the 4 mm zone or high values in coma (>0.32 μm) as a contraindication to implant MIOL. Although this has not yet been scientifically proven, many believe that exceeding these values leads to an increase in dysphotopsia.

Bifocal lens designs are generally no longer used because trifocal lenses provide better intermediate vision with equally good near and distance vision [10]. It is also known that bifocal IOL cause more photopic phenomena than trifocal MIOL. The decision whether monovision, EDOF lens or trifocal lens is the best choice must be made individually for each patient. A monovision with spherical, aspherical or aberration-correcting IOLs depending on the HOA of the cornea is the method of choice for patients for whom optical quality is the first priority. Patients who are not bothered by wearing reading glasses, drive a lot at night or who complain a lot about photopic phenomena preoperatively should also receive monovision if they wish to reduce the use of visual aids. Freedom from glasses cannot usually be achieved by this means (26% for monovision with 1D vs. 71% for multifocal lenses), [11] but patients manage without glasses a large part of their daily activities and report less impairment of vision quality and less discomfort than patients with multifocal lenses [12]. The advantage of a slight monovision (-0.75 to -1.25) is that it can be performed without negative consequences in almost any patient. Patients who, for example, have stronger higher order aberrations in one eye (>0.3 μm) should not receive multifocal lenses—but monovision in these cases, is still possible. On the other side however, mild spherical aberrations improve depth of field perception without clinically significant deterioration of visual quality. Presbyopia correction with the excimer laser makes use of this exact phenomenon.

Currently, there is still some controversy associated with EDOF lenses. Some surgeons regard EDOF lenses as simple multifocal lenses with a low near add and do not use them as their potential benefit for reducing optical phenomena (like halo or having an increased contrast sensitivity) is still very controversial. The current models based on spherical aberrations do not work on a sufficiently well enough, in the opinion of the authors, to be considered for patients who wish to have total spectacle independence. On the other hand, some surgeons claim that EDOF lenses make sense in patients for whom the intermediate area is particularly important in everyday life, because here these lenses are superior to monovision and trifocal lenses [13]. Similar to monovision, however, patients usually need reading glasses postoperatively. EDOF lenses are superior to monovision in the intermediate range and in terms of stereopsis, but the optical quality is usually somewhat poorer and the exclusion criteria much more extensive than with monovision. Therefore, their use in the usual target refraction (bilateral emmetropia) is rather limited, since patients who do not want to be completely free of glasses are usually better suited for monovision and patients who want to be completely free of glasses need trifocal lenses. The situation is different when EDOF lenses are combined with mini-monovision (non-dominant eye target refraction -0.75D). Patients have good distance vision, good intermediate vision and about 75% are completely spectacle-free. Correspondingly, patient satisfaction is also higher than in patients where both eyes were adjusted to distance [14]. Stereoscopic vision is better than classical monovision and patients are more often able to read a book or newspaper without glasses.

The great advantage of trifocal lenses is that they allow almost complete independence from glasses. For near vision in particular, it is superior to monovision and EDOF lenses. Unfortunately, it is also the option where contrast sensitivity is most likely to be reduced and where dysphotopsia, glare and halos tend to occur most frequently. Accordingly, the inclusion and exclusion criteria for the use of trifocal lenses must be strictly adhered to. Therefore, we recommend trifocal lenses only for patients who have no ocular pathologies, a regular corneal surface and a strong desire to be completely spectacle-free.

Multifocal IOLs in special situations

In amblyopia, most surgeons prefer not to implant multifocal IOLs and consider amblyopia as an absolute contraindication. If a surgeon wants to implant multifocal IOLs in a patient with amblyopia we prefer EDOF lenses over trifocal IOLs, although no studies exist currently to this subject. Furthermore, it is important to differentiate what the underlying cause is. Multifocal lenses can be used for refractive amblyopia, while multifocal lenses should be avoided for amblyopia caused by strabismus. In the literature there are two studies in which patients had amblyopia and MIOL were used. In both studies a multifocal lens was used in both eyes and both distance and near vision were good and binocular vision improved [15, 16].

The use of MIOLs must be evaluated very critically in patients with unilateral cataract. Patients in this group are typically, rather young and the patient will lose their ability to accommodate postoperatively. The use of multifocal lenses makes sense in principle. On the other hand, contrast sensitivity will probably be noticeably reduced compared to the healthy eye. The patient must be informed of this. In a study comparing the use of multifocal lenses with monofocal lenses in unilateral cataract, binocular near and intermediate vision was better in the multifocal group. The independence from glasses was also higher in the multifocal group, but contrast sensitivity was noticeably reduced [17].

Vrijiman and colleagues studied the vision of patients who had previously undergone laser corneal ablation to correct myopia or hyperopia. The IOL calculation after laser correction is more difficult, but the results did not differ significantly from previously published studies with monofocal lenses after laser correction. In the previously myopic patients, the postoperative spherical equivalent was -0.38 ± 0.78 dpt and 75% of the eyes were $\pm$ 0.5 dpt within the target refraction. However, if the patients were highly myopic (> 6 dpt) before laser ablation, the results were worse. [18]. In hyperopic patients, the visual outcome after MIOL implantation was independent of the degree of hyperopia before laser ablation [19]. However, since patients can be much more affected by residual refractive error when using multifocal lenses, the indication for the implantation of a multifocal lens in these cases should only be given by ophthalmologists who are used to the daily interpretation of corneoepithelial and corneal topographies and aberrometries.

Author's recommendation

For a detailed overview of multifocal IOLs we recommend to also read the book: "Multifocal Intraocular Lenses: The Art and the Practice" (Springer).

References

1. Vargas V, Radner W, Allan BD, Reinstein DZ, Burkhard Dick H, Alio JL, et al. Methods for the study of near, intermediate vision, and accommodation: an overview of subjective and objective approaches. Surv Ophthalmol. 2019;64(1):90–100.
2. Alio JL. Presbyopic lenses: evidence, masquerade news, and fake news. Asia Pac J Ophthalmol (Phila). 2019;8(4):273–4.
3. Fu Y, Kou J, Chen D, Wang D, Zhao Y, Hu M, et al. Influence of angle kappa and angle alpha on visual quality after implantation of multifocal intraocular lenses. J Cataract Refract Surg. 2019;45(9):1258–64.
4. Zhu X, He W, Zhang Y, Chen M, Du Y, Lu Y. Inferior decentration of multifocal intraocular lenses in myopic eyes. Am J Ophthalmol. 2018;188:1–8.
5. Tandogan T, Son HS, Choi CY, Knorz MC, Auffarth GU, Khoramnia R. Laboratory evaluation of the influence of decentration and pupil size on the optical performance of a Monofocal, bifocal, and trifocal intraocular lens. J Refract Surg. 2017;33(12):808–12.
6. Alio JL, Plaza-Puche AB, Fernandez-Buenaga R, Pikkel J, Maldonado M. Multifocal intraocular lenses: an overview. Surv Ophthalmol. 2017;62(5):611–34.
7. Rosen E, Alio JL, Dick HB, Dell S, Slade S. Efficacy and safety of multifocal intraocular lenses following cataract and refractive lens exchange: Metaanalysis of peer-reviewed publications. J Cataract Refract Surg. 2016;42(2):310–28.
8. Visser N, Berendschot TT, Verbakel F, de Brabander J, Nuijts RM. Comparability and repeatability of corneal astigmatism measurements using different measurement technologies. J Cataract Refract Surg. 2012;38(10):1764–70.
9. Tonn B, Klaproth OK, Kohnen T. Anterior surface-based keratometry compared with Scheimpflug tomography-based total corneal astigmatism. Invest Ophthalmol Vis Sci. 2014;56(1):291–8.
10. Kaymak H, Breyer D, Alio JL, Cochener B. Visual performance with bifocal and trifocal diffractive intraocular lenses: a prospective three-armed randomized multicenter clinical trial. J Refract Surg. 2017;33(10):655–62.
11. Wilkins MR, Allan BD, Rubin GS, Findl O, Hollick EJ, Bunce C, et al. Randomized trial of multifocal intraocular lenses versus monovision after bilateral cataract surgery. Ophthalmology. 2013;120(12):2449–55 e1.

12. Zhang F, Sugar A, Jacobsen G, Collins M. Visual function and patient satisfaction: comparison between bilateral diffractive multifocal intraocular lenses and monovision pseudophakia. J Cataract Refract Surg. 2011;37(3):446–53.
13. Webers VSC, Bauer NJC, Saelens IEY, Creten OJM, Berendschot T, van den Biggelaar F, et al. Comparison of the intermediate distance of a trifocal IOL with an extended depth-of-focus IOL: results of a prospective randomized trial. J Cataract Refract Surg. 2020;46(2):193–203.
14. Cochener B, Concerto Study G. Clinical outcomes of a new extended range of vision intraocular lens: International Multicenter Concerto Study. J Cataract Refract Surg. 2016;42 (9):1268-75.
15. de Wit DW, Diaz JM, Moore TC, Moore JE. Refractive lens exchange for a multifocal intraocular lens with a surface-embedded near section in mild to moderate anisometropic amblyopic patients. J Cataract Refract Surg. 2012;38(10):1796–801.
16. Petermeier K, Gekeler F, Spitzer MS, Szurman P. Implantation of the multifocal ReSTOR apodised diffractive intraocular lens in adult anisometropic patients with mild to moderate amblyopia. Br J Ophthalmol. 2009;93(10):1296–301.
17. Hayashi K, Manabe S, Yoshimura K, Hirata A. Binocular visual function with a diffractive multifocal intraocular lens in patients with unilateral cataract. J Cataract Refract Surg. 2013;39(6):851–8.
18. Vrijman V, van der Linden JW, van der Meulen IJE, Mourits MP, Lapid-Gortzak R. Multifocal intraocular lens implantation after previous corneal refractive laser surgery for myopia. J Cataract Refract Surg. 2017;43(7):909–14.
19. Vrijman V, van der Linden JW, van der Meulen IJE, Mourits MP, Lapid-Gortzak R. Multifocal intraocular lens implantation after previous hyperopic corneal refractive laser surgery. J Cataract Refract Surg. 2018;44(4):466–70.

Supplementary Intraocular Lenses

Michael Amon and Guenal Kahraman

Introduction

The "piggyback" technique, or polypseudophakia, refers to when in which at least two IOLs are implanted in the posterior chamber of the same eye. It was first described by Gayton and Sanders in 1993 for the treatment of high hyperopic errors, where the required lens power to achieve emmetropia was not available.

The aim was to achieve a total refractive power of 46 diopters, which at the time was not possible using a single intraocular lens. Both intraocular lenses were implanted into the capsular, but this implantation technique resulted in a relatively high rate of complications.

A common and significant complication associated with primary piggyback IOLs was interlenticular opacification (ILO), which usually occurred six months to two years post-implantation. This was a direct result of the interactions between both biconvex IOLs into the capsular bag.

Residual lens epithelial cell growth typically led to membrane formation between the surfaces of piggyback acrylic IOLs, leading to decreased vision, secondary postoperative hyperopic shift, as well as opacification [9, 16]. As a result, this approach for the most part has been abandoned. The modern piggyback approach avoids most of these issues by implanting the first IOL into the capsular

Supplementary Information The online version contains supplementary material available at https://doi.org/10.1007/978-3-031-05394-8_40. The videos can be accessed individually by clicking the DOI link in the accompanying figure caption or by scanning this link with the SN More Media App.

M. Amon (✉) · G. Kahraman
Krankenhaus der Barmherzigen Brüder Wien, Vienna, Austria
e-mail: michael.amon@bbwien.at; amon@augenchirurg.com

G. Kahraman
e-mail: guenal.kahraman@gmail.com

M. Shajari et al. (eds.), *Cataract and Lens Surgery*,
https://doi.org/10.1007/978-3-031-05394-8_40

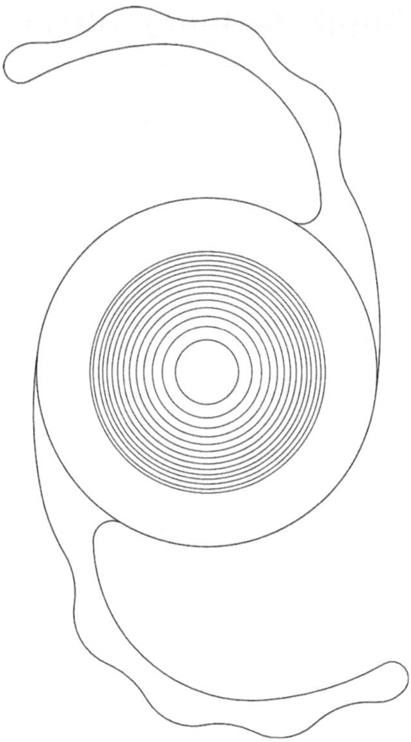

Fig. 1 Rayner Sulcoflex Trifocal Model IOL703F

bag and the second IOL into the ciliary sulcus, because the lens epithelial cell migration is blocked by the anterior capsular adhesion [15].

There are currently three companies producing supplementary intraocular lenses: Rayner Sulcoflex, Cristalens Reverso and 1stQ Supplementary IOL (Figs. 1, 2 and 3).

Versions range from trifocal to monofocal aspheric to the more complex multifocal, toric, and multifocal toric. It is important to note that these supplementary lenses are especially designed for pseudophakic eyes, and should not be implanted into aphakic or phakic eyes.

Another advantage of this method is its predictability. Power calculation for the supplementary IOL only depends on the patient's current refraction but the exact calculation should be carried out according to the manufacturer's recommendation.

Implantation

A supplementary intraocular lens is usually implanted under topical anesthesia with a well dilated pupil. A clear corneal incision of appropriate size (1.9 to 2.7 mm) is made and ophthalmic viscoelastic device (OVD) is injected under the iris to create space in the ciliary sulcus. Finally, the supplementary intraocular lens is injected

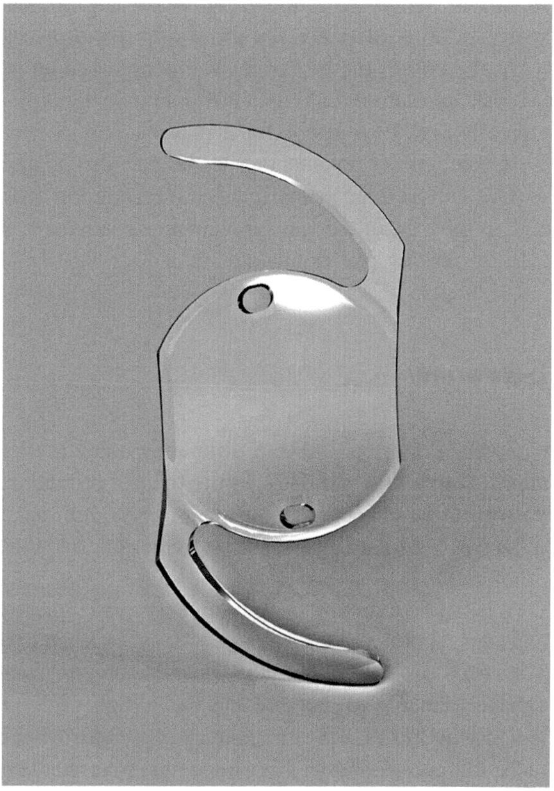

Fig. 2 Christalens Reverso

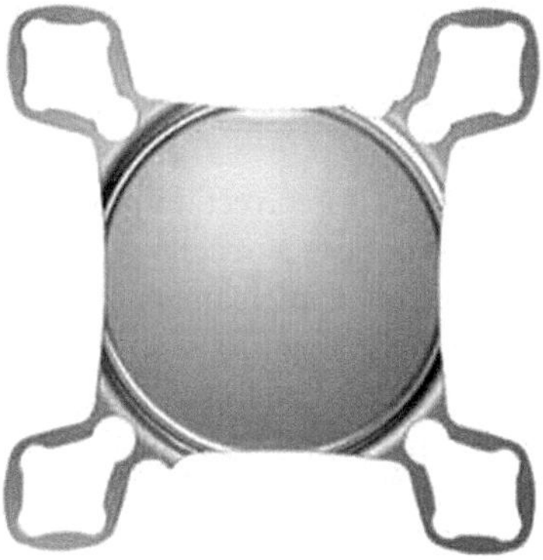

Fig. 3 1stq Addon IOL

and positioned in the ciliary sulcus. An upside-down implantation has to be avoided and can result in an iris capture.

Any type of OVD can be used for sulcus preparation but implantation using an anterior chamber maintainer is also possible. After the implantation, the OVD should be removed as much as possible, particularly from in the interlenticular space. In our experience, an iridectomy is not necessary.

At the end of the procedure we recommend an intracameral antibiotic to reduce the risk of endophthalmitis. Postoperative therapy consists of the application of topical NSAID eye drops for 2–4 weeks.

In principle, supplementary lenses can also be implanted during cataract surgery.

This can be done primarily after implantation of the first lens (Duet implantation, e.g., in the case of trifocal supplementary lenses) or as a secondary procedure in the case of existing pseudophakia.

Indications

One very important indication for supplementary lenses is secondary implantation after a "refractive surprise". In the field of refractive lens surgery, in particular, the postoperative expectations are extremely high and for an unhappy patient with a refractive surprise, a secondary lens can be an excellent option to solve the problem [11].

When encountering a refractive surprise, there are typically three options to consider, assuming that the patient does not wish to use spectacle or lens correction. The first option, refractive corneal surgery such as PRK or LASIK (laser enhancement) is predictable and has a high safety profile, though it is irreversible and correction is not immediately possible. Moreover, hyperopic outcomes are more difficult to correct with laser than myopic. The second option, IOL exchange can be considered but in cases where there are capsular defects (either due to capsular rupture or after Nd: YAG capsulotomy) this is more traumatic, and carries a higher risk of dehiscence of the zonular fibers, vitreous loss and subsequent retinal complications [3]. The third option, the implantation of a secondary IOL, is significantly less traumatic than a lens exchange and can avoid a refractive corneal intervention.

In addition to correcting postoperative ametropia, the introduction of toric and multifocal optics in recent years have widened the spectrum of indications for pseudophakic supplementary IOLs. Nowadays, toric supplementary lenses enable the correction of postoperative astigmatism, especially in pseudophakic patients after penetrating keratoplasty. One major advantage of this approach, compared to refractive laser surgery, is the reversibility and the much higher range of corrections available. IOL rotation, however, may occur more frequently than in toric capsular bag IOLs [12, 13] (Fig. 4).

Multifocal intraocular lenses offer an alternative to monofocal IOLs for patients who wish to be spectacle independent. However, this must always be weighed against the known disadvantages of multifocal IOLs, such as reduced contrast sensitivity and potential dysphotopsias (halos, glare, starburst). Despite careful consideration and patient selection, subjective complaints and multifocal intolerances can occur, which can make explantation of the capsular bag IOL necessary.

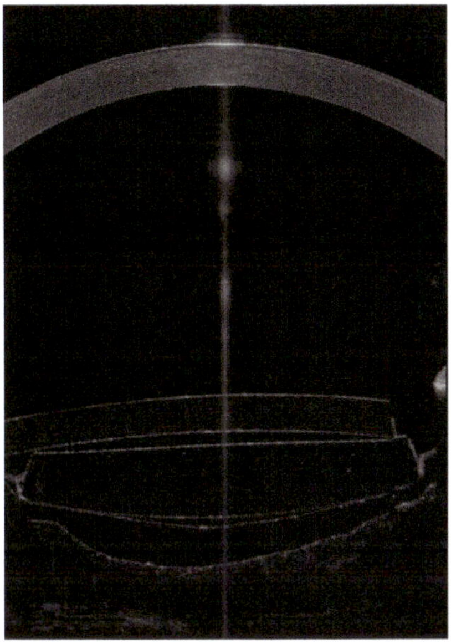

Fig. 4 Anterior OCT imaging shows nice distance between both IOLs

The implantation of a supplementary IOL with multifocal optics as part of cataract surgery (Duet implantation) provides a reversible option for presbyopia correction (Video 1). In the event of intolerance, supplementary IOL can easily be removed without disrupting the capsular bag [14] (Video 1).

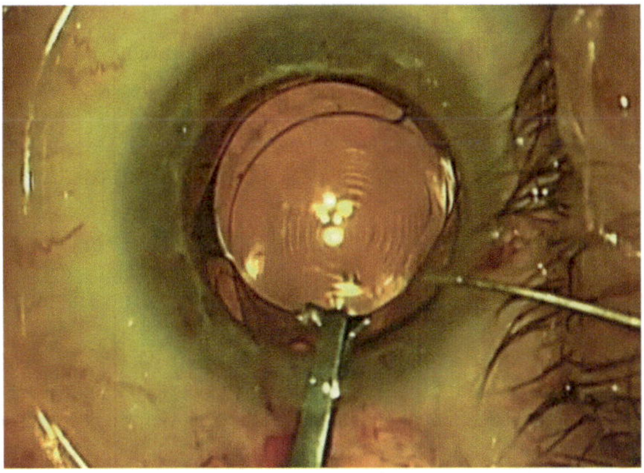

Video 1 Supplementary IOL explantation (▶ https://doi.org/10.1007/000-8d6)

It is also known that multifocal lenses are not advised in the presence of pathological retinal findings. Even in healthy eyes, later pathological changes (e.g., AMD, diabetic macular edema, etc.) can occur, therefore, the implantation of an additional "reversible" multifocal lens in the context of cataract surgery is a interesting alternative. If an eye disease occurs later in life, the sulcus-supported, multifocal, IOL can be removed with very little surgical trauma [6].

Another potential indication for a supplementary intraocular lens is in dynamic refraction cases, such as pediatric cataracts or after silicone oil filling [1]. One of the challenges of pediatric cataract surgery is predicting the postoperative refraction, which changes due to the further growth of the eye, which can cause significant myopic shift. The supplementary IOL can then be exchanged for the necessary refraction.

Note: The reversibility of the procedure, and the different optical options expand the range of indications for refractive cataract surgery.

Conclusion

The implantation of an add-on IOL is a simple and reversible procedure to optimize the refractive result in pseudophakic cases. Refractive results are predictable and based on preoperative refraction rather than lens calculation formulae.

References

1. Amon M, Kahraman G, Schrittwieser H. Supplementary intraocular lenses for pediatric cataract: Primary (Duett Implantation) or secondary implantation. *Spektrum der Augenheilkunde*. 2012.
2. Chang, Wellington H. et al. Pigmentary dispersion syndrome with a secondary piggyback 3-piece hydrophobic acrylic lens. Case report with clinicopathological correlation. J Cataract Refract Surg. 2007.
3. Dagres, Evgenios, Mushtaq A. Khan, Graham M. Kyle, David Clark. Perioperative complications of intraocular lens exchange in patients with opacified aqua-sense lenses. J Cataract Refract Surg. 2004.
4. Findl, Oliver et al. Morphological appearance and size of contact zones of piggyback intraocular lenses. J Cataract Refract Surg. 2001.
5. Gayton, Johnny L., Valerie N. Sanders. Implanting two posterior chamber intraocular lenses in a case of microphthalmos. J Cataract Refract Surg. 1993.
6. Gerten, Georg et al. Dual intraocular lens implantation: Monofocal lens in the bag and additional diffractive multifocal lens in the sulcus. J Cataract Refract Surg. 2009.
7. Hesse, Richard J. Refractive changes produced by capsule contraction after piggyback acrylic intraocular lens implantation. J Cataract Refract Surg. 2002.
8. Iwase, Takeshi, Nobushige Tanaka. Elevated intraocular pressure in secondary piggyback intraocular lens implantation. J Cataract Refract Surg. 2005.
9. Gayton JL et al. Interlenticular opacification: clinicopathological correlation of a complication of posterior chamber piggyback intraocular lenses. J Cataract Refract Surg. 2000.
10. Kahraman G, Dragostinoff N, Brezna W, Bernhart C, Amon M. Visual outcomes and patient satisfaction after bilateral sequential implantation of a capsular bag IOL and a supplementary sulcus-fixated trifocal IOL. J Refract Surg. 2021;37(2):105–11. https://doi.org/10.3928/1081597X-20201215-01.

11. Kahraman G, Amon M. New supplementary intraocular lens for refractive enhancement in pseudophakic patients. J Cataract Refract Surg. 2010; 36(7).
12. Linz K, Auffarth GU, Kretz FTA. Implantation of a sulcus-fixated toric supplementary intraocular lens in a case of high astigmatism after a triple procedure. Klinische Monatsblatter fur Augenheilkunde. 2014.
13. Meyer, Jay J, Bia Z Kim, Mohammed Ziaei, Charles NJ McGhee. Postoperative rotation of supplementary sulcus-supported toric intraocular lenses. J Cataract Refract Surg. 2017.
14. Munõz, Gonzalo, Ceśar Albarrán-Diego, Lurdes Belda, Stephanie Rohrweck. Add-on sulcus-based versus primary in-the-bag multifocal intraocular lens: intraindividual study. J Refract Surg. 2014.
15. Shugar, Joel K, Scott Keeler. Interpseudophakos intraocular lens surface opacification as a late complication of piggyback acrylic posterior chamber lens implantation. J Cataract Refract Surg. 2000.
16. Werner, Liliana et al. Analysis of elements of interlenticular opacification. Am J Ophthalm. 2002.

Considerations in Surgery of Eyes with Cataract and Vitreo-Retinal Diseases

Alvin Kwan-Ho Kwok

Sequential or Combined Cataract and Vitreous Surgery

It is not uncommon to encounter patients with both cataract and vitreo-retinal problems.

If the cataract is already visually significant for the patient or likely affecting the intraoperative surgical view of the posterior segment of the eye, then both cataract and vitreoretinal operations are indicated. The ideal and simplest scenario is combined cataract and vitreoretinal operations in the same setting by a posterior segment surgeon with or without the help of another cataract surgeon. In case the cataract surgery has to be performed first, the cataract surgeon needs a very detailed preoperative assessment and discussion with the patient, as posterior segment pathologies like dense vitreous hemorrhage, ocular hypotony, ocular inflammation, choroidal detachment, etc. might increase the risk of cataract surgery leading to failure of primary intraocular lens implantation, aggregation of posterior segment pathologies and hence more complex subsequent vitreo-retinal surgery.

If the cataract is not visually significant for the patient or unlikely affecting the intraoperative surgical view of the posterior segment of the eye, then whether the patient needs the cataract surgery largely depends on the age of patient and type of surgery. For young patients especially of pre-presbyopic age, we would like to avoid cataract surgery if possible, as rendering them the need of reading add after surgery is not welcoming from them (the discussion of the use of multifocal intraocular lens in this setting will be discussed). If the patient is planned for a scleral buckle, it is better to perform the cataract surgery later to avoid post-combined surgery refractive surprise. Nowadays, more and more vitreo-retinal problems are dealt with through pars planar vitrectomy. If the patient already has cataract or the age is 50 years old or above, we know that the patient has about 70% chance of

A. K.-H. Kwok (✉)
Hong Kong Sanatorium & Hospital, Hong Kong, China
e-mail: alvinkhkwok@netvigator.com

M. Shajari et al. (eds.), *Cataract and Lens Surgery*,
https://doi.org/10.1007/978-3-031-05394-8_41

receiving cataract surgery in the coming 2 years after pars planar vitrectomy [1, 2]. Hence for this group of patients, we have the choice of sequential (usually vitrectomy then cataract surgery) or simultaneous combined cataract and vitrectomy surgery (phaco-vitrectomy). In the USA, practice pattern and medico-legal concern might limit the choice of combined phaco-vitrectomy [3]. Elsewhere, phaco-vitrectomy has been more widely practiced, with the Royal College of Ophthalmologists (UK) database reporting combined phaco-vitrectomy in 49.9 and 40.5% of epiretinal membrane and macular hole surgeries, respectively [4, 5].

The advantages of combined phaco-vitrectomy over the sequential group include convenience for the patient, avoidance of second surgery, faster visual rehabilitation, less total operative time and cost [6]. Additionally there is an option of simultaneous posterior capsulotomy by vitrectomy, [7, 8] as combined phaco-vitrectomy was reported to have a higher rate of posterior capsular opacification than the cataract surgery group in a prospective study [9]. This is particular attractive for patients receiving vitrectomy for visually disturbing floaters. Otherwise, they have to face the future risk of seeing floaters again after receiving post-cataract surgery YAG capsulotomy. Interestingly, there was a retrospective study of posterior capsular opacification (PCO) among a combined procedure group (56 eyes), a sequential procedure group of pars plana vitrectomy and then cataract surgery (33 eyes) and a control group (130 eyes) who underwent cataract surgery alone [10]. The PCO rate checked at 1 year after cataract surgery was 12.5% in the combined surgery group, 24.2% in the sequential surgery group, and 4.6% in the control group. The differences in the PCO rate between the subgroups as well as among the 3 groups were statistically significant ($p < 0.05$). This study demonstrates that the PCO rate may be lower in patients who have a combined phaco-vitrectomy procedure than in those who have a sequential procedure.

A meta-analysis [11] aimed to compare the efficacy and incidence of complications between combined versus sequentially performed phacoemulsification and pars plana vitrectomy (phaco-vitrectomy) for any indication was recently published. Of the 5410 articles identified, 1 randomized controlled trial and 14 comparative studies were included, with 1407 and 951 eyes in the combined and sequential surgery groups, respectively. No significant differences were found in visual and refractive outcomes between combined and sequential groups, but the risks of macular hole non-closure or reopening (risk ratio [RR], 0.18; 95% confidence interval [CI], 0.03–0.93; $P = 0.04$) and posterior capsular tear (RR, 0.43; 95% CI, 0.25–0.73; $P = 0.002$) were significantly lower in the combined group. The cataract surgery may be more challenging after vitrectomy due to decreased vitreous and zonular support, and increased mobility of the posterior capsule [12]. However, the risks of synechiae formation (RR, 2.74; 95% CI, 1.83–4.11; $P < 0.001$), fibrin formation (RR, 2.81; 95% CI, 1.84–4.30; $P < 0.001$), and intraoperative or postoperative retinal detachment (RR, 2.65; 95% CI, 1.08–6.47; $P = 0.03$) were significantly higher after combined surgery. Although most evidence is derived from low- to moderate-quality retrospective studies, the above findings suggest that there may be more postoperative inflammation in the combined phaco-vitrectomy group. A two-round Delphi survey asked 28 international experts to rate both the inflammatory potential of different eye surgeries and their agreement with different treatment protocols. They rated combined phaco-vitrectomy as more inflammatory than cataract surgery [13]. However, the panel preferred the same treatment for combined phaco-vitrectomy, as for cataract surgery (topical non-steroid anti-inflammatory and corticosteroid three times a day for 1 month). The discrepancy between preferred treatment and perception of the eye's inflammatory status by the experts for combined vitreoretinal surgeries highlights the need for randomized control studies to establish treatment guidelines. I would recommend the use of topical non-steroid anti-inflammatory drop 3–4 times per day starting 3 days before surgery and topical non-steroid anti-inflammatory and corticosteroid 3–4 times per day for 1 month then gradually tapered, in such surgery. Regular monitoring of intraocular pressure, especially in myopic eyes, is strongly recommended.

Patients with Cataract and Epiretinal Membrane (ERM)

Ophthalmologists worry that the change of macular thickness after ERM surgery would lead to a significant refractive surprise after combined surgery, as compared to sequential one. In a single-center, retrospective study of 50 eyes that underwent combined phaco-vitrectomy and a control group of 50 eyes after cataract surgery over a 3-year period by a single anterior segment surgeon and a single posterior segment surgeon, they found that combined phaco-vitrectomy for concurrent cataract epiretinal membrane by experienced cataract and vitreoretinal surgeons seems to deliver as predictable refractive results as cataract surgery alone [14]. In a prospective clinical trial of 62 eyes, [15] the authors allocated phakic eyes with ERM to (1) cataract surgery and subsequent pars plana vitrectomy (PPV) (CAT group), (2) PPV and subsequent cataract surgery (VIT group) or (3) phaco-vitrectomy (COMBI group). In the immediate postoperative period, there was a higher incidence of CME in the CAT group. At 12 months follow-up, either phaco-vitrectomy or sequential surgery are equal approaches with respect to functional- (the difference between predicted and achieved spherical equivalence, best-corrected visual acuity) and anatomical outcomes (cystoid macular edema, central subfield macular thickness by optical coherent tomography test). Interestingly, if starting with cataract surgery, 17% of the cases may not need subsequent PPV.

Patients with Cataract and Age-Related Macular Degeneration

Cataracts and age-related macular degeneration (AMD) are common causes of visual impairment all over the world. With the growing aging population, these eye diseases become more prevalent causing visual disability, an increase in the risk of falls, fractures, depression, mortality and a decrease in quality of life [16, 17].

The advent of intravitreal anti-VEGF (vascular endothelial growth factor) injections has revolutionized the treatment of and improved the visual prognosis for patients with AMD. Prior to that, cataract surgery was believed to increase the risk of neovascular hemorrhage and leakage, resulting in worsening visual deterioration. In a prospective, multicenter, randomized controlled trial of nutritional supplements for treatment of AMD, the Age-Related Eye Disease Study 2, the visual acuity outcomes of a total of 1232 eyes of 793 participants with varying degrees of severity of age-related macular degeneration (AMD) and underwent cataract surgery were evaluated [18]. it showed that the mean visual acuities improved significantly after cataract surgery across varying degrees of AMD severity.

Whether blue-blocking intraocular lens (IOLs) protect against the development of AMD is controversial, despite they account for approximately 25% of IOLs implanted worldwide [19]. A register-based cohort study with data from the Swedish National Cataract Register and the Swedish Macula Register from 2010 to 2017 compared eyes with and without preoperative AMD that had undergone cataract surgery and was subsequently treated for wet AMD to eyes not treated within the study period. The only independent factor associated with postoperative treatment of wet AMD in both groups was female gender (67.3% vs. 58.8%, $p < 0.001$ and 66.4% vs. 60.6%, $p = 0.001$, respectively). Older age was an independent factor in eyes without preoperative AMD (78.4 ± 6.5 vs. 73.4 ± 9.6 years, $p < 0.001$). A blue-blocking IOL appeared to decrease the likelihood of subsequent wet AMD treatment slightly but not statistically significant in eyes with preoperative AMD (52.7% vs. 56.8%, $p = 0.110$) [20]. In a systematic review study, the authors show with moderate certainty that there is no clinically meaningful difference in short-term BCVA with the two types of IOLs. Further, these findings suggest that there is no clinically meaningful difference in short-term contrast sensitivity with the two interventions, although there was a low level of certainty for this outcome due to a small number of included studies and their inherent risk of bias. Based upon current, best-available research evidence, it is unclear whether blue-light filtering IOLs preserve macular health or alter risks associated with the development and progression of AMD, or both [21].

Studies investigating the risk of posterior capsular rupture (PCR) during cataract surgery in eyes with previous intravitreal injection (IVI) were published [22, 23]. The Moorfields Patient Administrative System and Open Eyes electronic databases were used to study all cataract surgery procedures undertaken between January 1, 2012 and August 31, 2015 in the Moorfields main and satellite sites. Among the 62,994 cataract surgery procedures undertaken over the study period, 1035 (1.64%)

were in eyes with previous intravitreal injection(s). PCR occurred in 650 (1.04%) eyes. After logistic regression, prior intravitreal injection was associated with an increased risk of PCR (P = 0.037), with an odds ratio of 1.66. The number of prior injections, indication for injections, and service undertaking the surgery were not associated with increased risk of PCR (P > 0.1) [22]. Another similar study in United Kingdom analyzed data for eyes undergoing cataract surgery from 20 hospitals using the same EMR for cases performed between 2004 and 2014. Among the 65,836 cataract operations, 1935 (2.9%) had undergone previous intravitreal therapy. In univariate regression analyses, patient age, advanced cataract, junior cataract surgeon grade, and number of previous intravitreal injections were significant predictors of PCR. By considering the number of previous intravitreal injections as a continuous variable, the odds ratio for PCR per intravitreal injection was 1.04 (P = 0.016) after adjusting for age, advanced cataract, and cataract surgeon grade. Repeat analysis considering intravitreal injections as a categoric variable showed 10 or more previous injections were associated with a 2.59 times higher likelihood of PCR (P = 0.003) after again adjusting for other significant independent predictors [23].

Patients with Cataract and Diabetic Retinopathy

Before surgery, patients should have good diabetic control and no evidence of ocular or periocular infection, as diabetics have a significantly higher prevalence of Staphylococcus aureus, Enterococci, certain Streptococci, and Klebsiella sp. than non-diabetics [24, 25]. Diabetic macular edema (DME) should be adequately treated before surgery as preexisting maculopathy may be aggravated postoperatively with associated poor visual outcome [26]. In patients with preexisting or treated DME, cataract surgery can increase the risk of progression or re-development of DME to 20%–50% [27, 28]. Similar to AMD, the advent of intravitreal anti-VEGF injections has revolutionized the treatment of DME and proliferative diabetic retinopathy [29, 30]. Additionally, perioperative antibiotics and anti-inflammatory agents should be considered, on top of strict intraoperative asepsis [31]. Combined phaco-vitrectomy can be considered in eyes with vitreous hemorrhage, traction retinal detachment and maculopathies.

Anterior capsular contraction after cataract surgery was greater in eyes of diabetic patients, especially in those with diabetic retinopathy and elevated aqueous flare intensity 12 months after surgery [32]. Ideally, the capsulorhexis size in eyes of diabetic patients should be slightly smaller than the optic diameter of IOL to balance the risk of anterior capsular phimosis and posterior capsular opacification. Anterior capsule phimosis and opacification were significantly less observed in the Technis IOLs (Abbott Medical Optics, Santa Ana, CA) with a continuous edge than in AcrySof IOLs (Alcon Laboratories, Fort Worth, TX) with an interrupted sharp optic edge [33, 34]. The aqueous humor and serum level of phosphorus in diabetics was significantly increased, especially in those with proliferative diabetic retinopathy. This result may be related to opacification of hydrophilic acrylic IOL [35]. Hydrophobic acrylic lenses have the lowest propensity for silicone oil adhesion and should be the IOL of choice in diabetic patients with potential need of complex vitreoretinal surgery [36]. Iris hooks, malyugin ring or other iris retractors should be prepared as there is a risk of poor pupillary dilatation related to pupillary parasympathetic supply damage in diabetic eyes [37]. As mentioned above, the risk of posterior capsular rupture during cataract surgery in eyes with previous intravitreal injection were increased [22, 23].

Multifocal IOL in Vitreo-Retinal Diseases

Multifocal IOLs may bring about unwanted visual disturbances such as glare, halo and reduced contrast sensitivity [38]. Posterior vitreous detachment, which is a common phenomenon seen in aging patients, is known to cause increase in light scattering, also resulting in a decrease in contrast sensitivity [39]. Macular diseases such as epiretinal membrane, age-related macular degeneration and diabetic maculopathy can progress after cataract surgery, resulting in a reduction in contrast sensitivity [40]. Another concern to the implantation of multifocal IOLs in previous vitrectomized eyes is a potential damage to the posterior capsule during previous posterior vitrectomies and a poor visualization of the posterior segment through the multifocal IOL [41]. Hence, presence of vitreoretinal diseases is a relative contraindication of implanting multifocal IOL due to the concern of further reduction in contrast sensitivity in these eyes. Careful patient selection, preoperative evaluation and counseling are very crucial in achieving the maximum potential of multifocal IOLs, with a warning of potential risk of IOL exchange. Our results show that the corrected distance visual acuity is improved after multifocal IOL implantation in eyes with vitrectomy done [42]. The near visual acuity of all eyes was also improved. The National Eye Institute Refractive Error Quality of Life Instrument-42 questionnaire also revealed very good subjective results reflecting a high subjective quality of life. Additionally, we found that visualization of the posterior segment was not compromised in eyes with any type multifocal IOLs implanted and we did not experience any intraoperative and postoperative complications. In general, patients with good visual potential of 20/20 vision after cataract and macular sparing vitreo-retinal surgeries, like vitreous opacification, uncomplicated vitreous hemorrhage and retinal detachment, may be given the option of full range of multifocal IOLs if they prefer no or less spectacle dependence. In patients with macular involving diseases like diabetic maculopathy, epiretinal membrane and macular hole, multifocal IOLs should only be considered if the predicted final vision after cataract and vitreo-retinal surgeries is to be 20/40 or better. In this group of eyes, extended depth of focus IOL, like Technis Symfony (Abbott Medical Optics, Santa Ana, CA) is safer and more forgiving than trifocal IOLs, as the former gives higher contrast sensitivity performance [43]. Extended depth of focus IOL, however, may not be able to provide adequate unaided near vision. To compensate for that, target refraction aiming at -0.5DS to -1DS may help. The same or other type of multifocal IOL can be considered in the fellow eye [44].

References

1. Jackson TL, Donachie PHJ, Sparrow JM, Johnston RL. United Kingdom National Ophthalmology Database Study of Vitreoretinal Surgery: report 1. Case mix, complications, and cataract. Eye (Basingstoke). 2013;27:644–51.
2. Melberg NS, Thomas MA. Nuclear sclerotic cataract after vitrectomy in patients younger than 50 years of age. Ophthalmology. 1995;102:1466–71.
3. Mompremier M, Adyanthaya R. Retina today - phacovitrectomy for the retina surgeon. In: Retina Today http://retinatoday.com/2014/10/phacovitrectomy-for-the-retina-surgeon/. Accessed 14 May 2019.
4. Jackson TL, Donachie PHJ, Williamson TH, et al. The royal college of ophthalmologists' national ophthalmology database study of vitreoretinal surgery: report 4, epiretinal membrane. Retina. 2015;35:1615–21.
5. Jackson TL, Donachie PHJ, Sparrow JM, Johnston RL. United Kingdom national ophthalmology database study of vitreoretinal surgery: report 2, macular hole. Ophthalmology. 2013;120(3):629–34.
6. Port AD, Nolan JG, Siegel NH, Chen X, Ness SD, Subramanian ML. Combined phaco-vitrectomy provides lower costs and greater area under the curve vision gains than sequential vitrectomy and phacoemulsification. Graefes Arch Clin Exp Ophthalmol. 2021;259 (1):45–52.
7. Shin KS, Park HJ, Jo YJ, Kim JY. Efficacy and safety of primary posterior capsulotomy in combined phaco-vitrectomy in rhegmatogenous retinal detachment. PLoS ONE. 2019;14(3): e0213457.
8. Aizawa N, Kunikata H, Abe T, Nakazawa T. Efficacy of combined 25-gauge microincision vitrectomy, intraocular lens implantation, and posterior capsulotomy. J Cataract Refract Surg. 2012;38(9):1602–7.
9. Toda J, Kato S, Oshika T, Sugita G. Posterior capsule opacification after combined cataract surgery and vitrectomy. J Cataract Refract Surg. 2007;33(1):104–7.
10. Roh JH, Sohn HJ, Lee DY, Shyn KH, Nam DH. Comparison of posterior capsular opacification between a combined procedure and a sequential procedure of pars plana vitrectomy and cataract surgery. Ophthalmologica. 2010;224(1):42–6.
11. Farahvash A, Popovic MM, Eshtiaghi A, Kertes PJ, Muni RH. Combined versus Sequential Phacoemulsification and Pars Plana Vitrectomy: A Meta-Analysis. Ophthalmol Retina. 2021;20:S2468–6530(21)00014–2.
12. Smiddy WE, Stark WJ, Michels RG, et al. Cataract extraction after vitrectomy. Ophthalmology. 1987;94:483–7.
13. Aptel F, Colin C, Kaderli S, Deloche C, Bron AM, Stewart MW, Chiquet C. OSIRIS group. Management of postoperative inflammation after cataract and complex ocular surgeries: a systematic review and Delphi survey. Br J Ophthalmol. 2017;101(11):1–10.
14. Shi L, Chang JS, Suh LH, Chang S. Differences in refractive outocmes between phacoemulsificaton for cataract alone and combined phacoemulsification and vitrectomy for epiretinal membrane. Retina. 2019;39(7):1410–5.
15. Hamoudi H, Correll Christensen U, La Cour M. Epiretinal membrane surgery: an analysis of 2-step sequential- or combined phacovitrectomy surgery on refraction and macular anatomy in a prospective trial. Acta Ophthalmol. 2018;96(3):243–50.

16. Tseng VL, Yu F, Lum F, Coleman AL. Risk of fractures following cataract surgery in Medicare beneficiaries. JAMA. 2012;308:493–501.
17. Brody BL, Gamst AC, Williams RA, et al. Depression, visual acuity, comorbidity, and disability associated with age-related macular degeneration. Ophthalmology. 2001;108:1893–900.
18. Age-Related Eye Disease Study 2 Research Group. Nancy Huynh, Benjamin P Nicholson, Elvira Agrón, et al. Visual acuity after cataract surgery in patients with age-related macular degeneration: age-related eye disease study 2 report number 5. Ophthalmology. 2014 ;121 (6):1229–1236.
19. Mainster MA, Turner PL. Blue-blocking IOLs vs. short-wavelength visible light: hypothesis-based vs. evidence-based medical practice. Ophthalmology 2011;118(1):1-2.
20. Westborg I, Albrecht S, Granstam E, et al. Treatment of age-related macular degeneration after cataract surgery: a study from the Swedish national cataract and macula registers. Acta Ophthalmol. 2021;99(1):e124–9.
21. Laura E Downie 1, Ljoudmila Busija, Peter R Keller. Blue-light filtering intraocular lenses (IOLs) for protecting macular health. Cochrane Database Syst Rev. 201822;5(5):CD011977.
22. Shalchi Z, Okada M, Whiting C, Hamilton R. Risk of posterior capsule rupture during cataract surgery in eyes with previous intravitreal jnjections. Am J Ophthalmol. 2017;177:77–80.
23. Aaron Y Lee, Alexander C Day, Catherine Egan, et al. United Kingdom Age-related Macular Degeneration and Diabetic Retinopathy Electronic Medical Records Users Group. Previous intravitreal therapy is associated with increased risk of posterior capsule rupture during cataract surgery. Ophthalmology. 2016;123(6):1252–6.
24. Kelkar A, Kelkar J, Mehta H, Amoaku W. Cataract surgery in diabetes mellitus: A systematic review. Indian J Ophthalmol. 2018;66(10):1401–10.
25. Fernández-Rubio ME, Rebolledo-Lara L, Martinez-García M, Alarcón-Tomás M, Cortés-Valdés C. The conjunctival bacterial pattern of diabetics undergoing cataract surgery. Eye. 2010;24(5):825–34.
26. Squirrell D, Bhola R, Bush J, Winder S, Talbot JF. A prospective, case controlled study of the natural history of diabetic retinopathy and maculopathy after uncomplicated phacoemulsification cataract surgery in patients with type 2 diabetes. Br J Ophthalmol. 2002;86(5):565–71.
27. Diabetic Retinopathy Clinical Research Network Authors/Writing Committee. Baker CW, Almukhtar T, Bressler NM, Glassman AR, Grover S, et al. Macular edema after cataract surgery in eyes without preoperative central-involved diabetic macular edema. JAMA Ophthalmol. 2013;131:870–879.
28. Chen XY, Song WJ, Cai HY, Zhao L. Macular edema after cataract surgery in diabetic eyes evaluated by optical coherence tomography. Int J Ophthalmol. 2016;9:81–5.
29. Wells JA, Glassman AR, Ayala AR, et al. Diabetic Retinopathy Clinical Research Network. Aflibercept, Bevacizumab, or Ranibizumab for Diabetic Macular Edema: Two-Year Results from a Comparative Effectiveness Randomized Clinical Trial. Ophthalmology. 2016;123 (6):1351–1359.
30. Gross JG, Glassman AR, Liu D, et al. Diabetic Retinopathy Clinical Research Network. Five-Year Outcomes of Panretinal Photocoagulation vs Intravitreous Ranibizumab for Proliferative Diabetic Retinopathy: A Randomized Clinical Trial. JAMA Ophthalmol. 2018;136(10):1138–48.
31. DeCroos FC, Afshari NA. Perioperative antibiotics and anti-inflammatory agents in cataract surgery. Curr Opin Ophthalmol. 2008;19(1):22–6.
32. Kato S, Oshika T, Numaga J, Hayashi Y, Oshiro M, Yuguchi T, et al. Anterior capsular contraction after cataract surgery in eyes of diabetic patients. Br J Ophthalmol. 2001;85:21–3.
33. Johansson B. Glistenings, anterior/posterior capsular opacification and incidence of Nd:YAG laser treatments with two aspheric hydrophobic acrylic intraocular lenses - a long-term intra-individual study. Acta Ophthalmol. 2017;95(7):671–7.

34. Kahraman G, Ferdinaro C, Wetzel B, et al. Intraindividual comparison of capsule behavior of 2 hydrophobic acrylic intraocular lenses during a 5-year follow-up. J Cataract Refract Surg. 2017;43:228–33.
35. Kim CJ, Choi SK. Analysis of aqueous humor calcium and phosphate from cataract eyes with and without diabetes mellitus. Korean J Ophthalmol. 2007;21(2):90–4.
36. Eaton AM, Jaffe GJ, McCuen BW 2nd, Mincey GJ. Condensation on the posterior surface of silicone intraocular lenses during fluid-air exchange. Ophthalmology. 1995;102:733–6.
37. Cahill M, Eustace P, de Jesus V. Pupillary autonomic denervation with increasing duration of diabetes mellitus. Br J Ophthalmol. 2001;85:1225–30.
38. Cao K, Friedman DS, Jin S, et al. Multifocal versus monofocal intraocular lenses for age-related cataract patients: a system review and meta-analysis based on randomized controlled trials. Surv Ophthalmol. 2019;64:647–58.
39. Sebag J, Yee KMP, Wa CA, Huang LC, Sadun AA. Vitrectomy for floaters: prospective efficacy analyses and retrospective safety profile. Retina. 2014;34(6):1062–8.
40. Liu L, Wang Y, Liu J, Liu W. Retinal-image quality and contrast sensitivity function in eyes with epiretinal membrane: a cross-sectional observational clinical study. BMC Ophthalmol. 2018; 18(1):290:1–6.
41. Hadayer A, Jusufbegovic D, Schaal S. Retinal detachment repair through multifocal intraocular lens- overcoming visualization challenge of the peripheral retina. Int J Ophthalmol. 2017;10(6):1008–10.
42. Chow LLWan, Fung NSK, Kwok AKH Alvin. Premium intraocular lens implantation in eyes with vitrectomy done. Int Ophthalmol. 2020 ;40(11):2949–56.
43. Mencucci R, Favuzza E, Caporossi O, Savastano A, Rizzo S. Comparative analysis of visual outcomes, reading skills, contrast sensitivity, and patient satisfaction with two models of trifocal diffractive intraocular lenses and an extended range of vision intraocular lens. Graefes Arch Clin Exp Ophthalmol. 2018;256(10):1913–22.
44. Black S. A clinical assessment of visual performance of combining the TECNIS Symfony Extended Range of Vision IOL (ZXR00) with the +3.25 D TECNIS Multifocal 1-piece IOL (ZLB00) in subjects undergoing bilateral cataract extraction. Clin Ophthalmol. 2018;12:2129–36.

Considerations in the Amblyopic Patient When Planning Cataract Surgery

Basak Bostanci

Amblyopia is a neuro-developmental disorder of the visual cortex and caused by disturbance in retinal image formation, by insufficient or inappropriate stimuli, during first years of life [1]. In the absence of any organic eye disease or refractive error being neutralized with lenses, a loss of visual acuity or impairment in stereopsis, position acuity and contrast sensitivity arise [2, 3].

Amblyopia is typically unilateral (but can be bilateral) and is estimated to affect between 1 and 4% of the general population [4, 5]. It is typically classified as strabismic, anisometropic, ametropic or deprivation amblyopia. Early treatment of amblyopia can improve vision, which may lead to a better prognosis for binocular vision development and a more stable alignment for strabismus surgery, if required [6]. It is believed that visual acuity and stereopsis in an amblyopic patient cannot be improved after a certain age (between 7 and 9) since the visual system is beyond the critical period for binocular vision development [7]. Studies conducted in the last 15 years, however, show that this is not true, as significant plasticity can be induced beyond a critical period if appropriate input is provided. The extent of recovery at this later stage, however, may be less complete [8].

When amblyopic patients develop cataract, it is not easy to decide when to perform the surgery. The low visual expectancy in the amblyopic eye may lead to delaying the operation, which may cause complications. On the other hand, the excellent visual acuity results obtained with today's cataract surgery may cause patients to have unrealistic expectations, and patients may even consider cataract surgery as a treatment option that will eliminate their amblyopia. At this point, the key to success is the correct timing of the surgery, informing patients about realistic

B. Bostanci (✉)
Cataract and Refractive Surgery Department, World Eye Hospital, Istanbul, Turkey
e-mail: drbbostanci@gmail.com

B. Bostanci
Ophthalmology Department, Bahcesehir University School of Medicine, Istanbul, Turkey

M. Shajari et al. (eds.), *Cataract and Lens Surgery*,
https://doi.org/10.1007/978-3-031-05394-8_42

results, and having a good knowledge of intraocular lenses (IOLs) that may be suitable for these patients.

The suppression of the visual information coming from the amblyopic eye can lead to the expectation that should a cataract develop in this eye, it will not significantly affect the patient's visual quality. There is more recent evidence however that amblyopic eyes are still very sensitive in detecting blur and glare, despite the reduced visual acuity and contrast sensitivity [9]. Even the most severe amblyopes can complete hard matching tasks that require edge sharpness matching, even though the spatial composition of these edges is outside the range of apparent resolution. This can be seen in both strabismus and anisometropic amblyopia.

A few studies have consistently reported visual improvement in adults with anisometropic amblyopia after refractive surgery [10, 11]. It is suggested that if the visual data flow between the eyes is balanced by correcting the refractive errors, the plasticity of the adult visual cortex can also be changed [12, 13]. Similar to refractive surgery, cataract extraction with intraocular lens implantation can improve vision in anisometropic amblyopic eyes through refractive correction and restoration of the clear optical medium.

In the 1997–1998 National Cataract Surgery Survey, 50% of amblyopic patients and 77% of those without amblyopia achieved 20/40 or better visual acuity. Although 11.5% of amblyopic eyes had white cataracts, it was present in only 3% of non-amblyopic eyes. In addition, 75% of the complications were observed in amblyopic eyes with white cataracts which serves as a reminder of the importance of carefully evaluating cataracts in amblyopic patients. Delaying surgery unnecessarily might increase the risk of complications associated with dense cataract [14].

Kwon et al. suggested that a large number of patients diagnosed with amblyopia may not have received the appropriate correction to ensure a favorable emmetropic condition [15]. The reduction caused by spectacles can be a source of visual impairment in patients with high spherical or cylindrical refractive errors [13]. The relative magnification of the image after correction that is performed on the corneal plane instead of the spectacle plane may contribute to the increase in postoperative vision in some cases after refractive surgery and may contribute to the increase in visual potential after surgery [16, 17]. Regardless of the mechanism, providing a clear optic media and eliminating high refractive errors are key for improving the visual potential in adult amblyopia, even in cases where the improvement in visual acuity is based on neuroplasticity alone.

Visual acuity is not the only factor that determines the visual quality of a patient and the extent of suppression on visual field due to amblyopia during binocular gaze is a matter of debate. This probably depends on the type and severity of amblyopia, but research suggests that, at least, the temporal crescent is preserved in most amblyopic eyes. The improvement in binocular vision of esotropic patients after strabismus operations may indicate that amblyopic eyes can also contribute to the visual field [18, 19].

In addition to the improvement in visual field, performing cataract surgery in the amblyopic eye is also important restoring binocular summation and stereopsis [20, 21]. However the effect on summation and stereopsis may be different in anisometropic amblyopic patients and strabismic cases with suppression. In anisometropic amblyopia, the correction of anisometropia may lead to the correction of the anisoconia which the patient has already adapted to, leading to a loss of fusion and decrease in binocular function. If the cataract surgery of the amblyopic eye is performed before the other eye, and the postoperative visual quality and acuity in the amblyopic eye becomes better than the other eye, and the so-called "fixation switch diplopia" may occur [22].

Fixation switch diplopia develops in a patient with a history of diplopia, strabismus, and / or amblyopia when the vision of the dominant eye is reduced, relative to the other, and may be difficult to treat and can cause significant morbidity [11]. As a result, extreme caution should be taken when planning the sequence of cataract surgery in those cases. There may be other reasons for diplopia following cataract surgery. In addition to the fixation switch diplopia, it may be caused by poor suppression, disruption of central fusion, or the onset of a concurrent systemic disease and can be seen in up to 3% of patients after cataract surgery [23, 24]. On the other hand, a cross-sectional study conducted in Wales showed that the awareness of diplopia after cataract surgery, and especially fixation shift diplopia, is not common among surgeons performing surgery [25]. When questioned, 34.4% of the surgeons participating in the study stated that they would operate the amblyopic eye first while planning cataract surgery, and 18.2% stated that they made this decision because they thought that any complication to occur in the amblyopic eye would be less important than the dominant eye. This not only increases chance of fixation switch diplopia, but also delays the treatment of the patient's main complaint, namely the visual impairment caused by the dominant eye.

Which Intraocular Lens to Use?

The choice of intraocular lens in patients with a history of amblyopia is another controversial topic. Particular caution must be taken when planning an amblyopic patient who expects complete independence from glasses after cataract surgery.

Firstly, it is important to know that the results of monovision are below the desired level in this group of patients. The major problem associated with monovision relates to the potential compromise in binocular visual function while trying to increase the depth of focus. The summation of the monocular range of clear vision is needed for each eye to achieve monovision, where the far focal point is set for far vision eye and the near focal point of the near vision eye and, as can be expected, maintaining acceptable stereovision in an already compromised setting is hard to manage. The main purpose of inducing monovision after cataract surgery is to reduce the dependence on glasses. In cases where the amblyopic eye is chosen as the near eye, no problem is expected in distance vision; however, the possibility of complete independence from the glasses is limited. When the healthy dominant eye has a strong ocular dominance, it lacks blur suppression for near and in cases of amblyopia, where strong ocular dominance is present, patients tend to suppress information originating from the non-dominant eye, which makes near vision blurry [26].

It should be noted that fixation switch diplopia can also occur when intentional or unintentional monovision modality is achieved after cataract surgery. Kushner reported this phenomenon in 16 adult patients with a history of strabismus [22]. Six of those patients developed diplopia secondary to their monovision correction after cataract surgery. Symptoms were eliminated when proper optical correction was instituted to encourage fixation with the dominant eye in all of those patients. Meridional amblyopia is a type of amblyopia which can be seen in individuals with high astigmatism (>3 D). Those patients show impaired vision despite optical correction in that astigmatic orientation. Some ophthalmologists do not recommend toric intraocular lenses for people with meridional amblyopia [27].

Although meridional amblyopia can be treated with optical correction in children up to school age, sometimes it may not be completely eliminated with glasses alone [28]. Children with astigmatism showed significantly lower best spectacle-corrected visual acuity (BCVA) compared to similarly treated amblyopes without astigmatism. Substantial distortion and suboptimal image quality can also be induced with spectacle correction of high astigmatism. In addition, the instability of the spectacle frame may contribute to the poor image quality [29].

Studies show that the improvement in visual acuity is higher following laser in situ keratomileusis (LASIK) in patients with meridional amblyopia than spectacle correction [11]. Arruabarrena et al. reported significant improvement in post-LASIK BCVA in meridional amblyopes (>3 D) [30]. Elimination of the meridional magnification secondary to vertex distance of the spectacle lens from the pupil and the decreased distortion of image quality secondary to limited stability of spectacle frame may be the main reasons for this improvement. Hence, by overcoming those factors, toric IOLs may induce similar improvements in post-operative visual acuity.

Multifocal IOL implantation in amblyopia is a controversial subject. Amblyopic patients lack the benefit of summation in binocular vision. Functionally, one-eyed patients should not expect to achieve the visual function that would result from bilateral multifocality. In addition, the decrease in contrast sensitivity caused by diffractive multifocal IOLs can further impair the quality of vision of these patients, since their second eyes do not have compensatory visual contribution [31]. Central vision in amblyopia should not be defined as a "reduced version" of normal foveal vision. The amblyopic condition includes a wide variety of visual deficiencies such as crowding, and misperception of grating signs [32]. These problems may disturb the complex neuroprocessing, the ability to interpret two images falling simultaneously on the retina, which is necessary during vision with multifocal lenses. Finally, amblyopic patients do not only suffer from misperceptions in the amblyopic eye, but they also frequently have subclinical deficits in the better eye [33].

On the other hand however, there are many studies which suggest that anisometropic amblyopic patients can actually benefit from the advantages of a multifocal IOLs. Petermeier et al. reported favorable visual outcomes in a non-controlled case series after implantation of the Restor diffractive multifocal IOL

(Alcon Laboratories, Inc.) in a small group of patients with mild to moderate amblyopia [34]. Their study suggested that stereo acuity was not correlated to visual acuity and preoperative suppression of the amblyopic eye. In addition, reduced performance in stereo tests or the degree of visual loss in the amblyopic eye was not a predictive factor for the postoperative binocular vision in such cases. Although amblyopic eyes' visual and stereo acuity achieved the level determined by the underlying amblyopia, dysphotopic problems, disturbed neuroprocessing of the separate images or interference with binocular contrast sensitivity were not encountered in the cases they reported. In contrast to non-amblyopic patients, where binocular visual acuity is usually one line better than monocular visual acuity after ReSTOR implantation, amblyopic patients' binocular visual acuity was not better than the monocular visual acuity in the better eye [35]. Similarly, de Wit et al. reported that there was no significant change in contrast sensitivity after Lentis Mplus multifocal IOL implantation in patients with mild to moderate anisometropic amblyopia, with binocular contrast sensitivity scores being equivalent to unilateral scores [36]. However, reading scores improved with binocular implantation in their group. They also found an improvement in binocular reading speed that surpassed the postoperative unilateral best acuity reading speed and explained this finding through a relative increase in Panum's fusional area in such patients.

It is worth emphasizing that the patients evaluated in both Petermeier's and de Wit's studies have mild to moderate amblyopia. Since it is hard to conduct comparative controlled clinical trials in such a group of patients, more objective evidence of long-term improvement in amblyopic patients' symptoms is required to advocate the use of any multifocal IOL in amblyopic patients. In addition, although there is no study about the use of enhanced monofocal IOLs in such patients their use may have promising results.

Ongoing investigations into the understanding of the neural basis of amblyopia and the use of new technology promise alternative and likely better treatments and cures in the future for this condition. Early work on perceptual learning and iPad-based dichoptic training have generated promising data for visual improvement in amblyopes [37–39]. Use of pharmaceutical augmentation with several therapeutic agents like levodopa and citicoline to neurosensitize the brain and enhance responsiveness to amblyopia therapy has also been investigated and promising results have been achieved [40, 41].

In conclusion, eyes with amblyopia can develop cataracts just like normal eyes. There is a need for more studies on the parameters to be evaluated when determining the indication or timing of cataract surgery in these eyes, the sequence to be followed in bilateral planning, the lenses that can be selected, and whether it is necessary to change the route in different types of amblyopia. However, current treatments to increase the visual potential in amblyopia show hope that in the future, satisfactory visual results will be obtained in patients with amblyopia after cataract surgery.

References

1. Holmes JM, Clarke MP. Amblyopia. Lancet. 2006, 22;367(9519):1343–51. https://doi.org/10.1016/S0140-6736(06)68581-4. PMID: 16631913.
2. Holmes JM, Repka MX, Kraker RT, Clarke MP. The treatment of amblyopia. Strabismus. 2006;14(1):37–42. https://doi.org/10.1080/09273970500536227 PMID: 16513568.
3. Levi DM. Visual processing in amblyopia: human studies. Strabismus. 2006;14(1):11–9. https://doi.org/10.1080/09273970500536243 PMID: 16513566.
4. Pai AS, Rose KA, Leone JF, Sharbini S, Burlutsky G, Varma R, Wong TY, Mitchell P. Amblyopia prevalence and risk factors in Australian preschool children. Ophthalmology. 2012;119:138–44.
5. McKean-Cowdin R, Cotter SA, Tarczy-Hornoch K, Wen G, Kim J, Borchert M, et al. Prevalence of amblyopia or strabismus in asian and non-Hispanic white preschool children: Multi-ethnic pediatric eye disease study. Ophthalmology. 2013;120:2117–24.
6. Demirci, Goktug, et al. "Do Amblyopic Eye First, Wait and Do Second Eye Cataract Surgery for Isoametropia, Accomodative Esotropic Amblyopia and Congenital Cataract Case." *American Journal of Medical Sciences and Medicine* 1.2 (2013): 21–23.
7. Wong AM. New concepts concerning the neural mechanisms of amblyopia and their clinical implications. Can J Ophthalmol. 2012;47(5):399–409.
8. Repka MX, Kraker RT, Beck RW, Birch E, Cotter SA, Holmes JM, Hertle RW, Hoover DL, Klimek DL, Marsh-Tootle W, Scheiman MM, Suh DW, Weakley DR. Pediatric eye disease investigator group. Treatment of severe amblyopia with weekend atropine: results from 2 randomized clinical trials. J AAPOS. 2009 Jun;13(3):258–63. https://doi.org/10.1016/j.jaapos.2009.03.002. PMID: 19541265; PMCID: PMC2713117.
9. Desai P, Minassian DC, Reidy A. National cataract surgery survey 1997–8: a report of the results of the clinical outcomes. Br J Ophthalmol. 1999;83:1336–40.
10. Cagil N, Ugurlu N, Cakmak HB, Ilker Kocamis S, Turak D, Simsek S. Photorefractive keratectomy in treatment of refractive amblyopia in the adult population. J Cataract Refract Surg. 2011;37(12):2167–74. https://doi.org/10.1016/j.jcrs.2011.06.026 PMID: 22108111.
11. Barequet IS, Wygnanski-Jaffe T, Hirsh A. Laser in situ keratomileusis improves visual acuity in some adult eyes with amblyopia. J Refract Surg. 2004 Jan-Feb;20(1):25–8. PMID: 14763467.
12. Simmers AJ, Bex PJ, Hess RF. Perceived blur in amblyopia. Invest Ophthalmol Vis Sci. 2003;44:1395–400.
13. Hale JE, Murjaneh S, Frost NA, Harrad RA. How should we manage an amblyopic patient with cataract? Br J Ophthalmol. 2006;90(2):132–3. https://doi.org/10.1136/bjo.2005.080689.PMID:16424518;PMCID:PMC1860192.
14. Desai P, Reidy A, Minassian DC. Profile of patients presenting for cataract surgery in the UK: national data collection. Br J Ophthalmol. 1999;83:893–6.
15. Kwon SW, Moon HS, Shyn KH. Visual improvement in high myopic amblyopic adult eyes following phakic anterior chamber intraocular lens implantation. Korean J Ophthalmol. 2006;20:87–92.
16. Sakatani K, Jabbur NS, O'Brien TP. Improvement in best corrected visual acuity in amblyopic adult eyes after laser in situ keratomileusis. J Cataract Refract Surg. 2004;30:2517–21.
17. Lanza M, Rosa N, Capasso L, Iaccarino G, Rossi S, Romano A. Can we utilize photorefractive keratectomy to improve visual acuity in adult amblyopic eyes? Ophthalmology. 2005;112:1684–91.
18. Kushner BJ. Binocular visual field expansion in adults after surgery for esotropia. Arch Ophthalmol. 1994;112:639–43.
19. Quah SA, Kaye SB. Binocular visual field changes after surgery in esotropic amblyopia. Invest Ophthalmol Vis Sci. 2004;45:1817–22.
20. Laidlaw A, Harrad R. Can second eye cataract surgery be justified? Eye. 1993;7(Pt 5):680–6.

21. Laidlaw DAH, Harrad RA, Hopper CD, et al. Randomised trial of effectiveness of second eye cataract surgery. Lancet. 1998;352:925–9.
22. Kushner BJ. Fixation switch diplopia. Arch Ophthalmol. 1995;113(7):896–9.
23. Nayak H, Kersey JP, Oystreck DT, Cline RA, Lyons CJ. Diplopia following cataract surgery: a review of 150 patients. Eye. 2008;22(8):1057–64.
24. Strominger MB. Diplopia following cataract extraction. Am Orthopt J. 2004;54:120–4.
25. Samuel Williams G, Radwan M, Menon J. Cataract surgery planning in amblyopic patients–which eye first? Awareness of the potential for post-operative diplopia amongst consultant ophthalmic surgeons in Wales. Ulster Med J. 2013 May;82(2):82–4. PMID: 24082284; PMCID: PMC3756863.
26. Schor C, Erickson P. Patterns of binocular suppression and accommodation in monovision. Am J Optom Physiol Opt. 1988 Nov;65(11):853–61. https://doi.org/10.1097/00006324-198811000-00001 PMID: 3252731.
27. Muthusamy K, Claoué C. Toric and toric multifocal IOLs in meridional amblyopia. Int J Ophthalmol. 2015 Jun 18;8(3):634. https://doi.org/10.3980/j.issn.2222-3959.2015.03.35.PMID:26086021;PMCID:PMC4458676.
28. Harvey EM. Development and treatment of astigmatism-related amblyopia. Optom VisSci. 2009;86(6):634–9.
29. Harvey EM, Dobson V, Miller JM, Clifford-Donaldson CE. Changes in visual function following optical treatment of astigmatism-related amblyopia. Vision Res. 2008;48(6):773–87.
30. Arruabarrena C, Teus MA, Hernández-Verdejo JL, Cañones R. Visual acuity after laser *in situ* keratomileusis to correct high astigmatism in adults with meridional amblyopia. Am J Ophthalmol. 2011;152(6):964-968.e1.
31. Braga-Mele R, Chang D, Dewey S, Foster G, Henderson BA, Hill W, Hoffman R, Little B, Mamalis N, Oetting T, Serafano D, Talley-Rostov A, Vasavada A, Yoo S; ASCRS Cataract Clinical Committee. Multifocal intraocular lenses: relative indications and contraindications for implantation. J Cataract Refract Surg. 2014 Feb;40(2):313–22.
32. McKee SP, Levi DM, Movshon JA. The pattern of visual deficits in amblyopia. J Vis. 2003;3:380–405.
33. Simons K. Amblyopia characterization, treatment, and prophylaxis. Surv Ophthalmol. 2005;50:123–66.
34. Petermeier K, Gekeler F, Spitzer MS, Szurman P. Implantation of the multifocal ReSTOR apodised diffractive intraocular lens in adult anisometropic patients with mild to moderate amblyopia. Br J Ophthalmol. 2009;93:1296–300.
35. Petermeier K, Szurman P. Subjektive und objektive Ergebnisse nach Implantation der apodisiert diffraktiven. AcrySof ReSTOR Ophthalmologe. 2007;104:399–408.
36. de Wit DW, Diaz JM, Moore TC, Moore JE. Refractive lens exchange for a multifocal intraocular lens with a surface-embedded near section in mild to moderate anisometropic amblyopic patients. J Cataract Refract Surg. 2012 Oct;38(10):1796–801. https://doi.org/10.1016/j.jcrs.2012.06.046 Epub 2012 Aug 21 PMID: 22920503.
37. Levi DM, Li RW. Perceptual learning as a potential treatment for amblyopia: a mini-review. Vision Res. 2009;49:2535–49. https://doi.org/10.1016/j.visres.2009.02.010.
38. Hess RF, Mansouri B, Thompson B. A new binocular approach to the treatment of amblyopia in adults well beyond the critical period of visual development. Restor Neurol Neurosci. 2010;28:793–802. https://doi.org/10.3233/RNN-2010-0550.
39. Žiak P, Holm A, Halička J, et al. Amblyopia treatment of adults with dichoptic training using the virtual reality oculus rift head mounted display: preliminary results. BMC Ophthalmol 2017;17:105. https://doi.org/10.1186/s12886-017-0501-8.
40. Sofi IA, Gupta SK, Bharti A, et al. Efficiency of the occlusion therapy with and without levodopa-carbidopa in amblyopic children-A tertiary care centre experience. Int J Health Sci. 2016;10:249–57.
41. Pawar PV, Mumbare SS, Patil MS, et al. Effectiveness of the addition of citicoline to patching in the treatment of amblyopia around visual maturity: a randomized controlled trial. Indian J Ophthalmol. 2014;62:124–9. https://doi.org/10.4103/0301-4738.128586.

Cataract Surgery—Considerations When Planning Monovision

Graham D. Barrett

Several pseudophakic options are available to surgeons who would like to offer a solution to their patients' presbyopia. These include spectacles combined with monofocal intraocular lenses (IOLs), multifocal IOLs, accommodating IOL's, and monovision.

Many surgeons attempt to custom fit a particular solution to an individual patient depending on factors such as his or her lifestyle, personality, and occupation. The approach recommended here is based on the authors experience and as such is believed to provide the greatest likelihood of success as defined by patients' satisfaction, with the least amount of compromise in their quality of vision. Despite many technological advances, modest monovision remains an excellent choice. It can be offered in the form of corrective laser surgery for phakic patients, but is most often performed as pseudophakic monovision in patients undergoing cataract surgery or in older patients with significant hyperopia undergoing refractive lens exchange.

Traditional Monovision Versus Modest Monovision

Monovision in pseudophakia is a term used to describe the intentional correction for distance vision or emmetropia in one eye and myopic defocus in the fellow eye for near. The term monovision encompasses a wide range of myopic defocus in the near eye and the terminology can be confusing. The term *mini monovision* may be used when the anisometropia is set at 0.75 D to 1.00 D; *modest monovision* at 1.25 D to 1.50 D; and *traditional monovision* at 1.75 D to 2.50 D. When even smaller amounts of myopic defocus such as −0.5D or less are targeted in one eye then the term *Micro monovision* would be appropriate.

G. D. Barrett (✉)
The University of Western Australia, Perth, Australia
e-mail: graham.barrett@uwa.edu.au

M. Shajari et al. (eds.), *Cataract and Lens Surgery*,
https://doi.org/10.1007/978-3-031-05394-8_43

Neurophysiology

The neurophysiology between the different levels of anisometropia is distinctive and whilst monovision is a suitable term for traditional Monovision, *Blended Vision* may be a better term for lower levels of anisometropia where binocular vision is retained with an increase in binocular depth of focus and decreased spectacle independence.

Monovision in pseudophakia was traditionally aimed at achieving emmetropia in the dominant eye but creating a myopic defocus for near vision in the non-dominant eye. Interocular suppression of the blurred image in this scenario is dependent on higher cortical function. The neurophysiology, however is quite distinctive between *traditional monovision*, where the level of myopia in the eye targeted for near vision is in the range of −2.00 D, and *modest monovision*, where the targeted degree of myopia is −1.25 D. −2 D myopic defocus in the near eye provides excellent unaided near vision and in a study published by Ito and Shimizu in 2009 provided better reading ability than refractive mutifocal IOLs [1]. The authors however, cautioned that careful patient selection was required with specific attention to issues of ocular dominance.

Contact lens studies have demonstrated that contrast sensitivity may be reduced with monovision. [2] With binocular viewing, the reduction in contrast for near increases as the myopic defocus approaches 2.0 dioptres and then improves again with higher levels. We can therefore minimize the reduction in contrast by limiting the myopic defocus to −1.5 dioptres.

A significant reduction of Titmus Stereoacuity test is evident in patients who have undergone refractive surgery and can be demonstrated at levels of anisometropia 2.00 dioptres and greater [3]. Once again this suggests that exceeding −1.5 dioptres of myopic defocus in the near eye should only be considered cautiously in patients considering monovision in pseudophakia. It is valuable to routinely assess stereocuity in patients with modest monovision and found that the impact is minor, 67 s (Modest Monovision) versus 63 s (Distance Vision Both eyes) of arc as long as the anisometropia is less than 1.5 Diopters.

Strong ocular dominance or rivalry may result in asthenopia, particularly when the anisometropia is greater than 2.0 D [4]. Strong rivalry may be problematic in monovision and once again we should limit the myopic defocus unless a patient has been a successful contact lens wearer at this level of monovision prior to cataract surgery to avoid this problem. Although total spectacle independence is less frequent with a lower level of myopia, limiting the anisometropia to approximately −1.25 D reduces the likelihood of a reduction in binocular contrast sensitivity, asthenopia, and loss of stereoacuity that can occur with higher levels of anisometropia. A clinical experimental study by Naeser et al. [5] suggested that −0.25 and −1.25 D pseudophakic monovision may be the optimal choice to provide spectacle independence and provided an extended range of clear vision for with the least compromise for binocular visual functions.

Neuroadapation is a term used to describe the period often required for patients to adapt to the nature of their vision and for the perception of dysphotosia to diminish after cataract surgery with multifocal implants. This phenomenon is less evident after modest monovision. The majority of patients hadapt within one week and problems in this respect are extremely rare. The reasons for the rapid adjustment to the nature of modest monovision is that the images are spatially congruent and therefore binocular fusion can occur which is more physiological than the monoptic suppression which is required to deal with the conflicting images which are inherent with multifocal vision.

Optics and IOLs

Spectacles

Monofocal intraocular lens implants provide a single plane of focus. If emmetropia is achieved for distance in both eyes, reading glasses with an add power ranging from two to three dioptres will be required for near vision after surgery. If we look critically at the quality of vision achieved with spectacles whether in the form of progressive, bifocal or separate reading glasses, they do provide excellent acuity with high contrast sensitivity, perfect stereo-acuity and do not create significant dysphotopsia or unwanted optical images. These patients, however, are functionally dependent on optical aides. Published data on the expectations of patients prior to cataract surgery suggests a paradox [6]. The vast majority do expect to wear reading glasses but a similar proportion rate spectacle independence as being very important following cataract surgery.

Multifocal Intraocular Lenses

One of the most widely practiced strategies to provide unaided distance and near vision following cataract surgery is the use of multifocal implants. These implants are based on diffractive or refractive optics that provide more than one focal plane. The optical principle is to provide simultaneous focus for near and distance vision. Central cortical processing allows most individuals to ignore the blurred image and concentrate on the image of regard. The superimposition of the defocused image, however, results in reduced contrast sensitivity compared to monofocal IOLs. A review of the literature comparing the results of multifocal IOLs [7] confirmed reduced contrast sensitivity as well as associated dysphotopsia, such as haloes, particularly when driving at night. Multifocal IOLs perform well in visual tasks when involving high contrast targets in photopic conditions such as the measurement of Snellen visual acuity but Intermediate acuity is deficient with earlier generations of bifocal multifocal IOLs. Redistribution of light energy from the near focus to the intermediate range has largely addressed this issue with trifocal multifocal IOLs. Trifocal IOLs are reported to be associated with fewer halos, less glare, and less loss of light energy to higher orders of diffraction than earlier bifocal multifocal designs. They therefore provide good Snellen acuity and Stereo-acuity but the modulation transfer function remains impaired and, together with dysphotopsia, remain important compromises compared to spectacles for near vision.

Accommodative Intraocular Lenses

An alternative to multifocal implants is accommodative intraocular lenses. These include lenses with hinged and anteriorly vaulted haptics as well as dual optic implants which have a greater potential for accommodation. In theory, these lenses would be an attractive alternative to multifocal implants as they do not have the same adverse effects on contrast sensitivity and incidence of dysphotopsia. The efficacy of this type of lens however is questionable. A comprehensive review [8] concluded that published objective data showed limited forward translation with accommodative lenses and that convincing psycho visual data demonstrating efficacy was lacking. Furthermore, the fixation characteristics and PCO prevention of many current accommodative lens designs has proved to be less predictable than conventional IOLs.

Monofocal IOLs

The defocus curve for a monofocal lens has a single focus for distance and provides reasonable intermediate acuity but inadequate unaided near vision. A diffractive mutifocal implant, in contrast, has two peaks providing good vision for distance and near, but lacks intermediate acuity. Monovision provides an additional focus for near in the second eye and the combined through focus curve is not dissimilar to the normal accommodative response.

In the absence of a true accommodating IOL, IOL monovision remains the preferred choice for many surgeons in the management of presbyopia among the cataract population. Annual ASCRS clinical surveys [9] indicate that IOL monovision is the number one modality for the management of presbyopia in cataract surgery. A recent thought-provoking article published in Eyeworld 2021 "What IOL would you Choose?" [10] discussed the results of a 29-question survey submitted to ophthalmic surgeons on which IOL they would select for themselves if they personally required cataract surgery. Despite the many articles on multifocal implants in the literature and high profile in meetings and new journals, the vast majority (93%) of respondents reported that quality was the most important criteria for their eye surgery. A monofocal (34.5%) intraocular lens was the IOL selected by the majority of surgeons for their own surgery followed by monovision (26.8%) as a close second. Although 67% of the respondents indicated they regularly used presbyopia correcting IOLs, only half of these respondents would have selected a presbyopia correcting IOL for themselves.

Extended Depth of Focus IOLs

The term Extended Depth of Focus (EDoF) was first coined by this author in 2012 to describe a modified monofocal lens design that utilised 4th and 6th order positive spherical aberration to extend the depth of focus whilst maintaining optical quality [11]. Positive spherical aberration (SA) and myopic defocus interact in a synergistic fashion such that the combined modulation transfer function (MTF) is enhanced. In addition, when combined with modest monovision of −1.25 D the defocus curves of the distant and near eye have a greater overlap maintaining the features of binocular vision and as well as providing greater near acuity for the same level of myopic defocus.

In recent years the term "extended depth of focus" has been applied to several IOLs based on different optical principles such as negative SA, low add diffractive bifocal and trifocal IOLs, and phase shift technology. The term therefore does not describe a homogeneous group of IOL models and features such as the presence or absence of dysphotopsia depends on the optical principles. In addition, not all of these IOLs are well suited for use in combination with myopic defocus as in monovision. Depending on the optical technology even minor myopic defocus can increase unwanted images or compromise MTF.

History

Monovision as a method of prescribing optical aids was first proposed in 1958 by Richard Westsmith, MD [12], and has been widely practiced with contact lenses since the 1960's with success in approximately 80% of cases [13]. Typically, two dioptres of induced myopia in the non-dominant eye is employed by practitioners who practice monovision with contact lens correction. From the contact lens literature, monovision presents several potential problems. Patients with high ocular dominance are often not able to fully suppress the blurred image. In particular high contrast, high frequency images proved to be troublesome particularly in low illumination. Finally there may be interference with monocular function and reduced stereo acuity.

Monovision is also widely practiced in patients undergoing refractive surgery. Generally, patients 40 years or older undergoing LASIK are offered monovision as an alternative to having both eyes corrected for distance. The experience of the author concurs with the results published in the literature which suggests that patients are highly satisfied with monovision correction after LASIK in the presbyopic age group [14]. Interestingly, the data suggests that patients corrected for distance in both eyes were equally happy to those who selected monovision emphasizing the importance of counseling patients and involving them in deciding what form of correction is most important.

Monovision can be an effective solution for unaided near vision for pseudophakic patients. Surprisingly there is a paucity of published studies in the literature but what is available demonstrates a very high success rate. In a study published by Greenbaum [15], 92% of patients achieved 20/30 and J1 unaided acuity with a 90% acceptance rate. This raises the question whether modifying the degree of intended myopia in monovision for pseudophakia could increase patients' satisfaction and the overall acceptance rate. As indicated previously, visual acuity testing with high contrast targets such as Snellen acuity is insufficient to explain patient satisfaction, so more information is required to identify the limitations and recommend which patients are eligible for monovision as a strategy in cataract surgery.

Required Myopic Defocus for Monovision in Pseudophakia:

We have all been surprised to encounter patients in the waiting room who have had bilateral monofocal intraocular lens implants and have excellent unaided distance acuity, quite happily reading the newspaper without glasses after cataract surgery. This observation piqued significant interest and when looking at the refractive outcome in a series of such patients to identify what degree of myopic defocus was required for adequate near vision. In this audit unaided near and distance acuity as well as the spherical equivalent refractive error was recorded. This study was performed approximately 20 years ago so this group of patients was intended to be emmetropic targeted with a minimal amount of residual myopia to assist with near vision. The mean spherical equivalent of myopia of this group of patients was −0.38 dioptres with the majority of patients clustered between 0 and −0.50 dioptres. This minor level of myopia provided excellent unaided distance acuity typically 20/20 or 20/25 which was expected but the unaided near vision N10 (J6) or decimal 0.33 to 0.4, which is the print size of novels and magazines was surprising.

Examination of the patients who ended up more myopic at −1.00 dioptres revealed that distance acuity was reduced to 20/30 or 20/40 but the unaided near vision improved to N5(J2) or 0.67 equivalent to the smallest type in general use. The results suggested that pseudo-accommodation with monofocal implants does exist and −1.00 to −1.50 dioptres of myopia should be sufficient for the majority of near vision tasks. Binocular summation is also a feature of monovision correction, in that near acuity improved by approximately one line with binocular compared to monocular testing. These results proved helpful in planning a strategy to avoid the limitations of traditional monovision which usually aims at a myopic defocus of −2.00 dioptres in the non-dominant eye.

In order to evaluate the strategy of modified monovision in more detail Barett and Finkelman conducted a prospective study on monovision in pseudophakia [16]. In this study the first eye was targeted for emmetropia and if achieved, the second eye had a target refraction of −1.25 dioptres. The important outcomes measured included the unaided near and distance acuity, spherical equivalent refractive error, as well as a modified V14 questionnaire to evaluate the level of spectacle independence and patient satisfaction after surgery. Despite the fact that only 27% achieve total spectacle independence, patients are rarely dissatisfied with their results.

The unaided acuity achieved was encouraging in that 80% of patients achieved N6 (J2) and 100% (J3) or better binocular near acuity. Similarly, the unaided distance acuity was excellent with 80% 20/20 and 100% 20/30 or better unaided binocular distance acuity. The mean spherical equivalent refractive error in the distance eye was −0.19 dioptres and for the near eye −1.36 dioptres.

To assess the need for glasses or contact lenses after surgery, patients were asked to rate their need for contact lenses or glasses after surgery. The scale runs from 0. to 10 where 0 is "I am completely free from glasses or contact lenses" and 10 is "totally dependent on glasses or contact lenses." The average score was 1.3 demonstrating that the vast majority of patients considered themselves spectacle independent. On a similar scale, patients were asked to estimate their satisfaction or dissatisfaction after surgery where 0 is "not satisfied at all" and 10 "very satisfied." An average score of 9.9 indicated that the vast majority of patients were highly satisfied with the refractive outcome.

In a prospective study comparing modest monovision to diffractive multifocal implants performed at Moorfields Eye Hospital in London [17], patients with multifocal IOLs reported a much higher level of total spectacle independence (71%) than those with modest monovision (25%), but 6% of patients in the study required a lens exchange—all in the multifocal group. It is interesting to speculate that one of the reasons for the disassociation of spectacle independence and satisfaction following multifocal implantation is that spectacles typically do not improve reading ability in the absence of significant refractive error. In contrast, reading glasses are of assistance to almost all patients with modest monovision for particular visual tasks.

It is possible that surgeons overestimate the importance of total spectacle independence as an index of patients' satisfaction after undergoing cataract surgery. Patients typically rank quality of vision and the avoidance of dysphotopsia as more important than total spectacle independence when judging their satisfaction after cataract surgery.

Incorporating Modest Monovision in Your Practice

Having offered modest monovision to all patients who are suitable for many years, one can therefore. often fail to appreciate that this could be daunting to surgeons who were unfamiliar with this technique. The principles are often not taught in a systematic fashion during training, courses are lacking and industry has not supported education in this area as there has not been a commercial product associated with modest monovision.

The requirements for achieving success with modest monovision include precise planning, skilled phaco surgery and postoperative care. These principles are common to all modern cataract surgery regardless of the type of implant. An unfortunate misconception is that residual astigmatism assists with extending focal range and this is particularly relevant to modest monovision [18, 19].

The best outcomes in terms of spectacle independence with modest monovision is when post op residual astigmatism is within 0.5 D. This is best achieved with Toric IOLs targeting close to zero residual astigmatism both for the emmetropic distance eye and the more myopic eye targeted for monovision. Patient satisfaction is very high but there are inherent limitations and compromises with any presbyopic solution and patients need to be counselled appropriately.

Patient selection is not restricted to the same extent as multifocal IOLs but remains an important consideration. Testing for dominance is not critical with the modest levels of anisometropia suggested for modest monovision when performing cataract surgery but should be considered in the context of clear lens extraction.

Contraindications are few but these must be understood to avoid patient dissatisfaction as well as strategies to address patient dissatisfaction.

Compromises

Perhaps the most important compromise with modest monovision with target of −1.25 D near eye is the occasional need for spectacles.

These are often required for reading small print and this should be clearly explained to patients when discussing the pseudophakic options to address presbyopia. In addition, to near visual tasks, spectacles may occasionally be required for driving, particularly at night. This is less common than the need for reading glasses and is largely dependent on the refractive outcome and acuity in the distance eye.

As mentioned earlier, total spectacle independence at the expense of quality of vision may not be a priority for many patients. There appears to be an increasing awareness of the value of preserving quality of vision, providing excellent unaided distance and intermediate acuity whilst accepting occasional correction for near vision with the popularity of extended depth of focus IOLs.

When considering the refractive target for near, a lens power may not be available for the exact target of −1.25 D as IOLs are often only available in 0.5 D steps. In this scenario one should typically select the next higher lens power e.g. targeting −1.35 D rather than accepting a target of −1.0 D but should also take the patient's expectations into account. Spectacle independence is more likely by targeting the slightly higher target for myopia in the near eye as in this example.

If a patient has worn contact lenses successfully, one should usually consider a slightly higher target of −1.5 D rather than −1.25 D, as they are more likely to be satisfied with the reading provided by this level of myopic defocus.

The strategy of an extended depth of focus IOL designed for modest monovision reduces the compromises associated with modest monovision as it provides additional near acuity for the same level of myopic defocus with less impact on distance acuity and steroacuity.

Patient Selection and Counselling

Attempting to explain to patients the impact of multifocal implants and screen for unsuitable patients is demanding, and not always successful. In contrast, the process is relatively straight forward with modest monovision—if 6/9 or better unaided vision for distance is obtained in the first eye the option of modest monovision can be easily demonstrated to patients with the addition of a +1.25 D spherical lens in the trial frame using their recently operated eye.

Occupation, personality, and refractive error are not critical screening factors in selecting patients suitable for modest monovision. Multifocal IOLs may not be well suited to discriminating individuals such as architects or engineers. These professions, however, are acceptable candidates for modest monovision, as are artists and truck drivers—spectacles can be worn, if necessary, for activities such as night driving, if required.

Minor levels of defocus created by astigmatism, posterior capsular opacification, and macular dysfunction have a limited impact on visual acuity with modest monovision compared with multifocal implants. Modest monovision is therefore a robust optical solution that is impacted less with the decline in macula function and the expected shift to ATR astigmatism that is inevitable with age. Visual acuity can always be improved with addition of spectacles in these circumstances if required.

Testing for Dominance

Tests for ocular dominance prior to cataract surgery can be classified as motor sighting dominance or sensory dominance tests.

A motor sighting test relies on patients' preference for one eye over the other when viewing a target—e.g. the "hole-in-the-card" test or "pointing at a target" test. The latter is the most straightforward test to use in the clinic. Simply ask the patient to point at a letter on the Snellen chart whilst lining up his vison with the pointing fingertip. Then cover each eye in turn and observe which eye the patient is using for this task by observing for fixation changes and asking the patient to observe if the image jump is greater when one or the other eye is covered.

Sensory dominance relies on patient comfort/preference when viewing through a 1.0 D lens with one eye or the other. Short-term viewing has little utility and a contact lens test for a two-week period is more informative. Contact lens testing can also be misleading as limited tolerance to the contact lens may be reported as discomfort unrelated to sensory perception.

More sophisticated testing using synoptophores with stereo-targets or Haidinger brushes can be considered but are not always practical in a clinical setting.

Sighting dominance [20, 21] has also been shown to be ambiguous and cross dominance is not uncommon. Furthermore testing for dominance in the presence of significant cataract can be unreliable so this is longer performed routinely. This is quite different when considering monovision in the context of refractive surgery in the 5th decade, or in a hyperopic patient considering clear lens extraction. In both of these scenarios dominance should be determined and a contact lens trial recommended.

One of the reasons for preferring modest monovision is that it does not appear that dominance is a critical issue with this level of defocus. Similarly, there was no preference for myopic defocus in the near eye rather than the distance eye (so called cross-dominance) in a clinical study of modest monovision published by Fuxiang Zhang [22].

Contraindications

Disruption of Binocular Fusion

Modest monovision is not an ideal term as indeed binocular function is maintained.

Situations where binocular fusion is absent or functionally impaired should therefore be avoided. These include motility disorders such as tropias, large phorias, monofixation syndrome and convergence insufficiency.

The presence of cataract may be referring physicians or optometrists rather than pre-existing diplopia due to a motility disorder. Monovision should be avoided as the symptoms will still be present and correction with prisms may be more difficult. The presence of dense cataracts may also reduce acuity to the extent that pre-existing diplopia is not noted and only become manifest after cataract surgery.

Screening for motility disorders is therefore important in cataract surgery and monovision avoided in this context. It is always worth checking the existing spectacles for prism and questioning the patient directly, if suspicious.

Extreme monovision, however, with a target of ~ -3.0 D in one eye can be considered as a method to manage intractable diplopia after cataract surgery where surgical alignment is not considered feasible or desirable [23].

Mild phoria is acceptable for monovision, but only if this is not associated with symptoms, and within 10 diopters of exophoria [24].

Modest levels of anisometropia may not be associated with amblyopia or monofixation syndrome but this may be masked in the presence of a dense cataract. Performing surgery initially in the suspect eye typically will reveal if this is a problem. Even when amblyopia is not evident if one eye has historically significantly been more myopic in the order of 2.0 D it is worth maintain this as the more myopic eye for near vision when considering modest monovision and targeting slightly more myopia than usual e.g. −1.50 D.

Monofixation syndrome refers to a small angle deviation with suppression of the deviated eye and the presence of binocular peripheral fusion [25]. The absence of foveal fusion that characterizes monofixation syndrome can occur in strabismic and orthotropic eyes [26]. Patients with monofixation may appear orthophoric, and diagnosis requires a stereopsis test, 4-diopter base out prism test and/or Worth 4-Dot fusion at a distance of 6 m is required to make the diagnosis. These tests may be difficult to perform in the presence of a dense cataract and poor vision. Questioning the patient about a history of diplopia, patching and avoiding selecting an eye which is reported as always been weaker may be helpful in inadvertently choosing a non-fixating eye for distance. Fixation switch diplopia can occur if monovision is performed and the balance of stable asymptomatic monofixation syndrome is disrupted.

Blowout fractures of the orbit may be associated with entrapment of the muscle. Even when treated surgically downgaze may elicit diplopia even though this may be absent in the primary position of gaze. These patients may therefore may not be suitable candidates for monovision.

In addition to more common phorias and tropias there are several systemic conditions that can involve the ocular muscles and may preclude consideration of monovision. These include Myasthenia Gravis, Graves' Disease and Multiple Sclerosis. Parkinson's disease can impact saccades as well as pursuit and is associated with convergence insufficiency.

Impaired Acuity

Modest monovision requires at least 6/9 unaided acuity in the distance eye and this can easily be determined after cataract surgery if the eye with the denser cataract has surgery performed initially. Reduced acuity due to amblyopia is considered a contraindication to modest monovision.

The vision may be impaired due to co-existing morbidity such as diabetic retinopathy, epiretinal membrane or age-related macular degeneration—these patients are not suitable candidates for monovision.

Glaucoma is not, in itself, a contraindication to modest monovision as long as the visual field is not significantly impaired. Extensive visual field defects due to glaucoma or stroke (including hemianopia) would exclude patients from being suitable for monovision.

The unaided acuity may be 6/12 or less due to an unintended refractive outcome in the first eye intended for distance vision and the majority of these patients will prefer to be targeted for distance in their second eye. Others, however, may find their distance vision quite adequate despite a small unintended residual myopia of ~ -0.5 D. They may desire more near vision and therefore be suitable for modest monovision.

Poor Comprehension

The most common situation where modest monovision should be avoided is circumstances where the patient may not fully understand the nature of the compromise involved. Situations where this may occur include dementia, language difficulties or simple lack of comprehension. These patients are likely not to recall why one eye is more blurred for distance and the other for near when each eye is occluded in turn.

Management of Dissatisfied Patients

Despite the contraindications listed for monovision, these are not frequently encountered and indeed are common to other presbyopia correcting IOLs such as multifocals. Although extremely uncommon, like any presbyopic solution there may be dissatisfied patients. In a period spanning two decades of monovision, the author has encountered only three cases where the decision had to be reversed.

(1) The First Case had bilateral cataract surgery performed elsewhere with an unexpected refractive outcome in the second eye. The refraction in the first eye (OD) was +0.05/−0.25 × 84° and in the second eye (OS) −3.50/−0.50 × 243°. Lasik was performed in the more myopic eye aiming for emmetropia and ended up with a satisfied and grateful patient with refraction of −0.25 sphere and unaided acuity of 6/5.

(2) The second case referred was a high myopc with a preoperative refraction of −14.25 spherical equivalent in both eyes. Despite ending up close to emmetropia in the dominant right eye (0.00/−0.50 × 26°) the patient never felt quite comfortable with the myopia in the second eye (−2.25/−1.75 × 155°). The patient had a dry eye and so the level of myopia in the myopic eye was reduced with PRK, eliminating the astigmatism with a final correction of −1.25 D. This proved to be sufficient for near vision and the patient was very happy with the outcome.

(3) The last case was a 42-year-old patient in whom Lasik was performed aiming for −1.00 in the non-dominant eye. This patient was slightly under corrected ending up more myopic than intended with −1.50 sphere in the non-dominant eye (OS). Her major problem, however, was distance acuity in the dominant eye which also ended more myopic than intended with −0.50/−0.50 × 230. The more myopic eye was re-treated aiming for emmetropia leaving the minor level of myopia in dominant eye to assist with near vision. Once again, the patient was very satisfied with the final result.

There are valuable lessons to be learned from each of these patients in regard to modest monovision.

The first case reinforced how important it is for the outcome of any presbyopic correction to meet or exceed patients' expectations. The second case is an example where anisometropia more than 2 diopters was problematic but reducing the level to −1.25 D proved to be successful. The final case is relevant to all presbyopic solutions and illustrates how the importance of achieving excellent unaided distance acuity in determining patient satisfaction. If modest monovision is targeted it is extremely rare to encounter dissatisfied patients and the examples illustrate the relative ease with which problems can be resolved.

Monovision is reversible with spectacle correction and patients understand these can be utilised at any time they feel necessary if they have trouble with small print or driving at night. In the rare instance where modest monovision is not adequately tolerated the refractive status can be reversed with laser correction as illustrated in these cases or alternatively with a piggyback IOL.

Surgeons who are often unaccustomed to using monovision in their practice are often uncertain as the best way to incorporate the solution in their practice. Many surgeons such as Zhang who practice monovision attempt to vary the myopic defocus according to the patient's hobbies, lifestyle or occupation [27]. Maloney suggested an approach where he classified functional vision into different zones and discusses with patients their preference in relation to these zones to help determine lens power selection and the degree of intended monovision [28]. Zone 1 consists of activities requiring small print whilst zone 5 emphasizes distance acuity with low illumination with recommendations of −2.00 dioptres for zone 1, −1 dioptres for zone 2 and −0.50 for zone 3.

This author's preference however is based on the principle that a monofocal lens provides additional depth of focus, −1.25 dioptres of myopic defocus is well tolerated for monovision and satisfies near vision requirements in the majority patients. The reality is that the expected outcome may vary from −1 to −1.50 D and this range is still likely to provide a useful range of intermediate and near vision.

If a patient is accustomed to monovision with contact lenses prior to cataract surgery then the targeted myopic defocus can be increased to −1.5 D. A slightly higher target level of myopic defocus of −1.5 D should also be considered for patients who were able to read unaided prior to cataract surgery due to longstanding myopia.

Surgeons planning pseudophakic monovision require accurate IOL power calculation methods that can be applied to both the distance eye and the near eye. Earlier studies have suggested that targeting a myopic outcome may be less accurate and we confirmed this in a recent study that demonstrated that reduced refractive accuracy can be anticipated to some extent when targeting a low level of myopia typical for monovision. The accuracy of prediction for myopic targets in our study varied with different formulae. The Barrett Universal II, Hill-RBF 2.0, and Holladay I formulas were the least affected by this phenomenon, but the Holladay I was less accurate overall for both distance and near eyes in this study [29].

The results of the study suggested that when planning a myopic outcome, cataract surgeons should use the Haigis, SRK/T, and Hoffer Q formulas with caution. The Barrett Universal II and Hill-RBF 2.0, however, offered a reliable option for a patient desiring a refractive outcome of myopia in one eye for monovision.

The approach is relatively simple and can be condensed to the "ABCDs of Monovision."

Address the Alternatives

First, address the alternatives. Tell patients that a monofocal implant provides the best quality of vision but requires reading glasses. Explain that a multifocal lens can provide spectacle independence but at the expense of contrast sensitivity and possibly with the induction of glare and halos. Conclude by saying that the outcome with accommodating lenses remains relatively unpredictable.

Broach Monovision

Then speak in further detail about the possibility of monovision and explain that optimal quality of vision can be obtained at any time, with spectacle correction. Although intermediate acuity is excellent, explain that typically some correction will be required for the sustained reading of small print. Caution patients that the option of modest monovision does require achieving excellent unaided distance acuity in the first eye.

Choose Distance

One should almost always operate on the eye with the denser cataract first and target emmetropia. Although correcting the dominant eye for distance is favourable, particularly for a refractive lens exchange, this is not a major issue for cataract patients. If a patient has the denser cataract in an eye that has always been significantly more myopic then one should still operate on this eye first but alter the routine and target myopic defocus, rather than alter the relative anisometropia to which the patient has become accustomed.

Demonstrate Defocus

If the first eye achieves at least 20/30 unaided visual acuity, one should then demonstrate the amount of myopic defocus with a +1.25 D lens and a trial frame. This is so that patients can appreciate the impact of the targeted myopia on their distance acuity as well as the level of near vision that they will achieve. In practice, more than 50% of patients elect to have modest monovision.

Conclusion

Modest monovision continues to be an attractive solution to presbyopia and should be considered a "premium" solution. It requires expert surgery and biometry, knowledgeable selection of IOLs, and the utilization of toric implants to reduce astigmatism. The popularity of the technique is increasing, and future complementary options include the concept of a monofocal IOL with an extended depth of focus. Together with a modest level of monovision, this technology could increase the level of spectacle independence while retaining the blended or binocular nature of modest monovision with less impact on stereoacuity.

References

1. Ito M, Shimizu K, Amano R, Handa T. Assessment of visual performance in pseudophakic monovision. J Cataract Refract Surg. 2009;35(4):710–4.
2. Pardhan S, Gilchrist J. The effect of monocular defocus on binocular contrast sensitivity. Ophthalmic Physiol Opt. 1990;10:33–6.
3. Wright et al. Binocular function and patient satisfaction after monovision induced by myopic PRK. JSCRS 1999;25:177–82.
4. Handa et al. Ocular dominance and patient satisfaction after monovision induced by lens implantation. JCSRS;30:769–74.
5. Naeser K, Hjortdal JØ, Harris WF. Pseudophakic monovision: optimal distribution of refractions. Acta Ophthalmol. 2014;92(3):270–5.
6. Hawker MJ et al. Expectations of patients having cataract surgery. JCRS;31:1970–52
7. Leyland M, Zinicola E. Multifocal vs monofocal lenses in cataract surgery: a systematic review. Ophthalmology. 2003;110:1789–98.
8. Dick BH. Accommodative intraocular lenses: current status. Curr Opin Ophthalmol. 2005;16:8–26.
9. ASCRS Clinical Survey 2019. EyeWorld supplement September 2020
10. "What IOL Would You Choose Doc? Hercules Logothetis, MD, Robert Feder, MD. EyeWorld. December, 2020.
11. "Zen and the Art of Monovision Maintenance"—Producer Graham D Barrett. In: ASCRS symposium on cataract, IOL and refractive surgery film festival, Chicago April 20–24, 2012.
12. Westsmith RA. Uses of a monocular contact lens. Am J Ophthalmol. 1958;46(1, Pt 1):78–81
13. Johannsdottir KR, Stelmach LB. Monovision: a review of the scientific literature. Optom Vis Sci. 2001;78(9).

14. Goldberg DB. Monovision with Lasik. JCRS. 2001;27.
15. Greenbaum S. Monovision with pseudophakia. JSCRS. 2002;28:1439–43.
16. Finkelman YM, Ng JQ, Barrett GD. Patient satisfaction and visual function after pseudophakic monovision. J Cataract Refract Surg. 2009;35(6):998–1002.
17. Wilkins MR, Allan BD, Rubin GS, et al. Moorfields IOL Study Group. Randomized trial of multifocal intraocular lenses versus monovision after bilateral cataract surgery. Ophthalmology. 2013; 120(12):2449–55.
18. Savage H, Rothstein M, Davuluri G, El Ghormli L, Zaetta DM, Mica. Myopic astigmatism and presbyopia trial. Am J Ophthalmol. 2003;135(5):628–32.
19. Lehmann RP, and Houtman. Visual Performance in Cataract Patients with Low Levels of Postoperative Astigmatism Full Correction Versus Spherical Equivalent Correction. Clinical Ophthalmology, 2012;6(Mar):333–8.
20. Seijas O, Gómez de Liaño P, Gómez de Liaño R, Roberts CJ, Piedrahita E, Diaz E. Ocular dominance diagnosis and its influence in monovision. Am J Ophthalmol. 2007;144 (2):209–216.
21. Charnwood L. Observations on ocular dominance. Optician. 1949;118:85–96.
22. Zhang F, Sugar A, Arbisser L, Jacobsen G, Artico J. Crossed versus conventional pseudophakic monovision: Patient satisfaction, visual function, and spectacle independence. J Cataract Refract Surg. 2015;41(9):1845–54.
23. Osher RH, Golnik KC, Barrett G, Shimizu K. Intentional extreme anisometropic pseudophakic monovision: new approach to the cataract patient with longstanding diplopia. J Cataract Refract Surg. 2012;38(8):1346–51.
24. Ito M, Shimizu K, Niida T, Amano R, Ishikawa H. Binocular function in patients with pseudophakic monovision. J Cataract Refract Surg. 2014;40(8):1349–54.
25. Parks MM. Th monofixation syndrome. Trans Am Ophthalmol Soc. 1969;67:609–57.
26. Weakley DR. The association between anisometropia, amblyopia, and binocularity in the absence of strabismus. Trans Am Ophthalmol Soc. 1999;97:987–1021.
27. Fuxiang Zhang MD, Alan Sugar MD, Graham D. Pseudophakic monovision—a clinical guide. Barrett MBBCh. Publisher: Thieme.
28. Maloney WF. Blended vision implants provide customized correction of presbyopia. Ocular Surgery News. 2003;15.
29. Turnbull AMJ, Hill WE, Barrett GD. Accuracy of intraocular lens power calculation methods when targeting low myopia in monovision. J Cataract Refract Surg. 2020;46(6):862–6.

Surgical Techniques

Phacodynamics

Shafak Toufeeq and Zaid Shalchi

Introduction

- Phacodynamics is the study of the physical principles that influence intraocular fluidics during phacoemulsification surgery.
- When challenges are anticipated or encountered, 'first principles' can be used to adapt surgical technique and machine settings to achieve optimal safety and ease of surgery.
- The two principles which comprise this discipline are phacofluidics and ultrasound energy.
- This chapter will explain these principles at a functional level and how they practically apply to machine settings during the stages of phacoemulsification.

Phacofluidics

- Phacofluidics describes the factors influencing the flow of fluid into, within, and out of the eye during phacoemulsification surgery.
- It is best understood as a three-part circuit comprising fluid inflow from an infusion system, flow within the anterior chamber (AC), and outflow from an aspiration system (Fig. 1).
- Irrigation and aspiration may be delivered either through a single probe with a coaxial handpiece, or separately with a bimanual configuration.
- Infusion is normally provided through two ports either side of an irrigation sleeve, which should be orientated in the plane of the iris to avoid trauma to the endothelium from the fluid current.

S. Toufeeq · Z. Shalchi (✉)
Royal Berkshire Hospitals NHS Foundation Trust, London Road, Reading RG1 5AN, UK
e-mail: zshalchi@gmail.com

S. Toufeeq
e-mail: shafak.toufeeq@nhs.net

M. Shajari et al. (eds.), *Cataract and Lens Surgery*,
https://doi.org/10.1007/978-3-031-05394-8_44

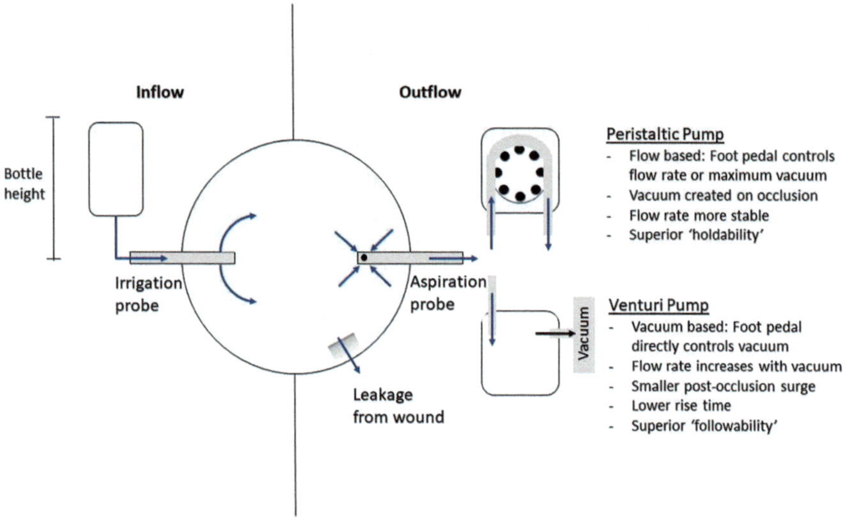

Fig. 1 The fluidics circuit

- This circuit is a primary determinant of the intraocular pressure (IOP), and consequently anterior chamber stability.
- The surgeon should aim to maintain a formed and stable anterior chamber, without excessively high IOP.

The fluidics circuit

- Flow occurs through the fluidics circuit when both irrigation and aspiration are active.
- Flow occurs along pressure gradients. The flow rate through this circuit is ultimately determined by the relative difference between irrigation and aspiration pressures.
- The aspiration flow rate (AFR) is usually expressed in cm^3/min. Pressure is expressed in mmHg.
- It is useful to consider the resultant IOP as the balance between AFR and fluid replacement via the infusion side of the system. So long as the infusion keeps up with the AFR, a steady state occurs in the AC and the flow rate is determined by the aspiration setting.

Dealing with a shallow anterior chamber

If the anterior chamber is found to shallow during the operation, it follows that either the irrigation pressure is insufficient, or aspiration pressure is excessive, to adequately keep the anterior chamber formed. Whilst it may be tempting to ameliorate this by simply increasing inflow, or decreasing the AFR, the following considerations should be made:

- Infusion: Check that the infusion line is not obstructed, and bottle is not empty.
- Aspiration: Check the integrity of the main wound and paracenteses, which are usually responsible for the majority of fluid outflow during surgery. A second instrument placed through a paracentesis that is too large will cause on-going leakage during surgery and cause eddy currents and AC instability. This significantly increases the risk of posterior capsular rupture and iris prolapse. Adjust your handling of the instruments to minimise leakage, and if possible, remove your second instrument.
- Be aware that a shallow anterior chamber can be caused by positive vitreous pressure, which is the anterior displacement of the lens-iris diaphragm as a result of raised pressure within the posterior segment. This can be recognised when the AC is shallow despite a high IOP, which can be quickly confirmed by palpating the globe to judge its firmness. Important causes of positive vitreous pressure include hydration of the vitreous by aqueous misdirection into the posterior segment, a tight lid speculum, a large body habitus, and a suprachoroidal haemorrhage.

Fluid inflow

- Fluid inflow is provided by an infusion system, which delivers fluid into the eye by way of either 'passive' or 'active' pressure from the fluid source.

Passive systems

Passive systems rely on the gravitational potential energy created by holding the bottle a certain height above that of the eye.

- Raising the 'bottle height' relative to the patient will increase the infusion pressure and therefore potential flow rate (subject to aspiration) but also increase the IOP.
- The infusion pressure is determined by bottle height less the flow resistance in the delivery tubing. For every **15 cms** of bottle height above the eye, there is a pressure increase of **11 mmHg**.
- The bottle height automatically changes to pre-set levels when switching the mode of phaco (for example sculpting to segment removal). It can also be changed using the interface settings.
- It should be noted that adjusting the height of the patient's head or operating table, for example to make room for the surgeon's legs when operating temporally, will also change effective bottle height.
- These systems are conceptually easy to understand and employ, but maximal flow rate is limited and changes to the settings are not implemented immediately.

Passive infusion without aspiration

When only irrigation is active, assuming no loss through incisions or ports, the IOP will quickly reach an equilibrium with the infusion pressure, while the flow rate will fall close to zero.

- In this circumstance there is a linear relationship between infusion pressure and IOP.
- Sustained raised IOP will create hydrostatic pressure within the eye. This may stress the zonular fibrils, hydrate the cornea which compromises visibility, and hydrate the vitreous which increases positive vitreous pressure, the latter of which may eventually shallow the anterior chamber. Furthermore, it can be painful for the patient as well as potentially worsening glaucomatous optic neuropathy if maintained for long periods.
- Therefore, avoid leaving irrigation active without aspiration for significant periods of time.

Active systems

Active systems generate pressure either from compressed air into a rigid bottle, or mechanical compression of a flexible infusion bag.

- This allows for higher potential flow rates, which may contribute to increased anterior chamber stability. However, this also causes a corresponding increase in IOP, particularly when aspiration is not active.
- They also can achieve near instantaneous adjustments of pressure, and some machines can be programmed to automatically maintain a target IOP (and therefore stable AC) as chosen by the surgeon by dynamically adjusting the infusion pressure.

Fluid outflow

- Aspiration systems create flow which draws material out of the anterior chamber.
- As the purpose of aspiration is not only to draw out fluid, but also lens matter or viscoelastic, the flow rate may not correspond to the vacuum level. For example, if the port is occluded with a lens fragment, the flow rate will fall to zero, whereas vacuum will rise. This may cause fluctuations in IOP as well as impacting the infusion flow rate, therefore affecting anterior chamber stability.
- There are two kinds of aspiration systems: peristaltic pumps and venturi pumps.

Peristaltic pumps

Peristaltic pumps utilise rollers to compress the outflow tubing as the pump rotates. This creates a 'milking' motion which draws fluid through the tubing.

- The tubing used is flexible, in order to be 'compliant' to the compression. The consequence of this is that when the aspiration is activated, there is a time taken to building the pre-set maximum vacuum to be reached once occlusion of the phaco tip has occurred. This is because the tubing itself constricts during the adjustment. This is called the **rise time**, and is influenced by the speed of the pump; The faster the pump, the quicker the rise time.
- When the occlusion is subsequently cleared, the flow rate momentarily surges as the sudden reformation of the tubing creates volume and therefore additional momentary vacuum beyond what the machine is set to. This is called the 'post-occlusion surge' and may cause sudden spikes in the flow rate, and thus affect anterior chamber stability.

Venturi pumps

- Venturi pumps operate by creating a vacuum using low pressure air within a rigid cassette with a fluid reservoir, which the fluid is drawn into.
- The tubing used is rigid, therefore rise time is generally lower.
- The surgeon can only control the vacuum, rather than the AFR directly, and therefore these are also liable to post-occlusion surges.

Aspiration settings

The aspiration settings between these two systems differ significantly.

- Peristaltic systems, by virtue of having physical rollers drawing the fluid, are considered 'flow based' and AFR remains relatively stable until occlusion. Only when occlusion occurs does vacuum significantly build, but they can achieve high vacuum at lower AFR than venturi systems. This can potentially allow for safer surgery, but also means these systems are not able to draw lens fragments towards the probe as easily. They can be configured to control either the AFR or maximal vacuum using the foot pedal at any one time, the other being adjustable on the machine interface. This potentially could be advantageous in the stop and chop technique, where high maximal vacuum should be combined with low AFR; note that the rise time will be slow in these circumstances.
- Venturi systems only allow control of vacuum, which directly affects the flow rate. They produce higher AFR at lower vacuum than peristaltic systems, but are also potentially less controllable. This creates faster flow within the anterior chamber and hence helps to draw in and hold onto lens fragments during segment removal, although can also inadvertently do the same for the iris or capsule. As such, venturi systems are classically considered to allow faster and more efficient surgery, albeit with greater potential for complications. Note that elevation of infusion bottle height will increase the AFR as well as IOP.

Phacoemulsification

- Phacoemulsification is the use of ultrasound energy transmitted by a phaco probe to fragment lens matter.
- This ultrasound energy is generated by running an electrical current through piezoelectric crystals, situated within the phaco probe, which then vibrate at a fixed high frequency.
- Ultrasound energy not absorbed by lens matter will dissipate as thermal energy within the surrounding media. If used excessively, this has the potential to cause corneal wound, iris or endothelial trauma. It is therefore important to minimise the cumulative dissipated energy (CDE).
- The irrigation sleeve plays a role in keeping the phaco tip cool.
- The surgeon's aim should be to efficiently fragment and aspirate lens matter whilst minimising thermal trauma to surrounding structures.
- Phaco can be delivered in 'continuous', 'pulsed' or 'burst' mode. In all, the phaco power is increased linearly with further foot depression. Pulsed mode, as the name suggests, delivers power in pulses when phaco is activated, whose duration as a proportion of the total time phaco is active is referred to as the duty cycle. In burst mode the maximum set phaco power is delivered in succession, the frequency of which is increased by depressing the pedal further down. This allows for more efficient use of power and produces less repulsive force (as described below) and allows time between pulses to dissipate heat from the phaco tip.
- The frequency of pulses is expressed as pulses per second (PPS).

Phaco needle movement

- The oscillations of the phaco probe conventionally occur in a longitudinal axis, whose distance of travel is referred to as the stroke length. Increasing the phaco power (normally expressed as a percentage of the maximum available) increases the stroke length and thus force delivered.
- In addition to emulsifying the lens, these movements may also cause repulsion of the fragments, pushing them away from the probe. If this overcomes the occlusion caused by the vacuum, the lens fragment may be rapidly thrust back and forth close to the tip of the phaco probe, which could be described as 'chattering'. This is highly inefficient and also compromises anterior chamber instability.
- Increasing phaco power facilitates emulsification but may make achieving occlusion more difficult and increases the amount of thermal energy produced.
- Newer phaco probe designs have incorporated torsional, for example the OZil handpiece (Alcon Inc.), and transverse ultrasound, for example the Ellips handpiece (AMO Inc.). As the movement is predominantly 'side-to-side', there is significantly reduced tip travel, and hence lower repulsive force. These are more efficient because the tip "cuts" in both directions of the oscillation and requires less vacuum for occlusion, and reduces the risk of thermal trauma.

Phaco needle design

The phaco tip significantly impacts the ease of certain intra-operative manoeuvres, and it is therefore important to become acquainted with the advantages and drawbacks of the various designs. It is also important to consider the required incision size for any given tip design.

- Needle size: Phaco probes usually come in 0.9 mm and 1.1 mm bore needles. Larger needles allow for an exponentially greater flow rate with the same level of vacuum, which allows for faster surgery, although at the risk of being potentially less controlled.
- Angle of bevel: Phaco tips which are significantly angled allow for easier sculpting and cracking of the lens, whilst blunter tips allow easier achievement of occlusion.
- Needle shape: Various designs are available which are suited to different operating techniques (Fig. 2). For example, the Kelman flared 45° phaco tip (Alcon Inc.), suited for torsional and longitudinal phaco, has an enlarged port to reduce post-occlusion surge, but can be subject to clogging. The angled end may make sculpting easier, but also pose a greater risk to the capsule and corneal endothelium.

Foot pedal control

The conventional 'linear' arrangement of foot pedal controls is outlined in Fig. 3. Note that the foot pedals can be configured in certain machines, such as Bausch and Lomb Stellaris, to control both aspiration and phaco power in independent linear modes by assigning either 'pitch' (depression of the pedal) and 'yaw' (transverse movement of the pedal) movements to one of each ('dual-linear' setting). Foot pedal controls usually also incorporate an auto-reflux control, by which flow can be reversed to release aspirated material back into the AC.

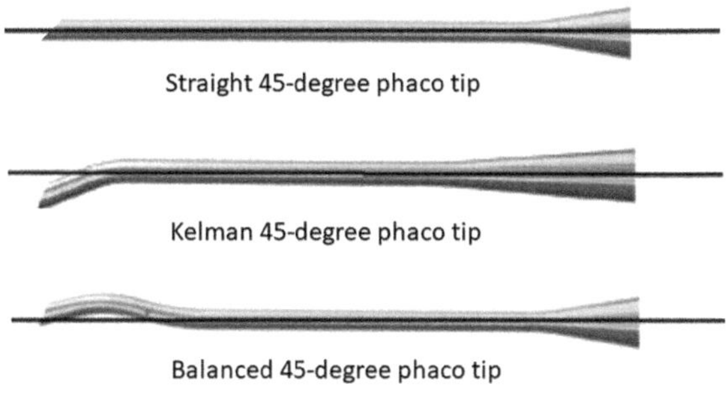

Fig. 2 Examples of phaco tip designs

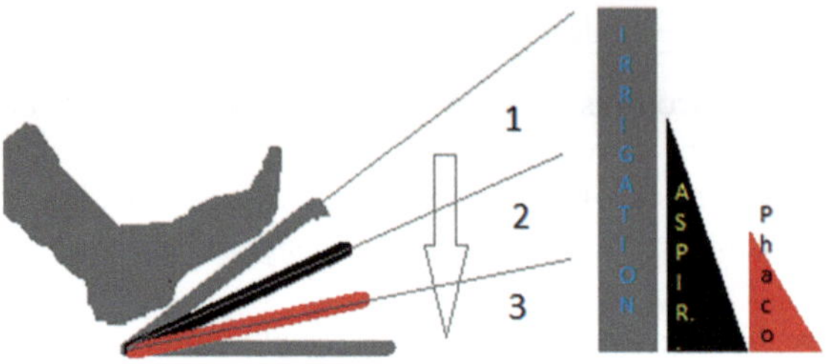

Fig. 3 Illustration of linear foot pedal control

- The irrigation (inflow) is activated by depression of the foot pedal to position 1 (see Fig. 3). The irrigation pressure is at a pre-set level which can only be adjusted on the machine panel.
- The aspiration is activated in position 2 and increases linearly up to its maximum pre-set limit by further depression of foot pedal. Be aware that if AFR exceeds the ability of the irrigation pressure to replace fluid loss, the AC will collapse. On the other hand, if aspiration ceases (in cases such as occluded outflow tubing or failed vacuum) during active phaco, then the AC will become cloudy with lens materials.
- The third position of the foot pedal actives phaco power. As with aspiration, this is usually set to a linear increase in power along with depression up to the pre-set maximum.

Fluidic settings

- Cataract surgeons should use their own machine settings for any specific cataract system. This establishes a 'baseline' of familiar phacodynamics, whose predictability suits the surgeon's technique.
- When deciding standard machine settings, the main variables to consider are the phaco technique being used, features of the handpiece/needle, and the wound size.
- The following table summarises the rationale for each stage and should serve as a guide for selecting your own standard phaco settings (Table 1).
- Note that with advances in phaco technology and automated fluidic management by phaco systems, surgery can be carried out with increasingly lower infusion and aspiration settings, and with reduced post-occlusion surge and other causes of anterior chamber instability.

Table 1 Suggested machine settings

Stage	Infusion (IOP)	Aspiration	Ultrasound power
Sculpting *Aim for minimal IOP required to keep AC formed, and minimal aspiration to clear AC of emulsified material*	Low • 50–55 mmHg *Minimise stress on zonules and risk of aqueous misdirection*	Low • Venturi: 40–75 mmHg • Peristaltic: max. vacuum 150 mmHg, AFR 25 cm^3/min *Keep the lens relatively static, and avoid inadvertent occlusion* *High AFR is not necessary, though may be increased if significant clouding from build-up of emulsified material in AC*	Variable • Continuous mode, linear phaco *Adjust according to density of nucleus. Higher power in continuous mode is more efficient* Variable
Chopping/Nuclear quadrant removal *Maintain deep and stable anterior chamber when pulling nuclear fragments towards anterior chamber*	Medium • 65 mmHg *Keep infusion sufficient to keep AC stable at AFR limit and negate the effect of post-occlusion surge. Note some modern phaco machines can automatically adjust infusion to maintain chosen IOP*	Medium • Venturi: 275–400 mmHg • Peristaltic: max. vacuum 250–300 mmHg, AFR 35 cm^3/min *'Followability' draws nuclear fragments towards phaco. Increasing flow, not vacuum itself, supports followability. The presence of a second instrument creates turbulence to the usual symmetrical flow of fluid within the AC, which affects movements of nuclear segments* *'Holdability' allows extraction of nuclear fragments from the capsule. This depends on achieving significant vacuum on occlusion with the probe. This is*	• Pulse or burst mode *Nuclear segments are mobile and therefore to avoid excessive 'chattering' whilst engaging horizontal phaco, ensure phaco power is balanced with adequate vacuum*

(continued)

Table 1 (continued)

Stage	Infusion (IOP)	Aspiration	Ultrasound power
		enhanced by increasing maximum vacuum, as well as increasing AFR to reduce rise time and thus more quickly achieve vacuum	
Cortical matter removal *Posterior capsule is liable to flap anteriorly if AC is unstable*	Medium • 65 mmHg *Maintain deep and stable anterior chamber for safer manoeuvring within the capsule*	High • Venturi: 500--600 mmHg • Peristaltic: Max. Vacuum 500 mmHg, AFR 35 cm^3/min *A higher AFR reduces the rise time, hence allowing faster achievement of vacuum and thus gripping of the cortical matter. However it also increases the risk of causing posterior capsular tears*	Not applicable

Acknowledgements We would like to thank Larry Benjamin for his kind review and great suggestions.

Bibliography

1. Benjamin L. Fluidics and rheology in phaco surgery: what matters and what is the hype? Eye (Lond). 2018;32(2):204–9. https://doi.org/10.1038/eye.2017.299.
2. Fishkind W, Wallace B, Henderson B, Colvard M, Devgan U, Serafano D, Chu R, Davis E, Gills J. Cataract and refractive surgery today. 2008. Online at https://crstoday.com/wp-content/themes/crst/assets/downloads/CRST0908_05.pdf.
3. Kent C. Phaco: know your fluidics options. Rev Ophthalmol. 2017. Online at https://www.reviewofophthalmology.com/article/phaco-know-your-fluidics-options.
4. Mckinney S. Phaco update: getting the right setting. Rev Ophthalmol. 2021. Online at https://www.reviewofophthalmology.com/article/phaco-update-getting-the-right-setting.
5. Seibel B. Phacodynamics, 4th ed. Slack Inc.; 2004.
6. Sullivan P, Benjamin L, Little B. Phacoemulsification surgery. Eyelearning ltd. 2019. Online at https://books.apple.com/.

General Cataract Surgery

Siegfried Priglinger, Thomas Kohnen, and Mehdi Shajari

In this chapter the individual steps of the cataract procedure are described. (Video 1 and Video 2).

Side Ports

In cataract surgery, the majority of the procedure is bimanual. The surgeon therefore needs at least one additional access point (side-port) in addition to the main incision, depending on the technique. Often, two side ports are made next to the main incision. These are smaller than the main incision and usually at an angle of 45–60° away from the main incision. A much larger angle would lead to an unnatural hand position and more difficult operation. If the angle is too close to the main incision, the side port and main incision can even merge during the operation creating a very unstable incision. This large incision would result in leakage and a significant loss of stability of the anterior chamber and an increased risk for complications.

Supplementary Information The online version contains supplementary material available at https://doi.org/10.1007/978-3-031-05394-8_45. The videos can be accessed individually by clicking the DOI link in the accompanying figure caption or by scanning this link with the SN More Media App.

S. Priglinger (✉) · T. Kohnen · M. Shajari
München, Germany
e-mail: s.priglinger@med.uni-muenchen.de

T. Kohnen
e-mail: thomas.kohnen@kgu.de

M. Shajari et al. (eds.), *Cataract and Lens Surgery*,
https://doi.org/10.1007/978-3-031-05394-8_45

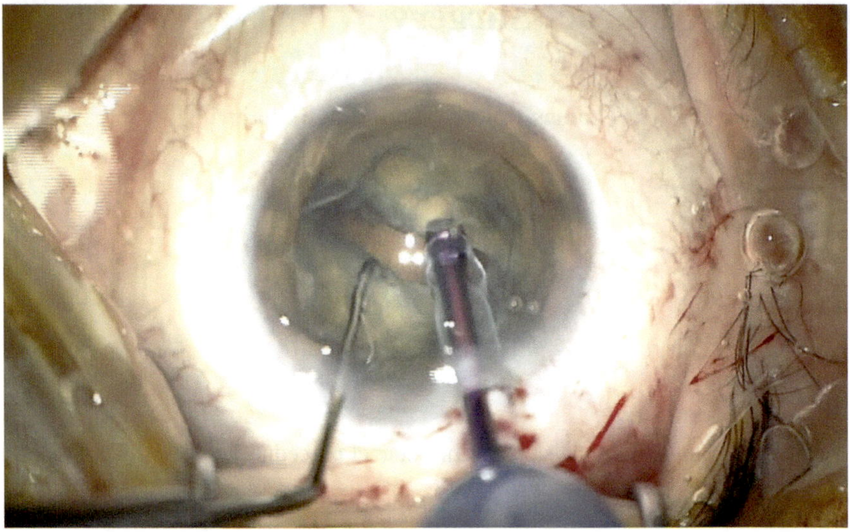

Video 1 In this unedited video a complete cataract procedure in phaco-chop technique with implantation of an artificial lens is shown (▶ https://doi.org/10.1007/000-8d8)

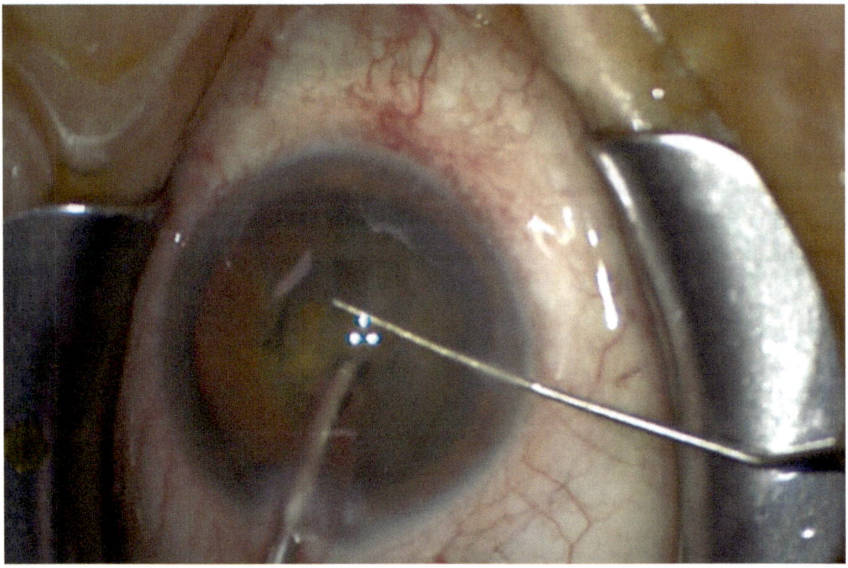

Video 2 As an alternative to the phaco-chop technique, many surgeons use the divide and conquer technique (▶ https://doi.org/10.1007/000-8d7)

The side ports are used to:

- inject pharmaceuticals for pupil dilatation, pain relief or anti-inflammatories
- inject OVD
- introduce a rhexis needle to perform the capsulorhexis
- introduce the chopper or other preferred second instrument to fragment the nucleus and rotate the lens
- remove cortex and OVD when using bimanual irrigation and aspiration
- position the IOL.

The side ports are usually placed immediately before or after the main incision is made. Even though the side ports can be placed very quickly, there are several sources of error in this apparently simple step. Possible errors and consequences when placing the side ports can include:

- Side port too wide: This is probably the most dangerous error. If the side port is too wide, more fluid can flow out of it. This leads to an unstable and flat anterior chamber and increases the probability of serious complications such as a capsular rupture. Although this problem can be partially compensated by increased fluid input (e.g. increasing the height of the bottle), an excessively wide incision will still influence anterior chamber flow and should be avoided.
- Side port too narrow: If the side port is too narrow, the instrument can only be inserted into the eye with greater force or not at all. If the instruments are forced into the eye against the high resistance, intraoperative descemet/deep stromal wrinkles can occur, which reduce the operative visibility and thus make the operation more difficult. The increased force can also damage the cornea and stretch the incisions, rendering them less water tight. Increased patient discomfort and postoperative local corneal oedema may occur.
- Side port too short (too steep): If the side port is too short, the opening will be easily deformed by inserted instruments. As a result, the wound closes more poorly and reflux is increased. In patients with IFIS (intraoperative floppy iris syndrome) in particular, or a very flat anterior chamber, this can lead to prolapse of iris tissue into the opening. The deformation of the side port also leads to poorer vision due to induction temporary corneal folds. In addition, the incision is harder to close by hydration at the end of the operation and suturing may even be necessary. Inadequate closure can lead to postoperative hypotension which allow easier entry of germs from the ocular surface, resulting in an increased risk of endophthalmitis.
- Side port too long (too flat): Side ports that are too long lead to increased shear forces on the cornea, when handling the instruments. This also leads to a local reduction of view. In addition, a delayed postoperative healing process can also occur. Very long incisions can also cause disturbing higher order aberrations, which may even affect the vision in the long-term.

Author's recommendation

In patients with IFIS, high hyperopia, high intraocular pressure or a very flat anterior chamber, a side port should be too long rather than too short in order to reduce the risk of prolapse of iris tissue.

Keypoint

The correct placement of the side port is crucial for safe surgery. A side port that is too wide or too short can lead to an unstable anterior chamber and serious complications like capsular rupture.

When placing the side port, it is important to differentiate whether the side port blade being used has one or two sharp sides (Fig. 1). If the instrument has only one sharp side, the cut will extend towards the sharp side when the instrument is inserted. This means that the puncture site will not be the center of the cut, but at the periphery of the opening. The instrument should be inserted at a flat angle, aiming towards the center of the pupil. A second instrument can be used as a counter-pressure is to stabilize the eye ball.

Author's recommendation

When operating from superior in particular, it can be difficult to perform flat side port incisions because of the prominent orbital bone, as the instruments are relatively long. In such situations they should be slightly bent so that the blade can be inserted at as flat an angle as possible.

To avoid a side port it is important to know how wide the instrument is at its widest point. It may be necessary to only partially insert the blade for an adequate cut. If the blade is not fully inserted, the outer opening of the incision at the corneal limbus margin is wider than the inner opening at the corneal endothelium, due to its conical form. It is the inner opening that determines whether the incision is too narrow or too wide.

When inserting and, above all, removing the instrument, it is important to ensure that no vertical pressure is exerted on the limbus. This would lead to gaping of the side port and increased outflow of anterior chamber fluid.

Main Incision

The main incision is usually made in the corneal periphery ("clear corneal incision") and is about 2.4 mm wide (smaller or larger depending on the lens model used). The main incision is mainly used for:

- The rhexis, if rhexis forceps is used.
- Inserting the phaco tip.

(A)

(B)

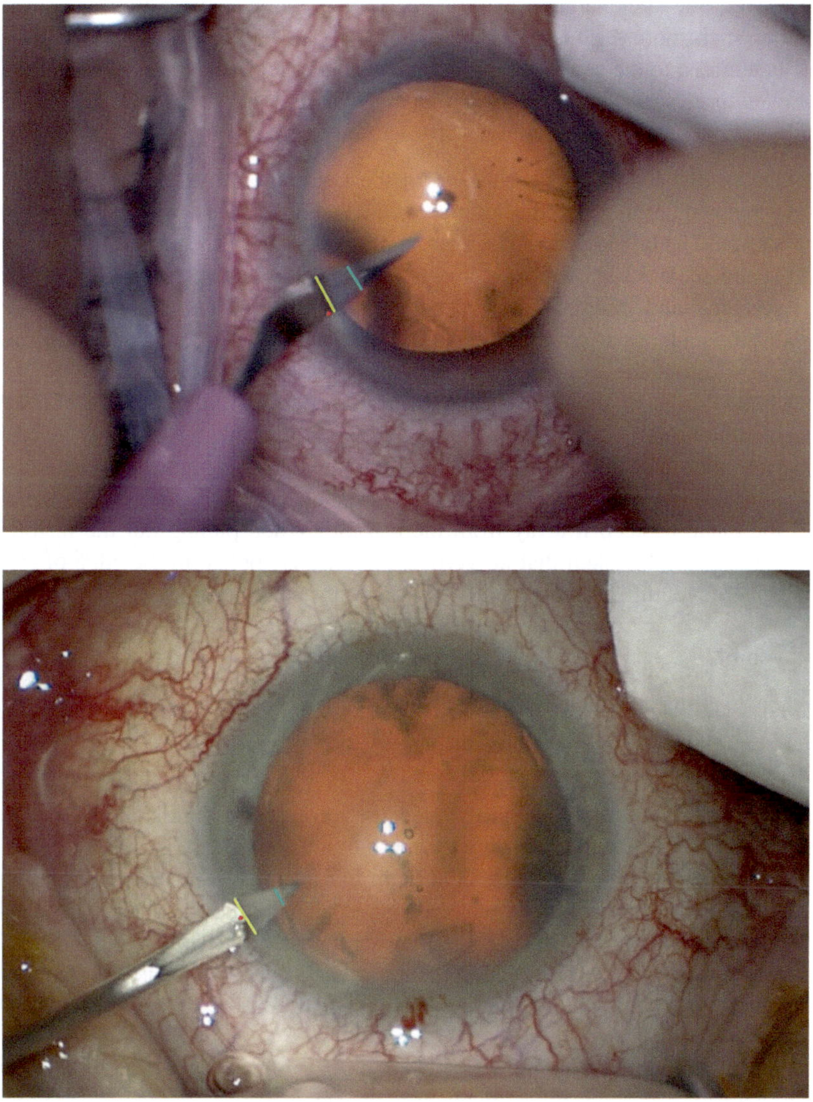

Fig. 1 **A** and **B**: (**A**) the opening of the cornea is shown with a blade with one sharp edge. The puncture point (arrow) is at the periphery of the opening. (**B**) a blade with two sharp sides is shown. The puncture point (arrow) is in the center of the opening

– The implantation of the intraocular lens.

Similar to the side port, the main incision can also be too tight, too wide, too short or too long. The consequences of the errors made during the incision are very similar to those of side port, e.g. increased reflux if the incision is too wide.

However, due to the larger size of the incision, possible complications are amplified and as such more serious.

In contrast to the side port, the main incision is not made in one step, but in two or even three steps. This creates an incision that, although it is much wider than the side port, is usually self-sealing.

1. In the first (optional) step, the tip of the keratome is used to make an incision perpendicular to the corneal surface, which should extend into the outer corneal stroma. The incision should be approximately as wide as the planned main incision.
2. In the second step, the keratome is placed flat—almost parallel to the corneal surface—and inserted with the tip pointing towards the corneal surface. The blade is advanced until the length of the incision corresponds approximately to the width of the incision.
3. in the third step, the tip of the keratome points downwards, so that the Descemet membrane is punctured and finally access to the anterior chamber is created. Care should be taken to advance the keratome to its maximum width through the incision ensure that the full tunnel is of equal width while observing the tip of the blade to keep it away from the capsule. When pulling out the instrument, care should be taken that no vertical pressure is applied to the edge of the cut, thus preventing increased outflow of anterior chamber fluid.

Keypoint

When making the main incision, at least two incision planes should be created (steps 2 and 3), thus reducing the probability of anterior chamber fluid leakage postoperatively.

It is important to stabilize the eye with the second hand during all three steps and to create a slight counter pressure during the incision.

It may be necessary to widen the main incision (e.g. if a different lens with a larger cartridge than originally planned is used). To do this, the blade should first be inserted completely into the eye via the existing main incision. When pulling out, the blade is turned towards the edge of the cut and the keratome is used to carefully expand the cut while pulling the instrument out carefully. Only cut when exiting the wound.

The characteristics of the main incision will influence the surgically induced astigmatism. The induced astigmatism is greater:

- the longer the main incision is
- the wider the main incision is
- the closer the main incision is to the center of the cornea (this accounts for why the induced astigmatism is greater in a superior approach than in a temporal approach, as the vertical corneal diameter is usually smaller than the horizontal).

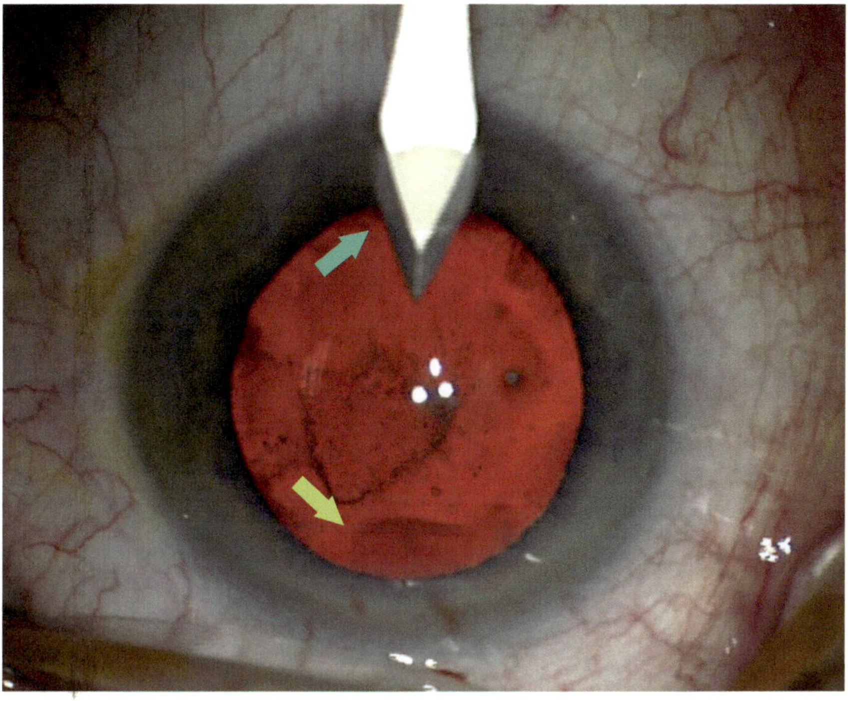

Fig. 2 Setting an "opposite clear corneal incision"—OCCI. The yellow arrow shows the already existing incision. The green arrow shows the OCCI

Author's recommendation

Patients with a total corneal astigmatism < 0.3D should be operated using a temporal approach to minimize surgically induced astigmatism. For preoperative astigmatism from 0.3D to 0.7D, surgery should be performed on the steep axis. If the steep axis is against the rule, temporal surgery is performed. With an astigmatism of 0.7 to 1.3D, a further incision can be made opposite to the main incision ("opposite clear corneal incision"—OCCI, Fig. 2). If the astigmatism is >1D, however, the option of a toric lens should also be discussed with the patient and is usually the preferred option for a good refractive result.

While it is debated, some authors believe that a slight residual astigmatism usually leads to a slightly improved depth of field in vision. This should be discussed with the patient before the operation and, depending on the patient's wishes, (be that the sharpest possible image in one distance or slightly increased depth of field) the surgeon should place the incisions accordingly.

Instead of the three incisions described so far (main incision and two side ports), it is also possible to operate with the MICS (Microincision Cataract Surgery) technique. Only two incisions are required in this scenario and the main incision is smaller than 1.8 mm (Video 3). The advantage of this technique is that the surgically induced astigmatism is negligible.

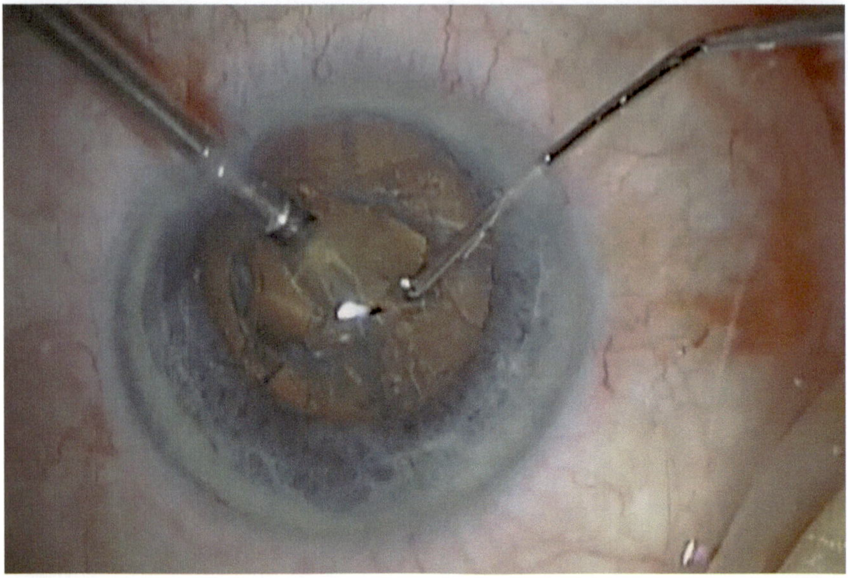

Video 3 With MICS the lens is implanted through a tunnel smaller than 1.8 mm (▶ https://doi.org/10.1007/000-8d9)

Rhexis

The creation of thc capsulorhexis is performed based on a technique originally described by Thomas Neuhann, Howard Gimbel and Kimiya Shimizu by most surgeons using an approach known as continuous curvilinear capsulorhexis (1). This circular construction is robust and the lens can then be safely and efficiently removed through it. Depending on personal taste and situation, either a rhexis forceps or a rhexis needle can be used for this purpose. While the rhexis needle can be inserted through the side port, most rhexis forceps are used through the main incision.

Author's recommendation

The shape (angle and length) of the rhexis needle should be adapted to the depth of the anterior chamber and the anatomy of the eye. The deeper the eye, the shorter the distal shaft should be and the greater the angle to the proximal shaft.

For the sake of simplicity, the following describes how to perform the capsulorhexis using the rhexis needle (Fig. 3):

1. The anterior chamber is filled with plenty of viscoelastic material. It is important to know that the more cohesive the viscoelastic material is, the slower the capsulorhexis can be performed afterwards.

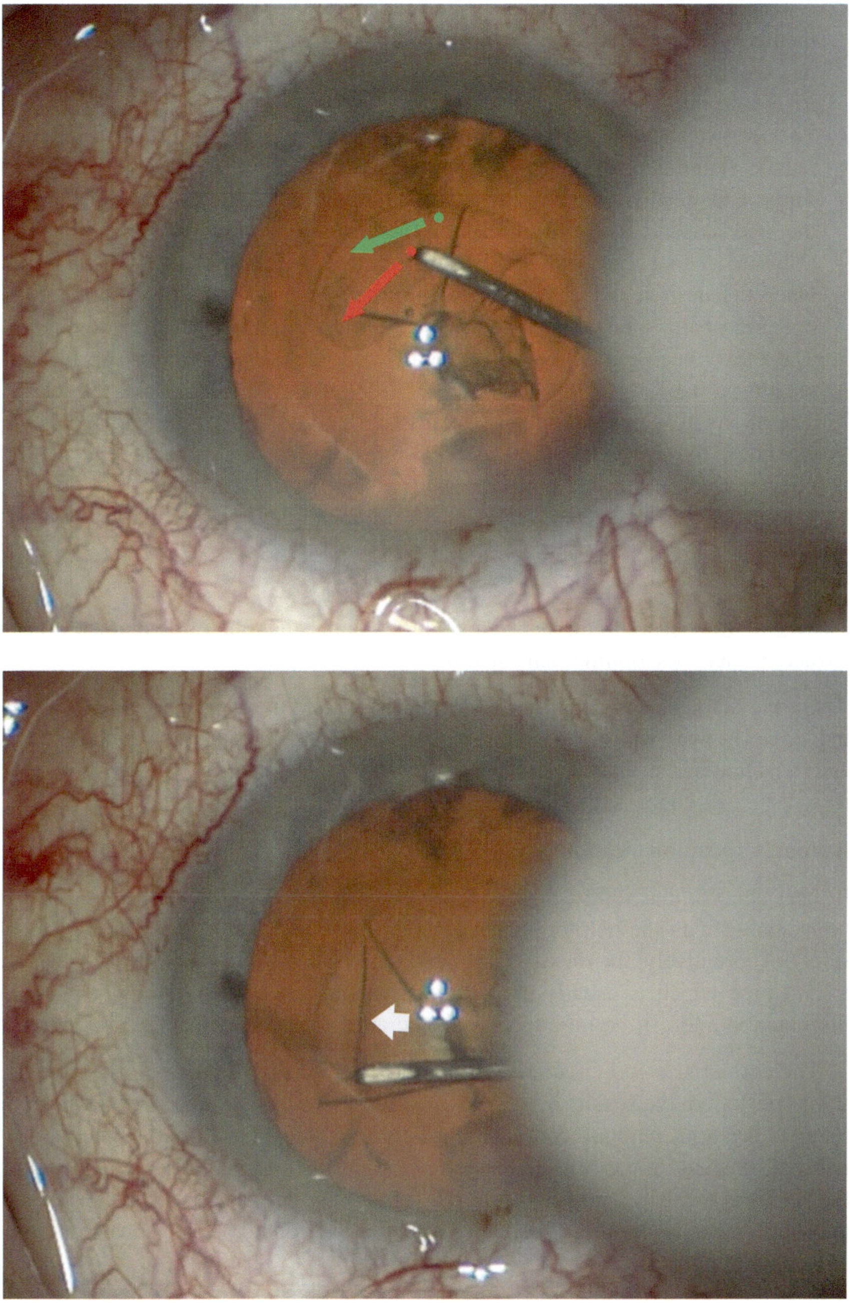

Fig. 3 Pulling at the wrong spot (red dot) and pulling the rhexis needle at the wrong angle for too much will create a stress line in the flap (white arrow), which can lead to tears. Ideally the needle should be placed further outside and near the edge (green point)

2. The rhexis needle is then inserted into the anterior chamber. It is important that the tip of the needle is inserted horizontally through the incision. This glides the instrument through the side port and reduces the risk of accidentally damaging iris tissue or the lens capsule.
3. The lens capsule is incised centrally, avoiding any light reflections that could reduce visibility.
4. The rhexis needle is guided towards the periphery and the resulting opening in the lens capsule is continued until the desired radius for capsulorhexis is achieved. This should be slightly smaller than the radius of the IOL optic.
5. Once the desired radius is reached, the rhexis needle is used to continue the opening of the anterior capsule at a perpendicular angle to the existing slit.
6. The rhexis needle is now used to fold over the exposed anterior capsule leaf, creating a flap.
7. The rhexis needle is placed peripherally, close to the fold of the flap and slowly extended by applying slight vertical pressure on the capsule and pulling counter-clockwise (or if preferred clockwise).
8. This process is repeated several times until a completely round flap is obtained.

Keypoint

The rhexis diameter should be sized slightly smaller than the optic diameter of the intraocular lens for optimal lens stability.

During all steps a clear red reflex should be visible in order to be able to see the flap edge. In eyes with a very cloudy lens, trypan blue should be injected into the anterior chamber so that the blue lens capsule stands out from the white, cloudy lens. When in doubt, stain the capsule.

Author's recommendation

If there is no fundus reflex, e.g. bin cases of vitreous hemorrhage, the contrast can be increased with the help of trypan blue and the rhexis can usually be performed safely. Alternatively, the rhexis margin and the flap can be visualized with the aid of a light pipe which is usually used in vitreoretinal surgery. This provides coaxial illumination and can be introduced into the anterior chamber via the side port.

The correct size and circularity of the rhexis are decisive factors for a good and stable postoperative result. If the rhexis is too small, it is much more difficult to remove the lens without complications, as the area of action is unnecessarily reduced. A small rhexis also increases the risk of postoperative rhexis phimosis. If the rhexis is too large, however, the IOL optic may lie outside of the capsule and may, for example, promote iris capture of the IOL or a UGH syndrome (uveitis glaucoma hyphema).

Mistakes are inevitable when learning capsulorhexis. However, negative consequences can be avoided in the majority of cases by correct management.

- Small rhexis before the capsulorhexis is completed: If the surgeon notices that the rhexis is becoming too small, an attempt can be made to continue the rhexis in an outwardly enlarging spiral.
- Small rhexis after the capsulorhexis is completed: With intraocular scissors, the edge of the rhexis should be incised at an angle of about 45° for 1–2 mm. With the rhexis forceps the flap is grasped and guided circularly until a larger capsulorhexis has been formed. In these cases, a forceps is typically easier than using the needle.
- Expanding opening: The most common causes for a rhexis "running out" are insufficient OVD, incorrect vector of pull or too much distance between the instrument and the flap edge when creating the capsulorhexis. If the rhexis is running out, the surgeon should first release the flap and insert more OVD. This is particularly important in eyes where there is a lot of pressure on the lens capsule, e.g. with a mature lens or "vis a tergo", where an OVD as cohesive as possible should be used. This creates a counter pressure and stabilizes the anterior chamber. The flap should be grasped close to the edge of the rhexis and slowly pulled back with a counter pull to the outgoing direction.
- Advanced rhexis opening: The "little technique" of capsulorhexis rescue can generally prevent further opening of the rhexis. (2) In this approach, the flap is first released and unfolded. Then, at a distance of about 0.5 mm from the edge of the rhexis, pull the rhexis against the outgoing direction and towards the center of the lens with the rhexis forceps.

Keypoint

During the capsulorrhexis, the anterior chamber should always be filled with viscoelastic material in order to be able to pull the flap in a controlled manner and to create a rhexis with high circularity.

Hydrodissection and Hydrodelineation

During the phacoemulsification step, the core of the cataract is usually divided into several pieces before they are removed individually. To do this, the lens has to be rotated several times and should be very mobile. Hydrodissection separates the lens from the capsule and allows it to be rotated freely.

For a successful hydrodissection and hydrodelineation several steps are necessary:

1. First, BSS (balanced salt solution) should be injected into the anterior chamber via the main incision so that the OVD is partially washed out
2. In the second step, a cannula is inserted approximately one millimeter below the rhexis edge and the tip is angled slightly upwards (Fig. 4). This should be done at a slight angle opposite to the main incision.

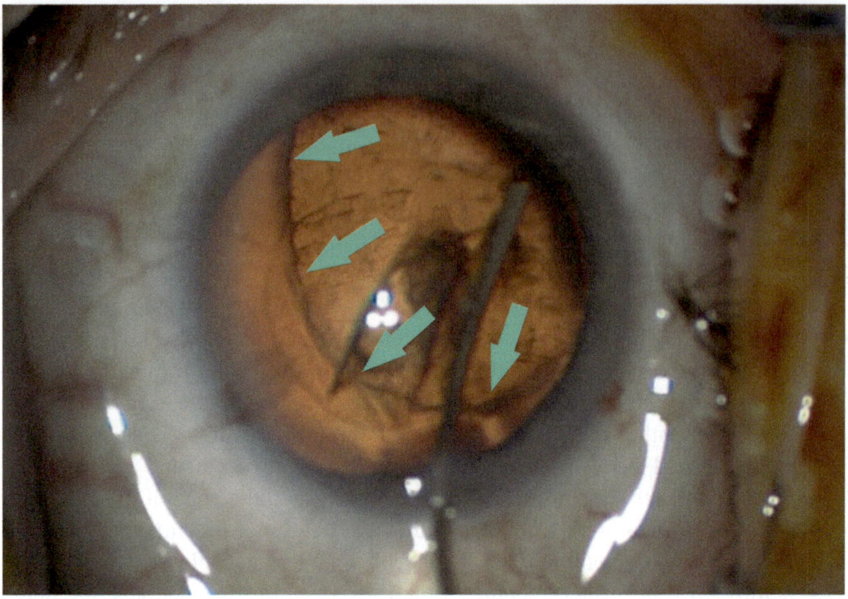

Fig. 4 The cannula opening is placed under the rhexis edge. Entered BSS separates the lens from the capsule and the BSS wavefront becomes visible

3. Liquid is then slowly injected under the capsule, separating the lens from the capsule. The wavefront of the fluid should be visible. While the liquid is being administered, the cannula should be pressed carefully on top of the lens so that the liquid can escape forward and does not collect behind the lens, pushing the lens forward out of the capsular bag or, in the worst case, causing a rupture of the capsule.

At this point, the cannula can be used to check whether the lens completely free. If not, the hydrodissection manoeuvre should be repeated elsewhere until the lens becomes mobile. In case of persistent adhesions, the lens can be carefully pressed down with the tip of the cannula in the area close to the main incision. This usually loosens persisting connections to the capsule. Rarely, this does not succeed due to massive adhesions to the capsule. In these cases it is recommended to continue with hydrodelineation before uncontrolled manoeuvres risk a capsular tear.

As soon as the lens can be rotated freely, a surgeon may then choose to insert the cannula and inject into the central periphery of the lens within a depth of approx. 1 mm. This separates the epinucleus from the nucleus and a "golden ring" becomes visible (hydrodelineation), though this is not always required.

Keypoint

Hydrodissection is one of the most important steps in cataract surgery and can be a hurdle for the inexperienced surgeon. It is advisable to invest a lot of time in this step, as a well performed hydrodissection with a freely rotating lens makes the further steps of cataract surgery much easier.

Phacoemulsification

Phacoemulsification enables the safe and efficient removal of the natural lens. The phacoemulsification technique depends on the personal preferences of the surgeon, technology available and the ocular conditions. In this section the most common techniques are presented. Regardless of the technique used, a dispersive viscoelastic agent should be applied before phacoemulsification is performed to minimize damage to the corneal endothelium.

Divide and Conquer

With "Divide and Conquer" surgical technique, two perpendicular fragments are created in the lens. This allows the lens to be divided into four quadrants (divide) by applying slight pressure and each quadrant is then removed (or conquered) separately.

1. Firstly, the "sleeve" of the probe should be checked to ensure that it is correctly positioned on the phaco handpiece, that the irrigation holes are horizontal and that both irrigation and phacoemulsification work. This is done by briefly pushing the foot pedal before entering the eye.
2. The phacotip is inserted into the anterior chamber with the help of a second instrument, which keeps the corneal incision open.
3. The superficial epinucleus is removed by rotating the phaco opening downwards and performing careful aspiration.
4. With the phaco-opening upwards (or slightly oblique), the first groove is now formed. The groove is started as vertically as possible near the proximal edge of the rhexis. The groove is extended distally in the direction of the main axis under application of ultrasonic energy until the opposite rhexis edge is reached. Apply as much phaco energy as is necessary to break up just enough lens material to be able to aspirate. Too much phaco energy could lead to uncontrolled emulsification of the lens, too little energy in turn would cause the lens to be pushed forward, which in turn would put unnecessary stress on the zonula fibres. When retracting the phaco-tip to the starting point of the groove, the foot pedal should be in position 1 (irrigation) to avoid damage from unnecessary ultrasound energy.
5. The groove is widened slightly on the surface so that the sleeve does not push the core down when digging deeper.
6. The groove is deepened up to 3/4–4/5 of the lens thickness.
7. The lens is then rotated by 90° using a second instrument, e.g. push–pull, and a groove is created again.
8. To complete the second groove, the lens is rotated once more, this time by 180° and the groove is extended distally again, so that finally two grooves in the shape of a cross are created within the lens.

9. A phaco spatula and the phaco-tip are then placed deep in the groove and gently separated. This creates a crack and two lens hemi-fragments are formed. As the opening of the phaco-tip is usually sloped, the phaco-tip should be rotated so that the longer side presses against the nucleus in order to have a better transmission of the separating forces.
10. The lens is rotated again and four lens fragments are created by opposing pressure.
11. The lens quadrants are individually pulled centrally and to the iris plane (by aspiration or manually) where they are removed by phacoemulsification and aspiration. A preserved epinucleus during quadrant removal can be advantageous as a protective layer in front of the lens capsule.
12. If epinucleus is still present at the end, it is carefully aspirated (without ultrasound energy) in the periphery, pulled into the center and aspirated there. The second instrument can help to mobilize the epinucleus during this process.

Author's recommendation

The phaco settings should be changed during the procedure so that each step can be worked on as efficiently as possible. When forming the groove, the sculpting should be carried out under low vacuum, moderate flow and continuous or pulsating ultrasound. The phacopower should be adjusted according to the hardness of the lens. For quadrant removal, the vacuum should now be increased to ensure a good grip of the fragments during quadrant removal. The ultrasonic energy should be applied in "pulsed" or "hyperpulsed" mode. When removing the epinucleus, the vacuum can be slightly reduced again. Ultrasonic energy should no longer be necessary.

The "divide and conquer" technique is a very safe method of lens removal and is usually the first technique that surgeons learn. Nevertheless, there are some typical beginner's mistakes which should be known before learning this method:

- The groove is started too centrally. As a result, the groove is too short and too central, too much hard lens material is still present. Breaking the lens into two fragments is therefore considerably more difficult or impossible.
- The groove is not deep enough at both ends. Beginners tend be very concerned with posterior capsular tears and do not to penetrate the lens steeply enough with the Phaco-tip. As a result, a lot of lens material remains on the periphery, which makes splitting the lens more difficult.
- Too little ultrasonic energy is used. This can be seen when the whole lens follows the movements of the phaco-tip during sculpting. This places unnecessary stress on the zonular fibers.
- When the phaco-tip moves backwards during the formation of the groove, the beginner sometimes continues using aspiration and ultrasonic energy. This exposes the eye to unnecessary ultrasonic energy and may even damage ocular tissue.

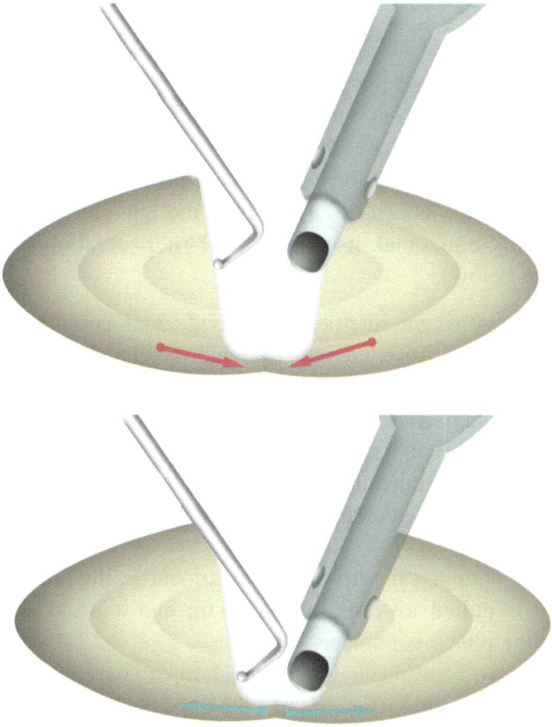

Fig. 5 In the upper graphic the instruments are placed too far up, so that when force is applied the lens may even be brought together in the bottom area. In the lower graph the instruments are placed deep enough inside the lens so that a minimal amount of force will split the lens

- The groove is not wide enough at the surface. The sleeve thus prevents the phaco-tip from dipping deeper into the lens. Therefore, the upper third of the groove should be widened a little before the groove is extended into the depth.
- The groove is not deep enough. The Phaco-tip is about 1 mm wide. The lens thickness is about 4 mm in the center. Accordingly, the groove can be about 3 times as deep as the Phaco-tip. Above all, when creating the groove, care should be taken to ensure that the red reflex and the lens fibers are not altered. The deeper the gap, the stronger the red reflex. Lens material should be removed until no more transverse lens (finger-print) fibers can be seen. Usually, it takes some time for the beginner to estimate the depth correctly, and accordingly an experienced surgeon should always assist the beginner.
- When splitting the groove, the instruments are not inserted deep enough into the groove. If the lens is moved too far apart at the top, the lens is compressed at the bottom so that no fragments can be created (Fig. 5).

Phaco-Chop

In 1993 Nagahara introduced the Phaco-Chop technique. Chopping is the process of bimanually breaking the lens into several fragments with the help of a second instrument, such as the Nagahara chopper. The phaco-tip is inserted into the lens core. The chopper is then carefully placed under the lens capsule and pulled from the lens periphery to the phaco-tip. This splits the lens into two parts. Since the movement is mainly horizontal, it is also called "horizontal chop" (as opposed to vertical chop, see below).

1. The first three steps are identical to "divide and conquer", i.e. the phaco handpiece is checked, inserted into the anterior chamber and superficial lens material is aspirated.
2. The phaco-tip is then inserted paracentral into the lens on the side of the main incision until the entire tip is within the lens core. The core is now held in place with the phaco-tip by sufficient vacuum.
3. The chopper is inserted with the tip horizontally under the lens capsule, opposite to the main incision.
4. By rotating the chopper, the tip of the instrument is aligned vertically.
5. The chopper is pulled towards the phaco-tip and a slight counterpressure is created with the phaco handpiece.
6. Just before the two instruments touch, the chopper is used to pull the nucleus to the left and the phaco-tip is used to push the opposite half of the lens to the right. This splits the lens.
7. Put the foot pedal on irrigation, rotate the lens and repeat the steps to further fragment the lens. This should produce four or six (or even eight in the case of particularly hard lenses) fragments.
8. Each fragment is individually pulled into the center and onto the iris plane with the phaco-tip and emulsified
9. Similar to "Divide and Conquer", a possible epinucleus is removed by aspiration in the last step. The second instrument can be used to mobilize the epinucleus.

Author's recommendation

The Phaco-Chop technique has proven to be particularly advantageous for hard lenses and for lenses with a relatively loose holding apparatus, as relatively little energy is required for the fragmentation of the lens and hardly any shear forces act on the zonular apparatus. When chopping, the vacuum should be relatively high and a low ultrasonic energy should be set in "burst mode". When removing the fragments, aspiration can be increased, the vacuum reduced and the fragments removed under higher ultrasonic energy in "pulsed mode" or "continuous mode" (more suitable for experienced surgeons). Some surgeons prefer to use the duo linear pedal adjustment for this technique, because vacuum and ultrasound can be used in a very controlled way.

As the whole procedure is bimanual and several points have to be considered at the same time, this technique may be a little more difficult for beginners to perform. Typical chopping mistakes are:

- Phaco-tip is not inserted deep enough into the nucleus. This means that there is no proper abutment for the chopper, and the lens cannot be split.
- The vacuum is too low and does not allow stable fixation of the lens.
- The chopper is guided vertically to the periphery and accidentally damages the anterior capsule when pressing on the lens.
- The chopper is not advanced far enough into the periphery. As a result, no proper pressure can be applied to the lens and instead of splitting the lens, only the surface of the lens is "scratched".
- When the last lens fragments are removed, the tip of the chopper points downwards and movements of the posterior capsule during aspiration through the phaco-tip cause the capsule to rupture. To prevent this, the tip of the instrument should be placed horizontally whenever it is not needed. When aspirating the last lens fragments, the chopper can also be replaced by a phaco spatula. The phaco spatula can then be held in the depth of the center, below the phaco-tip, to prevent accidental aspiration of the capsule with possible capsular rupture.
- The aspiration rate or ultrasonic energy is too high and, instead of having a firm hold of the lens by the phaco-tip, lens fragments are completely aspirated. In such a case, the aspiration rate and ultrasonic energy should be reduced and more attention should be paid to careful pressure on the foot pedal.
- There is too much pressure on the side port and the main incision. This leads to increased leakage of anterior chamber fluid and makes chopping much more difficult.

The "Stop and Chop" technique is a mixture of "Divide and Conquer" and "Phaco-Chop" techniques. Here the initial groove is created as in the "Divide and Conquer" technique and the lens is divided into two fragments. The two pieces are split into smaller fragments using the Chop technique.

Another modification of the Phaco-Chop is the "Phaco quick chop". Here, the lens is pulled upwards using a high vacuum and a pointed chopper is pressed into the lens, pulled to the phacotip and then pulled apart. Since vertical forces are mainly acting here, the method is also called "Vertical Chop". However, this method is not suitable for soft lenses.

Irrigation and Aspiration

During irrigation and aspiration, the remaining cortex is loosened and removed from the capsule. This can be done bimanually or coaxially (irrigation and aspiration in one handpiece). The bimanual method (for a right-handed person) is described here, but the same principles also apply to the coaxial technique.

1. The irrigation handpiece is introduced into the eye via the left side port under irrigation. The flow of irrigation should be in the direction of the capsular bag to push it away.
2. The aspiration handpiece is introduced through the right side port under continuous irrigation. Care must be taken to ensure that the opening of the instrument is always facing upwards.
3. The aspiration handpiece is placed 1–2 mm below the edge of the capsule. Under the edge of the capsule, the tip of the instrument is moved counter-clockwise (or clockwise) to capture as much cortex material as possible. This activates the aspiration and sucks in any residual cortex. The fact that there is material in the opening is usually indicated to the surgeon by the phaco machine changing its tone as the vacuum rises.
4. The aspiration is slowly increased under constant pressure on the foot pedal and the instrument is pulled into the center so that the material can be aspirated completely. This is repeated several times until about half of the capsule has been freed of cortex residues.
5. The aspiration handpiece is removed from the anterior chamber and then the irrigation handpiece under continuous irrigation.
6. The irrigation handpiece is inserted through the right side port under irrigation and the aspiration over the left side port.
7. The second half of the capsule is freed from the cortex material.
8. Both instruments are then removed from the eye. The posterior capsule is polished using a fine cannula and polishing it with BSS. This is best done via the main incision, as the greater outward flow pushes the posterior capsule upwards, allowing better tangential polishing.

Remember

Cortex removal is particularly efficient if the aspiration handpiece is guided sufficiently into the periphery, a clockwise/counterclockwise movement is made and the instrument is rotated slightly around its own axis. This makes it easier to "peel off" the cortex material and then aspirate it centrally.

Irrigation and aspiration may damage the capsular bag and zonulae, although the risk is reduced, compared to phacoemulsification. Every surgeon should be aware of the most common sources of error when learning this step:

- During cortex removal, the irrigation handpiece is accidentally pulled out of the eye. The beginner tends to focus only on the aspiration handpiece, as the main movement is performed with it. As a result, the irrigation port gradually "slides" out of the eye. It is important not to pull the aspiration handpiece out of the eye in such a moment, but to keep it in position and immediately take your foot off the pedal. Under irrigation, the irrigation handpiece is reinserted and the surgery is continued.

- When aspiration is activated, the opening of the instrument is not deep enough under the edge of the capsule and no circular movement is performed. This leads to a situation where not enough cortical material can be aspirated and the procedure takes unnecessarily longer.
- Instead of cortical material, the capsule is aspirated and pulling the handpiece centrally now damages the zonular apparatus or the capsule itself. Before increasing aspiration, always make sure that the opening is occluded by cortex and not by the capsule. The risk of aspiration of the capsule and chance of capsular rupture is significantly reduced with special aspiration handpieces for the coaxial technique, since the sleeve serves as a natural protection.
- The opening of the aspiration handpiece should not be pointed downwards during aspiration. This can lead to the posterior capsule being aspirated and to a capsular rupture.
- The irrigation opening points to the periphery instead of being directed towards the posterior capsule. In the worst case, this can cause fluid to migrate behind the capsule and increase the pressure behind the capsule, making the operation unnecessarily difficult.
- Minimal cortex remnants that cannot be aspirated. In such a case it should be checked whether the aspiration opening is deep enough below the edge of the capsule and corrected if necessary. If this does not work either, it is possible that the fibers are too thin to occlude the opening and create proper suction. It is then recommended that the fibers be flushed out with a fine cannula and BSS or, after implantation of the lens, to continue aspiration under the protection of the optic.

Implantation of the Iintraocular Lens

The intraocular lens is usually inserted into the capsular bag. The capsular bag is usually prepared to accept the lens by filling it and expanding it out. This can be done by OVD or, in the case of using implantation shooters, by irrigation via a side port. In the following section, the implantation technique with viscoelastic is described, as it is the safer option for beginners.

1. First, cohesive viscoelastic is placed in the capsular bag and in the lens cartridge.
2. The intraocular lens (IOL) should be check to ensure that it is placed correctly. Here the haptics form a "mirrored S" (Fig. 6).
3. The haptics are placed over the lens and the IOL is pushed into the cartridge.

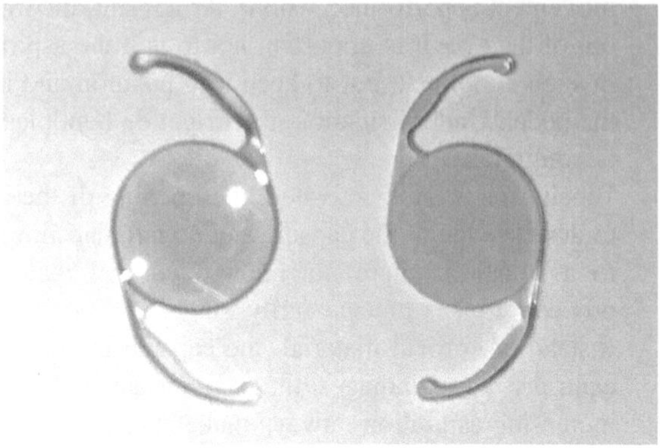

Fig. 6 The lens is correctly aligned on the left and forms a "mirrored S" through the haptics

4. The cartridge is fixed in the injector and by means of a press or screw movement on the injector the lens is pushed forward almost to the tip of the cartridge.
5. The tip of the cartridge is placed against the main incision and inserted into the anterior chamber by a sliding and rotating movement. The patient is asked to look opposite to the insertion movement to provide some counter traction.
6. The IOL is slowly inserted into the capsular bag, either by a pushing or a screwing motion, depending on the injector design.
7. A push–pull instrument can be used to place the IOL and its haptics into the capsular bag. The best way to do this is to turn the IOL clockwise at the optic-haptic junction and to apply slight downward pressure on the lens.
8. The viscoelastic material is then aspirated from in front of the lens using irrigation and aspiration.
9. The IOL is then tilted slightly so that the aspiration opening can be guided behind the lens and the remaining viscoelastic is aspirated. It is important to make sure that the opening is always pointing upwards so that the capsule is not inadvertently aspirated. Some surgeons to slide the lens side-to-side to release the OVD from behind the lens without having to aspirate directly behind it.
10. Finally, make sure that the IOL is correctly centered and not tilted before removing the aspiration handpiece and then the irrigation handpiece from the anterior chamber.

Reminder

The haptics of the IOL should always be seen as a "mirrored S", regardless of whether a one-piece or three-piece IOL is used.

The implantation of the intraocular lens and the aspiration of the viscoelastic are usually among the first steps in learning how to perform cataract surgery, as the risk of causing a serious complication is rather low. Nevertheless, there are some mistakes that should be avoided:

- The IOL is implanted "up-side-down". In this case the haptics are aligned to show an "S". This can cause a change in the effective lens position and may be associated with refractive errors. Furthermore, higher order aberrations can occur more frequently. If the IOL has been implanted "up-side-down", the lens is bimanually flipped under the protection of OVD. An instrument is first inserted under the lens and the lens is lifted. The second instrument is used to push the lens down and away on the opposite side. By moving the two instruments in opposite directions, the optic is flipped and the IOL is realigned.
- If the capsular bag is insufficiently filled with OVD and most of the OVD is rather in the anterior chamber than in the capsular bag. As a result, the anterior capsule is pushed backwards and the capsule is flattened, which makes the implantation of an intracapsular IOL considerably more difficult.
- If the haptics are not placed over the optic when placing the lens in the cartridge. This can lead to the IOL not being able to be pushed out of the cartridge or a haptic getting caught in the injector.
- If the tip of the injector is not placed deep enough into the anterior chamber. As a result, the IOL cannot be inserted into the anterior chamber and in the worst case it may even get stuck in the main incision. The IOL must be removed again by pulling it out with a forceps. This can damage the lens, and the incision.
- If the push-pull hook is removed and the instrument is not turned horizontally, it can get caught on the edge of the capsule and thus leads to a tear in the anterior capsule. In general, it is important to ensure that when inserting and removing instruments, the longer side is always aligned horizontally and thus parallel to the incision.
- If the OVD is not sufficiently removed, large quantities of viscoelastic material can accumulate behind the lens and lead to a postoperative increase in pressure. It is therefore essential to ensure that all viscoelastic material behind the lens is removed, either by careful lens sliding back and forth or direct aspiration behind the lens.
- If the IOL is not injected into the capsular bag but into the anterior chamber it needs to be repositioned. When putting the IOL into the eye, it is important to ensure that the injector is held at a relatively steep angle so that the IOL is guided safely towards the capsular bag. If the optic is partially inside the capsular bag, the angle can be slowly flattened before the IOL is slowly pushed further into the capsular bag to avoid unnecessary pressure (visible by capsule folds) on the posterior capsule.

Hydration

If the incision has been made correctly, the wound can usually be sealed with minimal hydration.

1. First the anterior chamber is filled with BSS and then the first side port is hydrated by "pushing" BSS into the corneal stroma. The stroma swells up and becomes whitish.

2. The second side port is closed similarly. If more fluid escapes from the first side port, it should be rehydrated.
3. Once both paracenteses are sealed, the position of the lens is checked again. If the lens is not centrally located in the capsular bag, the IOL is centered with irrigation, using the BSS cannula.
4. The main incision is then closed by hydration of both edges of the incision. Some surgeons skip this step as the main incision (if constructed properly) is usually self-sealing.
5. The intraocular pressure is checked by pressing on the sclera. If the pressure is too high, some fluid is removed via the side port.
6. Finally, an antibiotic is administered via a side port.

Reminder

It is essential that all cuts are sealed and no liquid can leak out. Otherwise, ocular hypotension and associated complications could occur. In the worst case, germs could also enter the eye through the open incision and increase the risk of endophthalmitis.

Before removing the eyelid retractor, some surgeons apply iodine-containing eye drops to prevent infection. After removing the eyelid retractor and the cover, the eyelids are cleaned and dried, an eye ointment containing steroids and antibiotics is applied and the eye is covered with an eye shield.

Author's recommendation

If the eye is hypotonic, the optics of the IOL may dislocate from the capsular bag and may even cause a "reverse optic capture" (haptics in the capsular bag, optic in front of the anterior rhexis). In such a case, all incisions should be very well hydrated. The IOL is then positioned in the capsular bag with irrigation using a fine cannula.

References

1. Neuhann T. Theory and surgical technic of capsulorhexis. Klin Monbl Ophthalmol. 1987;190 (6):542–5.
2. Little BC, Smith JH, Packer M. Little capsulorhexis tear-out rescue. J Cataract Refract Surg. 2006;32(9):1420–2.

Lens Surgery for Particularly Soft Lenses

Siegfried Priglinger, Sorcha Ní Dhubhghaill, and Mehdi Shajari

Many forms of cataract, e.g. a dense subcapsular cataract, a cortically accentuated cataract, a contusion rosette, etc., can significantly reduce visual acuity despite containing a soft lens core. In addition, the number of patients who do not have a cataract but who wish to have a surgical solution such as refractive lens exchange to achieve freedom from glasses due to presbyopia is constantly increasing. These soft lenses can usually be removed with very little use of ultrasound energy and surgery is therefore less harmful to the intraocular tissue. Nevertheless, there are a few points to consider in order to achieve an optimal result. The standard chopping or "divide and conquer" approaches rely on a firm lens to generate the vacuum and resistance for the required chop or groove formation. This is not typically possible in soft lenses.

The incision and capsulorhexis are performed in the same way as for standard cataracts. Two options are possible for hydrodissection.

Option 1: Hydrodissection is performed in the same way as for standard cataracts. The lens is carefully detached from the capsular bag using liquid. The surgeon presses the lens gently and repeatedly so that the fluid does not collect between the capsular bag and the lens. This loosens the lens but retains it in the capsular bag. Hydrodelineation is then carried out and a free rotation of the lens in the capsular bag is checked.

Option 2: During hydrodissection the lens is no longer pressed down. The fluid thus accumulates as a bolus between the lens and the lens capsule until the lens is prolapsed out of the capsular bag into the anterior chamber. In this scenario it is important that the rhexis is large enough so that the pressure on the anterior capsule stays at a low level.

S. Priglinger (✉) · S. N. Dhubhghaill · M. Shajari
Munich, Germany
e-mail: s.priglinger@med.uni-muenchen.de

S. N. Dhubhghaill
Antwerpen, Belgium

M. Shajari et al. (eds.), *Cataract and Lens Surgery*,
https://doi.org/10.1007/978-3-031-05394-8_46

The advantage of option 2 is that the lens is located in the anterior chamber, which means that the risk of a posterior capsule rupture during lens aspiration is very low. The disadvantage is that increased pressure is exerted on the anterior capsule sheet during lens extraction and any contact between the lens and endothelium could lead to minor endothelial damage.

Author's recommendation

Since the risk of a posterior capsule rupture is very low with soft lenses, we generally prefer the first option.

Aspiration is usually completely sufficient for removing the lens and therefore the application of ultrasonic energy should be avoided if possible. When aspirating the lens, the phaco handpiece can be inserted centrally and, if hydrodelineation is well carried out, the lens core can be aspirated first and then the epinucleus. This two-stage procedure has the advantage that the epinucleus acts as an additional protective barrier in front of the lens capsule when the nucleus is removed. Another approach to aspirating the lens is the so-called carousel technique. For this, the phaco handpiece is guided into the periphery of the lens and the handpiece is rotated by 90° so that the opening faces the lens core. Next, the tip of the Nagahara chopper is inserted into the center of the lens. By careful aspiration, the lens rotates around the chopper and can be slowly aspirated from the periphery to the center. This has the advantage that both instruments hardly need to be moved during lens removal.

The subsequent cortex removal and lens implantation does not differ from the standard cataract.

Surgical Techniques—Cataract Surgery in Very Hard Lenses

Abhay R. Vasavada, Vaishali Vasavada, Mehdi Shajari, and Siegfried Priglinger

Choice of Anaesthesia in Dense Cataract Surgery

The choice of anesthesia depends on several factors including the surgical technique (phacoemulsification versus ECCE), surgeon's preference as well as patient co-operation. However, as more and more surgeons perform phacoemulsification for dense cataracts, topical or subtenon's anaesthesia are often preferred over injection anesthesia.

Phacoemulsification in Dense Cataracts

Today, phacoemulsification is the standard of care for cataract extraction in most parts of the world. However, an encounter with a dense cataract can be demanding for both the surgeon and the patient, and it is for this reason that phacoemulsification is often not preferred in very dense cataracts. The major difficulties in successful phacoemulsification for hard cataracts are poor visibility, stressful rotation, and incomplete division of the leathery lens fibers. There is an increased risk of

Supplementary Information The online version contains supplementary material available at https://doi.org/10.1007/978-3-031-05394-8_47. The videos can be accessed individually by clicking the DOI link in the accompanying figure caption or by scanning this link with the SN More Media App.

A. R. Vasavada (✉) · V. Vasavada · M. Shajari · S. Priglinger
Vadodara, India
e-mail: icirc@abhayvasavada.com

V. Vasavada
e-mail: vaishali@raghudeepeyeclinic.com

S. Priglinger
e-mail: s.priglinger@med.uni-muenchen.de

M. Shajari et al. (eds.), *Cataract and Lens Surgery*,
https://doi.org/10.1007/978-3-031-05394-8_47

wound site thermal injury and corneal endothelial damage due to the use of excessive ultrasound energy, as well as hard fragments repeatedly hitting the endothelium [1]. The key factors that will often define outcomes in dense cataract emulsification are: achieving a complete division of the leathery lens fibers, maintaining a posterior plane of emulsification, and judicious use of ultrasound energy. To achieve these, the procedure should be governed by the following paradigms:

Incision and Anterior Capsulorhexis

A square or nearly square configuration of the main incision is crucial in order to for it to be self-sealing. Incision size depends on the phaco tip-sleeve configuration as well as planned intraocular lens. Often, in very hard cataracts, the red reflex is poor, and in such cases, staining the anterior capsule with a capsular dye like trypan blue improves visualization of the capsular flap. Anterior capsulorhexis (ACCC) sizing also needs meticulous attention—a very small capsulorhexis may increase the chances of anterior capsule split during subsequent maneuvers with the chopper or phaco probe. On the other hand, too large a capsulorhexis may result in fluid current induced propulsion of the divided fragments out of the bag, sometimes dangerously close to the endothelium. Surgeons should aim for an ACCC around 5 to 5.5 mm in diameter, since this would confine the mobile nuclear fragments within the capsular bag and facilitate posterior plane emulsification.

Cortical cleaving hydrodissection:

In hard cataracts, the nucleus is bulky, and often there is not much space within the capsular bag. A forceful cortical cleaving hydrodissection can lead to sudden blow-out of the posterior capsule [2], since the bulky nucleus does not allow egress of the fluid, especially in eyes where the capsulorhexis is small [3]. In these eyes, careful and gentle cortical-cleaving hydrodissection should be performed. Furthermore, dense cataracts may have strong corticocapsular adhesions [4], making rotation difficult and potentially stressful on the capsulozonular complex. Performing multi-quadrant hydrodissection helps surgeons to cleave the cortico-capsular adhesions without causing a sudden rise in hydraulic pressure, thereby making nucleus rotation easier.

Principles for nucleus division and fragment removal:

Surgeons need to divide the entire process into distinct phases e.g. sculpting, chopping, and fragment removal. This will help surgeons to utilize a different set of ultrasound and fluidic parameters, depending on the need during that phase. Chop techniques, both horizontal and vertical, and their many modifications are very effective for dense cataract emulsification, since they allow complete division of the nuclear fibers.

Sculpting:

The anterior chamber is formed by injecting ophthalmic viscosurgical device (OVD). We prefer the soft shell technique [5], where a dispersive OVD is injected first, followed by a cohesive OVD, which pushes the dispersive OVD towards the corneal endothelium. This helps to protect the endothelium from damage caused by energy dissipation or mechanical trauma. Sculpting creates a central groove in the bulky nucleus that acts as a recess for emulsifying the initial fragments within its confines. An ideal groove is deep, wide, and steep walled with a very thin posterior plate and is confined within the area of the capsulorhexis. While carrying out sculpting, it is advisable not to mechanically push the nucleus but to scrape the layers gently using optimal energy. A bent tip is better suited to achieve a deep sculpting without undue zonular stress, since it minimizes incision distortion when sculpting is performed in the depths of the crater.

We prefer the to use ultrasound (U/S) energy, whether longitudinal or torsional in interrupted delivery mode (either burst or pulse mode) during all phases of the surgery. During sculpting, U/S energy is used with linear foot pedal control and a preset amplitude of 70–80%. It is important that the surgeon intermittently change the foot-pedal position from the 3rd to the 2nd position, in order to allow cooling of the phaco tip. The aspiration flow rate is preset to 25–30 cm^3/min. The end point of sculpting is indicated by a red glow that is visible through the thinned out posterior plate. An adequate sculpting with a deep, central space is the sheet anchor for dense cataract emulsification.

Chopping:

A dense cataract characteristically has extraordinarily tenacious and cohesive leathery fibers that are difficult to separate. Separation of these fibers with forceful lateral movements may produce stress on the capsular bag and the zonules. Also, incomplete separation results in multiple fragments held together like the petals of a flower. Fragments attached centrally make posterior plane emulsification extremely difficult, and risky, and increase the possibility of anterior capsular split, posterior capsular rupture, and prolonged U/S energy dissipation close to the endothelium.

Direct Chop

The direct, or horizontal chop, originally described by Nagahara, is a very effective technique for division of dense nuclei [6]. No sculpting or trenching is required here. The phaco tip is impaled beyond the midpoint of the nucleus and a complete vacuum seal is achieved. A sharp tipped chopper is introduced underneath the capsulorhexis margin beyond the lens equator. Once preset vacuum is achieved, the chopper is then moved towards the phaco tip to initiate a crack. However, we have found that using a blunt tipped chopper is equally effective, and yet reduces the risk of mechanical injury to the equatorial posterior capsule. It is important that maximal or supramaximal vacuum is used alongwith appropriate U/S energy for achieving an effective vacuum seal.

Step-by-step chop in situ and separation technique

Our technique of division [7] involves a judicious combination of chop in situ and lateral separating movements. This technique comprises of five steps:

Step 1: Vacuum seal—Following a small central sculpt, the foot pedal is depressed to the third position and the phaco tip is buried inside the trench. If the wall of the trench is arbitrarily divided into 3 equal parts, the tip is buried at the junction of the anterior 1/3 and posterior 2/3 of the trench (Fig. 1). The footpedal immediately switches from the third position to the second position and remains there till occlusion (indicated by the machine audio) is achieved.

Chop in situ: Initiating a crack—The chopper is placed within the capsulorhexis, just in front of and lateral to the phaco tip. The vertical element of the chopper is depressed posteriorly (toward the optic nerve) (Fig. 1). The aim is to only initiate a partial thickness crack and not to divide the nucleus at a single stroke.

Lateral separation: In hard cataracts, the initial crack seldom reaches the bottom. Therefore, the chopper is progressively repositioned in the depths of the cracked nucleus (Fig. 1) and also repositioned from periphery to the centre. Thus, the crack is gently extended from superficial to deep and from periphery to the centre. This maneuver allows complete separation of the nuclear fragments without undue zonular stress.

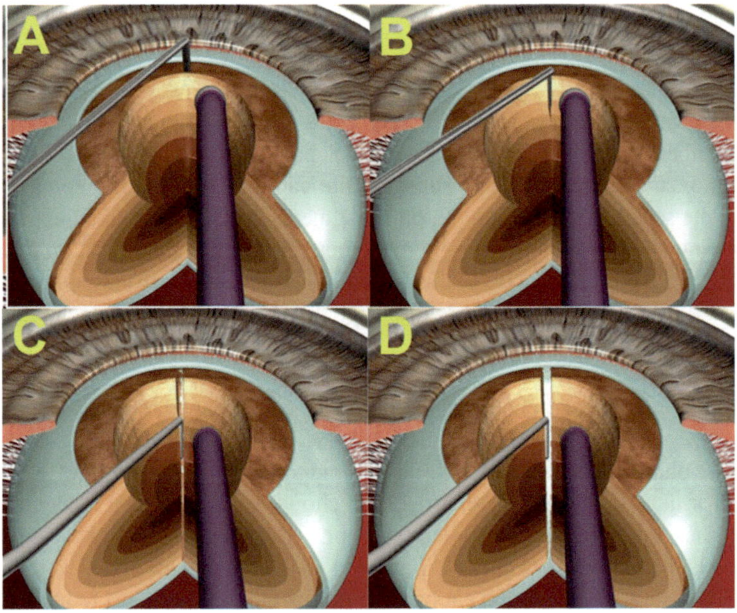

Fig. 1 (**A**) Phaco tip buried in the vertical wall of the trench. (**B**) Chopper being placed just in front of and lateral to the phaco tip. (**C**) Initial vertical movement of chopper, aimed at creating a partial thickness crack. (**D**) The chopper is positioned in the depth of the crack and lateral separating movements are performed

Multilevel chopping:

Often the very dense cataracts will resist complete division of nuclear fragments. In such cases, a multilevel chop technique comes in very handy [8]. For techniques using modifications of the vertical chop technique, an initial crack is initiated, and no attempt is made to extend the crack to the depth. Subsequently, the phaco tip is occluded at a deeper plane, and with each occlusion, fibres adjacent to the tip are chopped with minimal lateral separating movements. This progressive deeper occlusion of the phaco tip allows a better vacuum seal and division of the nucleus adjacent to the tip. This facilitates complete division of posterior plate without the need for excessive separation movements. Multiple fragments can be created by repeating this technique every 1–2 clock hours. (Video 1). The advantages of this technique are safety and efficacy in division of dense, leathery cataracts. The same technique can also be used with direct chop. Here, the phaco tip is first impaled in the periphery and a crack initiated with horizontal movement of the chopper (Fig. 2). Subsequently, the phaco tip is brought centrally and occlusion is achieved. The crack that was initiated is then extended centrally. The technique can also be employed in cataracts with weak zonules, pseudoexfoliation, subluxated cataracts, hypermature cataracts, as well as in small pupils.

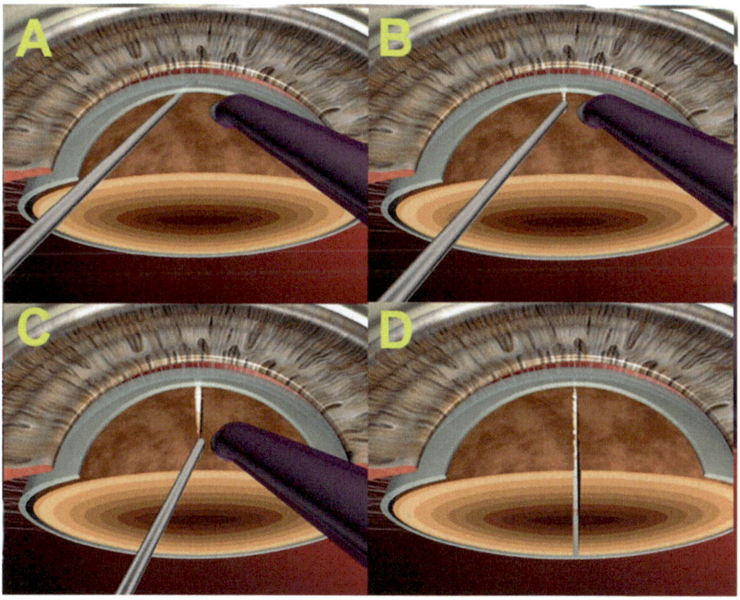

Fig. 2 Multiple, small fragments which become easy to remove during phacoemulsification

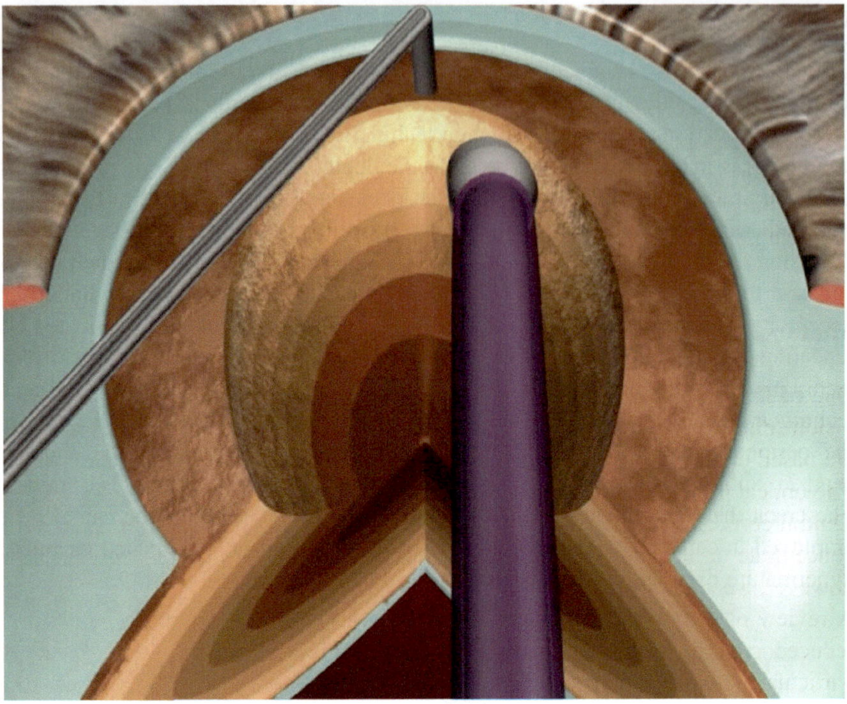

Video 1 Technique to separate fragments in a dense cataract (▶ https://doi.org/10.1007/000-8db)

Nuclear Fragment Removal:

Creating as many small fragments as possible allows surgeons to emulsify them easily (Fig. 3). Surgeons must try to perform emulsification at a posterior plane, in order to avoid thermal and mechanical damage to the corneal endothelium (Fig. 4). However, emulsification in the posterior plane increases the risk of inadvertent aspiration of the posterior capsule and iris, especially if a very high vacuum and aspiration flow rate (AFR) are used while removing the last fragments or epinucleus. Therefore, we suggest lowering the vacuum and AFR as progressively more fragments are removed and the posterior capsule is exposed [9, 10]. This allows surgeons to continue emulsifying at a posterior plane without the risk for posterior capsule rupture (Fig. 5).

Optimal utilization of U/S energy is important for efficient and safe emulsification. Whether longitudinal or torsional ultrasound is used, it is advisable to use interrupted energy as compared to continuous energy. This allows intermittent cooling of the phaco tip, which reduces the chances of wound site thermal injury and corneal endothelial injury. With longitudinal ultrasound, there is a conflict between aspiration forces on one hand which attract the nuclear material, and U/S

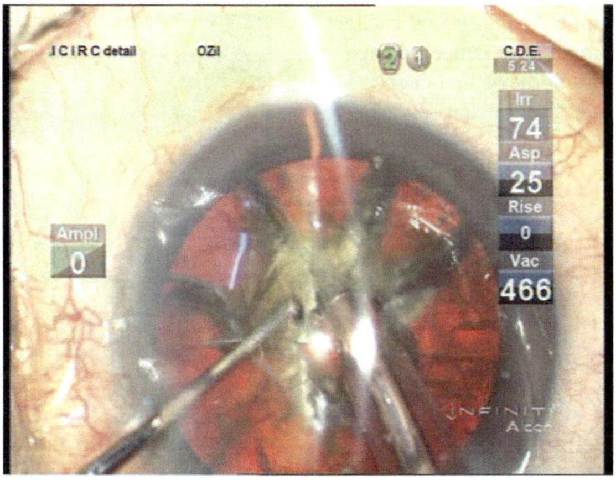

Fig. 3 Horizontal multilevel chopping. The phaco tip is first impaled beyond the centre of the nucleus and a crack initiated. Subsequently, the tip is occluded more centrally, and the crack is extended centrally, to achieve complete nucleus division without undue capsulozonular stress

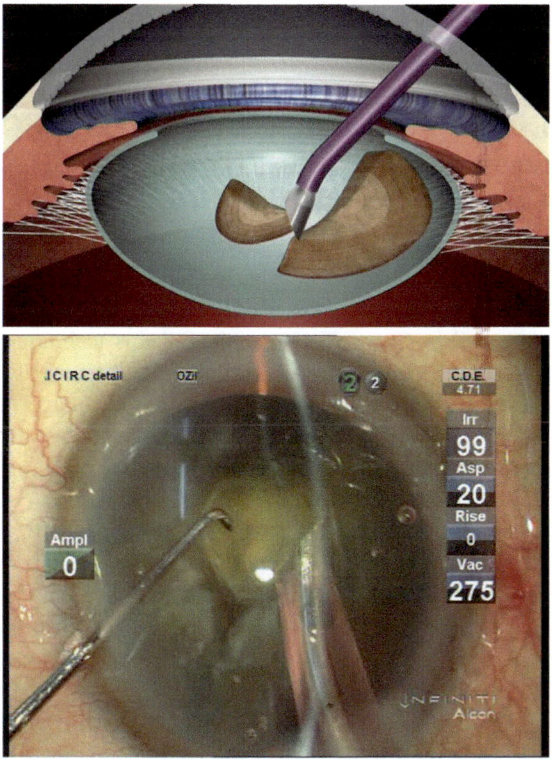

Fig. 4 (**A** and **B**) Animation and clinical picture showing dense nuclear fragment being removed away from the corneal endothelium

energy on the other, which tends to repel the fragments. However, with the torsional ultrasound, since there is a constant oscillatory motion at the phaco tip, there is a seamless cutting with minimal repulsion (chatter) of lens material which makes the U/S energy more efficient, especially in hard cataracts [11, 12]. Whatever the

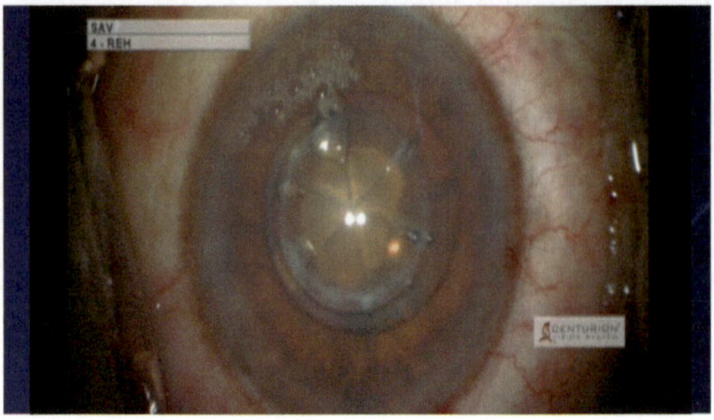

Fig. 5 Femtosecond cataract surgery in a dense cataract, capsulorhexis and chop pattern of nucleus division performed

technique or technology used, it is very important to repeatedly inject dispersive OVD during fragment removal to protect the corneal endothelium. It is of utmost importance to closely inspect the incision at the end of surgery to look out for incision distortion/WSTI. In case of doubt, the incision should be sutured.

Extracapsular Cataract Extraction (ECCE) and Manual Small Incision Cataract Surgery (MSICS) for Dense Cataract Emulsification

Despite the advances in phacoemulsification techniques, there still is a place for ECCE, especially in removal of the very hard cataracts. This technique is further discussed in Chap. 55. Not only can this technique be a fallback in cases where phacoemulsification poses difficulties, but it can also be the primary technique of choice in these difficult cases. The disadvantage of ECCE is the large incision required, inability to maintain a closed chamber during surgery and the need for multiple sutures, with resultant postoperative astigmatism.

On the other hand, with MSICS, a self-sealing, 5 to 6 mm scleral tunnel incision is created. The incision maybe superior or temporal. Following a relatively large ACCC, the nucleus is prolapsed into the anterior chamber and subsequently removed from the eye. Now, several modifications such as the use of irrigating wire Vectis, nuclear snare, nucleus glides, visco-expression, nucleus fracture and nucleus bisection are employed by surgeons in order to reduce the size of the nucleus and make delivery out of the eye easier and safer.

There are several published studies in literature that compare outcomes following MSICS and phacoemulsification, and most of the recent ones show that both techniques are safe and effective [13–21]. MSICS and ECCE, however, are more cost effective than phacoemulsification and not dependent on technology. This is the reason why these techniques are often favoured in developing nations. Therefore, it would be left to the surgeon's surgical skill and experience, availability of machines, as well as economic viability to choose which is the best surgical strategy in their hands.

Newer Techniques/Devices for Dense Cataract Surgery

Endocapsular Manual Nucleus fragmentation in Phacoemulsification

Recently, the miLoop, a disposable manual device has been introduced for endocapsular manual nuclear fragmentation during cataract surgery. Initial reports suggest that this device is safe and effective and that corneal endothelial cell loss as well as intraoperative complications are comparable when performing traditional phacoemulsification versus using the miLoop device [22, 23].

Femtosecond Laser Assisted Cataract Surgery (FLACS)—Role in Dense Cataract Removal

With the advent of femtosecond laser technology for cataract surgery, it has been approved for creating corneal incisions, capsulotomy and nuclear division. Both the temporal incision and paracenteses incisions can be customized and positioned based on real-time anterior segment optical coherence tomography. A centered anterior capsulotomy of a desired size can be created, even in the absence of a good red reflex. Contrary to the initial expectations from the laser, FLACS is able to create various patterns of nucleus division, and even though the division may not extend to the complete depth in very leathery cataracts, it may be useful in reducing the U/S energy consumption during sculpting and chopping. Thus, as this technology continues to evolve, and becomes more cost effective, it may find more use in the surgeons' armamentarium, especially to manage dense cataracts [24–26].

Complications During Dense Cataract Surgery

Common complications that might arise during dense cataract surgery are enlisted below. Although most of them can occur with any technique, some are specific to phacoemulsification or extracapsular cataract surgery:

- Corneal endothelial trauma: surgery in dense cataracts can potentially cause increased endothelial cell loss or even corneal decompensation causes for excessive endothelial cell loss include excessive and continuous use of U/S energy during phacoemulsification, as well as mechanical trauma caused by nuclear fragments/entire nucleus rubbing with the corneal endothelium.
  Preventive Measures: repeated use of dispersive OVD to coat the corneal endothelium, being conscious about the plane of emulsification, and the use of interrupted U/S energy delivery/torsional U/S.

- Incisional Thermal Damage: caused by excessive and continuous use of U/S energy, especially with a tight wound construction. In ECCE/MSICS, an irregular wound construction can lead to collagen distortion and irregular wound healing.
  Preventive Measures: During phacoemulsification, surgeons must make sure to use interrupted U/S energy, which allows for intermittent cooling of the phaco tip. Further a higher AFR should be used during sculpting, so as to allow continuous cooling of the phaco tip. Also, it is very important to create an incision that is not too tight. There should be no compression of the phaco tip at the incision, so that the irrigation flow around the phaco tip is not compressed. For e.g. if a surgeon uses 2.2 mm incision routinely, he should perform a 2.4mm incision to avoid oar locking and tight wound geometry.
- Posterior Capsule Rupture: often occurs due to the use of very high flow rate and vacuum settings in these eyes which may have fragile capsular bags to begin with.
  Preventive measures: adhering to the principles of closed chamber technique and the use of modestly low vacuum and AFR settings will allow the surgeon to avoid inadvertent rupture of the posterior capsule as well as injury to the iris tissue.
- Zonular dialysis/weakness: dense cataracts are very often associated with pre-existing zonular weakness. Also, stressful surgical maneuvers such as nucleus rotation, excessive lateral separation movements or forceful nucleus delivery during phacoemulsification/ECCE/MSICS may lead to iatrogenic zonular defects. Many times, dense cataracts maybe associated with comorbidities such as glaucoma or pseudoexfoliation syndrome which can further predispose to zonular weakness.
  Preventive measures: it is important for surgeons to detect any zonular weakness preoperatively by performing a thorough and full dilated slitlamp evaluation.

Considerations in an intumescent cataract

Not every mature cataract is the same (Video 2). During the slit-lamp examination, the doctor should pay particular attention to whether slight shading, colour differences or patterns are still visible in the front surface of the lens. This would indicate that the lens has not yet liquefied in the periphery.

If differentiation is not possible and everything is relatively uniformly white, the most likely cause is an intumescent cataract. In an intumescent (lat. Intumescencia —swelling) cataract, the lens cortex is partially liquefied. According to Figueiredo et al., three compartments can form within the lens capsule:

- Liquid anterior layer
- Hard middle layer
- Liquid back layer

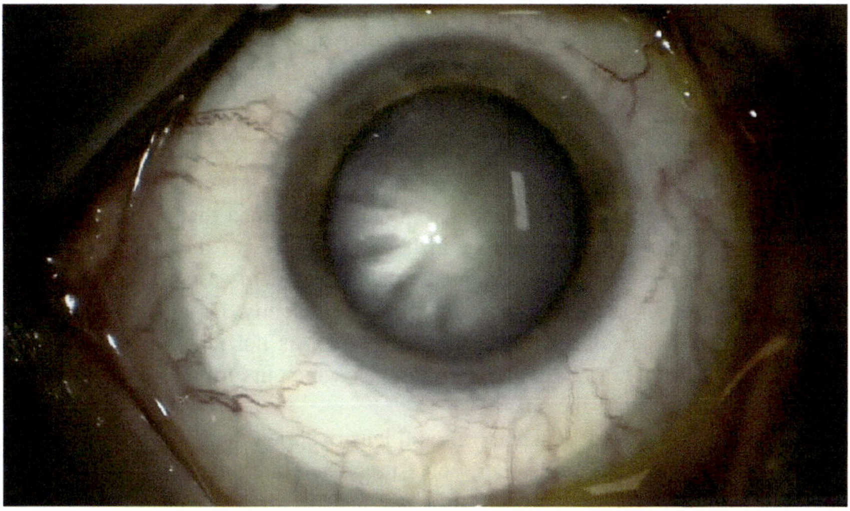

Video 2 Unedited video of mature cataract removal (▶ https://doi.org/10.1007/000-8da)

If the central non-liquefied lens layer in the periphery is still in contact with the lens capsule, there can be no exchange between the anterior and posterior compartments. If the capsule is now opened during capsulorhexis, liquefied lens material will escape from the anterior compartment into the anterior chamber. The liquefied cortex in the posterior compartment is under increased pressure and presses the middle lens layer against the anterior capsule. This can cause the capsulorhexis to leak out or even lead to a so-called "Argentinian flag sign" (blue coloured anterior capsule sheet left and right of the white lens).

Capsulorhexis can therefore be a challenge in an intumescent cataract. However, there are also further considerations required in the ongoing steps which should be considered when removing an intumescent cataract.

1. Incisions: First of all, only a paracentesis should be made in order to maximize stability of the anterior chamber so that the rhexis is performed under high pressure. The relatively small incision reduces the risk of viscoelastic material escaping and thus a high anterior chamber pressure can be maintained.
2. After the administration of an anaesthetic and, if needed, a mydriatic, the capsule is stained with trypan blue. It is important to note that especially in the case of a pathology of the corneal endothelium, such as Fuchs' endothelial dystrophy, the cornea is also stained to a greater extent, which may reduce vision during the operation. The insertion of an air bubble in front of the dye reduces this undesirable side effect. After staining, the trypan blue is washed out of the anterior chamber with BSS.

3. A highly cohesive viscoelastic is injected into the anterior chamber. This allows the high intracameral pressure to counteract the high intracapsular pressure. This significantly reduces the probability of tearing and further peripheral leakage of the rhexis.
4. The rhexis needle is used to open the capsule centrally. Now two strategies can be considered:

    a. If no liquid lens material emerges, it can be assumed that a stable situation prevails and a capsulorhexis can be performed with the rhexis needle or rhexis forceps inserted through the paracentesis. In cases of a mature cataract it is essential that the rhexis is sufficiently large (at least 5 mm diameter). Capsulorhexis via a main incision is not recommended, as this can lead to increased leakage of the OVD, which in turn increases the risk of an uncontrollable rhexis.
    b. If there is increased leakage of liquid lens material, there still may be higher intracapsular than intracameral pressure. There are now several options for the surgeon in order to perform a safe capsulorhexis

        i. The first option is to aspirate liquid lens material using a cannula. The tip of the instrument is carefully pressed onto the lens core in a way that ideally, liquid lens material behind the hard lens can also be aspirated. Afterwards, capsulorhexis is performed with the help of a rhexis forceps and a low intracapsular pressure.
        ii. First a capsulorhexis with a small diameter (about 2 mm) is created and lens material is aspirated as far as possible. The lens capsule is now no longer under pressure. The rhexis needle (or capsular scissors) is used to cut at the edge of the rhexis and then the rhexis diameter is enlarged to 5 mm or more with a forceps.
        iii. Via a second paracentesis, viscoelastic is slowly and steadily applied centrally with the left hand and the rhexis needle is used to perform the capsulorhexis. This way the centrally applied viscoelastic displaces liquid lens material from the field of vision and ensures that the intracameral pressure remains high throughout the capsulorhexis.

5. The main incision is now made and the viscoelastic is removed using BSS. When using older phaco devices, care should be taken to ensure that the main incision is slightly larger than in a standard cataract. This allows fluid to escape at the edge of the incision during phacoemulsification and reduces the risk of burns in the area of the main incision caused by the slightly increased fluid escape. However, it is important to mention that this might also destabilize the anterior chamber.
6. In many cases, the lens core is already well mobile due to the lens liquefaction and usually no hydrodissection is necessary. Should this nevertheless have to be

carried out, BSS should only be introduced very slowly under the capsule, as the lens capsule has already been under tension due to the originally large lens volume and the risk of a posterior capsule tear due to too much fluid is not insignificant.

7. The next step is to insert dispersive viscoelastic and then the phako handpiece.
8. A phaco chop technique is useful for fragmentation of the lens, as this requires less ultrasonic energy than the Divide & Conquer technique. It is important to sink the tip of the phaco handpiece deep into the lens core using sufficient ultrasound energy and then fix the lens core with a high vacuum to then divide the lens core with the chopper guided over the equator of the lens. This technique makes it possible to exert maximum force on the lens, thus facilitating the splitting into two fragments. To actually cross the equator of the lens, some surgeons lift the lens out of the capsular bag at one point. This reduces the risk of rupture by the chopper and facilitates separation of the posterior parts of the lens. The prerequisite for this is a sufficiently large capsulorhexis. If necessary, during phacoemulsification, a dispersive viscoelastic should be applied again to protect the cornea i. Some surgeons also apply a dispersive viscoelastic into the capsular bag, since in a mature lens the epinucleus is liquefied and therefore cannot act as a protective layer between the capsular bag and the phaco handpiece.
9. If there are still cortex residues, these are removed by irrigation and aspiration. Often, adhesions or fibrotic thickening of the capsular bag are visible in mature lenses. These should not be removed as the risk of a capsule tear is too high. Instead, it is recommended to open the capsular bag at a later stage by YAG capsulotomy.

Finally, the capsular bag is filled with cohesive viscoelastic material, the lens is inserted and centered, and the viscoelastic material removed before the incisions are closed by hydration.

Conclusion

Dense cataract management has improved dramatically over time. However, technique and technology must compliment each other for consistent and predictable outcomes. Surgeons need to be extra careful during preoperative evaluation, paying special attention to the corneal endothelial health, pupillary dilatation and zonular weakness. During surgery, the judicious use of U/S energy, adhering to posterior plane phacoemulsification, optimal use of U/S energy such as the use of torsional U/S, interrupted energy and repeated use of dispersive OVDs will ensure intraoperative efficacy and safety and good postoperative outcomes.

References

1. Singh R, Vasavada AR. Phacoemulsification of brunescent and black cataracts. J Cataract Refract Surg. 2001;27:1762–9.
2. Fine IH. Cortical cleaving hydrodissection. J Cataract Refract Surg. 1992;18:508–12.
3. Yeoh R. The 'pupil snap' sign of posterior capsule rupture with hydrodissection in phacoemulsification (letter). Br J Ophthalmol. 1996;80:486.
4. Vasavada AR, Goyal D, Shastri L, Singh R. Cortico capsular adhesions and their effect during cataract surgery. J Cataract Refract Surg. 2003;29:1–6.
5. Arshinoff SA. Dispersive-cohesive viscoelastic soft shell technique. J Cataract Refract Surg. 1999;25:167–73.
6. Can I, Takmaz T, Cakici F, Ozgul M. Comparison of Nagahara phaco-chop and stop-and-chop phacoemulsification nucleotomy techniques. J Cataract Refract Surg. 2004;30:663–8.
7. Singh R, Vasavada AR. Step-by-step chop in situ and separation of very dense cataracts. J Cataract Refract Surg. 1998;24:156–9.
8. Vasavada AR, Raj SM. Multilevel chop technique. J Cataract Refract Surg. 2011;37:2092–4.
9. Vasavada AR, Raj S. Step down technique. J Cataract Refract Surg. 2003;29:1077–9.
10. Osher RH. Slow motion phacoemulsification approach. J Cataract Refract Surg. 1993;19:667.
11. Liu Y, Zeng M, Liu X, et al. Torsional mode versus conventional ultrasound mode phacoemulsification: randomized comparative clinical study. J Cataract Refract Surg. 2007;33:287–92.
12. Vasavada AR, Raj SM, Patel U, et al. Comparison of torsional (Ozil) versus microburst longitudinal (traditional) phacoemulsification—a prospective, randomized, masked clinical trial. Ophthalmic Surg Lasers and Imaging. In press.
13. Minassian DC, Rosen P, Dart JK, Reidy A, Desai P, Sidhu M. Extracapsular cataract extraction compared with small incision surgery by phacoemulsification: a randomised trial. Br J Ophthalmol. 2001;85:822–9.
14. Gogate PM, Wormald RP, Deshpande M, Deshpande R, Kulkarni SR. Extracapsular cataract surgery compared with manual small incision cataract surgery in community eye care setting in Western India: a randomized controlled trial. Br J Ophthalmol. 2003;87:673–9.
15. Gogate PM, Wormald RP, Deshpande M. Is manual small incision cataract surgery affordable in the developing countries? A cost comparison with extracapsular cataract extraction. Br J Ophthalmol. 2003;87:841–4.
16. Gogate PM, Kulkarni SR, Krishnaiah S, Deshpande RD, Joshi SA, Palimkar A, et al. Safety and efficacy of phacoemulsification compared with manual small incision cataract surgery by a randomized controlled clinical trial: six weeks results. Ophthalmology. 2005;112:869–74.
17. Gogate PM, Deshpande MD, Nirmalan P. Why do phacoemulsification? Manual small incision cataract surgery is almost as effective and more economical. Ophthalmology. 2007;114:965–8.
18. Venkatesh R, Muralikrishnan R, Balent LC, Prakash SK, Prajna V. Outcomes of high volume cataract surgeries in a developing country. Br J Ophthalmol. 2005;89:1079–83.
19. Madurai NG. Manual small incision cataract surgery: an alternative technique to instrumental phacoemulsification. Aravind Publication; 2000. Dec.
20. Henning A, Kumar J, Yorston D, Foster A. Sutureless cataract surgery with nucleus extraction: outcome of a prospective study in Nepal. Br J Ophthalmol. 2003;87:266–70.
21. Ruit S, Tabin G, Chang D, Bajracharya L, Kline DC, Richheimer R, et al. A prospective randomized clinical trial of phacoemulsification vs. manual sutureless small incision extracapsular cataract surgery in Nepal. Am J Ophthalmol. 2007;143:32–8.
22. Ianchulev T, Chang DF, Koo E, MacDonald S, Calvo E, Tyson FT, Vasquez A, Ahmed IIK. Microinterventional ensocapsular nucleus disassembly: novel technique and results of first-in human randomized controlled study. Br J Ophthalmol. 2019;103(2):176–80.

23. Ianchulev T, Chang DF, Koo E, MacDonald S. Microinterventional endocapsular nucleus disassembly for phacoemulsification-free full-thickness fragmentation. J Cataract Refract Surg. 2018;44(8):932–4.
24. Roberts HW, Day AC, O'Brart DP. Femtosecond laser-assisted cataract surgery: a review. Eur J Ophthalmol. 2020;30(3):417–29.
25. Chen X, Xiao W, Ye S, Chen W, Liu Y. Efficacy and safety of femtosecond laser-assisted cataract surgery versus conventional phacoemulsification for cataract: a meta-analysis of randomized controlled trials. Sci Rep. 2015;13(5):13123.
26. Taravella MJ, Meghpara B, Frank G, Gensheimer W, Davidson R. Femtosecond laser-assisted cataract surgery in complex cases. J Cataract Refract Surg 2016;42(6):813–6.

Posterior Subcapsular Cataract

Jesper Hjortdal

Posterior subcapsular cataract is the least common of the three main types of cataracts related to aging, but often the most rapidly progressive form of cataract [1]. In addition to a rapid and pronounced deterioration of visual acuity, it can lead to striking glare sensitivity, monocular double images and visual phenomena such as halo-like scattered light particularly when backlit [2]. Histopathologically, it occurs when lens epithelial cells migrate from the lens equator to the normally epithelial cell-free posterior pole. Here they proliferate and enlarge to form Wedl cells. The pathophysiology appears to be very similar to the development of proliferative posterior capsule opacification [3].

While posterior subcapsular cataract is related to aging, it can also occur due to trauma, systemic, topical, or intraocular corticosteroid use [4], to inflammation, exposure to ionizing radiation, and due to alcoholism. Isolated posterior subcapsular opacities typically occur in younger patients (40 years and younger). In older patients, posterior subcapsular cataract is almost always combined with some nuclear and cortical cataract. In these cases, cataract surgery follows the usual principles.

Pre-operative Considerations

Challenges may occur in relation to the young patient with isolated posterior subcapsular cataract. Firstly, one must be aware that optimal results are very important to these patients, as they are usually of working age and likely to wish to continue driving. As with any patient, the risk of complications should be min-

J. Hjortdal (✉)
Department of Ophthalmology, Aarhus University Hospital, Aarhus N, Denmark
e-mail: jesphjor@rm.dk

Department of Clinical Medicine, Aarhus University, Aarhus N, Denmark

M. Shajari et al. (eds.), *Cataract and Lens Surgery*,
https://doi.org/10.1007/978-3-031-05394-8_48

imised, and special attention should also be paid to the refractive outcome and preoperative counselling. Young patients with shell opacities should not be operated by novices and certainly belong in the hands of an experienced surgeon. It should also be considered that some of these patients are not yet presbyopic and have at least some relevant residual accommodation that they will lose postoperatively. Accordingly, there is an increased need for explanation during the preliminary discussion and explanation before surgery. In addition, as always with younger patients, it should be considered and discussed whether optimal cooperation for topical/intracameral anaesthesia can be ensured or whether general anaesthesia would be preferred and medically indicated.

Keypoint

Taking cortisone preparations can cause or promote the development of posterior subcapsular opacities. While in such cases they may be referred to as a "steroid cataract" one should remember that such early cataracts can also be observed without a history of steroid use.

Operative Technique

When considering the intraoperative strategies and risks, it is particularly important that the surgeon is aware of what kind of eye it is and draws conclusions for the procedure. These cataracts are usually seen in younger eyes with soft lens nuclei. The lens capsule should be expected to be relatively elastic. Making a perfectly sized and centred rhexis can be challenging because these capsules tend to "run out" during the rhexis as a result of the elasticity and therefore turn out slightly larger than planned. It is therefore important to ensure perfect anterior chamber stability during the rhexis by adding extra ophthalmic viscosurgical device (OVD) to completely flatten the capsule. Next, start the rhexis a little too small in order to be able to correct it outwards. When continuing the rhexis, it is best to pull the "flap" a little more towards the centre than usual in order to prevent spiral leakage. Be prepared to grasp and regrasp more than normal as this will improve control over the tearing forces. If the anterior chamber becomes shallower during the rhexis due to OVD leakage, it should definitely be made deeper again by refilling. A personal trick is not to perform the rhexis with the forceps but completely with the curved needle (cystotome). In doing so, the cystotome can be used on top of the OVD syringe so that the anterior chamber can be continuously kept deep with OVD without having to change instruments.

Even when removing the lens nucleus and epinucleus, one must be aware that these parts of the lens may not show any signs of cataract at all. The opacity is usually purely subcapsular, although of course there can be mixed forms. The surgeon must expect the lens nucleus and epinucleus to be "age normal", i.e. soft with little structure. Traditional methods such as divide-and-conquer, phaco chop or stop-and-chop are therefore not suitable in these cases.

Author's recommendation

If the lens is very soft, the correct surgical approach is lens aspiration with very little to no ultrasound energy. This requires a gentle but thorough hydrodissection. Some surgeons recommend hydrodelineation. After hydrodelineation, the nucleus can be removed without risk to the capsule, but the removal of the epinucleus shell is then all the more tedious. This often "sucks" itself into the capsular bag and can only be removed by manipulations that are not always well controlled. I therefore advise against hydrodelineation.

There are two possible approaches for removing the core:

(1) If the core is not too soft and reasonably structured, then the normal standard technique should be used, but the parameters of the phaco machine should be optimised for soft cores. The maximum phaco power should be reduced which will allow for more controlled work. However, it is important to explicitly warn against an additional increase of the vacuum, even if semi-solid material could be aspirated more efficiently by doing so. Increasing the vacuum also increases the risk of the "surge" phenomenon occurring; when the semi-soft material occludes the phaco tip, a negative pressure is created in the tubing system, which can lead to an abrupt increase in vacuum in the anterior chamber when the occlusion is (suddenly) released. This must be avoided at all costs. (2) If the nucleus is really very soft, then a pure lens aspiration can be performed. After a good hydrodissection, the soft nucleus is aspirated with the I/A instruments.

Author's recommendation

I would advise against dislocating the core into the pupillary plane. Of course, the soft nucleus can be aspirated there without any problem. But with this technique the surgeon loses track of where exactly the rhexis rim and the anterior capsule are and this is an unnecessary loss of control!

After removal of the nucleus and cortex, the posterior shell opacity often remains as a central membrane on the posterior capsule and can be easily removed with the I/A instruments or the polishing needle. Sometimes this requires some patience, and it can be helpful to select the "capsule polishing" settings with less vacuum and more flow on the phaco machine. A good option is also what the Anglo-Saxons call "turbo polishing": The hydrodissection cannula is inserted into the eye via the main incision and the posterior capsule is cleaned of epithelial cells under a constant, directed water jet.

Author's recommendation

As always with turbidity on or in the rear capsule, "Perfect is the enemy of the good!" If these residual opacities cannot be removed safely, then by all means leave them. There is nothing more frustrating than a posterior capsular rupture at this late stage of surgery! And a laser capsulotomy two or three months postoperatively is very safe and will give a very good result.

Conclusion

Posterior capsular opacities must be clearly distinguished from posterior polar cataract or traumatic cataract already in the consultation. In the case of polar cataract, the opacities are not located under the posterior capsule, but often very substantially IN the posterior capsule. The development and findings are completely different and accordingly these cases must be approached surgically in a different way. If there is uncertainty about the classification in a specific case, a more experienced colleague must be consulted. Under certain circumstances, an OCT can also help to distinguish between the two entities.

References

1. Hashemi H, Pakzad R, Yekta A, Aghamirsalim M, Pakbin M, Ramin S, Khabazkhoob M. Global and regional prevalence of age-related cataract: a comprehensive systematic review and meta-analysis. Eye (Lond). 2020;34(8):1357–70.
2. Gholami S, Reus NJ, van den Berg TJTP. Changes in intraocular straylight and visual acuity with age in cataracts of different morphologies. J Ophthalmol. 2017:5649532.
3. Martinez G, de Iongh RU. The lens epithelium in ocular health and disease. Int J Biochem Cell Biol. 2010;42(12):1945–63.
4. James ER. The etiology of steroid cataract. J Ocul Pharmacol Ther. 2007;23(5):403–20.

Cataract Surgery in Short and Long Eyes

Michael J. daSilva, Austin Woolley, and Uday Devgan

Hyperopes

Preoperative Discussion, Examination, and Planning

Hyperopic eyes present a unique challenge to cataract surgeons, and require distinct preoperative and intraoperative considerations. Axial lengths are usually shorter in hyperopic eyes, and may be less than 22 mm. Inaccurate measurements of the axial length will result in larger refractive errors compared to eyes with more common dimensions. An axial length that is 0.5 mm off may result in missing the target by 1.0 to 1.5 diopters in a normal eye; in a hyperopic eye, this could result in an error of 2.0 to 3.0 diopters. Optical means of assessing the axial length are preferred.

There are several ways to mitigate the risk of refractive surprise in hyperopic cataract surgery. Many surgeons prefer to operate on the non dominant eye first. Many also use multiple formulas and compare predicted and postoperative refractions to determine the most accurate formula, using this information to guide the lens selection for the dominant eye. Lens calculations in the axial hyperope are affected primarily by the estimated effective lens position (ELP). Because a high-power lens will commonly be implanted in a hyperope, changes in ELP will have greater refractive consequences. A variety of approaches are used to predict the ELP. Of the third generation formulas, the Hoffer Q is accepted as being more accurate in eyes with axial lengths less than 22 mm [1, 2]. Fourth and fifth generation formulas, such as the Ladas Super Formula, Haigis, Barrett II, Hill-RBF,

Supplementary Information The online version contains supplementary material available at https://doi.org/10.1007/978-3-031-05394-8_49. The videos can be accessed individually by clicking the DOI link in the accompanying figure caption or by scanning this link with the SN More Media App.

M. J. daSilva (✉) · A. Woolley · U. Devgan
Los Angeles, USA
e-mail: dasilva6532@gmail.com

M. Shajari et al. (eds.), *Cataract and Lens Surgery*,
https://doi.org/10.1007/978-3-031-05394-8_49

Kane, and Holladay 2, are considered accurate in hyperopes because they use additional variables to predict the ELP; these include anterior chamber depth, age, horizontal white-to-white, lens thickness, and preoperative refraction [1].

Lens selection is important when operating on hyperopic eyes. Flexible haptics are preferable in a small capsular bag, and can be found in single-piece acrylic lenses, or 3 piece acrylic or silicone lenses. Hyperopic eyes require higher power lenses, and every effort should be made to use a single lens with the appropriate power. The surgeon may need to special order a lens outside of their regular consignment; one such example is the single-piece acrylic AcrySof SA60AT, which has powers available up to +40D in the United States. If the required power is greater than +40D, it may be necessary to "piggyback" using two separate intraocular lenses (IOLs.) This is best accomplished by implanting the higher power IOL in the capsular bag, letting the eye heal, selecting the second IOL based on the postoperative refractive results, and implanting the corresponding second IOL in the sulcus space. Using two acrylic lenses is thought to increase the risk of interlenticular opacification, so the surgeon should consider using two silicone lenses or mixing materials [3]. Care should also be taken when considering a piggyback technique to ensure that there is sufficient space in the posterior chamber to avoid uveitis-glaucoma-hyphema (UGH) syndrome.

Shorter eyes tend to have narrow anterior chambers, with a depth of 2 mm or less. The growth of a cataract can further shallow the anterior chamber, putting the corneal endothelial cells at increased risk during cataract surgery. Therefore, a thorough preoperative examination of the cornea, with attention to the endothelium, is warranted. Specular microscopy can be employed to quantify endothelial cell density in suspicious cases; this may help in preoperative counseling if it reveals an increased risk of pseudophakic corneal edema.

Intraoperative Considerations

It can be more difficult to maneuver inside a narrow anterior chamber, leading to a higher risk of trauma to the iris or corneal endothelium during hyperopic cataract surgery. A dispersive viscoelastic may be used to coat the corneal endothelium, followed by a cohesive viscoelastic to deepen the anterior chamber. The surgeon can also consider increasing the intraocular pressure infusion settings, as well as lowering the aspiration rate, to maintain a larger working space in the eye. If an anterior chamber is extremely narrow, preoperative mannitol may be administered to dehydrate the vitreous; care should be taken that the patient does not have any contraindications to mannitol, and the patient should be monitored closely with the help of anesthesiology. If these interventions fail to deepen the chamber adequately, a limited pars plana vitrectomy may be performed, removing 0.2–0.3 cm^3 of retro-lental vitreous with a 25-gauge cutter [4].

Care should be taken throughout the cataract surgery to keep the chamber as deep as possible. This may require refilling the eye with viscoelastic to prevent run out of the capsulorrhexis. Extra dispersive viscoelastic may be injected prior to phacoemulsification to further protect corneal endothelial cells.

Due to the proximity of the corneal endothelial cells in narrow chambers, phacoemulsification performed in the capsular bag is preferred to supracapsular techniques in order to prevent excessive corneal edema. A more anterior corneal incision may be beneficial in preventing iris prolapse. It is also important to note that standard corneal incisions on smaller eyes have a larger relative area and arc length, which can increase the astigmatic effect of the incisions, and may also prevent sufficient sealing of the wounds. Nanophthalmic eyes (AL < 20.5) have an increased risk of intraoperative and postoperative uveal effusions, and the surgeon may need to use scleral windows as a preventative measure [5]. While rare, choroidal hemorrhages are more common in smaller eyes.

Postoperative Follow Up

Hyperopic eyes are at greater risk for aqueous misdirection, which may not manifest immediately. The cataract surgeon should advise patients to call if they develop pain, or if their vision becomes progressively more blurry, as increasing myopia may be a sign of insidious aqueous misdirection. Hyperopic patients are at higher risk of corneal decompensation, and postoperative corneal edema should be monitored closely. If a piggyback technique is used, the surgeon should watch for the development of interlenticular fibrosis. Due to the higher risk of refractive surprises, a careful postoperative refraction should be performed with appropriate counseling on corrective procedures if desired. If a patient is to undergo cataract surgery in their second eye, the refractive outcome from the first surgery should help guide the selection of the lens for the second eye.

Myopes

Preoperative Discussion, Examination, and Planning

High myopia has profound effects on ocular health, and on outcomes after cataract surgery. It is therefore important for the surgeon to have a frank discussion with the patient about the general and individual risks of surgery. Of particular importance is the risk of rhegmatogenous retinal detachment (RRD.) At the initial evaluation, the patient should be counseled about the association of high axial length and retinal detachment [6, 7] Younger age, male sex, and vitreous loss during surgery are also reported risk factors for RRD after cataract extraction [6], and the confluence of these variables can make RRD significantly more likely in certain axial myopes. The patient should be taught the symptoms of retinal tear or detachment, including new floaters, flashing lights, and curtain-like visual field deficit. The patient should seek immediate care if any of these symptoms develop.

Long eyes with cataract are at high risk for comorbidities of the retina and optic nerve. Conditions associated with myopia include amblyopia, RRD, open angle glaucoma, and myopic macular degeneration with or without choroidal neovascularization [8, 9]. The cataract surgeon should perform a complete preoperative examination with attention to the macula, optic nerve, and retinal periphery. If significant myopic morphology is apparent, such as peripapillary atrophy, oval-shaped tilted disc, or degenerative changes of the macula, further testing is warranted. This testing should be based on the individual characteristics of the eye being evaluated. Testing may include optical coherence tomography (OCT) of the macula and nerve, visual field testing, and fluorescein angiography if choroidal neovascularization is suspected. If posterior staphylomatous changes are present B-scan ocular ultrasound should be obtained to assess the shape of the eye, which may affect foveation and the optically measured axial length. The cataract surgeon should not hesitate to refer to a retina specialist colleague for a scleral depressed examination of the periphery. Prophylactic laser retinopexy may be necessary if any symptomatic holes, tufts, or tears are present.

Lens calculations in the axial myope are affected primarily by corneal contour and the axial length. Because a low-power lens will be implanted, changes in effective lens position (ELP) have less refractive consequence. In a simple example, a lens with zero diopters of power has no vergence, and will not change with ELP. Similarly, low power positive or negative lenses are minimally affected by changes in ELP; however, very deep anterior chambers greater than 4 mm may impact the IOL calculation. It is important to have accurate measurements of the corneal curvature (K values,) but the greatest challenge in high axial myopia is often to obtain an accurate axial length (AL.) Again, optical means of measuring AL are preferred. Here the patient is instructed to fixate on a target, which aligns the biometer measurement beam with the fovea. Care should be taken with directly applying the AL value produced by an optical biometer, as biometers generally assume a constant refractive index of the eye. This assumption does not remain accurate in extremely long eyes, in which the vitreous cavity may represent a higher proportion of the measurement beam path. With older generation two-variable formulas, it was advisable for the surgeon to adjust AL measurements greater than 25 mm using the formula proposed by Wang and Koch [10]. Newer generation formulas such as the Ladas, Barrett Universal II, and Hill-RBF automatically account for measurement characteristics in long eyes.

Highly myopic eyes will need a low-power or even negative-power lens. The geometry of the lens implant changes at very low or negative powers. The most popular U.S. lens platforms begin at +5 to +6 diopters. Lenses below this power, or negative power lenses, are likely to employ a meniscus design. These lenses are commonly produced in one-diopter increments. Meniscus geometry shifts the optical principal plane relative to standard biconvex design, and thereby alters the effective lens position. Meniscus lens geometry is compared to biconvex designs in Fig. 1.

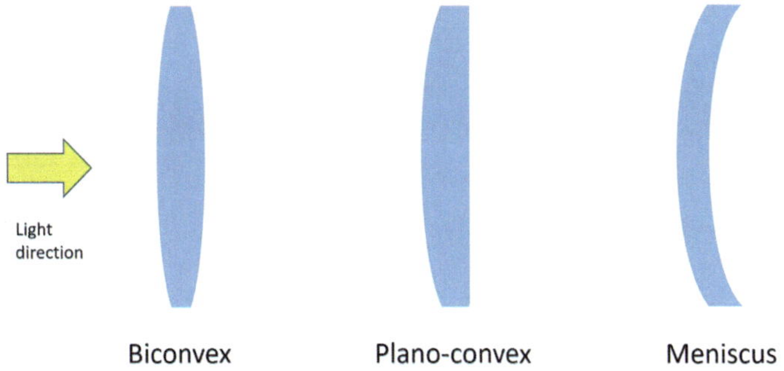

Fig. 1 Lens geometry of common IOL designs

Various means of adjusting lens calculation equations for high axial myopia have been employed. One strategy is to adjust the lens A-constant with each step in dioptric power of a meniscus lens platform [11, 12]. These optimized A-constants can be accessed at the User Group for Laser Interference Biometry (ULIB) online, and can be applied to standard formulae. A second proposed strategy is to adjust the axial length, using a formula that accounts for the effect of a longer biometry measurement beam path through the vitreous cavity [10, 13] Studies of axial myopes note that two variable formulae with axial length adjustment have lens power calculation accuracy comparable to fourth generation formulae [14, 15]. One study noted that the incidence of small hyperopic outcomes was reduced by using the Wang-Koch AL adjustment when compared to fourth-generation formulae [16]. Fourth-generation formulae use additional variables, such as anterior chamber depth or lens thickness, to increase accuracy in all eyes. The accuracy of these modern formulae have been analyzed repeatedly in the setting of high axial myopia. Excellent results have been achieved using the Barrett Universal II [15–19]. Hill-RBF [16, 19] and Olsen [17] formulae among others. One study of Chinese patients with extreme axial myopia found the Haigis less accurate in the subgroup with AL >30 mm [17]. For practical purposes, the authors recommend the surgeon become familiar with one or two modern formulas and apply it as intended by its creator(s), as not all formulae require measurement data adjustment of any kind. High quality outcomes can be achieved with several formulae, but all the above-referenced studies indicate high performance of the Barrett Universal II in high myopia.

Consider targeting residual myopia in patients with high axial length. Despite the advancement of biometry and lens calculation, it is still possible to end up with an unintentional hyperopic outcome if measurement error is introduced to any variables. The patient is habituated to myopia, and may appreciate the finer near vision afforded by low degrees of myopia. The surgeon should freely discuss the option of targeting near vision. In the past, it has been common practice to target one to two diopters of residual myopia. Given the advancement of lens calculation and formulas which use anterior chamber depth as a variable, the authors recommend targeting only 0.5 to one diopter of residual myopia if an emmetropic result is desired.

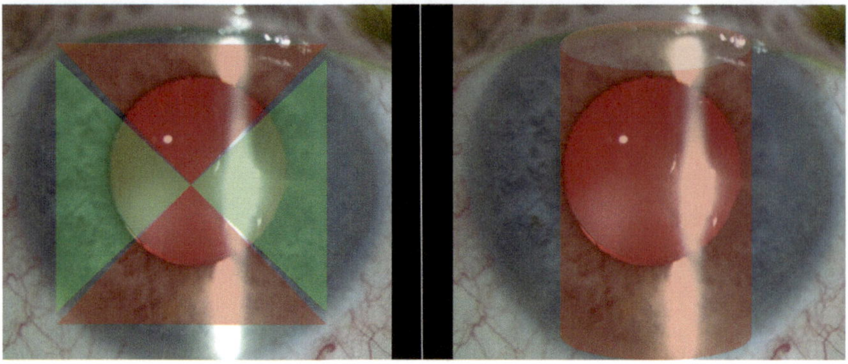

Fig. 2 The left image depicts an eye with postoperative refraction +1.00 −2.00×090. The excimer laser would steepen the horizontal axis, and flatten the vertical axis. The surgeon should avoid this situation, or consider postoperative limbal relaxing incisions. The right image depicts an eye with postoperative refraction plano −2.00 × 090, simplifying the ablation pattern

The approach to astigmatism management in extreme axial myopes differs from the general population. Toric intraocular lenses are only available down to +5 or +6 diopters depending on the manufacturer. Astigmatism management patients may therefore require cornea-based treatment. The surgeon can perform intra- or post-operative astigmatic keratotomy or limbal relaxing incisions. Another option is to plan postoperative laser vision correction, termed bioptics by the refractive surgery community. If bioptics are planned, it is beneficial to leave the astigmatic patient with pure myopic astigmatism, and not with mixed astigmatism. Outcomes from excimer laser ablation are more predictable and durable for myopic treatment, so a spherical equivalent in excess of one half the corneal astigmatism should be targeted. This gives the laser a simple ablation pattern, as outlined in Fig. 2. If a spherical equivalent of plano is targeted, resulting in mixed astigmatism, the laser would attempt to steepen one axis while flattening the other; this situation should be avoided if possible. A final consideration is the Light Adjustable Lens (LAL,) which has been reported to be efficacious in astigmatism management in axial myopes [20]. This platform is currently limited by its dioptric range, which extends from +10.0 to +30.0 diopters, and may therefore not be suitable for extreme axial myopes. The LAL is able to correct up to two diopters of cylinder.

Intraoperative Considerations

Elongated eyes are likely to be larger in several dimensions, and may have a white-to-white corneal measurement of 13 mm or more. Myopic eyes may also dilate excessively. If the surgeon proceeds to create a continuous curvilinear capsulorhexis (CCC) gauged by the pupil size, it may become larger than the IOL optic. The authors recommend one of two means of ensuring a consistent capsulorhexis size. One common method is to use a ring guide to indent and thereby lightly mark the cornea; the ring guide takes into account the twenty percent magnification of the anterior lens capsule that is produced by the cornea itself. The rhexis can then simply trace the mark. Another method is to mark the 2.5 and 5 mm distances from the tip of the capsulorhexis forceps, to visualize the intended rhexis size prior to its creation. Before CCC, the surgeon should be aware that a larger amount of ophthalmic viscosurgical device (OVD) may be needed to adequately form the chamber and flatten the anterior lens capsule. Further alternatives include the use of a nanopulse vacuum capsulotomy device or femtosecond laser-assisted capsulorhexis.

The lens capsule in highly myopic eyes is prone to large anteroposterior movements, which may heighten the risk of capsular rupture. Supracapsular lens disassembly can mitigate this risk. Some surgeons favor prolapsing the lens nucleus into the anterior chamber (AC). Due to typically larger AC, safe distance can be maintained from the corneal endothelium while the nucleus is then chopped and emulsified in the AC. In addition to capsular movement, many surgeons have noted qualitatively that zonular laxity is common in extreme axial myopia. Decades of research into the genetics of myopia have indeed found polymorphisms in proteoglycan synthesis and cell signaling pathways, which would be expected to interact with zonular strength; some of these include PAX6, WNT, and Decorin mutations [21]. It is therefore wise to avoid stressing the zonules. Some surgeons prefer chop techniques for nucleus disassembly. Most agree that thorough hydrodissection can reduce zonular trauma. It is also wise to have assistive devices such as capsular tension rings, capsular tension segments, and capsular hooks readily available in the operating room.

Lens-iris diaphragm retropulsion syndrome (LIDRS) refers to posterior movement of the iris and lens capsule complex. This typically occurs in myopic eyes during cataract surgery. It is caused by a reverse pupillary block, when fluid can no longer travel out of the posterior chamber. In addition to being painful for the patient, it may stress the zonules. The reverse pupillary block can be broken either by gently lifting the underside of the iris or by depressing the anterior capsule to re-establish fluid flow into the retro-irideal space. For persistent reverse pupillary block, an alternative that is rarely necessary is to place a single nasal iris hook.

Care should be taken throughout lens removal, and especially between steps which require removal of the handpiece, to prevent collapse of the anterior chamber. The first important step is to create an adequately long corneal incision, the architecture of which limits fluid egress. The surgeon should next lower the infusion pressure; high infusion pressure can deepen the anterior chamber excessively in myopic eyes, which causes more anteroposterior movement upon depressurization. The surgeon can also use his or her second hand to inject viscoelastic while the handpiece is still in the eye on position one, prior to removal of the handpiece at the end of cortical cleanup. Likewise, after implantation of the intraocular lens and removal of the viscoelastic, balanced saline can be injected in the paracentesis during removal of the handpiece. These extra steps aimed at preventing chamber collapse can reduce anterior movement of the vitreous base, which may theoretically reduce the risk of vitreous traction and subsequent retinal tears.

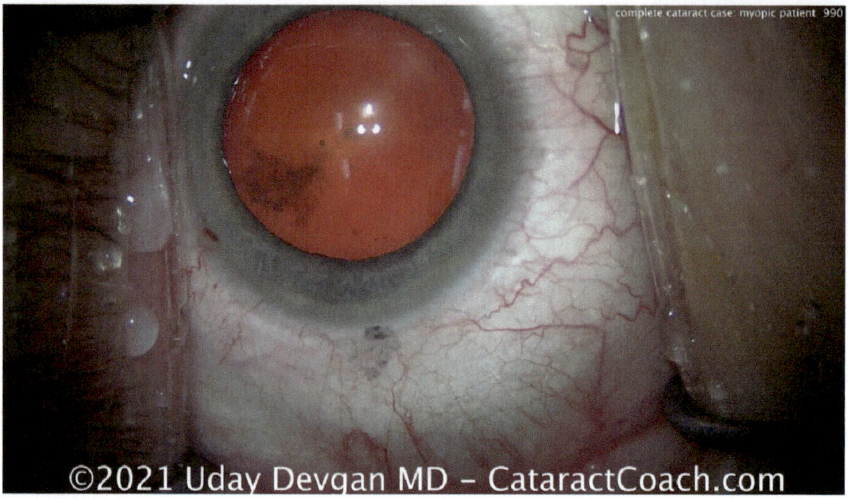

Video 1 Cataract surgery in a highly myopic eye. Cataract Coach original video #990 (▶ https://doi.org/10.1007/000-8dc)

Postoperative Follow Up

In the postoperative period the cataract surgeon should again carefully counsel the patient regarding the symptoms of retinal tears, and of retinal detachment (RD.)The patient should resume care with their habitual retina specialist, ideally one who examined their eyes prior to surgery. Retrospective studies have found variable rates of retinal detachment in myopic eyes after cataract surgery. A large retrospective review of eyes with axial length greater than 27 mm found no increased risk of RD after cataract surgery through two years, when compared to reported idiopathic incidence [22]. A smaller retrospective study sorted their study population into subgroups, and found a high rate of retinal detachment in eyes with lattice degeneration who first developed posterior vitreous detachment (PVD) in the postoperative period; among this smaller group, the rate of RD was reported to be 21% at five years [23]. This same study noted a low rate of RD (0.70%) in patients who had neither lattice nor preoperative PVD. Though the exact incidence of retinal tear or detachment is unclear, and certainly varies depending on what group is selected, evidence distinctly recommends close follow up.

Myopic patients may require prompt sequential surgery, within two weeks, due to intolerable degrees of aniseikonia. Patients should be alerted preoperatively, so they may plan on sequential surgery. The visual disturbance of aniseikonia is likely to be mitigated by the high residual myopia in the partner eye. An alternative to prompt sequential surgery, if the patient can tolerate their degree of aniseikonia, is contact lens use.

Author's recommendations

Hyperopes

1. Preoperative examination and counseling should focus on anterior chamber depth, axial length, and the health of the corneal endothelium.
2. Lens calculations are greatly affected by effective lens position (ELP). We recommend using Hoffer Q in conjunction with fourth and fifth generation formulae, including Barrett II, Kane, Holladay II, and Ladas Super Formula.
3. High powered lenses are not often on consignment and may need to be specially ordered. Piggy-backing lenses may be required.
4. Actions to deepen the anterior chamber include preoperative mannitol, increasing the intraocular pressure on the phaco machine, using a liberal amount of dispersive viscoelastic throughout the case, and performing a limited vitrectomy.
5. Intracapsular nucleus disassembly and frequent use of dispersive viscoelastic can prevent excessive corneal endothelial cell loss.
6. Postoperative counseling and examination should include monitoring for aqueous misdirection, corneal decompensation, and refractive error.

Myopes

1. Preoperative examination and counseling should focus on common retinal and optic nerve comorbidities.
2. Lens calculations are affected mainly by keratometry. We recommend becoming acquainted with fourth generation formulae; the Barret Universal II performs well in high myopes. Consider targeting residual myopia of −0.5 to −1.0 diopters.
3. Intraoperative steps to reduce fluctuation in the anterior chamber include making longer incisions, lowering bottle height, supracapsular nucleus disassembly, and replacing fluids before withdrawing infusion.
4. Postoperative counseling and examination should highlight the risk of retinal detachment.

References

1. Xia T, Martinez C, Tsai L. Update on Intraocular Lens Formulas and Calculations. Asia-Pac J Ophthalmol. 2020;9(3):186–93.
2. Doshi D, Limdi P, Gohil N, et al. A comparative study to assess the predictability of different IOL power calculation formulas in eyes of short and long axial length. Journal of Clinical and Diagnostic Research. 2017;11(1):NC01–4.
3. Werner L, Mamalis N, Stevens S, Hunter B, Chew JJ, Vargas LG. Interlenticular opacification: dual-optic versus piggyback intraocular lenses. J Cataract Refract Surg. 2006;32(4):655–61. https://doi.org/10.1016/j.jcrs.2006.01.022 PMID: 16698490.

4. Chalam KV, Gupta SK, Agarwal S, Shah VA. Sutureless limited vitrectomy for positive vitreous pressure in cataract surgery. Ophthalmic Surg Lasers Imaging. 2005;36(6):518–22. PMID: 16355960.
5. Brockhurst RJ. Cataract surgery in nanophthalmic eyes. Arch Ophthalmol. 1990;108(7):965–7. https://doi.org/10.1001/archopht.1990.01070090067041.
6. Qureshi MH, Steel DHW. Retinal detachment following cataract phacoemulsification-a review of the literature. Eye (Lond). 2020;34(4):616–31. https://doi.org/10.1038/s41433-019-0575-z. Epub 2019 Oct 1. Erratum in: Eye (Lond). 2019 Oct 28;: PMID: 31576027; PMCID: PMC7093479.
7. Sheu SJ, Ger LP, Chen JF. Axial myopia is an extremely significant risk factor for young-aged pseudophakic retinal detachment in taiwan. Retina. 2006;26(3):322–7. https://doi.org/10.1097/00006982-200603000-00011 PMID: 16508433.
8. Haarman AEG, Enthoven CA, Tideman JWL, Tedja MS, Verhoeven VJM, Klaver CCW. The complications of myopia: a review and meta-analysis. Invest Ophthalmol Vis Sci. 2020;61 (4):49. https://doi.org/10.1167/iovs.61.4.49.PMID:32347918;PMCID:PMC7401976.
9. Marcus MW, de Vries MM, Junoy Montolio FG, Jansonius NM. Myopia as a risk factor for open-angle glaucoma: a systematic review and meta-analysis. Ophthalmology. 2011;118 (10):1989-1994.e2. https://doi.org/10.1016/j.ophtha.2011.03.012 PMID: 21684603.
10. Wang L, Shirayama M, Ma XJ, Kohnen T, Koch DD. Optimizing intraocular lens power calculations in eyes with axial lengths above 25.0 mm. J Cataract Refract Surg. 2011 Nov;37 (11):2018–27. https://doi.org/10.1016/j.jcrs.2011.05.042. PMID: 22018365.
11. Haigis W. Biometry and intraocular lens calculation in extreme myopia. Acta Clin Croat. 2012;51(Suppl 1):65–9 PMID: 23431727.
12. Petermeier K, Gekeler F, Messias A, Spitzer MS, Haigis W, Szurman P. Intraocular lens power calculation and optimized constants for highly myopic eyes. J Cataract Refract Surg. 2009;35:1575–81.
13. Preussner P-R. Intraocular lens calculation in extreme myopia. [letter] J Cataract Refract Surg 2010;36:531–2, reply by W Haigis, 532–4.
14. Zhang J, Tan X, Wang W, Yang G, Xu J, Ruan X, Gu X, Luo L. Effect of axial length adjustment methods on intraocular lens power calculation in highly myopic eyes. Am J Ophthalmol. 2020;214:110–8. https://doi.org/10.1016/j.ajo.2020.02.023 Epub 2020 Mar 12 PMID: 32171766.
15. Abulafia A, Barrett GD, Rotenberg M, Kleinmann G, Levy A, Reitblat O, Koch DD, Wang L, Assia EI. Intraocular lens power calculation for eyes with an axial length greater than 26.0 mm: comparison of formulas and methods. J Cataract Refract Surg. 2015 Mar;41(3):548–6. https://doi.org/10.1016/j.jcrs.2014.06.033. Epub 2015 Feb 21. PMID: 25708208.
16. Liu J, Wang L, Chai F, Han Y, Qian S, Koch DD, Weikert MP. Comparison of intraocular lens power calculation formulas in Chinese eyes with axial myopia. J Cataract Refract Surg. 2019;45(6):725–31. https://doi.org/10.1016/j.jcrs.2019.01.018 PMID: 31146930.
17. Rong X, He W, Zhu Q, Qian D, Lu Y, Zhu X. Intraocular lens power calculation in eyes with extreme myopia: comparison of Barrett Universal II, Haigis, and Olsen formulas. J Cataract Refract Surg. 2019;45(6):732–7. https://doi.org/10.1016/j.jcrs.2018.12.025 Epub 2019 Mar 12 PMID: 30876784.
18. Zhou D, Sun Z, Deng G. Accuracy of the refractive prediction determined by intraocular lens power calculation formulas in high myopia. Indian J Ophthalmol. 2019;67(4):484-–9. https://doi.org/10.4103/ijo.IJO_937_18. PMID: 30900579; PMCID: PMC6446621.
19. Wan KH, Lam TCH, Yu MCY, Chan TCY. Accuracy and precision of intraocular lens calculations using the new hill-RBF version 2.0 in eyes with high axial myopia. Am J Ophthalmol. 2019;205:66–73. https://doi.org/10.1016/j.ajo.2019.04.019. Epub 2019 May 10. PMID: 31078534.
20. Hengerer FH, Hütz WW, Dick HB, Conrad-Hengerer I. Combined correction of sphere and astigmatism using the light-adjustable intraocular lens in eyes with axial myopia. J Cataract Refract Surg. 2011;37(2):317–23. https://doi.org/10.1016/j.jcrs.2010.08.037 PMID: 21241915.

21. Cai XB, Shen SR, Chen DF, Zhang Q, Jin ZB. An overview of myopia genetics. Exp Eye Res. 2019;188: 107778. https://doi.org/10.1016/j.exer.2019.107778 Epub 2019 Aug 28 PMID: 31472110.
22. Neuhann IM, Neuhann TF, Heimann H, Schmickler S, Gerl RH, Foerster MH. Retinal detachment after phacoemulsification in high myopia: analysis of 2356 cases. J Cataract Refract Surg. 2008;34(10):1644–57. https://doi.org/10.1016/j.jcrs.2008.06.022 PMID: 18812113.
23. Ripandelli G, Coppé AM, Parisi V, Olzi D, Scassa C, Chiaravalloti A, Stirpe M. Posterior vitreous detachment and retinal detachment after cataract surgery. Ophthalmology. 2007;114 (4):692–7. https://doi.org/10.1016/j.ophtha.2006.08.045. Epub 2007 Jan 17. PMID: 17208303.2006.08.045. Epub 2007 Jan 17. PMID: 17208303.

21. [illegible] ... An overview of myopia policies ... [illegible] 2014 Aug 28. [illegible]
22. [illegible] M, [illegible] [illegible] ... [illegible]

Reduction of Astigmatism by Corneal Incisions

Catarina Pedrosa and Filomena Ribeiro

The surgical success of cataract surgery relies on reducing postoperative spectacle dependence and maximizing uncorrected distance visual acuity. The goal for visual function improvement is emmetropia, comprising the correction of preexisting astigmatism along with a controlled surgically induced astigmatism. The correction of residual astigmatism is possible either with the implantation of a toric intraocular lens (IOL), use of limbal relaxing incisions, astigmatic keratotomy or excimer laser refractive surgery. The effect of the wound on the existing astigmatism should also be considered.

This chapter will focus on the correction of low-to-moderate astigmatism during cataract surgery using corneal incisions which include limbal relaxing incisions, paired opposite clear corneal incisions and arcuate keratotomy.

Limbal relaxing incisions (LRI), also named peripheral corneal relaxing incisions reduce the astigmatism by flattening the steep axis of the cornea. LRIs are a cost effective and convenient alternative in small amounts of astigmatism, from 0.50D up to 1–1.25 D, and also in eyes without capsular support for a toric IOL or in patients with residual astigmatism after cataract surgery. Corneal optical features are preserved with this method and visual stability is achieved in a short-term follow-up.

LRIs may be placed in the beginning or in the conclusion of cataract surgery, and also postoperatively, in the operating room or even on the slit lamp. It is important to consider how the surgically induced cylinder will affect the patient's preexisting astigmatism. Incisions may be manual, using a guarded diamond knife set at a defined depth, or using femtosecond laser.

Accurate corneal astigmatism assessment is a key step for successful surgical outcomes. The astigmatism of the posterior corneal surface influences total corneal

C. Pedrosa (✉) · F. Ribeiro
Lisbon, Portugal
e-mail: pedrosa.catarina@gmail.com

M. Shajari et al. (eds.), *Cataract and Lens Surgery*,
https://doi.org/10.1007/978-3-031-05394-8_50

astigmatism (TCA) and is a major source of error when not considered in preoperative measurements. The authors found in a previous study that the percentage of eyes with posterior corneal astigmatism superior to 0.5D and the differences between anterior and total corneal astigmatism are higher than that previously reported in the literature [5]. To avoid this error TCA may be directly measured or there are currently available nomograms to consider the posterior corneal surface, based on data from Scheimpflug cameras, Color Led Topography or Optical Coherence Tomography.

There are several methods of measuring corneal astigmatism. Manual keratometry is less precise when compared with the following, although it allows an accurate identification of the steep axis by requiring the crosshairs alignment. Autokeratometry using devices such as IOLMaster (Carl Zeiss Meditec) and LenStar (Haag-Streit), corneal topography and corneal elevating mapping are other useful methods to preoperatively assess the astigmatism. In addition, ORA (Alcon) enables intraoperative astigmatic measuring. Furthermore, the use of antique tools such as the keratoscope (Fig. 1a and b, Video 1), although inaccurate, may be helpful for the astigmatic assessment during or after cataract surgery in selected cases.

Video 1 The use of keratoscope for compensating the postoperative corneal astigmatism with the adjustment of the main incision suture. This patient had surgery of phakic IOL explantation followed by phacoemulsification and in-the-sulcus IOL implantation. The final residual astigmatism was 0.5D.

Surface disease may interfere in the corneal astigmatic assessment and should be evaluated and treated before surgical planning. Patients with corneal pathology or irregular astigmatism are not good candidates for LRIs due to the unpredictability of the surgical results.

Once regular corneal astigmatism is determined in magnitude and axis, the surgeon consults a nomogram to determine the length and location of LRIs and may also use the online www.lricalculator.com. There are several available nomograms, including Nichamin (Table 1a and b) and Donnenfeld (Table 2), to determine the

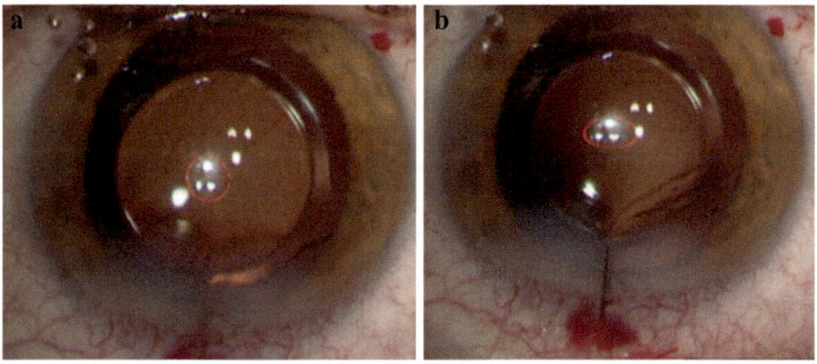

Fig. 1 (**a** and **b**) The use of keratoscope as a tool to aid astigmatism correction by incision suture adjustment

Table 1 Nichamin LRI nomogram to correct keratometric astigmatism during cataract surgery

(a) With-the-rule astigmatism (steep axis 45–145°)

Preoperative cylinder (D)	N. Incisions[a]	Degrees of arc to be incised by age						
		30–40 y	41–50 y	51–60 y	61–70 y	71–80 y	81–90 y	>90 y
1.00–1.50	2[b]	50	45	40	35	30	–	–
	2[b]	60	55	50	45	40	35	30
	2[b]	70	65	60	55	50	45	40
	2[b]	80	75	70	65	60	55	45

(b) Against-the-rule astigmatism (steep axis 0–30°/150–180°)

Preoperative cylinder (D)	N. Incisions	Degrees of arc to be incised by age						
		30–40 y	41–50 y	51–60 y	61–70 y	71–80 y	81–90 y	>90 y
0.75–1.25	1 nasal	–	–	–	–	–	35	–
0.75–1.25	2[a, b]	55	50	45	40	35	–	–
1.50–2.00	2[a, b]	70	65	60	55	45	40	35
2.25–2.75	2[a, b]	90	80	70	60	50	45	40
3.00–3.75	2[a, b]	o.z. to 8 mm	o.z. to 8 mm	85	70	60	50	45

[a] Neutral temporal clear corneal incision
[b] Paired limbal arcs on steep axis
y = years

length and location of LRIs. Most nomograms are based on age and preoperative corneal astigmatism. According to results, the surgeon may modify nomograms, creating his or her own nomogram tailored to the preferred surgical approach and the patient individual visual demands. LRIs may be single or paired depending on the amount of existing astigmatism. To avoid cyclotorsion, the patient's eye is previously marked on the slit lamp with the patient upright and looking straight ahead and during the procedure a marked fixation ring, astigmatic ruler or arcuate axis marker is centered on these marks to identify the corneal axis. Intraoperative aberrometry with devices such as ORA (WaveTec Vision) or digital marking such as Callisto eye (Carl Zeiss Meditec) or Verion (Alcon) may be used to determine the steep axis.

Table 2 Donnenfeld nomogram (DONO) for LRIs

Preoperative astigmatism	Number of incisions[a]	Length of incisions, (clock hours)[b]
0.5	1	1.5
0.75	2	1
1.5	2	2
3	2	3

[a] All incisions are placed 0.5mm from the limbus in the correct axis
[b] Patients who have against-the-rule astigmatism or who are less than 45 years old may benefit from slightly longer incisions. Shorter incisions may be indicated for patients older than 65 years

LRIs are located in the steep meridian at the most peripheral area of clear cornea, just inside the limbal vessels. Incision depth is most often set at 550 or 600 micra and length varies with the needed correction. Length is more accurate when measured by degrees, instead of millimeters, due to the variability in patient's corneal diameter. Results rely on surgical planning, surgeon technique and patient healing factors. Number of incisions (1 or 2), length, depth and location and also distance to the limbus, amount of preexisting astigmatism, corneal diameter and age are factors affecting the final outcome.

Arcuate keratotomy (AK) is another effective and low-cost alternative method of reducing astigmatism at the time of cataract surgery. While predictability is believed to be lower than that of toric IOLs, laser AK has improved the precision of incision parameters. There is limited published data regarding arcuate keratotomy for the correction of low-to-moderate corneal astigmatism at the time of cataract surgery.

Overcorrections are rare with LRIs while under-corrections are mainly related with incision depth. Inversion of the axis of astigmatism should be avoided since it is not well tolerated by the patient. Complications also include infection, wound leak, pain and foreign body sensation. Corneal trauma induced by the incisions can lead to dry eye by disrupting the normal corneal innervation and significantly reducing corneal sensitivity. This is a major limitation of LRIs which may be more severe when using femtosecond laser. LRIs are also associated with less predictability when compared to toric IOLs.

LRIs are commonly partial-depth arcuate incisions. However, during cataract surgery the clear corneal incision, placed on the steep corneal meridian, may be paired with a second full thickness corneal incision directly opposite. This method is called paired opposite clear corneal incisions. The second incision can be performed after the IOL implantation; before viscosurgical device aspiration, in the end of phacoemulsification; and/or using a second instrument to maintain the anterior chamber stability (Fig. 2). In the end of cataract surgery both incisions are hydrated. These paired phaco incisions are both on the same meridian, are self-sealing, require no extra surgical equipment and may achieve an enhanced flattening effect. Devgan [15] suggested a nomogram for paired phaco incisions with 2.8 mm in width, placed at the limbal vessels, stating that the astigmatic benefit was 0.7D of flattening for against-the-rule placement and 1.0 D of flattening for with-the-rule placement. Therefore, the flattening effect depends on the location (distance to limbus), length, and tunnel features. Digital marking, such as Callisto eye shown in Fig. 2, is a useful tool to enhance the precision of this method since it allows the identification of the steep axis and also the incision length and distance to limbus.

Author's recommendation

Paired opposite clear corneal incisions are an effective choice for correction of preexisting low to moderate astigmatism at the time of cataract surgery in cases where toric IOL implantation is not suitable or possible.

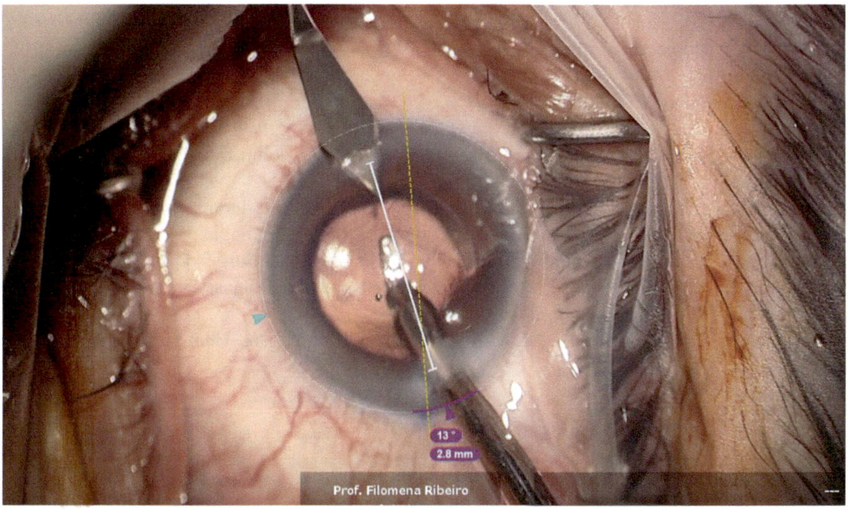

Fig. 2 Paired opposite clear corneal incisions of 2.75–2.80 mm treating astigmatism at the time of cataract surgery, using Callisto eye (Carl Zeiss Meditec). The patient had pseudoesfoliation syndrome and cataract with against-the-rule TCA of 0.98 D at 13°. The postoperative residual astigmatism was 0.25D

References

1. Roberts HW, Wagh VK, Sullivan DL, Archer TJ, O'Brart DPS. Refractive outcomes after limbal relaxing incisions or femtosecond laser arcuate keratotomy to manage corneal astigmatism at the time of cataract surgery. J Cataract Refract Surg. 2018;44(8):955–63.
2. Ferreira TB, Ribeiro FJ, Pinheiro J, Ribeiro P, O'Neill JG. Comparison of surgically induced astigmatism and morphologic features resulting from femtosecond laser and manual clear corneal incisions for cataract surgery. J Refract Surg. 2018;34(5):322–9.
3. Visco DM, Bedi R, Packer M. Femtosecond laser-assisted arcuate keratotomy at the time of cataract surgery for the management of preexisting astigmatism. J Cataract Refract Surg. 2019;45(12):1762–9.
4. Lake JC, Victor G, Clare G, Porfírio GJ, Kernohan A, Evans JR. Toric intraocular lens versus limbal relaxing incisions for corneal astigmatism after phacoemulsification. Cochrane Database Syst Rev. 2019;12(12):CD012801.
5. Mendes J, Ribeiro FJ, Ferreira TB. Evaluation of posterior and total corneal astigmatism with colour-LED topography. Eye (Lond). 2020.
6. Ferreira TB, Ribeiro FJ. Comparability and repeatability of different methods of corneal astigmatism assessment. Clin Ophthalmol. 2017;20(12):29–34.
7. Rho CR, Joo CK. Effects of steep meridian incision on corneal astigmatism in phacoemulsification cataract surgery. J Cataract Refract Surg. 2012;38(4):666–71.
8. Nichamin LD. Nomogram for limbal relaxing incisions. J Cataract Refract Surg. 2006;32 (9):1408.
9. Khanal S, Tomlinson A, Esakowitz L, Bhatt P, Jones D, Nabili S, Mukerji S. Changes in corneal sensitivity and tear physiology after phacoemulsification. Ophthalmic Physiol Opt. 2008;28(2):127–34.

10. Rubenstein JB, Raciti M, Management of astigmatism: LRIs. Int Ophthalmol Clin. 2012;52 (2):31–40, Lippincott Williams & Wilkins.
11. Amesbury EC, Miller KM. Correction of astigmatism at the time of cataract surgery. Curr Opin Ophthalmol. 2009;20(1):19–24.
12. Khokhar S, Lohiya P, Murugiesan V, Panda A. Corneal astigmatism correction with opposite clear corneal incisions or single clear corneal incision: comparative analysis. J Cataract Refract Surg. 2006;32(9):1432–7.
13. Ribeiro F. Cirurgia incisional na correção do astigmatismo durante a facoemulsificação. Presbiopia, 2019; pp. 69–72. Sociedade Portuguesa de Oftalmologia.
14. Eric D. Donnenfeld. The importance of LRIs. Cataract Refract Surg Today. 2008. pp. 49–50.
15. Cristóbal JA, Mateo A, Faus F, Belmonte J, Cirugía incisional. Incisiones relajantes limbares. Correccion del astigmatismo, 2006. pp. 197–221.
16. Devgan U. Paired phaco incisions can treat corneal astigmatism. Heal Ophthalmol. 2019.

Special Surgical Features When Using Toric and Multifocal Intraocular Lenses

Wolfgang J. Mayer and Rudy Nuijts

Special Surgical Features of Using Toric Intraocular Lenses

Lens surgery with toric intraocular lens implantation is essentially the same procedure as standard minimal invasive phacoemulsification cataract surgery. The difference is primarily related to the preoperative marking of the patient's eye for intraoperative axial alignment and the subsequent surgical alignment of the toric lens within the capsular bag. For this purpose, all toric IOLs have markings on the edge of the optic.

The influence of "surgical induced astigmatism" (SIA) is also an important aspect to consider. Where possible, the surgeon's own SIA should be included in the calculation of the toric lens power in order avoid an unintended influence on the refractive result. An alternative approach is to use temporal access for the main incision as the influence of this incision on corneal astigmatism is very low.

Important: After lens implantation and axial alignment, the remaining viscoleastic material should be removed with great care to prevent the possibility of inadvertent postoperative lens rotation.

Supplementary Information The online version contains supplementary material available at https://doi.org/10.1007/978-3-031-05394-8_51. The videos can be accessed individually by clicking the DOI link in the accompanying figure caption or by scanning this link with the SN More Media App.

W. J. Mayer (✉)
University Eye Hospital Munich, Munich, Germany
e-mail: wolfgang.j.mayer@med.uni-muenchen.de

R. Nuijts
Maastricht University Medical Center (MUMC), Maastricht, The Netherlands
e-mail: rudy.nuijts@mumc.nl

M. Shajari et al. (eds.), *Cataract and Lens Surgery*,
https://doi.org/10.1007/978-3-031-05394-8_51

Author's recommendation

When using hydrophilic IOL models, it is also possible to implant the lens in a bimanual technique under irrigation without the use of viscoelastics. The lens can then be turned into the appropriate position even under irrigation.

The use of a cascade tension ring to stabilize the lens geometry in the capsular bag to reduce the possibility of rotation of the lens after surgery is controversial and is not a primary indication for toric lens implantation [1].

Marking and axis alignment: manual versus digital

Preoperative exact corneal marking is crucial to effectively align the toric lens. Manual marking [2] uses various corneal markers (dye marking), which either mark a reference axis (0 degree axis), which is then used to align the lens intraoperatively using a ring gauge, or allow direct marking of the torus axis (Video 1).

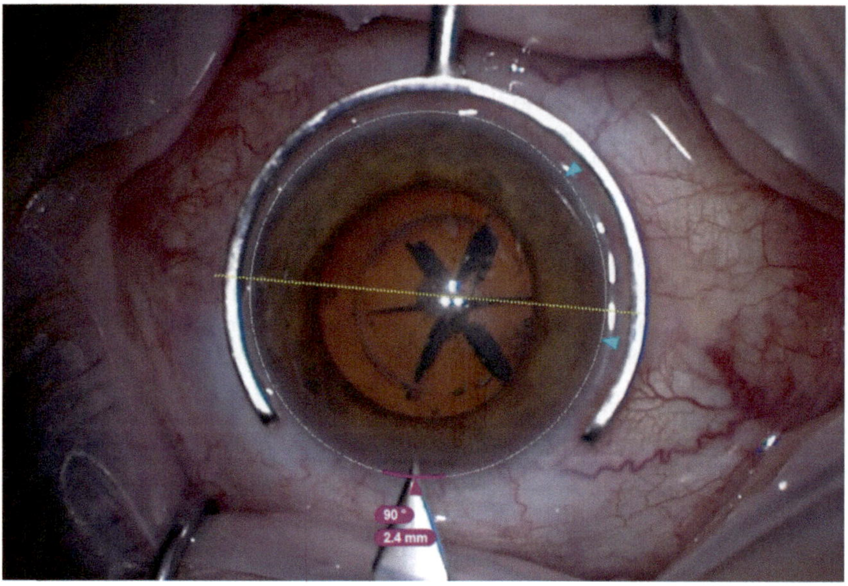

Video 1 A multifocal toric IOL is inserted under irrigation using digital axis marking after femtosecond laser-assisted lens surgery. For the lens power calculation, a SIA of 0.5 D was included and the superior incision was set accordingly. The steep axis is also indicated by digital visualisation so that the incision is made at the correct position despite cyclotorsion (M4V 56396 kb) (▶ https://doi.org/10.1007/000-8dh)

Keypoint

The manual marking should always be performed preoperatively in the upright position of the patient in order to reduce the influence of cyclotorsion of the eye while lying down during the surgery

Modern surgical assistance systems allow digital tracking of vessels in the limbus area of the cornea on the basis of a digitally generated reference image of the eye. Therefore, dye marking in an upright position is not necessary. Surgical assistance systems enable digital axis insertion via the surgical microscope. Current studies prove a more exact alignment and effectiveness of toric IOLs though the visual acuities in both groups are comparable [3, 4].

Author's recommendation

For combined surgery with vitrectomy, e.g. within the scope of a membrane peeling, a toric lens can also be implanted in case of regular astigmatism within the indication area. In this case a "myopic shift" due to the vitrectomy should be included in the calculation [5].

Special Surgical Features When Using Multifocal Intraocular Lenses

Multifocal or multifocal-toric optics are used in cataract surgery but also when performing refractive lens exchange with a clear phakic lens. Meanwhile, there also "add-on" multifocal and multifocal-toric systems exist which can be implanted into the sulcus if the patient is already pseudophakic [6, 7].

Great care must be taken when performing lens surgery with implantation of multifocal systems. Any deviation from the surgical technique on the tissue can lead to changes in the optical principle and perception (capsule injury, iris injury, corneal endothelial injury, etc.). For an optimal surgical course, care must be taken when performing corneal incisions. The main incision should be performed astigmatism neutral from the temporal side, or better yet, by calculating SIA for the main incision. The rhexis should be neither too large nor too small and should be chosen in such a way that a small overlap to the optics is created. This prevents early capsule constriction or posterior capsule opacification, regardless of the lens material used. The use of dispersive viscoelastics is recommended to protect the corneal endothelium during surgery. The effective phaco time should also be kept low during phacoemulsification using a femtosecond laser or chop techniques for harder lens nuclei. The implantation of hydrophilic multifocal optics can be performed under irrigation, but should be performed under strict control of irrigation, especially for lens rotations. Otherwise, filling the capsule bag with viscoelastic is the method of choice here.

Among the key factors that must be taken into account in order to achieve optimal results are the optics of the different axes of the eye, the characteristics of the specific implants and their interaction with the anatomy of the eye.

One goal of IOL surgery is to align the IOL as well as possible along the visual axis of the eye, with the real challenge to predict its position at the time of surgery. Strategic considerations in this regard should already be taken into account for capsulorhexis. Modern surgical microscopes allow a coaxial light reflex imaging of the corneal vertex.

The decisive factor here is whether the IOL remains in the same position if the capsule narrows by about 14% in diameter in the first three months after surgery, which could cause decentration and tilting of the IOL [8–10].

Spherical and aspherical IOLs

Spherical and aspherically neutral IOLs are most resistant to the negative effects of improper centration. Consequently, the shift of their centration axis from the centre of the pupil does not have as much effect on the optics of these lenses as in multifocal IOLs. Nevertheless, some experts now suggest that aspherical IOLs work best when they are shifted to a centering axis that is between 0.3 and 0.6 mm supronasally from the pupil axis [11].

Multifocal IOLs

The place of perfect centration and effective position for multifocal diffractive IOLs is still the subject of numerous prospective studies. Experts advise that multifocal lenses should be centred as close as possible to the entrance pupil, as they require a balanced incidence of light to create two focal points by constructive interference of diffracted light.

However, like most conventional IOLs, these lenses centre themselves in the capsular bag after implantation [12, 13].

Author's recommendation

For IOL alignment the coaxial light source of the surgical microscope should be used to align both corneal and lenticular Purkinje images (with patient-assisted fixation). The integrity and preservation of the lens capsule after optimal capsulorhexis, which allows a small overlap of the lens optics, is essential for the functional principle of modern intraocular lenses.

References

1. Vokrojova M, Havlickova L, Brozkova M, Hlinomazova Z. Effect of capsular tension ring implantation on postoperative rotational stability of a toric intraocular lens. J Refract Surg. 2020;36(3):186–92.
2. Lipsky L, Barrett G. Comparison of toric intraocular lens alignment error with different toric markers. J Cataract Refract Surg. 2019;45(11):1597–601.
3. Mayer WJ, Kreutzer T, Dirisamer M, Kern C, Kortuem K, Vounotrypidis E, et al. Comparison of visual outcomes, alignment accuracy, and surgical time between 2 methods of corneal marking for toric intraocular lens implantation. J Cataract Refract Surg. 2017;43(10):1281–6.
4. webers VSC, Bauer NJC, Visser N, Berendschot T, van den Biggelaar F, Nuijts R. Image-guided system versus manual marking for toric intraocular lens alignment in cataract surgery. J Cataract Refract Surg. 2017;43(6):781–8.

5. Vounotrypidis E, Shajari M, Muth DR, Hirnschall N, Findl O, Priglinger S, et al. Refractive outcomes of 8 biometric formulas in combined phacovitrectomy with internal limiting membrane peeling for epiretinal membrane. J Cataract Refract Surg. 2020;46(4):591–7.
6. Cassagne M, Porterie M, Gauthier L, Chapotot E, Soler V, Malecaze F, et al. Primary sulcus implantation of a diffractive multifocal pseudophakic piggyback intraocular lens. J Cataract Refract Surg. 2018;44(3):266–73.
7. Khoramnia R, Yildirim TM, Son HS, Labuz G, Mayer CS, Auffarth GU. [Duet procedure to achieve reversible trifocality]. Ophthalmologist. 2020.
8. 8th Liu X, Xie L, Huang Y. Effects of decentration and tilt at different orientations on the optical performance of a rotationally asymmetric multifocal intraocular lens. J Cataract Refract Surg. 2019;45(4):507–14.
9. 9th Meng J, He W, Rong X, Miao A, Lu Y, Zhu X. Decentration and tilt of plate-haptic multifocal intraocular lenses in myopic eyes. Eye Vis (Lond). 2020;7:17.
10. 10th Zhu X, He W, Zhang Y, Chen M, Du Y, Lu Y. Inferior Decentration of Multifocal Intraocular Lenses in Myopic Eyes. At J Ophthalmol. 2018;188:1–8.
11. 11th Hayashi K, Hayashi H, Nakao F, Hayashi F. Correlation between pupillary size and intraocular lens decentration and visual acuity of a zonal-progressive multifocal lens and a monofocal lens. Ophthalmology. 2001;108(11):2011–7.
12. Findl O, Hirnschall N, Draschl P, Wiesinger J. Effect of manual capsulorhexis size and position on intraocular lens tilt, centration, and axial position. J Cataract Refract Surg. 2017;43(7):902–8.
13. Montes-Mico R, Cervino A, Ferrer-Blasco T. Intraocular lens centration and stability: efficacy of current technique and technology. Curr Opin Ophthalmol. 2009;20(1):33–6.

Corneal Complications and Management Associated with Cataract Surgery

Martin Grüterich

In most cases, the cataract lens is accessed via incisions in the cornea. Phacoemulsification of the nucleus and aspiration of the cortical material are performed only a few millimeters away from the delicate corneal endothelium. The intraocular lens is also implanted only a small distance away from the back surface of the cornea. Due to the layer structure of the cornea, the potential damage that can be caused during cataract surgery can be divided into three areas: ocular surface disorders, stromal scarring and endothelial cell loss/failure.

What are the particular features of the cornea that should be considered and examined before planning a cataract operation?

Is there preexisting dry eye? If so, is it due to a lack of aqueous tears or due to meibomian gland dysfunction? Is there a preexisting condition with a compromised corneal endothelium, such as cornea guttata, PEX or previous glaucoma surgery? How hard does the lens nucleus appear? Is a long phacoemulsification time expected? Is a higher viscosity viscoelastic required? Are the anterior chamber conditions particularly narrow or extremely deep?

Dry Eye

Surgical interventions of the cornea such as phototherapeutic keratectomy (PTK), laser in situ keratomileusis (LASIK) are known to lead to partial denervation and thus disruption of the corneal innervation. The incisions performed during cataract

Supplementary Information The online version contains supplementary material available at https://doi.org/10.1007/978-3-031-05394-8_52. The videos can be accessed individually by clicking the DOI link in the accompanying figure caption or by scanning this link with the SN More Media App.

M. Grüterich (✉)
München, Germany
e-mail: grueterich@augen-arzt-muenchen.de

M. Shajari et al. (eds.), *Cataract and Lens Surgery*,
https://doi.org/10.1007/978-3-031-05394-8_52

surgery can do the same. As a result, there is an increased release of inflammatory mediators and reduced lacrimal functional unit input, which in turn reduces tear production and distribution as well as an increased epithelial permeability and prolonged epithelial wound healing [1–4].

Basically, a distinction has to be made between patients who already suffer from dry eye prior to cataract surgery and those who develop dry eye after an eye operation. The former should be treated according to the guidelines of the TFOS Dry Eye Workshop (DEWS) II Report prior to a surgical intervention [5]. Depending on the type of dry eye, these measures comprise intensive eyelid care, tear substitution, anti-inflammatory therapy with local steroids or local immunomodulators such as cyclosporine A. As it can be assumed that the symptoms will worsen postoperatively and will return to the preoperative state at the earliest 3 months after surgery, dry eye therapy should be discussed and emphasized to the patient and be continued peri—and postoperatively. Patients who developed dry eyes only postoperatively should be treated with topical drop therapy until they are free of symptoms. Local antisepsis with povidone iodine, the local anesthetics as well as the creation of the tunnel incision and the paracentesis can all lead to a damage of the sensitive corneal nerves and contribute to postoperative dry eye. Kato et al. reported that dry eye disorders that in the worst-case scenario led to corneal perforations (extremely rare) with postoperative use of topical non-steroidal anti-inflammatory drugs and suggests that this treatment should be carefully administered to patients with cystoid macular edema or to steroid responders. Close monitoring is recommended [6].

Keypoint

Dry eye is a relatively frequent complication after cataract surgery. In addition to discomfort, it often leads to impairment of postoperative visual acuity and thus to patient dissatisfaction—particularly when using multifocal intraocular lens implants. Postoperatively, intense dry eye therapy should be added to the standard ant-inflammatory and antibiotic treatment regimen. Patients with a pre-existing dry eye should continue their established therapy and be informed that their symptoms are likely to worsen temporarily after surgery. (see Chap. 79; Messmer).

Incision-Associated Complications

The corneal incisions required for cataract surgery (clear cornea incision, paracentesis) can result in complications if they are not properly sided and positioned. If the incision is too short, wound leakage or (in the case of a floppy iris syndrome) recurrent iris incarceration can occur. There is also an increased risk of post operative endophthalmitis. Leakage of the tunnel incision may be caused by heat damage from the phacotip (Phako-burn). Phaco-burns almost always leak despite copious stromal hydration usual require a suture to assure a watertight closure. These wounds are best closed with a non-resorbable suture as the wound healing can take a long time and prolonged leakage postoperatively can occur. In addition to suture closure, the use of fibrin glue, conjunctiva flaps or the introduction of an air bubble into the anterior chamber of the eye have also been used. With the latter, however, the risk of a pupillary block must be taken into account [7, 8]. The pupil should not be completely covered by the air bubble or a peripheral iridectomy/iridotomy should be performed to prevent pupillary block.

Long lamellar incisions, reaching the midperiphery of the cornea, can produce irregular astigmatism, induce higher order aberrations and scarring resulting in low postoperative visual acuity. There is no curative treatment (except perforating keratoplasty) available.

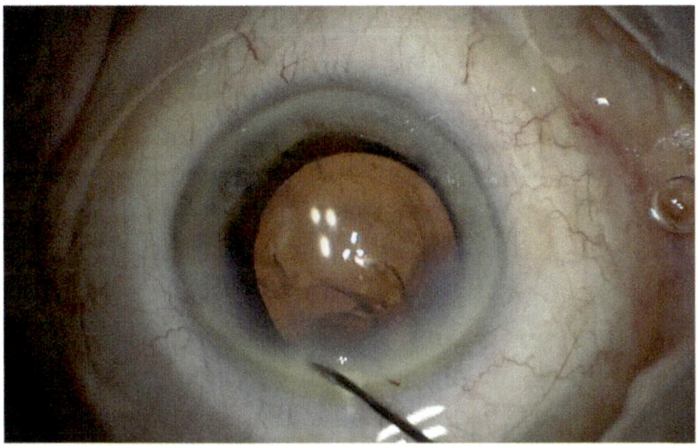

Video 1 Tear in Descemet membrane (▶ https://doi.org/10.1007/000-8kk)

Corneal Endothelial Damage

Corneal endothelial damage has been one of the dreaded complications since the beginning of cataract surgery. The extent of damage has been significantly reduced through the improvement of the surgical technique over time, but even today, despite modern techniques and the greatest experience of each surgeon it is still not completely eliminated. The damaging effect on the endothelium may be through a direct accidental manipulation with the instruments, by liquid as it flows through the anterior chamber, by the ultrasonic phacoemulsification energy, by the temperature increase of the phacotip as well as by the implantation of the intraocular lens. As a result, the pump function of the endothelial cells can reach its limits, some of the endothelial cells can be directly damaged or the Descemet membrane (including the endothelial cells) detach from the stroma. The latter complication is also known as descemetolysis. If the Descemet membrane does not reattach to its anatomical position, endothelial decompensation occurs and the transparency of the cornea can no longer be maintained.

Intraoperative endothelial cell decompensation with stroma edema and resulting visual impairment usually occurs on a background of preexisting endothelial cell damage (i.e. cornea guttata, low endothelial cell density of other origin or PEX). A long operating time with a correspondingly high fluid flow through or a long phacoemulsification time in the case of a hard lens nucleus intensify such a condition. When operating on eyes with a hazy cornea, short-term improvement of visualization can be achieved by a combination of epithelial abrasion and deswelling of the stroma using a hypertonic glucose or mannitol solution [9]. The effect only lasts about 30 minutes but this is normally sufficient to safely finish the cataract procedure.

A Descemetolysis is a particular complication that is worth specific attention. About 43% of clinically detectable postoperative Descemetolysis are found after cataract surgery. However, only a small proportion of these are clinically relevant [10] (N. Sharma et al., 2015b). Recent studies by Ti et al. and Kumar et al. cite an incidence of the occurrence of a visual acuity-relevant descent membrane detachment after phacoemulsification of 0.044% and 0.52% respectively [11, 12]. Preoperative risk factors for descemetolysis are an age above 65, an existing Fuchs endothelial dystrophy or a history of ocular trauma such as a chemical burn [13].

Intraoperative risk factors for Descemetolysis are direct trauma to the endothelium, irregular or inclined inner cut edges of the incisions by blunt instruments as well as a long phaco emulsification time and high phacoemulsification energy. Moreover, with each insertion of instruments (phacotip, manipulators, irrigation cannula or the intraocular lens) a small circumscribed descemetolysis can be increased and extended. Interestingly, a history of DMEK does not increase the risk of descemetolysis. To the contrary, the transplanted Descemet-endothelium-complex appears to form a more solid stromal attachment compared to the natural conditions [14, 15]. Clinically, descemetolysis can appear very differently. Circumscribed detachments near the incisions without visual impairment are relatively frequently observed whereas a large descemetolysis with central corneal edema rarely occur (Fig. 1) [16].

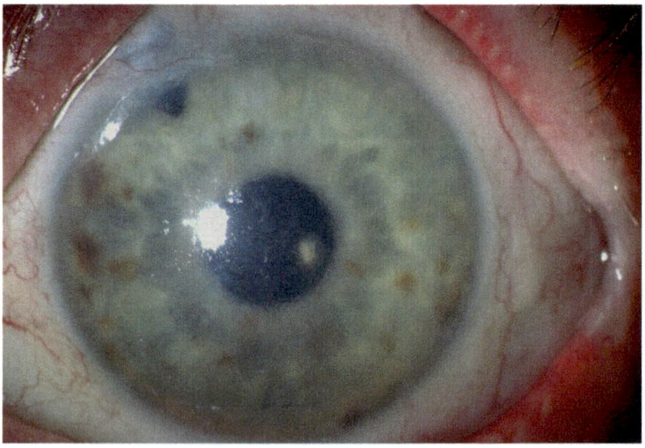

Fig. 1 Diffuse corneal edema after cataract surgery with posterior chamber lens implantation

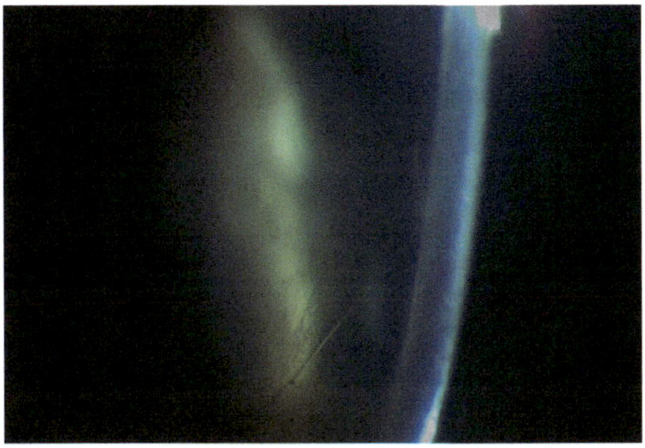

Fig. 2 A peripheral, circumscribed Descemetolysis can be seen in a narrow lslit

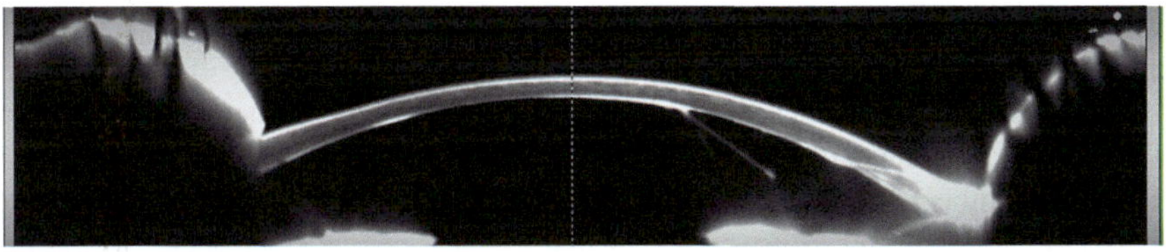

Fig. 3 Pentacam imaging of a peripheral Descemetolysis

At high magnification and with a narrow slit-lamp beam Descemetolysis can usually be detected (Fig. 2). However, this is not always possible if the corneal edema is severe. In these situations, imaging the anterior segment using Scheimpflug images or OCT can be helpful to determine the extent and shape of the Descemet detachment (Fig. 3). Ultrasound biomicroscopy (UBM) can also make Descemetolysis visible, but it is less widespread and technically more complex than the aforementioned methods.

There are a number of approaches to classify Descemetolysis with corresponding treatment algorithms [12, 16]. Action is required whenever the Descemetolysis extends over 50% of the total corneal endothelial surface area, or if visual acuity impairing stromal edema is present. In situations with a circumscribed shallowDescemet detachment without curled edges observation for spontaneous reattachment for 1–2 weeks is feasible. In the case of bullous detachments with partially rolled up edges and central corneal edema, we consider rapid interventional reattachment by so called re-bubbling.

For the reattachment of a detached Descemet membrane, the introduction of an air or gas bubble in the anterior chamber is the recommended procedure. This technique was first described by Sparks in 1967 and is called Descemetopexy [17]. The principle of this method is to press and support the detached membrane section

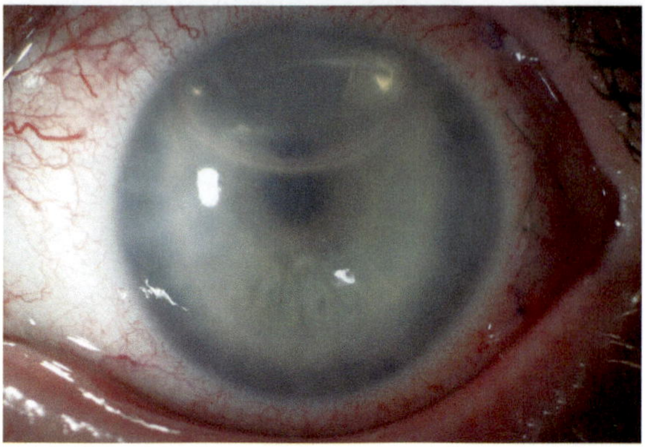

Fig. 4 Air filled anterior chamber, edematous cornea after Descemetolysis

by air or a non-expanding gas concentration (20% SF6 or 14% C3F8), until it can self-adhere [18–20]. This technique was later adopted as the standard procedure for DMEK transplantation (Fig. 4). An air bubble is introduced into the anterior chamber of the eye in an area where the Descemet membrane is still attached and, by means of blunt manipulation on the limbus or the central cornea, is brought into position so that the detached area is pushed against the posterior stroma. The anterior chamber should then be filled with air/gas to such an extent that the edematous corneal area is covered, but that the preoperative peripheral iridotomy remains open. After administration of 250 mg acetazolamide p.o. and lying on the back for about 30 min, the air can be partially deflated. The iridotomy as well as the administration of acetazolamide prevents a pupillary block. The more complex the Descemetolysis is, the longer the air/gas bubble should remain in the anterior chamber. SF6 and C3F8 remain in the anterior chamber longer than sterile air. According to our own experience, the use of sterile air is usually sufficient. If the visibility is reduced due to epithelial and/or stromal edema preventing a safe application and positioning of the bubble, an epithelial abrasion and the administration of a hypertonic topical solution as described above may be required. In this situation, a soft contact lens should also be placed at the end of the procedure to reduce the postoperative pain.

The edema should subside within 4 weeks, as long as there are still sufficient viable endothelial cells. Postoperative therapy includes the topical administration of steroids, hyperosmolar eye drops and acetazolamide as long as the pupil is covered by the air bubble. If a therapeutic contact lens was used, a topical antibiotic should be considered. If the corneal edema ultimately does not clear, it must be reevaluated whether the Descemet membrane has detached again or whether the endothelial cell damage is irreversible. In the latter case, a corneal endothelial transplantation may be required.

Keypoint

Both temporary and irreversible endothelial decompensation is a serious complication that can occur after cataract surgery. Transient edema in previously normal corneas usually recover with conservative treatment. If the endothelium is compromised prior to the surgery due to other pathologies, an endothelial keratoplasty is often required in the long term. Descemetolysis is a special form of corneal complication. If it is less complex, the prognosis after Descemetopexy is good. If the findings are pronounced and the cornea does not tend to clear up, endothelial keratoplasty is the treatment of choice.

References

1. Belmonte C, Acosta MC, Gallar J. Neural basis of sensation in intact and injured corneas. Exp Eye Res. 2004;78(3):513–25. https://doi.org/10.1016/j.exer.2003.09.023.
2. Bron AJ, de Paiva CS, Chauhan SK, Bonini S, Gabison EE, Jain S, et al. TFOS DEWS II pathophysiology report. Ocul Surf. 2017;15(3):438–510. https://doi.org/10.1016/j.jtos.2017.05.011.
3. Cho YK, Kim MS. Dry eye after cataract surgery and associated intraoperative risk factors. Korean J Ophthalmol. 2009;23(2):65–73. https://doi.org/10.3341/kjo.2009.23.2.65.
4. Oh T, Jung Y, Chang D, Kim J, Kim H. Changes in the tear film and ocular surface after cataract surgery. Jpn J Ophthalmol. 2012;56(2):113–8. https://doi.org/10.1007/s10384-012-0117-8.
5. Jones L, Downie LE, Korb D, Benitez-Del-Castillo JM, Dana R, Deng SX, et al. TFOS DEWS II management and therapy report. Ocul Surf. 2017;15(3):575–628. https://doi.org/10.1016/j.jtos.2017.05.006.
6. Kato K, Miyake K, Hirano K, Kondo M. Management of postoperative inflammation and dry eye after cataract surgery. Cornea. 2019;38(Suppl 1):S25–33. https://doi.org/10.1097/ICO.0000000000002125.
7. Berdahl JP, DeStafeno JJ, Kim T. Corneal wound architecture and integrity after phacoemulsification evaluation of coaxial, microincision coaxial, and microincision bimanual techniques. J Cataract Refract Surg. 2007;33(3):510–5. https://doi.org/10.1016/j.jcrs.2006.11.012.
8. Sippel KC, Pineda R Jr. Phacoemulsification and thermal wound injury. Semin Ophthalmol. 2002;17(3–4):102–9. https://doi.org/10.1076/soph.17.3.102.14776.
9. Böke WDG. Operation on the lens. 1992. p. 88–89.
10. Sharma N, Gupta S, Maharana P, Shanmugam P, Nagpal R, Vajpayee RB. Anterior segment optical coherence tomography-guided management algorithm for descemet membrane detachment after intraocular surgery. Cornea. 2015;34(9):1170–4.
11. Ti SE, Chee SP, Tan DT, Yang YN, Shuang SL. Descemet membrane detachment after phacoemulsification surgery: risk factors and success of air bubble tamponade. Cornea. 2013;32(4):454–9. https://doi.org/10.1097/ICO.0b013e318254c045.
12. Kumar DA, Agarwal A, Sivanganam S, Chandrasekar R. Height-, extent-, length-, and pupil-based (HELP) algorithm to manage post-phacoemulsification Descemet membrane detachment. J Cataract Refract Surg. 2015;41(9):1945–53. https://doi.org/10.1016/j.jcrs.2015.01.020.
13. Benatti CA, Tsao JZ, Afshari NA. Descemet membrane detachment during cataract surgery: etiology and management. Curr Opin Ophthalmol. 2017;28(1):35–41. https://doi.org/10.1097/ICU.0000000000000332.
14. Dapena I, Ham L, Tabak S, Balachandran C, Melles G. Phacoemulsification after Descemet membrane endothelial keratoplasty. J Cataract Refract Surg. 2009;35(7):1314–5. https://doi.org/10.1016/j.jcrs.2008.12.050.

15. Musa FU, Cabrerizo J, Quilendrino R, Dapena I, Ham L, Melles GR. Outcomes of phacoemulsification after Descemet membrane endothelial keratoplasty. J Cataract Refract Surg. 2013;39(6):836–40. https://doi.org/10.1016/j.jcrs.2012.12.032.
16. Singhal D, Sahay P, Goel S, Asif MI, Maharana PK, Sharma N. Descemet membrane detachment. Surv Ophthalmol. 2020;65(3):279–93. https://doi.org/10.1016/j.survophthal.2019.12.006.
17. Sparks GM. Descemetopexy. Surgical reattachment of stripped Descemet's membrane. Arch Ophthalmol. 1967;78(1):31–4. https://doi.org/10.1001/archopht.1967.00980030033006.
18. Kremer I, Stiebel H, Yassur Y, Weinberger D. Sulfur hexafluoride injection for Descemet's membrane detachment in cataract surgery. J Cataract Refract Surg. 1997;23(10):1449–53. https://doi.org/10.1016/s0886-3350(97)80013-2.
19. Odayappan A, Shivananda N, Ramakrishnan S, Krishnan T, Nachiappan S, Krishnamurthy S. A retrospective study on the incidence of post-cataract surgery Descemet's membrane detachment and outcome of air descemetopexy. Br J Ophthalmol. 2018;102(2):182–6. https://doi.org/10.1136/bjophthalmol-2016-309766.
20. Sharma A, Singh SK, Bhutia PL, Pant R. Perfluoropropane (C3F8) injection for Descemet's membrane detachment in cataract surgery. Nepal J Ophthalmol. 2015;7(1): 74–8. https://www.ncbi.nlm.nih.gov/pubmed/27479993. https://doi.org/10.1097/ICO.0000000000000514.

Iris Complications and Management in Cataract Surgery

Peter Szurman

Serious Complications of the Iris During Cataract Surgery

Direct injuries to the iris such as phaco bites, hemorrhage, iris touch, and iris prolapse lead to significant problems with prolonged irritation, iris transillumination defects, and irreparable iris sphincter injury, resulting in unfavorable visual and cosmetic results such as de-rounded or mydriatic pupils. Conversely, a narrow pupil is a common cause of a complicating course of cataract surgery. Several pupil dilation strategies are described below. It is crucial to distinguish between a narrow, rigid pupil and a narrow, atonic pupil, as the timing and nature of the problems, as well as their management, are different.

Memo
The simplicity of a cataract operation depends critically on the size of the pupil and the rigidity of the iris

The Narrow, Rigid Pupil

A narrow, rigid pupil affects the entire surgical process. This type of pupil problem can arise from PEX, diabetes, uveitis, injuries, or glaucoma medication. Posterior synechiae or a fibrosis ring at the pupillary margin are common. With a rigid pupil

Supplementary Information The online version contains supplementary material available at https://doi.org/10.1007/978-3-031-05394-8_53. The videos can be accessed individually by clicking the DOI link in the accompanying figure caption or by scanning this link with the SN More Media App.

P. Szurman (✉)
Sulzbach, Germany
e-mail: Peter.Szurman@kksaar.de

M. Shajari et al. (eds.), *Cataract and Lens Surgery*,
https://doi.org/10.1007/978-3-031-05394-8_53

size of less than 3–4 mm, depending on the experience of the surgeon, all steps of the surgery are difficult-from capsulorhexis to nuclear fragmentation to intraocular lens implantation. Therefore, a pupil dilation strategy is needed in these cases.

As early as the preoperative stage, maximum drug-induced mydriasis should be ensured. Intraoperative application of epinephrine (0.3 ml, 1:1000) intracamerally [11] and in the irrigation solution (0.5 ml of 1:1000 epinephrine and 500 ml BSS) have been shown to be effective [8]. The second step is viscodilation, in most cases, a simple deepening of the anterior chamber with a cohesive viscoelastic results in pupil dilation sufficient for capsulorhexis.

Surgical Management of Narrow, Rigid Pupils

Before the pupil is mechanically dilated, the presence of synechiae or a fibrosis ring must first be excluded. Loosening of synechiae can be achieved with a push–pull hook, but care must be taken not to overstretch the iris sphincter. It is not uncommon to find a fine fibrosis ring at the pupillary rim, typically in uveitis eyes, and especially in JIA-associated uveitis in children [12]. This ring must not be pulled off under any circumstances; doing so would injure the thin iris sphincter muscle (Videos 1 and 2). Instead, segmentation is performed with approx. 12–16 radial incisions (e.g., with 23 g vitreous scissors; better: curved diabetic scissors). The incisions must not injure the iris sphincter (see Fig. 1). More extensive mechanical pupil dilation strategies are ambivalent because all mechanical aids overstretch the iris sphincter and leave permanent damage.

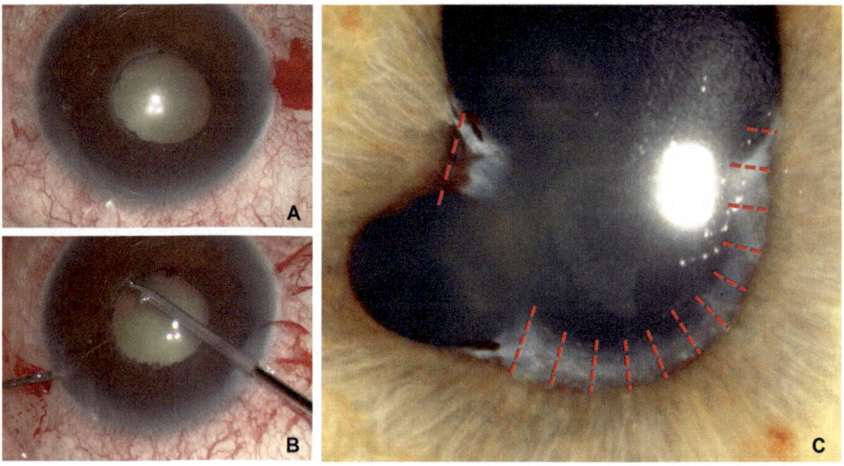

Fig. 1 Segmentation of fibrosis ring in uveitis. **A** Fibrotic ring **B** Radial incisions **C** Where incisions should be placed

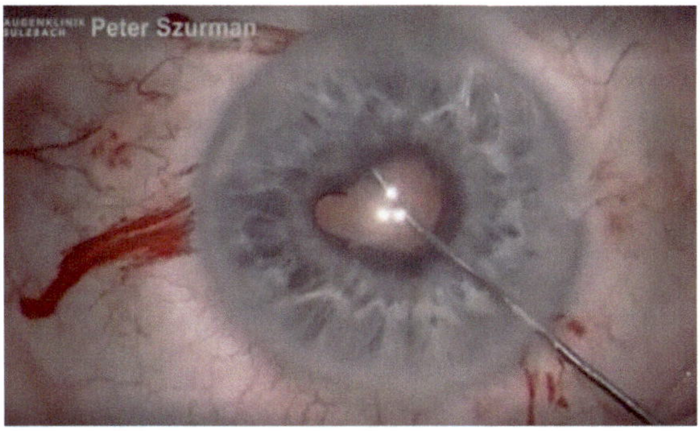

Video 1 Segmentation of fibrosis ring in uveitis (▶ https://doi.org/10.1007/000-8dm)

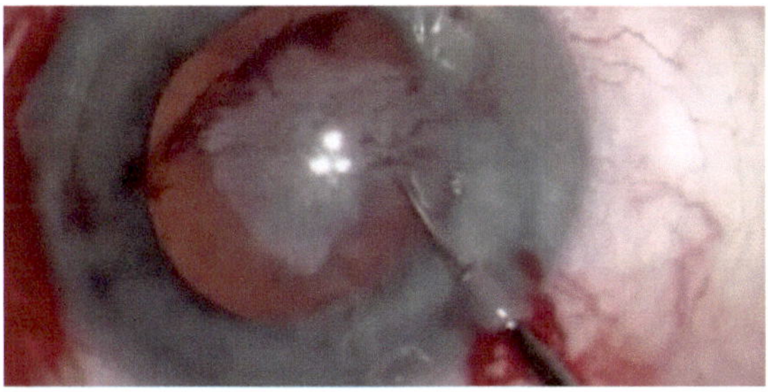

Video 2 Removal of a pupillary membrane in uveitis (▶ https://doi.org/10.1007/000-8dk)

Iris stretching is particularly critical: two push–pull hooks are hooked over opposite paracenteses in the pupil margin and pulled against each other. The slightly dilated pupil is then atonic and complicates rather than facilitates the further course of surgery [7].

Iris retractors have a similar effect. For this purpose, four retractors are inserted via paracentesis, hooked into the pupil margin, and pulled outwards (Video 3). This results in a quadrangular dilated pupil. Aside from the permanent damage caused by sphincter tears (see Fig. 2), there is another disadvantage: iris retractors not only pull the pupil outwards but also pull the entire iris diaphragm upwards, which promotes prolapse of the iris base [13].

Pupil expanders such as the Malyugin ring are comparatively gentler. They lead to a more rounded pupil configuration and keep the iris diaphragm at the natural level (see Video 4). They can be easily implanted via the tunnel incision and explanted in the same manner (see Fig. 3). Postoperatively, an atonic pupil is rare, but microsphincter tears can still lead to permanent atony [9].

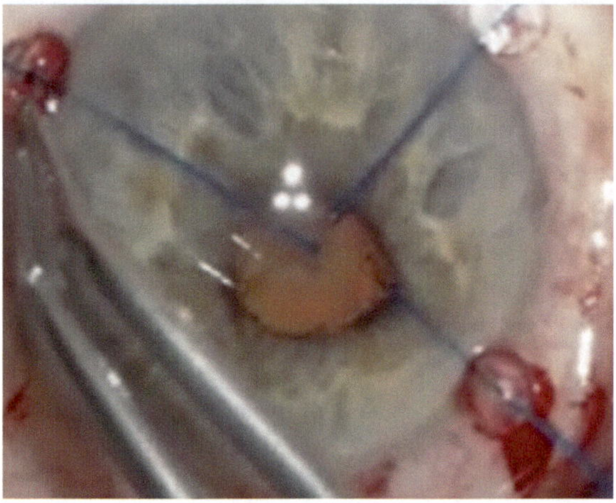

Video 3 Iris retractors with a narrow pupil (▶ https://doi.org/10.1007/000-8dj)

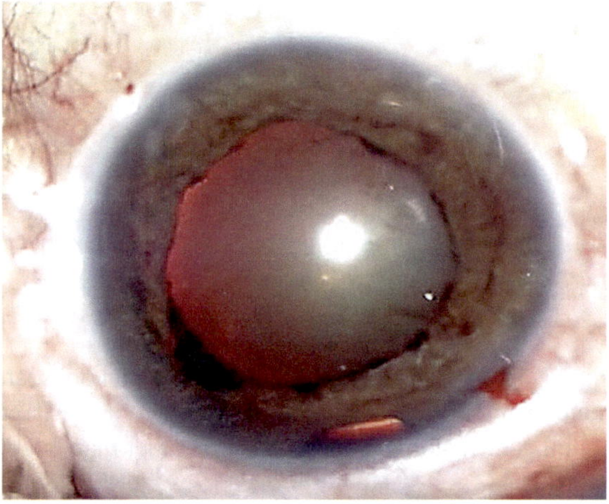

Fig. 2 Significant de-rounding after removal of iris retractors with permanent damage to the iris sphincter.

Therefore, experienced surgeons will avoid mechanical pupil dilation whenever possible and perform the surgery gently with a narrow or moderately dilated pupil. After intracamerally injecting epinephrine and subsequent viscodilation, often combined with various soft-shell techniques, a pupil width of 3.5-4 mm is almost always achieved, which is sufficient. It is then crucial that the capsulorhexis is created with a normal size. For this purpose, the capsulorhexis is guided under the iris, which is easier with a needle than with forceps (see Fig. 4). Phacoemulsification is performed in the capsular bag using a chop technique, which reduces the risk of iris aspiration.

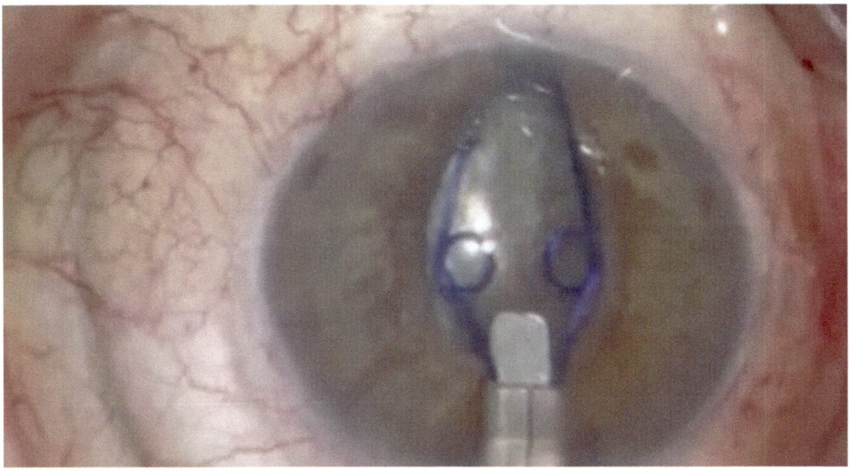

Video 4 Malyugin pupil expander in the case of a narrow pupil (▶ https://doi.org/10.1007/000-8dn)

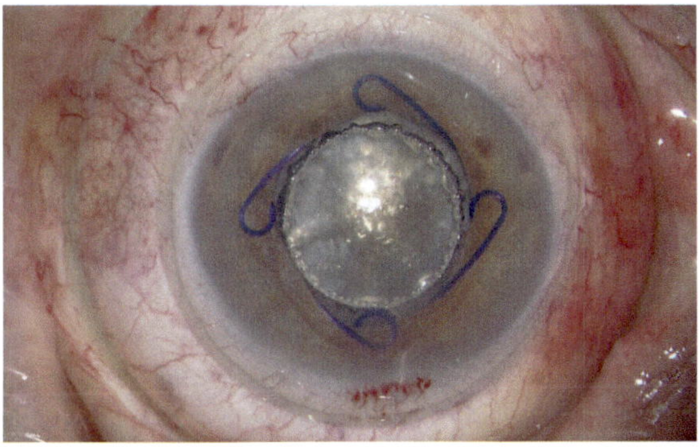

Fig. 3 Malyugin pupil expander in femto-assisted cataract surgery.

Author's recommendation

Mechanical pupil expanders can be helpful in selected cases. However, foregoing their use and performing the surgery when the pupil is not ideally dilated is the only way to spare the iris sphincter muscle.

The Narrow, Atonic Pupil in IFIS

Performing surgery on narrow, atonic pupils is entirely different, both with respect to the causative pathomechanism and the nature of the intraoperative problems. This type of pupil occurs mainly in IFIS, which was first described in 2005 in the context of tamsulosin [3]. Other drugs have since been reported to have similar

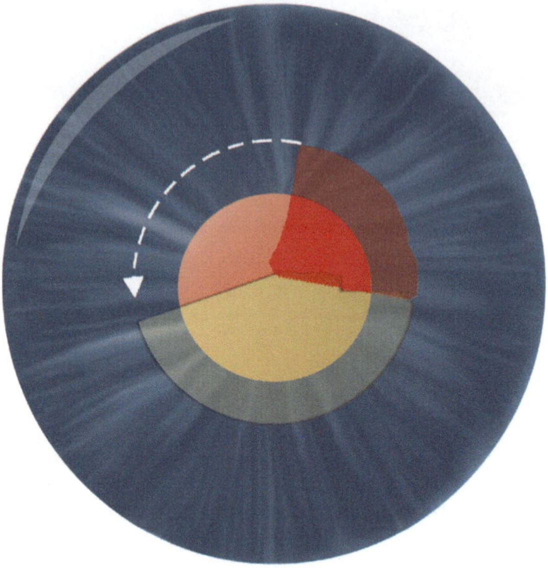

Fig. 4 Scheme of capsulorhexis underneath the iris without pupil expander with miotic pupil.

effects, but to a lesser extent. In addition to poor preoperative pupillary dilation, IFIS has a triad of typical intraoperative pathologies:

(1) Atonic, floppy iris
(2) Iris prolapse in tunnel incision and paracenteses
(3) Progressive intraoperative miosis

The severity of IFIS is variable, with only 10% of all tamsulosin patients showing no IFIS signs at all, while half show a severe manifestation. Large studies show a twofold increase in the rate of severe postoperative complications [2]. Typically, the pupil and iris appear reasonably wide or stable at the beginning of surgery, but become increasingly atonic and floppy as the surgery progresses, therefore, most complications occur later in the surgery.

This slow onset and then markedly escalating course illustrates well why prevention is more important than management in IFIS. With the appropriate measures and preoperative identification of patients at risk, we can often prevent the most severe course and the complications that follow.

A patient's history should not only be screened for tamsulosin but also for other drugs with similar effects. It should be considered that women are increasingly treated with tamsulosin for urinary tract problems [5]. The most important prognostic warning sign for a severe course is poor preoperative mydriasis, while mild and moderate degrees of severity usually show sufficient mydriasis at the beginning and progressive miosis only during the course of surgery. Unfortunately, studies have shown that preoperative discontinuation of tamsulosin is ineffective [6].

Surgical Management of IFIS

To date, there is no proven protocol for preventing IFIS. However, several measures can significantly reduce the risk. Preoperatively, maximum dilatation should be attempted. In some studies, atropine has also been shown to be additively effective [10]. Even if the pupil does not dilate, this form of prophylaxis stiffens the iris tissue, reduces fluctuation, and decreases the risk for progressive intraoperative miosis later in the surgical procedure.

The same effect is achieved by the intracameral injection of alpha agonists such as phenylephrine or epinephrine. We use 1:000 epinephrine along with the intracameral local anesthetic lidocaine, which has a supportive effect. Mydrane® (tropicamide 0.02% + phenyephrine 0.31% + lidocaine 1%, Thea Pharma) is a new on-label drug that also achieves this effect. In addition, adding epinephrine to the irrigation fluid has a beneficial effect [4], for dosage details, see above.

The onset of surgery is mostly free of complications. The pupil is usually moderately dilated, and in the viscoelastic-filled anterior chamber the atonic iris tissue is unproblematic. This time must be used for the largest possible capsulorhexis, which is pulled under the iris (see Fig. 4).

Here, it is important to understand the mechanism of how both iris flaccidity and miosis develop during surgery. The crucial factor is the irritation of the iris, which continuously increases during the course of the surgery. Two mechanisms are causative:

- One mechanism is continuous fluid convection, which irritates the iris. Therefore, it is crucial to keep irrigation low, with plenty of occlusion and little suction; a phaco chop requires less irrigation than a groove technique. In particular, the tunnel incision should be smaller than usual to completely seal the phaco tip, at the potential cost of mild corneal burn. Also, the paracenteses should be created flatter and more corneal than usual in order to make iris prolapse more difficult.
- Second, any contact with the iris must be prevented. For this very reason, mechanical pupil dilation strategies are largely contraindicated. In particular, iris stretching provokes iris irritation and is more likely to result in reactive miosis rather than dilation. Similarly, iris retractors that additionally pull the iris diaphragm upwards promote prolapse of the iris base and make iris contact by the phaco tip or bimanual I/A instruments more likely.

Only pupil expanders such as the Malyugin ring are still popular in IFIS surgery, but their beneficial effect is small because the iris stimulus promotes the fluctuation of the peripheral iris. In other words, a Malyugin ring does not prevent prolapse of the iris base, but it does prevent complete iris prolapse.

The reduction of flow parameters is an important factor in preventing iris damage. When the pupil is narrow, the iris tissue is closer to the zone of high fluid flow. Therefore, the phaco tip and I/A instruments should be held in a central position with minimal movement to prevent iris damage. Many surgeons perform the core fragmentation completely inside the capsular bag because this allows the fluidic flow to be localized inside the capsular bag. Other surgeons argue the converse and advocate an anterior chamber phaco because the fluid flow pushes the iris backwards. The tri-soft-shell technique may have some value here in stabilizing the iris diaphragm and limiting the flow dynamics [1].

Author's recommendation

In IFIS surgery, the maximum possible mechanical pupil dilation is not the decisive factor. Much more important is an iris-preserving surgical procedure with little fluid convection; tight, anteriorly created incisions; and motionless nucleus processing with controlled, centrally held instruments without iris contact (Video 5).

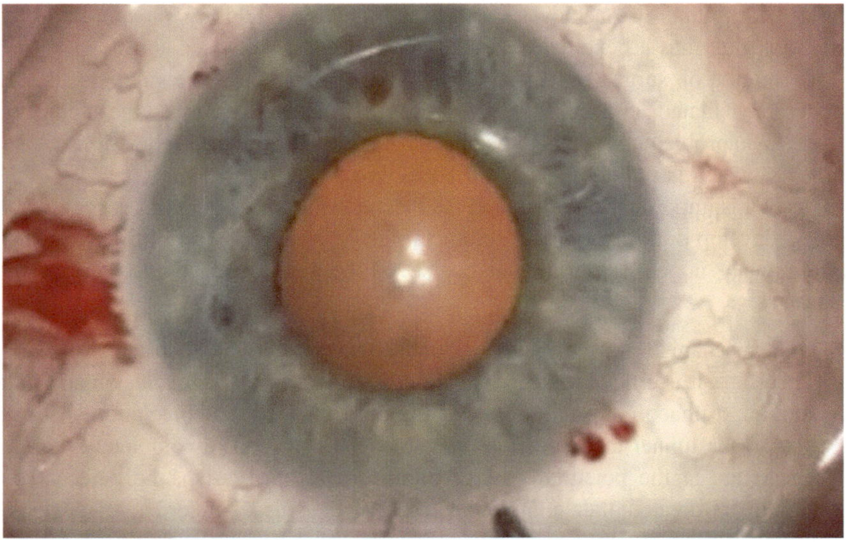

Video 5 Surgery for IFIS without pupil expander (▶ https://doi.org/10.1007/000-8dp)

Iris Prolapse

Iris prolapse is a serious complication that cataract surgeons seek to avoid. Causes may include tunnel incisions that are too wide and too short, or vitreous pressure, but iris prolapse most commonly occurs in the setting of IFIS, typically later in the course of cataract surgery. Recurrent prolapse, as is typical with IFIS, results in serious, permanent damage with iris transillumination, pupil de-rounding, and atony. Therefore, the above-mentioned prevention strategies are of paramount importance. However, once iris prolapse has occurred, rapid and consistent action is required.

The immediate generation of hypotension is crucial for management: switching off the infusion, draining fluid by applying pressure to the paracenteses, and flattening the anterior chamber. Only then may the phaco tip be removed and the iris repositioned. Often the iris falls back on its own as a result of the hypotony; if not, the iris should not be actively pushed back. This can be done more gently by carefully tapping on the tunnel lip or carefully pushing it back with a viscoelastic. Only in the case of failure should the iris be rubbed back from the inside.

With IFIS, the phaco should not be continued in the same manner afterwards. The hope for a one-off event is usually in vain. In IFIS, an iris prolapse will occur progressively with increasing frequency and extension, as the prolapse-related iris irritation further intensifies the atony. Supporting measures for the iris base, such as placing a viscoelastic depot under the tunnel or iris retractors next to the tunnel, are also not sustainable. The best solution is a consistent "new start' by suturing the tunnel incision and creating a new tunnel incision at a different site—one that is more corneal, longer, and tighter. Repeated intracameral administration of epinephrine and lidocaine is helpful, but it does not solve the problem at this stage. The subsequent implantation of a pupil expander is also hardly helpful here, but in severe cases it can at least protect the pupillary margin. The conscientious control of the fluid dynamics in the further course with low infusion pressure is more important, along with attentiveness towards the direction of the irrigation jet and rapid completion of the surgery.

Memo
Careful attention to fluid dynamics can prevent this frustrating complication.

Direct Injuries to the Iris

A mechanical injury to the iris typically occurs as a result of narrow pupils with or without IFIS and also inattention. Touching or aspiration of the iris into a handpiece without ultrasound energy usually causes minor iris defects, and significantly greater damage is done when aspirating with ultrasound activation. In these cases, immediate hypotension helps, and only then, if necessary, aspiration with a second instrument. Possible bleeding usually stops when the anterior chamber pressure is increased and only rarely needs to be coagulated.

In the damaged area, usually only the frayed iris fibrils remain, which repeatedly leads to further aspiration. In these cases, a pupil expander such as the Malyugin ring is useful.

Author's recommendation

If, in rare cases, an extensive iris defect or tissue loss occurs, a two-step approach to iris reconstruction is preferable. In simultaneous procedures, the irritation caused by iris injury and iris reconstruction potentiate and reinforce each other (see Chap. 57).

Conclusion

Cataract surgery for narrow and especially atonic pupils is challenging. Most surgical maneuvers for pupil dilation are not reliable and cause microtears in the iris sphincter. Therefore, primary prevention is by far the preferable measure and usually prevents a severe course. As always in iris surgery, the gentlest route is usually the best.

References

1. Arshinoff SA, Norman R. Tri-soft shell technique. J Cataract Refract Surg. 2013;39:1196–203.
2. Bell CM, Hatch WV, Fischer HD, et al. Association between tamsulosin and serious ophthalmic adverse events in older men following cataract surgery. JAMA. 2009;301:1991–6.
3. Chang DF, Campbell JR. Intraoperative floppy iris syndrome associated with tamsulosin. J Cataract Refract Surg. 2005;31:664–73.
4. Chang DF, Campbell JR, Colin J, et al. Intraoperative floppy iris syndrome severity with tamsulosin versus alfusosin. Ophthalmology. 2014;121:829–34.
5. Chang SJ, Chiang IN, Yu HJ. The effectiveness of tamsulosin in treating women with voiding difficulty. Int J Urol. 2008;15:981–5.
6. Chang DF, Osher RH, Wang L, et al. Prospective multicenter evaluation of cataract surgery in patients taking tamsulosin (Flomax). Ophthalmology. 2007;114:957–64.
7. Dinsmore SC. Modified stretch technique for small pupil phacoemulsification with topical anesthesia. J Cataract Refract Surg. 1996;22:27–30.
8. Lorente R, de Rojas V, Vázquez de Parga P, et al. Intracameral phenylephrine 1.5% for prophylaxis against intraoperative floppy iris syndrome: prospective, randomized fellow eye study. Ophthalmology. 2012;119:2053–8.
9. Malyugin B. Small pupil phaco surgery: a new technique. Ann Ophthalmol. 2007;39:185–93.
10. Nuzzi R, Arnoffi P, Tridico F. Best prophylactic strategy in groups at risk of intraoperative floppy iris syndrome development: comparison between atropine instillation and adrenaline intracameral injection. Open Ophthalmol J. 2018;12:34–40.
11. Shugar JK. Intracameral epinephrine for prophylaxis of IFIS. J Cataract Refract Surg. 2006;32:1074–5.
12. Szurman P, Heiligenhaus A, Hettlich HJ, et al. Kataraktchirurgie bei Uveitis im Kindesalter. Klin Monatsbl Augenheilkd. 2007;224:532–7.
13. Yuguchi T, Oshika T, Sawaguchi S, et al. Pupillary functions after cataract surgery using flexible iris retractor in patients with small pupil. Jpn J Ophthalmol. 1999;43:20–4.

Zonular Disorders and Management in Cataract Surgery

Thomas C. Kreutzer and Jeffrey Caspar

Introduction

Preexisting phacodonesis or intraoperative development of a zonular dehiscence can be challenging, even for the most experienced anterior segment surgeon. Risk factors for zonular insufficiency during cataract surgery include high myopia, advanced age, pseudoexfoliation syndrome, connective tissue diseases such as Marfan syndrome, prior ophthalmic procedures such as vitrectomy, intravitreal injections or trabeculectomy and eyes suffering from previous trauma. Surgeons noting preoperative phacodonesis should know that they are in for a challenging surgery. This chapter discusses surgical options to better manage these technically demanding cases.

Pre-existing phacodonesis visible at the slit lamp or a clearly dislocated crystalline lens confirm the presence of zonular damage. Other, more subtle signs such as chronic mydriasis after trauma or a shallow anterior chamber in the setting of pseudoexfoliation syndrome should also alert the surgeon to likely zonular weakness. In such cases, consideration should be made for possible peribulbar, retrobulbar or general anesthesia during the procedure to allow for maximum flexibility of techniques. Appropriate surgical devices such as capsular retention hooks, capsular tension rings and ring segments as well as proper suture and lens implants to allow for possible scleral or iris fixation should be available. IOL calculations should be prepared in anticipation for a possible scleral sutured, iris fixated or anterior chamber lens implant. Ideally, any clear corneal surgical approach should be chosen in a way

Supplementary Information The online version contains supplementary material available at https://doi.org/10.1007/978-3-031-05394-8_54. The videos can be accessed individually by clicking the DOI link in the accompanying figure caption or by scanning this link with the SN More Media App.

T. C. Kreutzer (✉) · J. Caspar
München, Germany
e-mail: thomas.kreutzer@med.uni-muenchen.de

M. Shajari et al. (eds.), *Cataract and Lens Surgery*,
https://doi.org/10.1007/978-3-031-05394-8_54

such that conversion to a sclero-corneal approach remains possible, if needed as a backup. Alternatively, phacoemulsification can be performed using a sclero-corneal incision primarily, which can then be enlarged if necessary. Intraoperatively, zonular weakness typically becomes apparent during capsulorhexis with increased mobility of the lens and capsular wrinkling due to laxity. Care must be taken to ensure that the capsulorhexis is not too small, at least 5.5 mm in diameter, to avoid additional stress and further damage to the weakened zonules during lens manipulation and to increase the success of subsequent hydrodissection and hydrodelineation. A small capsulorhexis can also contribute to postoperative capsular phimosis, which can result in further capsular contraction and stress to the zonules.

Author's recommendation

The capsulorhexis should initially be started in the area of intact zonular fibers, tearing toward the weakened zonules. Starting the capsulorhexis through the paracentesis leaves the option of choosing the location of the primary surgical incision later if the lens turns out to be too mobile for safe removal via phacoemulsification. It also provides for a more stable and deeper anterior chamber during capsulorhexis.

Mastering a "horizontal phaco chop" and "cross chop" technique for medium-hard and hard lens material or the "phaco roll" technique for soft lenses reduces the stress on the zonules during phacoemulsification [1]. During irrigation/aspiration of the cortex material, the use of a dispersive viscoelastic to inflate the capsular bag can serve as a "third hand", supporting the capsule and reducing stress on the zonules. Aspirating and peeling the cortex tangential to the capsulorhexis helps to protect the remaining zonular fibers by spreading the force over a larger area, when compared to peeling radially [2]. In case of sectorial zonular defects of less than three clock hours, it is usually sufficient to place one of the haptics of the intraocular lens in the area of the zonular defect to achieve sufficient capsular support. A three-piece IOL with more rigid haptics provides better capsular support than a one-piece style lens. Slowly opening hydrophobic, one-piece lens implants, however, allow for a gentler implantation with less capsular stress. In larger zonular defects of up to 5 clock hours with an associated decentration of the capsular bag, at a minimum, a capsular tension ring should be used to support the capsular equator and help center the lens implant (Video 1). A bimanual technique of implantation, directing the tip of the ring with a second instrument, can be useful to preserve the remaining zonular fibers during implantation.

Zonular dehiscence of greater than 5 h usually requires capsular fixation techniques. One option is the use of a Cionni modified capsular tension ring, which can stabilize the affected hemisphere when fixated with a 10.0, or better yet, 9.0 prolene suture to the sclera. As introduction of a Cionni modified capsular tension ring into an unstable capsular bag can be quite challenging, an alternative approach is the use of an Ahmed capsular tension segment (Video 2) [3]. These can be gently implanted under viscoelastic through the clear corneal incision and then scleral fixated with suture without significant stress on the remaining zonules.

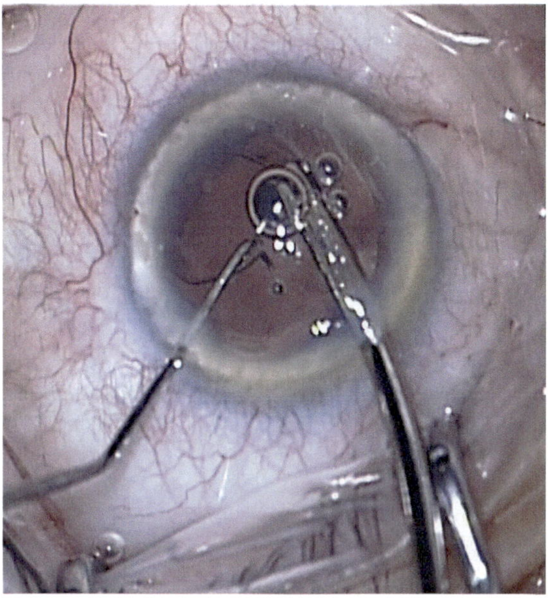

Video 1 Bimanual implantation of a capsule tension ring in sectorial zonulolysis (▶ https://doi.org/10.1007/000-8dr)

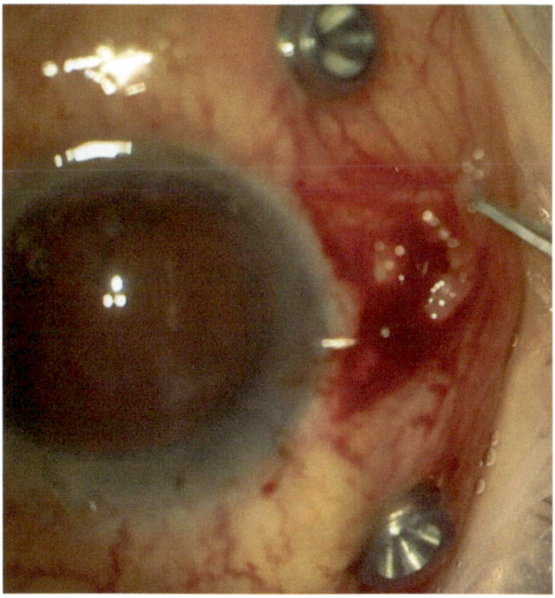

Video 2 Use of an Ahmed capsular tension segment in a case of five clock hours of zonular dehiscence after blunt trauma (▶ https://doi.org/10.1007/000-8dq)

A capsular tension ring can be extremely useful in difficult situations (Video 3). However, if it becomes apparent during surgery that safe phacoemulsification is not possible due to significant mobility of the crystalline lens, other surgical options should be considered. The capsular bag can be stabilized during phacoemulsification by using special capsular holding hooks or even iris hooks placed within the capsulotomy. Alternatively, it is possible to switch to an ECCE or ICCE procedure. This requires a sufficiently large sclero-corneal incision of up to 10 mm, depending on the approach and whether or not bisection of the lens nucleus could be accomplished. The mobile lens and corneal endothelium should be cushioned with a dispersive viscoelastic. If vitreous prolapse has also occurred, this should be managed first before lens removal.

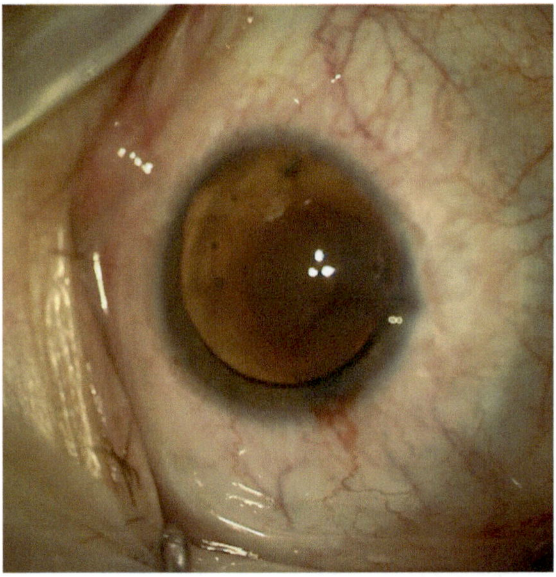

Video 3 Phacoemulsification with pronounced phacodonesis with an iris-choroidal coloboma and implantation of a capsular tension ring (▶ https://doi.org/10.1007/000-8ds)

The likelihood of capsular complications, especially posterior capsular rupture, is significantly increased in cases of zonular dehiscence. Due to possible fluid flow through the area of zonular weakness into the vitreous cavity, sudden forward displacement of the posterior capsule can occur, or the capsular bag can collapse (Aqueous Misdirection Syndrome), especially at the time of final lens fragment removal. The risk of fluid misdirection is increased with high bottle heights or intraocular pressure settings. The targeted use of a dispersive or viscoadaptive viscoelastics into the capsular bag and at the area of zonular weakness can reduce the risk by keeping the capsule away from the phacoemulsification tip and while resisting aspiration. If a capsular rupture does occur, a capsular tension ring implantation should not be considered unless the posterior capsular rupture can be contained with a stable posterior capsulotomy. However, in situations of significant zonular weakness, a posterior capsulotomy can be extremely difficult. Another problem associated with posterior capsular rupture is that stable sulcus implantation of the lens implant may not be possible. If sulcus placement of the lens is considered, the optic of the lens implant should a be captured in the anterior rhexis to achieve more stable fixation. The haptics should be placed in the sulcus 90 degrees away from the area of zonular dehiscence and the optic captured first in the area of zonular weakness and then put behind the intact rhexis at the area of stable zonules. In case of doubt, in these then highly complex cases, implantation of a lens implant may be omitted, a complete anterior vitrectomy performed, the incision closed, and implantation of a lens implant left for a second operation. This can be a suitably planned anterior chamber lens, iris claw lens or scleral fixated lens implant.

In cases of zonular dehiscence, the use of trypan blue can be associated with an unpleasant surprise. The dye can migrate into the vitreous cavity through the zonular dehiscence during injection into the anterior chamber, resulting in a sudden loss of the red reflex. Therefore, if zonular dehiscence is suspected, it is advisable, to either refrain from using such dyes or to carefully inject it only into the anterior chamber after use of viscoelastic as a shield in the area of zonular dehiscence. This migration in the vitreous itself is not dangerous but does make for a very difficult surgery.

Keypoint

Weaknesses of the zonules supporting the crystalline can make cataract surgery a challenging situation even for experienced surgeons. The success of such operations is often decided during the capsulorhexis. Therefore, a well-considered and controlled procedure is crucial in these challenging cases.

Author's recommendation

A sufficiently large rhexis of at least 5.5 mm is the foundation of a successful removal of the lens in cases of zonular weakness. In these cases, it is therefore advisable to construct the necessary wound for removal of the lens after opening of the capsule, as the stability of the zonules can usually be assessed at this step.

References

1. Jacob S. Different methods of chopping in cataract surgery. Curr Opin Ophthalmol. 2019;30(1):25–38.
2. Nakano CT, Motta AF, Hida WT, Nakamura CM, Tzelikis PF, Ruiz Alves M, et al. hurricane cortical aspiration technique: one-step continuous circular aspiration maneuver. J Cataract Refract Surg. 2014;40(4):514–6.
3. Hasanee K, Butler M, Ahmed II. Capsular tension rings and related devices: current concepts. Curr Opin Ophthalmol. 2006;17(1):31–41.

Complication Management in Case of Damage to the Lens Capsule or Loss of Lens Fragments

Thomas C. Kreutzer and Sorcha Ní Dhubhghaill

Introduction

The posterior capsular rupture (PCR) has an incidence of 0.4–7%, depending on the study [1]. While radial tears in the anterior capsule are the most common form, if they do not extend behind to the posterior capsule, they are usually relatively easy to manage and far less problematic. Factors that influence the incidence of PCR are mainly the experience of the cataract surgeon and the complexity of the surgery (including PEX, diabetes, hardness of the lens) [2, 3]. If lens fragments fall through the rupture into the vitreous cavity, a second vitreoretinal surgery is usually necessary. This chapter describes measures and techniques for managing capsular defects and avoiding the problematic loss of lens fragments.

Radial tears in the anterior lens capsule, are much more frequent than posterior capsular ruptures though are typically far more benign. These can occur as a result of instrument contact (e.g. the chopper) during lens removal, while performing the capsulorhexis with a cystotome and the rhexis edge running out, as a mechanical tear during anterior capsular polishing (especially with reusable instruments) or in incomplete capsulorhexis created by a femtosecond laser. If these radial tears do not run out past the equator to the posterior capsule, they can usually be rounded off to create a somewhat larger, but continuous curvilinear capsulorhexis. In these cases, implantation of the intraocular lens implant in the capsular bag can usually be achieved but the implantation of plate haptic lenses should be avoided if an unstable radial tear is present.

Supplementary Information The online version contains supplementary material available at https://doi.org/10.1007/978-3-031-05394-8_55. The videos can be accessed individually by clicking the DOI link in the accompanying figure caption or by scanning this link with the SN More Media App.

T. C. Kreutzer (✉) · S. N. Dhubhghaill
München, Germany
e-mail: thomas.kreutzer@med.uni-muenchen.de

M. Shajari et al. (eds.), *Cataract and Lens Surgery*,
https://doi.org/10.1007/978-3-031-05394-8_55

If a radial tear occurs, an attempt should always be made to convert it into a stable form. If the edge of the tear is visible, this can be achieved by using a capsular rhexis forceps and grasping the edge of the capsular flap and pulling opposite to the course of the tear (Little's rhexis rescue technique). Alternatively, incising the anterior capsule elsewhere and creating a new break in the opposite direction of the tear, and widening the capsulorhexis can be helpful. The idea is to integrate the original tear into this newer capsulorhexis edge and can result in a strange triangle pointing inwards shape, but a safe rhexis overall.

If the outer edge of the tear is no longer visible, the surgery can and must continue but it is important to continue as carefully as possible. A gentle but complete hydrodissection, reduced infusion pressure, as well as a phaco chop technique, which allows the tension to run perpendicular to the tears edge and not across it, and the consistent use of viscoelastic are valuable options to help prevent extension of the tear posteriorly. In most cases, the natural lens can be removed without extending the radial tear to the posterior capsule. During irrigation and aspiration, the cortex in the area of the tear should be approached last and suction of cortex parts should always be performed pulling towards the tear, and not away from it. Before an intraocular lens is implanted, a prolapse of vitreous in the area of the tear must be excluded. A slowly opening hydrophopic one-piece intraocular lenses is well suited for implantation in such a capsular bag. The haptics should be at 90° away from the tear to maximize stable positioning of the implant. Here too, slow and controlled implantation is crucial. When a radial tear does run out onto the posterior capsule, the resulting damage to the bag renders it incompatible with standard intraocular lens implantation (without additional fixation techniques). After the necessary anterior vitrectomy, a firm, secure position for the implant in the sulcus ciliaris is usually not guaranteed either. It is then recommended that an alternative implant be selected; an anterior chamber lens, iris claw lens or scleral fixated lens are all excellent options but in the event that this is not possible or the surgeon too inexperienced, it is always acceptable to perform a thorough anterior vitrectomy, close all incisions and leave the eye aphakic until the lens can be placed in a secondary step, under controlled conditions.

Remember

A posterior capsular rupture is indicated by a sudden deepening of the anterior chamber which then becomes shallow and unstable.

The posterior capsular rupture is indicated by a sudden deepening of the anterior chamber followed by sudden shallow and unstable anterior chamber. When this occurs, it is important to avoid the "burn hand reflex" and not to remove the infusion abruptly from the eye. Doing so usually leads to an immediate prolapse of vitreous body material and extension of the tear. Instead, the surgeon should remain calm and attempt to stabilize the anterior chamber. Lowering the infusion pressure reduces the mechanical stress on the posterior capsule, replacing the second hand instrument with a viscoelastic cannula and gently filling the anterior chamber with viscoelastic allows initial stabilization of the anterior chamber. The instruments can then be removed and the extent of problem inspected. By cushioning the remaining lens fragments with a dispersive or viscoadaptive viscoelastic, a loss of lens material into the vitreous cavity can be counteracted. If a vitreous prolapse is present, it must first of course be removed. Staining the vitreous in the anterior chamber with triamcinolone acetate can act like a "sheet over the ghost" and greatly aid in visualizing the extent of the vitreal prolapse but also reduces contrast due to the diffuse opacification of the vitreous cavity with triamcinolone crystals. The remaining lens fragments can then be phacoemulsified by adding viscoelastic. In doing so, it is important to ensure that vitreous material is kept away from the phaco-tip. After the lens fragments have been removed, the irrigation/aspiration of cortex remnants is performed. This can be carried out with a vitreous cutter and, at the same time enables the removal of any vitreous strands that may prolapse in the anterior chamber during the cleaning. It is important to note that the infusion should only be removed after stabilization of the anterior chamber with viscoelastic in order to counteract any subsequent surge and displacement of vitreous and thus, possible widening of the posterior capsule tear. After the cortex has been removed and a remaining prolapse of vitreous material managed, the chamber should then be reformed with viscoelastic. Now the extent of the posterior capsular tear determines further maneuvers. In the case of a small posterior tear, an attempt can be made to convert it into a stable, round posterior capsular opening with a capsulorhexis forceps. If the tear can be successfully converted into a posterior capsulorhexis with a size of ≤ 5 mm, very careful implantation of the artificial lens into the capsular bag is possible. It is important to remove vitreous material behind the enlarged posterior opening, as the incarceration of vitreous material between posterior capsular rhexis and lens optic significantly increases the later occurrence of a retinal detachment. If the posterior capsular tear cannot be stabilized and the anterior capsulorhexis is intact, a suitable intraocular lens can be implanted in the ciliary sulcus. Here, three-piece intraocular lens models are preferred due to their usually larger diameter and the possibility of capturing the optic in the anterior capsulorhexis (optic capture), or both anterior and posterior capsulorhexis (posterior optic buttonholing). This way a permanently stable and centered lens positioning can be achieved in a centered capsulorhexis. The refractive power of the artificial lens must be reduced accordingly, when positioned in the ciliary sulcus compared to a capsular bag implantation. A helpful estimate on the extend of power reduction when implanting a lens into the sulcus as opposed to in the bag implantation can be found on the website of Dr. Warren Hill. [4] We advise printing out this guide and storing it together with the stock of 3-piece IOLs. A stable positioning of the artificial lens in the ciliary sulcus is also important because the posterior capsule rupture significantly increases the risk of further complications such as retinal detachment and postoperative endophthalmitis (Video 1). With a stable, well-positioned intraocular lens vitreoretinal surgery becomes less complicated.

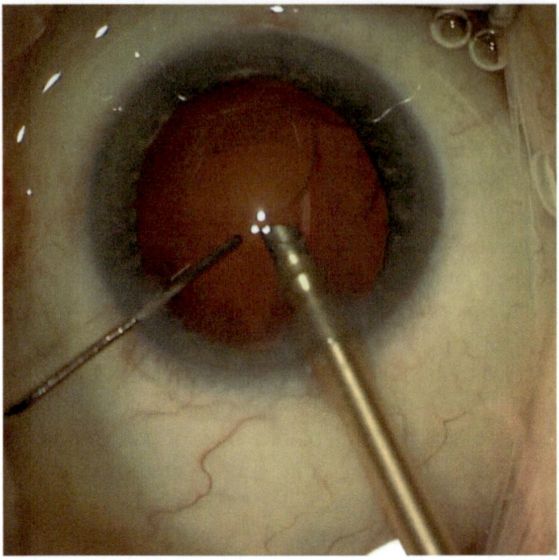

Video 1 Posterior capsule rupture and treatment during lens surgery of a mature cataract (▶ https://doi.org/10.1007/000-8dv)

Careless management decisions of the anterior segment surgeon make further treatment by the vitreoretinal surgeon more difficult e.g. an unstable positioned artificial lens that falls into the posterior segment. Although clear data on this is lacking, the author, who is also a vitreoretinal surgeon, recommends not to implant lenses composed of silicone optics on the basis of his own experience in the treatment of complications after lens surgery, as these often tend to get clouded optics during complex retinal surgery.

Posterior capsular rupture is the most common serious complication of lens surgery, but it can still result in a good outcome for the patient, provided, it is done in a controlled manner (Video 2). In such complicated cases it is essential to remain calm. It is important to realize that although the posterior capsular rupture may be a personal defeat, any hasted and uncontrolled surgical step can prevent a good result for the patient. Therefore, further measures should always be taken in honest consideration of one's own experience and complication management skills. Stabilization of the situation with removal of prolapsed vitreous and termination of the surgery despite remaining lens fragments and sealing of the operation wounds should not be seen as a "failure" by a young surgeon and enables a surgeon experienced in the management of complication to achieve a good result in a second surgery [5]. Rushed and uncontrolled phacoemulsification of lens fragments with prolapsed vitreous, uncontrolled dilation of a corneal incision and extrusion of lens fragments with subsequent insufficient suturing can lead to irreversible damage. The most important factors are the preservation of anterior chamber stability and a pressurized eye, the consistent removal of prolapsed vitreous material and only then the removal of lens components. The loss of lens material into the vitreous chamber

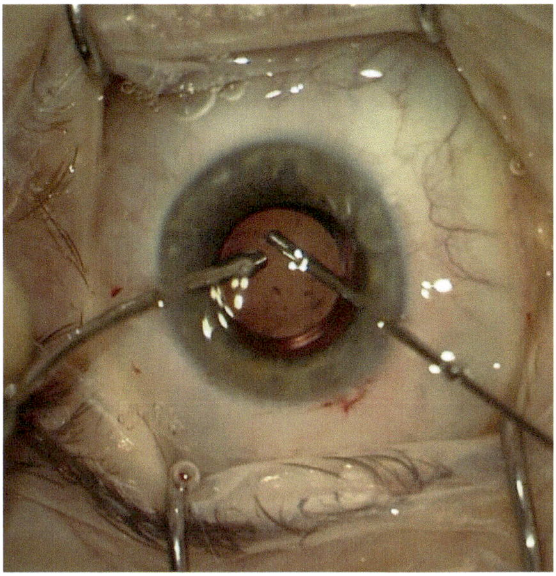

Video 2 Posterior capsular rupture after artificial lens implantation. Artificial lens exchange and management (▶ https://doi.org/10.1007/000-8dt)

through the posterior capsular tear usually requires further treatment by a vitreoretinal surgeon. While it may appear tempting, the anterior segment surgeon should never try to fish them out. The aim is to stabilize the eye using vitrectomy and sutures and to refer the patient. The author is of the opinion that a lens implantation should not be carried out if further treatment is necessary anyway, as this gives the second surgeon all options. It is then helpful to provide the patient with biometric results to the level of the primary surgery.

Author's recommendation

The posterior capsular rupture is a complication that can occur even with the most experienced surgeon. It is crucial to remain calm and to carefully perform the necessary steps of complication management. A rushed procedure or measures taken in haste or uncertainty can cause unnecessary and permanent damage to the eye.

References

1. Grinton M, Sandhu J, Shwe-Tin A, Steel DHW, Ting DSJ, North East Trainee Research in Ophthalmology N. Incidence, characteristics, outcomes and confidence in managing posterior capsular rupture during cataract surgery in the UK: an ophthalmology trainees' perspective Eye. 2020.
2. Rutar T, Porco TC, Naseri A. Risk factors for intraoperative complications in resident-performed phacoemulsification surgery. Ophthalmology. 2009;116(3):431–6. https://doi.org/10.1016/j.ophtha.2008.10.028 Epub 2009 Jan 22 PMID: 19167084.

3. Zare M, Javadi MA, Einollahi B, Baradaran-Rafii AR, Feizi S, Kiavash V. Risk Factors for Posterior Capsule Rupture and Vitreous Loss during Phacoemulsification. J Ophthalmic Vis Res. 2009 Oct;4(4):208–12. PMID: 23198076; PMCID: PMC3498858.
4. Hill W. Calculating bag vs Sulcus IOL Power. Website. https://doctor-hill.com/iol-power-calculations/bag-vs-sulcus/ (2021)
5. Hong AR, Sheybani A, Huang AJ. Intraoperative management of posterior capsular rupture. Curr Opin Ophthalmol. 2015;26(1):16–21. https://doi.org/10.1097/ICU.0000000000000113 PMID: 25390858.

Extracapsular and Intracapsular Cataract Extraction

Thomas C. Kreutzer

Introduction

Thanks to modern phacoemulsification machines, the ECCE and ICCE expression of the natural lens has become very rare in western industrialized countries. Through the targeted use of modern viscoelastics in conjunction with current phacoemulsification machines and phaco chop techniques, even some of the hardest lens nuclei can be removed successfully and the loss of endothelial cell scan be prevented even via small incision surgery. Hard lens nuclei in combination with a loose zonula apparatus are particularly problematic however. Here the possible conversion of phacoemulsification to ECCE or ICCE or even primary ICCE technique can still play an important role so it is important for cataract surgeons to understand the fundamentals of these techniques. The training of surgeons in the correct construction of a sclero-corneal tunnel which necessary in these techniques is of great importance but usually only takes place in large surgical centers or university hospitals with a frequent occurrence of such complex cases. However, it is extremely useful for every lens surgeon to master the preparation of a sclero-corneal tunnel (Video 1).

Supplementary Information The online version contains supplementary material available at https://doi.org/10.1007/978-3-031-05394-8_56. The videos can be accessed individually by clicking the DOI link in the accompanying figure caption or by scanning this link with the SN More Media App.

T. C. Kreutzer (✉)
München, Germany
e-mail: thomas.kreutzer@med.uni-muenchen.de

M. Shajari et al. (eds.), *Cataract and Lens Surgery*,
https://doi.org/10.1007/978-3-031-05394-8_56

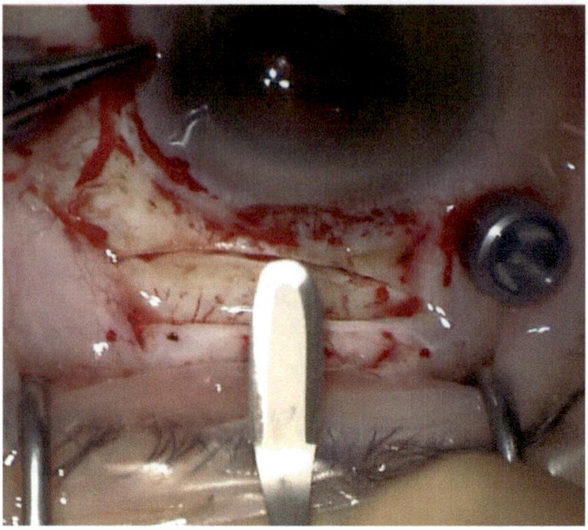

Video 1 Preparation of a large sclero-corneal tunnel before ICCE
(▶ https://doi.org/10.1007/000-8dx)

The basis of an ECCE or ICCE is a sclero-corneal approach. Although a sclero-corneal tunnel induces less astigmatism when compared to clear corneal incisions of equal size, in these cases, the incision is likely to be far larger than the standard clear corneal cataract incision. While the greater distance from the optical centre can be helpful in sclero-corneal tunnels, the sheer size of the means that attention should be paid to their astigmatic effect [1]. Approaching from the temporal side, where possible, further reduces induced astigmatism. While a superior approach can offer additional protection for the wound by the eyelids, the negative effect for future glaucoma surgery should be considered.

When creating a sclero-corneal incision, first, the conjunctiva and tenons capsule are opened at the limbus according to the required width of the access and bluntly dissected from the sclera in a posterior direction. For larger tunnel width, the conjunctiva and tenon's capsule can be incised wider to achieve better access. Episcleral bleeding is reduced by cauterisation. A sufficiently wide scleral groove (ECCE min. 6–7 mm, ICCE (min. 10 mm) of 30–50% of the sclera is incised approx. 2 mm post-limbally with the 15° blade.

An arched "frown-shaped" incision reduces the astigmatic effect compared to a straight construction and also has a higher probability of watertightness [2]. The sclera is then split along the lamellae in the direction of the cornea with a tunnel knife to create a scleral pocket terminating about 1 mm intra-corneally. Care should be taken to ensure that the eye is well pressurized (if necessary, by injecting a viscoelastic into the anterior chamber via a paracentesis) and that the eye is held firmly in position during preparation with a toothed forceps. The preparation is started centrally and then widened on both sides with attention being paid to the position of the tunnel knife in relation to the curve of the scleral wall during lateral preparation in order to avoid cutting through the upper scleral flap (buttenhole, scleral tear). This also applies to the central preparation. If the pocket preparation is too steep, the anterior chamber is penetrated too early through the sclera and not through the cornea. This in turn results in a significantly increased tendency of iris prolapse and bleeding during the subsequent surgery. The central opening of the tunnel is then carried out with a clear cornea incision knife. The cornea is incised initially centrally and can then be extended sideways. The inner lip of the tunnel can be made larger than the outer lip to ensure easier removal of lens material. If the construction is clean, sclero-corneal wounds up to 6 mm are usually watertight, if larger or in case of doubt a suture should be made at the end. It is always better to have an unnecessary suture than a wound that leaks. A further advantage of the sclero-corneal tunnel is the possibility to create a sufficiently large opening for the phaco tip with the clear cornea incision knife, which is only opened further if it is necessary to switch to an ECCE or ICCE technique. The widening of clear corneal incisions to 5–6 mm, which the author repeatedly experiences in the context of management of complications, does not constitute proof of surgical skill.

In ECCE (Video 2), the anterior chamber is opened and, if necessary, stabilized with viscoelastic.

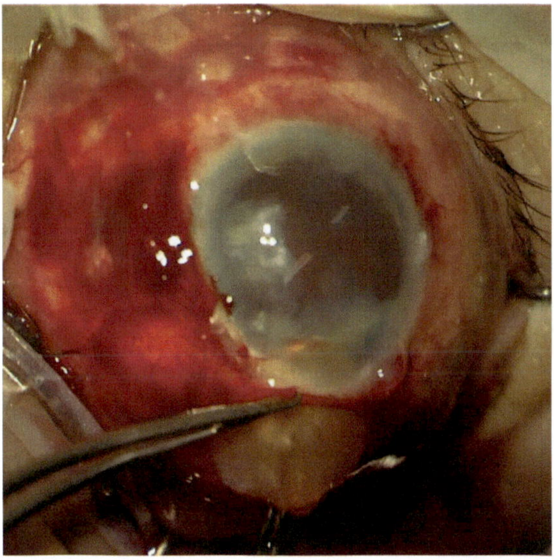

Video 2 ECCE extraction of the lens after changing from clear cornea incision to ECCE in a case of mature cataract, secondary narrow-angle glaucoma and zonulolysis (▶ https://doi.org/10.1007/000-8dw)

This is followed by the capsulorhexis, which in the case of ECCE must be at least 5.5 to 6 mm in size to express hard nuclei. During hydrodissection, the capsule content is luxated into the anterior chamber with a Sauter or lacrimal cannula and by careful hydrodissection. A small amount of viscoelastic material is then injected between the cornea and the lens material, to protect the endothelium. The lens can then be expressed out of the eye by holding the upper lip of the scleral flap at the central point with the toothed forceps and inserting an irrigation loop (Irrigating Vectis) under the lens material and applying pressure with the connected 5 mL syringe to the rear lower part of the lip. The loop should be slightly tilted in a superior direction. Care must be taken not to build up too much pressure, which could break the capsule or cause an iris prolapse with possible iris disruption. The risk is higher if the tunnel is too short. Further maneuvers of irrigation/aspiration of cortex remains is similar to the steps of a normal phacoemulsification. The artificial lens can be inserted into the capsular bag folded or unfolded and pushed through the tunnel using an implantation forceps. After removal of the residual viscoelastic, the eye is pressurized with hydration of the paracentheses and the sclero-corneal tunnel with balanced salt solution. If self-sealing and watertight, no suture is necessary. Otherwise, a suture should be placed with either a 9.0 or 7.0 Vicryl or a 9.0 or 10.0 nylon thread. The conjunctiva above the tunnel is then closed with a Vicryl thread or by spot cauterisation.

For ICCE (Video 3) a larger tunnel of at least 10 mm width is necessary. In the case of a loose zonulae, the entire lens can be luxated into the anterior chamber by using viscoelastic and a phaco spatula. It can then be pushed out of the eye with the rinsing loop, similar to the ECCE. Alternatively, the lens capsule can be frozen with a cryoprobe after viscoelastic application and extracted from the eye, attached to the probe. With ICCE, an anterior vitrectomy is always necessary afterwards. A lens implantation is carried out either in the anterior chamber (anterior chamber lens), as an iris claw lens (pre- or retropupillary) or in the form of a scleral-fixed artificial lens. Standard in-the-bag lens placement is never possible after and ICCE.

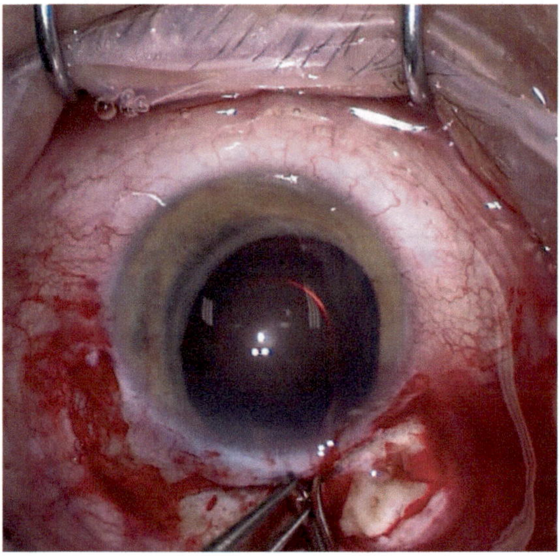

Video 3 ICCE extraction of a cataracta brunescens with subluxation followed by retropupillary fixation of an iris claw artificial lens (▶ https://doi.org/10.1007/000-8dy)

Keypoint
To master ECCE/ICCE—techniques construction of a sclero-corneal tunnel is of crucial importance. A clear corneal incision is possible in principle, but has major

disadvantages concerning stability, induction of astigmatism and increased risk of postoperative leakage, even when sutured.

Author's recommendation

In cases of severe pseudoexfolation or lentodonesis or eyes after trauma, it is advisable to only place the paracenteses and see how the capsulorhexis proceeds. If the mobility of the lens is already clearly visible, a primary sclero-corneal tunnel can be created for the removal of the lens. The presence of a clear corneal incision always makes the subsequent creation of a sclero-corneal tunnel more difficult.

References

1. Archana S, Khurana AK, Chawla U. A comparative study of sclero-corneal and clear corneal tunnel incision in manual small-incision cataract surgery. Nepalese J Ophthalmol Biannual peer-reviewed Acad J Nepal Ophthalmic Soc NEPJOPH. 201(1)–22.
2. Haldipurkar SS, Shikari HT, Gokhale V. Wound construction in manual small incision cataract surgery. Indian J Ophthalmol. 2009;57(1):9–13.

Biaxial (Bimanual) Microincisional Cataract Surgery

İzzet Can and Basak Bostanci Ceran

In the preface of 2010 book "Minimizing Incisions and Maximizing Outcomes in Cataract Surgery", editors Jorge L. Alio and I. Howard Fine stated the following—"Throughout this process, the history of cataract surgery has been related to the decrease in incision size" [1]. After Kelman's invention of phacoemulsification in 1967 [2], the technical advances in phaco devices and the ability to implant foldable intraocular lenses (IOLs) through small incisions, cataract surgery which was performed through 7.0 mm incisions in the 1970s, was reduced to 4.0 mm incisions in the 1990s down to the modern 2.2 mm and smaller incisions since the 2000s. Small incision surgeries have made great contributions to cataract surgery in terms of safety, functionality and effectiveness. These include shorter recovery time [3], less wound closure problems [4], less inflammation [5], less endophthalmitis risk [6], less risk of perioperative complications and haemorrhage [7], better protection of prolate shape and biomechanics of cornea and visual quality [8], as well as less surgically induced astigmatism [9–11] and higher-order aberrations [12].

Since this time, surgeries performed with 2.2 mm or smaller incisions were referred to as "microincisional cataract surgery" (MICS). MICS can be performed by two different methods. (1) Biaxial (=Bimanual) MICS, and (2) Microcoaxial MICS.

Biaxial MICS maintained its popularity with its advantages over microcoaxial MICS from the early 2000s to the mid-2010s, but in the following period, it lost its prominence as a result of the developments in the field of microcoaxial MICS, but it is worth mentioning that the smallest incisional cataract surgery in history was performed using the biaxial MICS method. Amar Agarwal performed pha-

Supplementary Information The online version contains supplementary material available at https://doi.org/10.1007/978-3-031-05394-8_57. The videos can be accessed individually by clicking the DOI link in the accompanying figure caption or by scanning this link with the SN More Media App.

İ. Can (✉) · B. B. Ceran
Ankara, Turkey
e-mail: izzetcan@yahoo.com

M. Shajari et al. (eds.), *Cataract and Lens Surgery*,
https://doi.org/10.1007/978-3-031-05394-8_57

coemulsification surgery in 2005 with the biaxial method through a 0.7 mm incision and called this operation "microphaconit" [13].

Biaxial Small Incisional Cataract Surgery Technique:

A. **Preparation and Anesthesia:** Anesthesia does not differ from standard phaco surgery. It can be performed under topical or peribulbar anesthesia, and intracameral anesthetic agents can be used. Agarwal has even applied this technique completely without anesthesia [14]. In our practice; cyclopentolate hydrochloride 1%, phenylephrine HCl and ketorolac tromethamine 0.5% are applied 3 times at five-minute intervals 30 min before surgery, and lidocaine HCl + adrenaline with bupivacaine hydrochloride soaked sponges are placed in the upper and lower fornixes and left for approximately 20 min. Anti-sepsis is provided by application of 5% povidone iodine solution into the conjunctival fornix for 3 min.
B. **Incision:** It is necessary to make 2 incisions to insert the chopper (which also provides irrigation), and the sleeveless phaco tip. The most common incision type is the 20 G incision, but 19 G incisions are also used. 22 G (0.7 mm) is the size of the incision recommended in the "microphaconit" technique [13]. For Biaxial-MICS, 2 incisions are made approximately 3–4 clock hour (90–110°) apart. Since one of the incisions will be enlarged for IOL insertion at the end of the surgery, this can be made on the steep axis at the beginning of the surgery. There are blades specially designed for this job, targeting 2 or 3 step wound site architecture to prevent leakage from the wound site and iris prolapse and the wound shape should be trapezoidal. The internal edge of the 20 G incision in the anterior chamber should be 1.2 mm wide and the outer edge should be 1.4 mm [15] (Fig. 1).

C. **Capsulorhexis:** Standard capsulorhexis forceps will not be suitable because the incision entrances are too small. Capsulorhexis is performed either with a needle, a cystotome device or using 23 G capsulorhexis forceps. (Fig. 2a–b). A problem that can be experienced with micro forceps is that the connection point behind the end of the forceps may be tucked inside the wound while passing near the incision site, reducing the maneuverability (oarlocking effect). A capsulorhexis of similar size to the traditional technique (4.5–5 mm) is made.

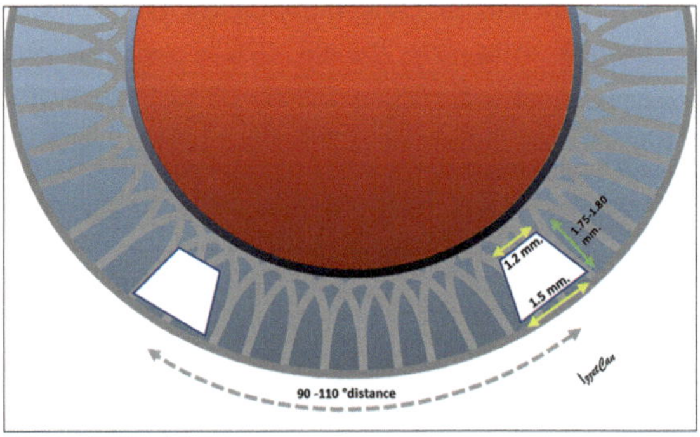

Fig. 1 Schematic view of a 20 G trapezoidal corneal incision

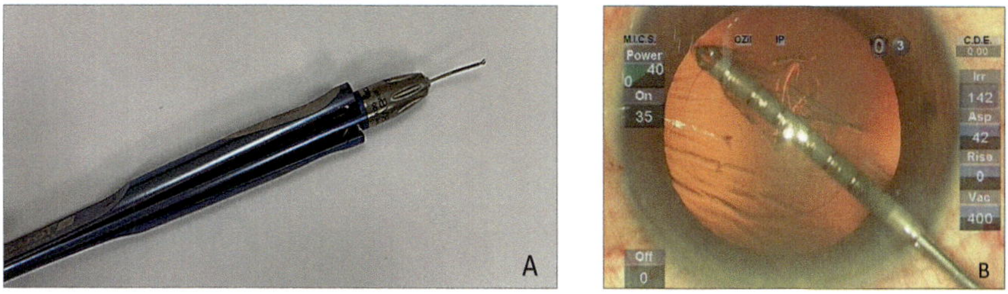

Fig. 2 **A** 23 G. microcapsulorhexis forceps (MST, USA). **B** The ideal size capsulorhexis is performed by verifying with the markings on the forceps

D. **Hydrodissection and Hydrodelineation:** Because of the small incisions in biaxial-MICS, a procedure that will load fluid into the eye can be risky. It would be beneficial to allow the release of the same volume of viscoelastic material by applying BSS on the lens before hydrodelineation or hydrodissection.

If the distal end of the nucleus prolapses forward through the capsulorhexis opening lens will be prepared for horizontal chopping procedure. This method was described by us as "Half-moon supranuclear phacoemulsification" [16].

E. **Nucleofractis:** All nucleofractis techniques, from "divide and conquer" to "chopping", can be used in Biaxial-MICS. When starting the phaco procedure, first the chopper providing the irrigation is inserted into the anterior chamber, followed by the the phaco tip.

One of the potentially important complications of Biaxial-MICS is wound burn. It is generally accepted that the temperature at the wound site should not exceed 45 °C [17]. Therefore, nucleofractis techniques that minimize the use of U/S energy are advantageous [18, 19]. Use of cold BSS (+4°), a preference for "microflow" phaco tips with grooves on the outer surface, placing a cut sleeve on the outer part of the phaco tip, making a slightly wider incision than the phaco tip, and using hyperpulse or microburst type power modulation systems are among the methods applied that can help prevent thermal burns.

F. **Quadrant removal:** One of the two main problems that can develop during quadrant removal in the biaxial-MICS technique is the "surge" phenomenon due to the insufficient inflow and the posterior capsular rupture. To increase the inflow; methods such as infusion with external gas pressure, infusion with internal gas pressure, using an A/C maintainer and increasing the height of the infusion bottle have been proposed. However, the main improvement that made the inflow sufficient was irrigation choppers and the Duet system.

In order to perform biaxial-MICS safely, the inflow should be at least 50 mL/min. The basic law of maintaining a balanced fluid circulation in the anterior chamber, called, microphacodynamics always states that a greater inflow than outflow is required. Therefore, if an irrigating chopper with an inner diameter of

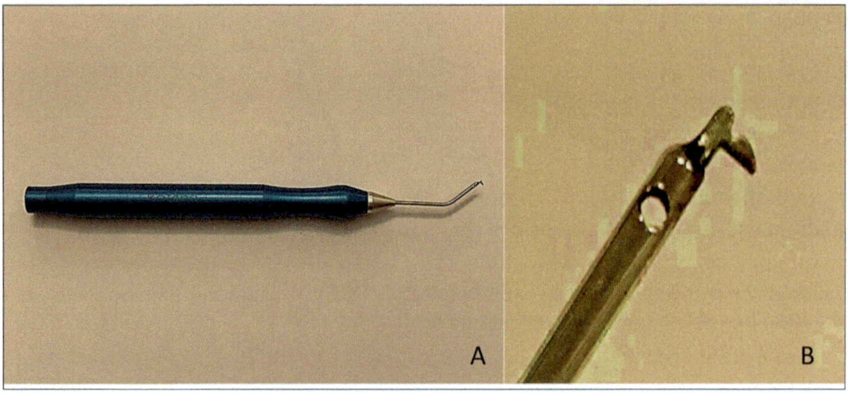

Fig. 3 **A, B** Double side-opening irrigating chopper (Katena, USA)

19 G. is used, a 20 G. phaco tip should be used. Or, for a 20 G. irrigation, an aspiration system with an inner diameter of 21 G. would be appropriate (Fig. 3a, b).

Another task of an irrigator chopper is to retract the iris when the pupil is small or irregular. In floppy iris cases especially, the fluid flow is used to push the iris back. The most important advantage of Biaxial-MICS compared to coaxial or microcoaxial cases is that the nuclear parts which are stuck in the depths of the angle, sulcus, sub-incision area or capsule can be directed towards the phaco end by the help of this decoupled flow of fluid. Briefly, the Biaxial-MICS technique is a method that increases the efficiency of the phacoemulsification process by increasing the followability of the material by providing irrigation from a different angle. With the help of the irrigation choppers, (one of the most important advantages of the Biaxial-MICS technique) the liquid flow is used as an invisible additional instrument. The fluid flow from the irrigating chopper should always be directed downward (towards the posterior capsule) at a right angle to facilitate the transport of materials towards the phaco tip, and to enable a safe surgery by keeping the posterior capsule away. The fluid should not be directed directly towards the phaco tip since this will keep the materials away (Fig. 4). In floppy iris syndrome, if

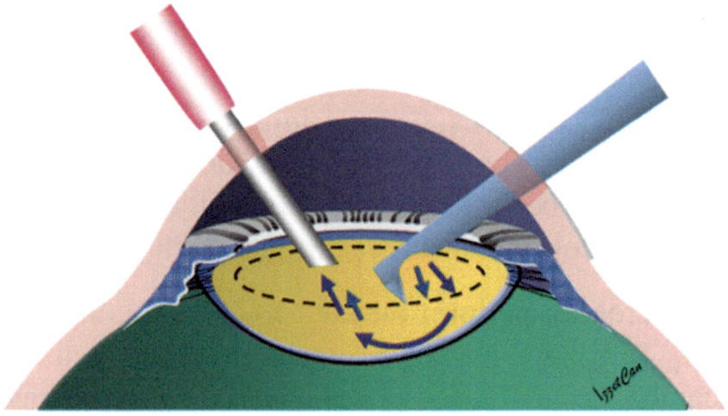

Fig. 4 In the Biaxial-MICS technique, the proper use position of the irrigating chopper to provide the ideal direction of fluid flow

the fluid is directed back too far, the returning fluid will move the iris forward, causing it to incarcerate in the wound.

The phaco settings we use in Biaxial-MICS are as follows. Using the Alcon Infiniti device and the Fine-Nagahara irrigator chopper (MST), with the "half-moon supra capsular nucleofractis" technique, after the lens is broken, chop is applied, while in burst mode, US power is 40% Linear (L) (on 30 ms, off time 5 ms), Vacuum 300 mmHg F (fix), AAH 25 cc/min. F, bottle height is 110 cm. Cortex cleaning after removal of the epinucleus with Duet set Vacuum 600 mmHg L, AAH 60 cc/min.L, bottle height 110 cm.

G. **Cortex cleaning:** The irrigation aspiration cannulas chosen for the infusion/ aspiration (I/A) procedure should be compatible with each other in terms of their inner diameter, and the irrigation cannula should always have a larger diameter. Cannulas with 0.3- or 0.4-mm aperture are used most.
H. **Intraocular Lens (IOL) Implantation:** The postoperative incision, completed with an incision of approximately 1.4 mm, is expanded to the required diameter of the IOL to be inserted. With lenses implanted through incisions of 1.8 mm or less, extremely successful results can be obtained in terms of safety and functionality [9−12].

Comparison of biaxial-MICS and Micro-coaxial-MICS:

The main difference of both techniques is that they have different fluidics characters. In all coaxial techniques, U/S and irrigation are repulsive forces, while aspiration and incisional outflow are attractive forces. In the biaxial technique, while the repulsive force is only the U/S, the irrigative chopper uses all other forces (irrigation, aspiration and outflow from the main incision) attractively. BSS coming out of the chopper directs the material towards the phaco tip rather than pushing it.

The publications reporting the superiority of the biaxial-MICS technique mainly emphasize the increase in efficiency [20−24]. Less BSS is reported to be used with biaxial-MICS, also, effective phaco time and total operation times are significantly shorter.

However, some disadvantages of biaxial-MICS are also present. These are mostly reporting about the safety of the incision site and the insufficient sealing efficiency of the incisions [25–27]. There is also data stating that the microcoaxial technique is more successful in terms of efficiency [28, 29] and may be better for the corneal endothelium [24, 30].

In our study performed with AS-OCT comparing the biaxial-MICS and Microcoaxial-MICS techniques, we observed that the microcoaxial group had a safer arcuate healing model compared to biaxial phaco [4].

Why has the biaxial technique lost its popularity?

It can be said that the competition between micro-coaxial and biaxial techniques has turned in favor of the micro-coaxial technique since the mid-2010s with the effect of advances in microcoaxial technique and also as a result of difficulties in performing the biaxial technique.

Torsional or elliptical phaco technology has solved the problems of microcoaxial technique such as fluidics and phacodynamics. Active fluidics technology (Centrion, Alcon labs), which provides intraocular pressure control during surgery, enables the surgeons to perform safer surgeries. In addition, coaxial approaches are the procedures that surgeons usually learn first and feel familiar.

Although the biaxial technique allows phaco surgery to be completed with incisions smaller than 2.2 mm, nowadays, surgeries performed with 2.2 mm incisions with microcoaxial technique also yield sufficient results in terms of achieving the goals of refractive cataract surgery. In spite of all these, the biaxial technique may take the stage again when customized IOLs are being implanted in the future since these surgeries have the least effect on the cornea.

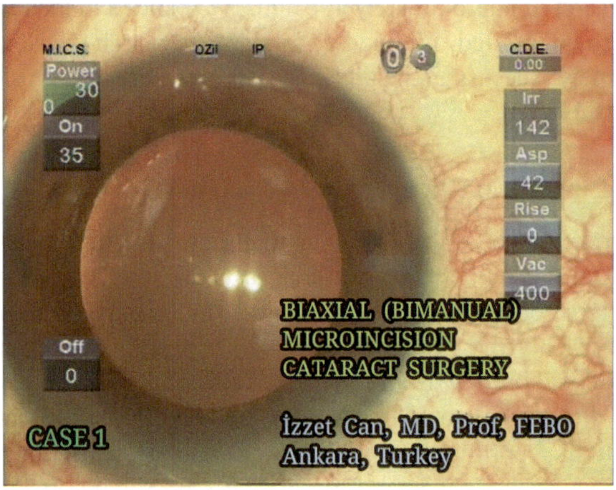

Video presentation of 2 cases completed with biaxial (bimanual) cataract surgery technique (▶ https://doi.org/10.1007/000-8dz)

References

1. Alio JL, Fine IH. Preface. In: Alio JL, Fine IH, editors. Minimizing ıncisions and maximizing outcomes in cataract surgery. Heidelberg: Springer;. 2010. p. Vii–viii.
2. Kelman CD. Phaco-emulsification and aspiration; a new technique of cataract removal; a preliminary report. Am J Ophthalmol. 1967;64:23–35.
3. Can İ, Takmaz T, Yıldız Y, Bayhan HA, Soyugelen G, Bostancı B. Coaxial, microcoaxial, and biaxial microincision cataract surgery: prospective comparative study. J Cataract Refract Surg. 2010;36:740–6.
4. Can İ, Bayhan HA, Çelik H, Bostancı CB. Anterior segment optical coherence tomography evaluation and comparison of main clear corneal incisions in microcoaxial and biaxial cataract surgery. J Cataract Refract Surg. 2011;37:490–500.
5. Alio J, Rodriguez-Prats JL, Galal A. Advances in microincision cataract surgery intraocular lenses. Curr Opin Ophthalmol. 2006;17:80–93.

6. Chee S-P, Bacsal K. Endophthalmitis after microincision cataract surgery. J Cataract Refract Surg. 2005;31:1834–5.
7. Alio JL. What does MICS require? In: Alio JL, Rodriguez Prats JL, Galal A, editors. MICS micro-incision cataract surgery. Miami: Highlights of Ophthalmology; 2004. p. 1–4.
8. Elkady B, Alio J, Ortiz D, Montalban R. Corneal aberrations aftermicroincision cataract surgery. J Cataract Refract Surg. 2008;34:40–5.
9. Can İ, Takmaz T, Bayhan HA, Bostancı CB. Aspheric microincision intraocular lens implantation with biaxial microincision cataract surgery: efficacy and reliability. J Cataract Refract Surg. 2010;36:1905–11.
10. Can İ, Bostancı Ceran B, Soyugelen G, Takmaz T. Clinical outcomes of two different small incision diffractive multifocal intraocular lenses: comparative study. J Cataract Refract Surg. 2012;38:60–7.
11. Can İ, Bostancı CB. Micro-incision intraocular lenses (review). Ophthalmol Int. 2011;6:74–9.
12. Can İ, Bayhan HA, Çelik H, Bostancı CB. Comparison of corneal aberrations after biaxial micro-incision and micro-coaxial cataract surgeries: a prospective study. Curr Eye Res. 2012;37:18–24.
13. Agarwal A, Trivedi RH, Jacop S, et al. Microphakonit: 700 micron cataract surgery. Clin Ophthalmol. 2007;13:323–5.
14. Pandey SK, Werner L, Agarwal A, Agarwal S, Agarwal A, Apple D. No anesthesia cataract surgery. J Cataract Refract Surg. 2001;28:1710.
15. Berdahl JP, DeStafano JJ. Corneal wound architecture and integrity after phacoemulsification evaluation of coaxial, microincision coaxial, and microincision bimanual techniques. J RefractCataract Surg. 2007;33:510–5.
16. Can İ, Takmaz T, Genç İ. Half-moon supracapsular nucleofractis phacoemulsification: safety, efficacy, and functionality. J Cataract Refract Surg. 2008;34:1958–65.
17. Soscia W, Howard JG, Olson RH. Bimanual phacoemulsification through 2 stab incisions; a wound-temperature study. J Cataract Refract Surg. 2002;28:1039–43.
18. Can İ, Takmaz T, Çakıcı F, Özgül M. Comparison of Nagahara phaco-chop and stop-and-chop phacoemulsification nucleotomy techniques. J Cataract Refract Surg.2004;30:663–8.
19. Alio JL, Klonowsky P, Rodriguez Pratz JL, El Kady B. MICS (Microincision cataract surgery) In: Garg A, Fine IH, Alio JL et al. Mastering the techniques of advanced phacosurgery. New Delhi, India: Jaypee Brothers; 2008. p. 121–36.
20. . Tsuneoka H, Shiba T, Takahashi Y. Ultrasonic phacoemulsification using a 1.4 mm incision: clinical results. J Cataract Refract Surg. 2002;28:81–6.
21. Alio J, Rodriguez- JL, Galal A, Ramzy M. Outcomes of microincisional cataract surgery versus coaxial phacoemulsification. Ophthalmology. 2005;112:1997–2003.
22. Kurz S, Krummenauer F, Gabriel P, Pfeiffer N, Dick HB. Biaxial microincision versus coaxial small-incision clear cornea cataract surgery. Ophthalmology. 2006;113:1818–26.
23. Cavallini GM, Campi L, Masini C, Pelloni S, Pupino A. Bimanual microphacoemulsification: prospective study. J Cataract Refract Surg. 2007;33:387–92.
24. Kahraman G, Amon M, Franz C, Prinz A, Abela-Formanek C. Intraindividual comparison of surgical trauma after bimanual microincision and conventional small-incision coaxialphacoemulsification. J Cataract Refract Surg. 2007;33:618–22.
25. Praveen MR, Vasavada AR, Gajjar D, Pandita D, Vasavada VA, Vasavada MS, Raj MS. Comparative quantification of ingress of trypan blue into the anterior chamber aftermicro-coaxial, standard coaxial, and bimanual phacoemulsification randomized clinical trial. J Cataract Refract Surg. 2008;34:1007–12.
26. Johar SR, Vasavada AR, Praveen MR, Pandita D, Nihalani B, Patel U, Vemuganti G. Histomorphological and immunofluorescence evaluation of bimanual and coaxial phacoemulsification incisions in rabbits. J Cataract Refract Surg. 2008;34:670–6.
27. Gajjar D, Praveen MR, Vasavada AR, Pandita D, Vasavada VA, Patel DB, Johar K, Raj S. Ingress of bacterial inoculum into the anterior chamber after bimanual and microcoaxial phacoemulsification in rabbits. J Cataract Refract Surg. 2007;33:2129–34.

28. Osher RH, Injev VP. Microcoaxial phacoemulsification Part 1: laboratory studies. J Cataract Refract Surg. 2007;33:401–7.
29. Osher RH. Microcoaxial phacoemulsification Part 2: clinical study. J Cataract Refract Surg. 2007;33:408–12.
30. Crema AS, Walsh A, Yamane Y, Nose W. Comparative study of coaxial phacoemulsification and microincision cataract surgery one year follow-up. J Cataract Refract Surg. 2007;33:1014–8.

Exchange of Intraocular Lenses

Thomas C. Kreutzer and Sorcha Ní Dhubhghaill

Introduction

There are many reasons to exchange an intraocular implant, including lens subluxation or total luxation into the vitreous cavity and intraocular lens opacification [1]. It may also be required in cases of refractive surprise where the implanted IOL is not of the correct refractive power (and cannot be managed in a simpler way). The surgical strategy is determined by the status and stability of the capsular bag apparatus and the position of the intraocular lens, the material of the intraocular lens and the anatomical conditions of the respective eye.

The most common cause of subluxation and dislocation of intraocular lens implants is pseudoexfoliation syndrome with an estimated rate of 1–2% after 25 years [2]. Other causes include trauma or pre-existing trauma prior to the cataract surgery, connective tissue diseases such as Marfan or Ehlers-Danlos syndrome or zonula defects in the context of anatomical variations, e.g. in colobomas. Subluxation can also occur after ophthalmological interventions (e.g. vitrectomy). When considering the surgical management of subluxated artificial lenses, the capsular bag cannot be reliably used to support the replacement IOL so alternative refixation strategies such as iris or scleral fixation should be performed.

The status of the posterior capsular bag is one of the most important preoperative prognostic factors for the surgery. Patients with a prior capsulotomy are at an increased risk for difficult mobilization of the IOL out of the capsular bag, vitreous

Supplementary Information The online version contains supplementary material available at https://doi.org/10.1007/978-3-031-05394-8_58. The videos can be accessed individually by clicking the DOI link in the accompanying figure caption or by scanning this link with the SN More Media App.

T. C. Kreutzer (✉) · S. Ní Dhubhghaill
Munich, Germany
e-mail: thomas.kreutzer@med.uni-muenchen.de

M. Shajari et al. (eds.), *Cataract and Lens Surgery*,
https://doi.org/10.1007/978-3-031-05394-8_58

prolapse and associated complications, while those with an intact bag typically have a more predictable surgery. Examining the status of the capsular bag preoperatively can be particularly difficult in the cases of opacified lenses and in these cases a detailed history and examination of the patients' medical records may reveal whether a laser capsulotomy was performed or not.

The material of the artificial lens also determines the surgical approach, so a thorough understanding of the history of IOL materials and identification of the IOL is important when considering an IOL explantation. Today, acrylic and silicone lenses can be removed through a 3.0 mm clear cornea incision when cut into half with scissors. Artificial lenses with optics made of polymethmethylacrylate (PMMA) however, cannot be cut and usually require a sclero-corneal tunnel of about 6 mm, for removal from the eye. If the capsular bag and the posterior capsule are preserved, the new artificial lens can be reimplanted into the capsular bag. If the posterior capsule leaf is torn, a sulcus implantation should then be considered and this can include the capture of the optic into the rhexis (optic capture). If the capsular apparatus is defective and the zonular complex unstable, the replacement lens cannot be implanted in the bag or the sulcus and should be in the form of an anterior chamber lens, an iris claw lens (anterior chamber, retroiridally fixed) or a sclerally fixated lens.

Keypoint

Before replacing an artificial lens from the capsular bag, it should be known what lens implant it was and whether a posterior capsulotomy has already been performed. An opening in the posterior capsular bag makes the exchange much more difficult.

Explanting the Lens from the Capsular Bag

In order to exchange an artificial lens from the capsular bag, the first step should be to mobilise implant within the bag. Two paracentheses are useful for this. The anterior chamber should stabilised with viscoelastic material, though it is important not to overfill the bag, as additional OVD will be required in the capsular bag itself. An overfilled anterior chamber can put pressure on the zonulae and increase the chance of a posterior capsular tear in cases where a capsulotomy has been performed. Next, the anterior capsular rhexis margin is separated from the lens optic with a blunt instrument, e.g. a phaco spatula, positioned between anterior capsular edge and the anterior lens optic. As soon as a sufficient gap between the lens optic and the lens capsule has been achieved, viscoelastic is injected into the space to further viscodissect the capsule from implant. A bimanual approach where the non-dominant hand is used to lift the capsular edge while the OVD is injected into the space using the dominant hand can reduce the stress and forces placed on the bag. This separation is very important and should also be carried out in the area of the haptics very thoroughly. If the posterior capsule is intact and the viscodissection sufficient, the lens optic can be lifted forward and out of the capsular bag. Using the bimanual technique, the artificial lens is rotated with the rotating lens hook and a blunt instrument on the capsular bag (e.g. phaco spatula) from the capsular bag into the anterior chamber. During this maneuver, care must be taken not to apply too much viscoelastic or to repeatedly decompress some viscoelastic to counteract high pressure and possible iris prolapse. As soon as the old artificial lens is placed in the anterior chamber, the posterior capsule should be assessed. If this is intact, the next step is the removal of the artificial lens (Video 1).

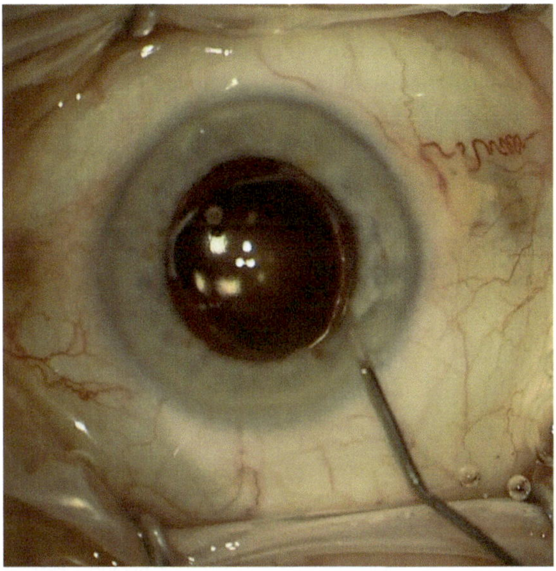

Video 1 Exchange of an opacified intraocular lens from the capsular bag and implantation of a hydrophobic IOL into the capsular bag (▶ https://doi.org/10.1007/000-8e1)

If the posterior capsule is open, the authors recommend an anterior vitrectomy via the paracenthesis, behind the IOL in the anterior chamber to prevent vitreous prolapse during removal of the implant. After this has been done, a main incision can be made for the removal of the implant. In the case of cuttable artificial lenses, a 2.8–3 mm clear cornea incision is usually sufficient. Ideally, this should be made on the steep axis, in the case of low corneal astigmatism and astigmatism against the rule temporally. The lens implant can be cut through the incision, either in three thirds, two halves or half of the optic is incised. The lens pieces can then be accessed with a forceps at the cut margin and is rotated out of the eye through the incision. If the implant has been completely cut, the various parts can directly be removed with a forceps. Hydrophilic artificial lenses can often be pulled out directly through a 3.0 mm incision without dissection. After removal, if necessary, anterior vitrectomy should be performed and then implantation of the new intraocular lens follows.

For intraocular lenses subluxated in the capsular bag, the authors recommend placing a vitrectomy infusion trocar temporally inferior (Video 2). The capsular bag-lens complex can then be supported with an instrument (e.g. phaco spatula) through this trocar and easily moved into the anterior chamber with counterpressure by a viscoelastic given through a paracentheses on the iris. Afterwards two options remain: Removal of the complex with subsequent implantation of an anterior chamber lens, iris claw lens or a scleral-fixed artificial lens, or freeing the artificial lens from capsule material with a vitrectomy cutter and subsequent refixation to the sclera, which is an option especially for three-piece artificial lenses. The latter is advantageous, particularly when the optic of the intraocular lens is made of PMMA material and therefore cannot be cut. These lenses require a large sclero-corneal tunnel access to be removed. However, it must be taken into account that haptics of artificial lenses that have remained in the capsular bag for a long time often undergo change of material tension and stability of the haptics. A secondary scleral fixation, e.g. as described by Yamane and Scharioth, can be associated with a postoperative tilt or re-dislocation of the implant (see also chapter "Zonular Disorders and Management in Cataract Surgery"). It is the authors experience, that replacement with a new intraocular lens is usually more reliable and preferable.

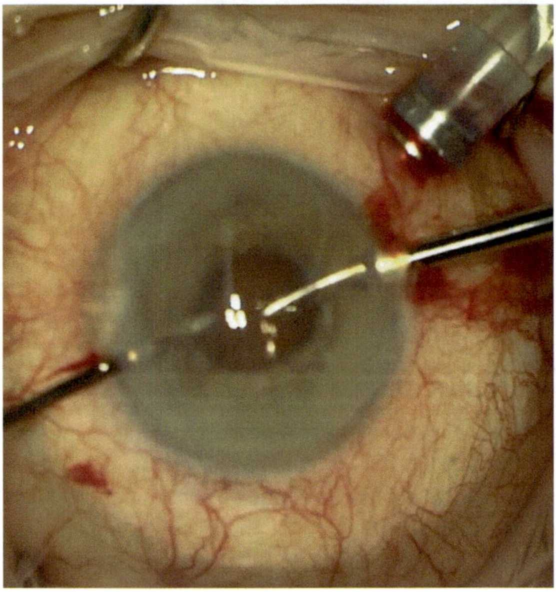

Video 2 Exchange of a three-piece artificial lens subluxated in the capsular bag (▶ https://doi.org/10.1007/000-8e0)

If an exchange is carried out, it is possible to extract the entire capsule/artificial lens complex via a 6 mm sclero-corneal tunnel. The advantage is that the luxated material can be quickly removed via this access. The disadvantages are the higher risk of astigmatism and invasiveness of the procedure.

A second possibility, with acrylate artificial lenses and silicone lenses, is to cut the capsule-lens complex as described above. It is important to know that in the case of significant amounts of regenerative cataract, these can be difficult to be removed with difficulty using a vitrectomy cutter. It is therefore recommended that an anterior vitrectomy be performed first, behind the capsular bag-lens-complex located in the anterior chamber, ideally with a placed infusion trocar in the vitreous cavity (Video 3). This makes it easier to flush this regenerative cataract material out of the eye after dissection with an intraocular scissor and extracting them via the CCI as they are less likely to sink into the vitreous chamber due to BSS flow coming from behind the iris. This can usually be successfully achieved by opening the CCI by lifting the anterior CCI lip with a kolibri toothed forceps with a phaco spatula on the lower lip.

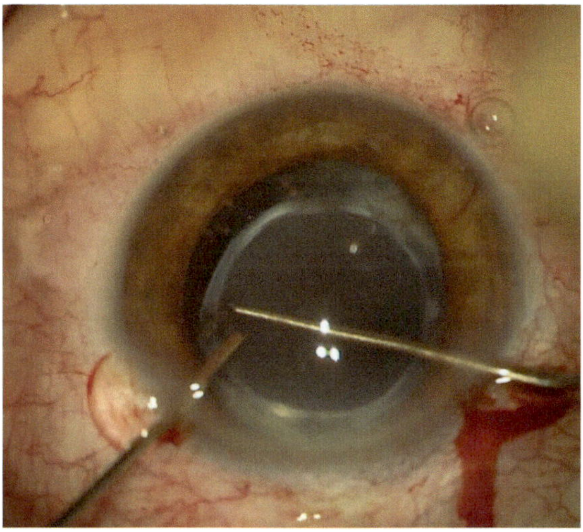

Video 3 Replacement of a clouded three-piece artificial lens from the capsular bag and implantation of a new three-piece artificial lens in the sulcus (▶ https://doi.org/10.1007/000-8e2)

Once the capsular bag-implant complex has been completely removed, the anterior vitrectomy is completed, if necessary. The implantation of the new artificial lens via a CCI incision is then performed as a scleral-fixed lens.

Author's recommendation

Preoperative strategic planning is important for the exchange of intraocular lenses. This can significantly reduce the likelihood of difficulties during surgery. The exchange is therefore often minimally invasive and can provide a good refractive result.

References

1. Goemaere J, Trigaux C, Denissen L, Dragnea D, Hua MT, Tassignon MJ, Dhubhghaill SN. Fifteen years of IOL exchange: indications, outcomes, and complications. J Cataract Refract Surg. 2020;46(12):1596–603. https://doi.org/10.1097/j.jcrs.0000000000000349 PMID: 33259388.
2. Ascaso FJ, Huerva V, Grzybowski A. Epidemiology, etiology, and prevention of late IOL-capsular bag complex dislocation: review of the literature. J Ophthalmol. 2015;2015: 805706.

Implantation of Anterior Chamber Lenses

Carl Clemente and Thomas Neuhann

Introduction

The angle-supported anterior chamber lens (ACL), historically, was one of the earliest approaches to intraocular lens implantation but has lost popularity in recent years. ACLs are still used from time to time by some surgeons when capsular support is completely absent. With correct case selection and if a few points are taken into account, implantation is relatively easy and can be carried out in a controlled manner without much time, leading to a good functional result.

About the Anterior Chamber Lens

The first anterior chamber lenses came onto the market in the 1950s. However, implantation often had disastrous consequences due to bullous keratopathy, uveitis, bleeding and glaucoma. Manufacturing defects and defects in haptic design were identified as the primary causes. Even much later models of anterior chamber lenses, however, still showed unacceptable complications.

Basically, the chamber angle, with its structures uveal tissue, trabecular meshwork and corneal endothelium is a very sensitive anatomical region and as a result, the condition of the implant is of crucial importance [1].

Over the years, the findings of Peter Choyce, David Apple and Peter Clemente contributed significantly to the understanding of the anterior chamber lens supported by the chamber angle and to clinical safety [2]. A flexible haptic with wide, smooth foot plates in the contact area proved to be essential. Perforations, such as positioning holes, must not be present in the footplates and, while polymethyl

C. Clemente (✉) · T. Neuhann
München, Germany
e-mail: dr.clemente@neuhann.de

M. Shajari et al. (eds.), *Cataract and Lens Surgery*,
https://doi.org/10.1007/978-3-031-05394-8_59

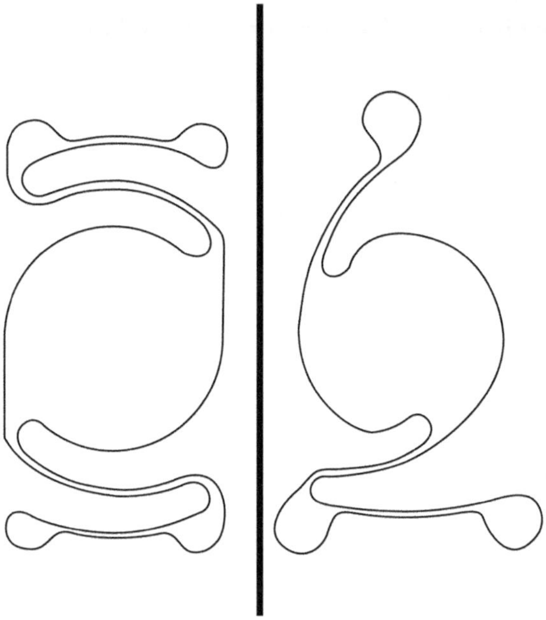

Fig. 1 Schematic drawing of ACLs with four-point and three-point haptic

methacrylate (PMMA) is a safe material, such footplates tend to elicit the formation of a fibrous membrane [3]. The complication risk of such an ACL model, especially the risk of chronic corneal endothelial damage with decompensation, is low [4].

In Germany, models from Bausch + Lomb (L122UV), AJL Ophthalmic (A601250) and EyeKon Medical (P125, P130) are currently available on the market. Regrettably, some well-tried products disappeared not long ago: models from Alcon (MTA3UO, MTA4UO) und Zeiss (CT13A). Maybe these exemplars are still in some shelfs also. The significant difference between the Zeiss IOL and the others is the number of haptic contact points (Fig. 1). The Zeiss model is equipped with three contact points instead of four. The origin of the three-point haptic design goes back to Charles Kelman, to his anterior chamber lens model Omnifit. It has a more size-independent fitting behavior [5].

Prerequisites for Implantation

- Weighing up indications

Because the performance of a later endothelial keratoplasty would be made more difficult by an ACL, they should be avoided in cases of low endothelial cell counts or other forms of endothelial pathology. In these cases, iris-fixated lenses or transscleral fixation of a posterior chamber lenses are better options.

Extensive anterior synechia are also a contraindication to anterior chamber lens implantation. A chronically hypotonic eye pressure situation also excludes the use of an anterior chamber lens due to unstable anterior chamber conditions.

- Size adjustment

It is particularly important that the implant does not rotate in the anterior chamber. Therefore, the lens must not be too small in relation to the anterior chamber width (size). According to the product information, the MTA3UO (total diameter 12.5 mm, Alcon) is suitable for anterior chamber sizes 11.5–11.9 mm, the MTA4UO (total diameter 13.0 mm, Alcon) for sizes 12.0–12.4 mm. The L122UV (total diameter 13.75 mm, Bausch + Lomb) is suitable for sizes from 11.50 to 12.25 mm. The P125 (total diameter 12.5 mm, EyeKon Medical) is suitable for anterior chamber sizes 11.0–12.5 mm, the P130 (total diameter 13.0 mm, EyeKon Medical) for sizes 11.5–13.0 mm. The anterior chamber size is equated to the horizontal corneal diameter, measured as "white-to-white" distance (WTW).

The WTW value is also usually given by modern optical biometry devices.

For the lens CT13 A (total diameter 13.3 mm, Zeiss) the manufacturer does not specify any size ranges. In our long-standing experience with this model, it can be recommended for WTW from 11.0 to 12.6 mm.

- Controlled initial situation

The question of the anterior chamber lens often arises in the course of a complicated cataract operation. The cornea must also permit sufficient visibility for ACL implantation. Prolapse of vitreous material must be controlled and removed by vitrectomy and a thorough anterior vitrectomy should be performed prior to implantation. In case of doubt, thorough vitrectomy and watertight wound closure should be ensure. A properly planned secondary lens implantation can then be arranged, where the required implant and instrumentation can be ensured to be present in the operating room.

Preparation of the Implantation

- Incision 6.0 mm

In the case of pre-planned implantation, a sclerocorneal tunnel incision is recommended, ideally in the steepest meridian for refractive reasons. If the ACL implantation is unexpectedly performed as part of the cataract surgery, the initial incision can simply be widened. In this case, sufficient time should be taken for meticulous incision preparation to avoid further complications. Alternatively, the clear corneal incision can be closed, and a proper sclerocorneal tunnel be constructed 90 degrees from the clear corneal incision.

- Injection of miotic agent

The miosis considerably facilitates the performance of iridectomy and lens implantation.

- Peripheral iridectomy (IE)

To avoid a pupillary block, a generous peripheral iridotomy is mandatory (e.g. with the vitreous cutter). To prevent the iris hole from being occluded by vitreous material, it is also recommended that the space behind the iridectomy also should be vitrectomized.

Implantation

- Viscoelastic injection

Use tweezers to grasp the lens on the optic (Fig. 2a)

It is essential to pay attention to the correct orientation: if there is an optic-haptic angulation the haptics of the lens are angled backwards, i.e. towards the iris.

- Insert the haptics (Fig. 2b)

If the lens has a three-point haptic, it is recommended that you insert the haptic with the two contact points first. Caution: PMMA is not scratch-resistant and not unbreakable!

- Insert the second haptic (Fig. 2c)

A suitable instrument (e.g. a "Y-hook") should be used for the trailing haptic bar to guide it inwards and posteriorly under the incision lip. If you suspect that the iris is trapped, the lens or haptic must be lifted again with an instrument to free the iris.

- Wound closure with suture (Fig. 2d)

The implantation wound must be securely closed with a 10/0 nylon suture if it is located at the clear cornea. After this, the anterior chamber should be carefully checked once again to ensure the absence of persisting vitreous strands.

- Gonioscopic check (Fig. 2e)

It is recommended that the fit of the lens should be checked gonioscopically at the end of surgery. The haptic contact points must sit on the ciliary body band, with sufficient distance from the iridectomy. Otherwise, the lens must be turned a little

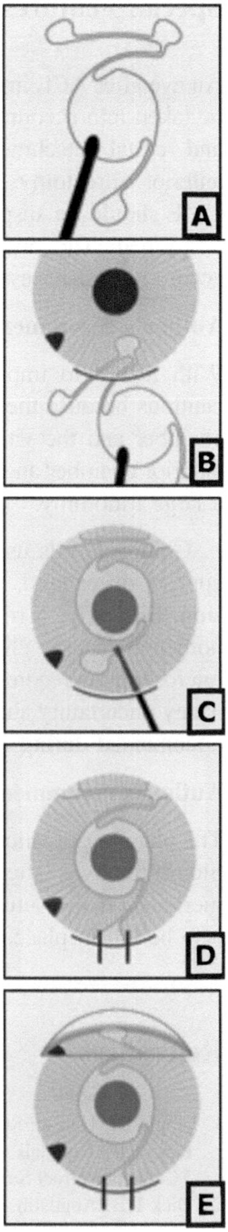

Fig. 2 Steps of the implantation (the schematic drawings show a lens with three-point haptics)

more or the haptic contact points raised respectively. Pupil and lens should be as well centred as possible when the eye is pressurized to avoid inadvertent postoperative rotation.

Special Features of Postoperative Follow-Up Care

An eye after ACL implantation naturally has a more complicated history. This must be taken into account in postoperative diagnostics. Cystoid macular edema (CME) and retinal detachment are more common in post-operative conditions following anterior vitrectomy. In cases where the resulting visual acuity is unsatisfactory, CME should be suspected and an ocular coherence tomography (OCT) should be performed. The postoperative anti-inflammatory medication should be adjusted accordingly if necessary.

Author's recommendation

With regard to implantation of slow releasing steroid implants, one should be cautious because the ACL does not form a significant barrier between the anterior chamber and the vitreous cavity. As a result, such implants can migrate into the anterior chamber and damage the corneal endothelium. This can also occur through a large iridotomy.

Gonioscopy is useful for checking the fit of the lens, especially if the implant appears off-centred. A haptic dislocation in the iridectomy needs immediate revision. Similarly, a rotating lens is not tolerable. A rotating ACL (propeller phenomenon) causes chronic endothelial damage and must be removed. Endothelial microscopy is recommended at regular intervals to assess the endothelium. If there is any uncertainty about the stability, the position of the haptics should be precisely documented during examinations to detect implant rotation in follow-up visits.

Author's recommendation

The planning of suture removal should take into account the resulting astigmatism. Suture removal (after four weeks at the earliest) flattens the cornea in the relevant meridian. If the sutures are subconjunctival after sclerocorneal incision, they can also be left in place.

References

1. Apple DJ, Hansen SO, Richards SC, Ellis GW, Kavka-Van Norman D, Tetz MR, Pepper BR, Park RB, Crandall AS, Olson RJ Anterior chamber lenses. Part II: A laboratory study. J Cataract Refract Surg. 1987;13(2):175–189. https://doi.org/10.1016/S0886-3350(87)80132-3.
2. Dick HB, Augustin AJ. Lens implant selection with absence of capsular support. Curr Opin Ophthalmol. 2001;12(1):47–57. https://doi.org/10.1097/00055735-200102000-00009.
3. Zaugg B, Kleinmann G, Apple DJ. The Evolution of intraocular lenses. In: Kleinmann G, Assia EI, Apple DJ, (eds.). Premium and specialized intraocular lenses. 2014. p. 3–20. https://doi.org/10.2174/97816080583271140101.

4. Hennig A, Johnson GJ, Evans JR, Lagnado R, Poulson A, Pradhan D, Foster A, Wormald RP. Long term clinical outcome of a randomised controlled trial of anterior chamber lensesafter high volume intracapsular cataract surgery. Br J Ophthalmol. 2001;85:11–7. https://doi.org/10.1136/bjo.85.1.11.
5. Bleckmann H, Conrad R. Surgical techniques for lens implantation. In: Intraocular lenses and their implantation. Berlin, New York: de Gryter; 1986. p. 40–92.

Sulcus IOLs

Michael Amon and Barbara Wetzel

Introduction

The ideal anatomical position for optimal placement of an intraocular lens (IOL) is in the capsular bag. This is not always possible, however, and as a result, the second most common method of anchoring an IOL is by placement in the ciliary sulcus. Ciliary sulcus implantation can be performed primarily, usually as part of a surgical complication or can be performed secondarily, as in the case of aphakia or intraocular lens exchange [8].

Indications/Contraindications

The ciliary sulcus is an excellent option for the support of an intraocular lens in a wide range of clinical scenarios. The main indications are abnormal anatomical conditions of the iris-lens apparatus such as defects and tears in the anterior and

Supplementary Information The online version contains supplementary material available at https://doi.org/10.1007/978-3-031-05394-8_60. The videos can be accessed individually by clicking the DOI link in the accompanying figure caption or by scanning this link with the SN More Media App.

M. Amon · B. Wetzel (✉)
Department of Ophthalmology, Academic Teaching Hospital of St. John of God, Vienna, Austria
e-mail: babsi.wetzel@gmail.com

M. Amon
e-mail: amon@augenchirurg.com

M. Amon · B. Wetzel
Medical Faculty, Sigmund Freud University, Johannes von Gott Platz 1, 1020 Vienna, Austria

M. Shajari et al. (eds.), *Cataract and Lens Surgery*,
https://doi.org/10.1007/978-3-031-05394-8_60

posterior layers of the capsular bag. While less common, cases of aphakia with a phimotic capsular bag or a lens exchange combined with capsular defects may also create a situation where sulcus implantation the most suitable choice for the lens position [4]. Another frequent indication for sulcus lens placement is in the field of phakic refractive surgery. In these patients seeking spectacle-free vision, a phakic IOL is implanted in the sulcus in over the natural crystalline lens. Implanting a "add-on" lens in the ciliary sulcus to correct a refractive surprise is yet another application of sulcus placement in the so called "piggy-back" technique [1, 2]. Similarly, sulcus lens placement can be beneficial in the management of negative dysphotopsias, where a "reverse optic capture" with relocation of the optic to the level of the sulcus can be carried out to good therapeutic effect [7].

In the event of extensive zonular dialysis, in patients with pseudoexfoliation, Marfan's syndrome or after trauma for example, IOL implantation in the sulcus should be preferred since placement of the lens in the capsular bag carries a higher risk of IOL dislocation in the vitreous space. As a aside, the use of a capsular tension ring should always be considered in such cases [6].

For a safe implantation of an IOL in the ciliary sulcus, certain anatomical structures of the iris-lens capsule apparatus must be at least partially present, in particular the anteriorly delimiting iris tissue and at least parts of the posteriorly stabilizing lens capsule. If sufficient "capsular support" is missing, alternative fixation techniques such as iris fixation or scleral fixation must be used as the sulcus itself may not be capable of reliably supporting the lens [3].

Surgery Technique

The technique of IOL implantation in the sulcus depends mainly on the given anatomical conditions and the lenses available for sulcus placement. Both the implantation technique and its degree of difficulty differ depending on the surgical setting (planned secondary IOL implantation versus intraoperative complication).

If an IOL has not yet been implanted or the IOL currently in the eye can be left in place, the current access sites (CCI tunnel and lateral paracenteses) are usually sufficient. However, if the IOL has to be explanted, it may be necessary to widen the incision. In cases where a PMMA IOL must be removed, an incision larger than the lens is required, as these IOLs are not flexible and cannot be cut. If time has passed since the primary operation, a new corneal tunnel must be prepared. If necessary, a suture can be placed at the end of the operation [11].

When implanting a three-piece IOL in the sulcus, it is recommended to use an ophthalmic viscoelastic device (OVD) for stabilization and preparation of the space between the iris and the anterior capsule. If the anterior capsule is stable, the leading haptic can be positioned directly into the sulcus, then the trailing haptic is rotated and dialed in. Another possibility is to first insert the IOL into the anterior chamber with subsequent rotation and placement of the haptics in the sulcus using a second instrument, for example push–pull hooks.

In the event of an intraoperative capsular rupture, the residual capsular structure should be carefully examined to determine whether there is sufficient stability to ensure stable placement of the IOL in the sulcus. If the anterior rhexis is intact, sulcus placement can be carried out and augmented using "optic capture", despite the defective posterior capsule. Here the haptics remain in the sulcus, the optic of the IOL is pushed posteriorly through the rhexis and thus placed at the "level" of the posterior capsule. The aim of this method is to reach an optimal functional and refractive visual result.

A three-piece lens with posterior angulation and a corresponding overall diameter is recommended as the implant in these situations, as it is known that one-piece lenses can lead to "iris chafing" and pigment dispersion with further complications [5, 9]. Also, it has to be kept in mind that the lens position is a little more anterior which should be considered when choosing the lens power. When converting a lens power from capsular bag placement to sulcus placement, the IOL power should be adapted but this adaptation depends on the original power of the lens. We recommend the website of Dr Warren Hill as it provides a diagram for conversion. This can be printed out and stored with the 3 piece IOLs for such an emergency.

When implanting a sulcus IOL as part of a secondary operation, preparation of the rhexis or its enlargement may be necessary in order to achieve "optic capture". This can be done through radial incisions, either preoperatively using an Nd: YAG laser or intraoperatively using microscissors or a capsular forceps. If fixation of the IOL using "optic capture" is not possible, the entire IOL can also be anchored in the sulcus, but with less rotational stability. This procedure is recommended, for example, if the posterior capsule is intact, but the anterior part of the capsule has a major defect, which makes stable fixation in the capsular bag impossible.

One of the main goals of a sulcus IOL implantation is to avoid vitreous prolapse. (Randleman JB, Ahmed IIK 2016) The use of dispersive viscoelastics is recommended for intraoperative tamponade in order to better tamponade the vitreous. If the capsule ruptures, it should be applied before the phaco needle or the I/A system is removed [8]. In the case of accidental vitreous prolapse, all herniated vitreous strands must be removed. Marking the vitreous with triamcinolone can extremely be helpful here.

Choice of IOL

The best options for implantation in the sulcus are one-piece PMMA IOLs and three-piece IOLs with posteriorly angled haptics so that the optics can maintain a sufficient distance from the iris [6].

The optic should have a smooth surface with rounded edges and a diameter of at least 6 mm. The total diameter from haptic to haptic should be at least 13 mm to enable a well-centered position of the IOL. Among the three-piece IOLs available on the market, one can choose between acrylic and silicone, although acrylic is preferred for eyes with a ruptured capsule after trauma, as these patients have a higher risk of developing retinal detachment at a later point in time. Traumatic eyes with retinal detachments often have to be filled with silicone oil and in these cases silicone oil may be deposited on the silicone optic of the IOL [6].

Nowadays the one-piece PMMA IOLs mentioned above are more of a second choice, as they require an incision size of 6–7 mm due to the rigid, non-foldable optic. The configuration and thin nature of the haptics of this IOL, however, allow safe implantation both in the sulcus and in the capsular bag Ahmed [10]. One-piece, foldable acrylic lenses are not recommended for implantation in the sulcus due to their optic and haptic design. The IOL diameter is too small, the posterior angulation is missing and the haptics are too thick, which significantly increases the risk of friction at the edge of the IOL with associated "iris chafing" and the resulting complications [3].

Complications

The selection of an appropriate IOL is the key factor for avoiding the occurrence of severe complications after IOL placement in the ciliary sulcus. According to current literature, one-piece acrylic lenses in the sulcus mainly lead to secondary pigment dispersion syndrome (83%), increased intraocular pressure (33%) with consecutive secondary pigment glaucoma, intraocular bleeding (23%) and "iris chafing" with transillumination defects (80%) (Figs. 1 and 2). Furthermore, one-piece sulcus IOLs can lead to recurrent iridocyclitis, uveitis-glaucoma-hyphema syndrome, vitreous hemorrhage, cystoid macular edema, or, often, decentration of the IOL (Fig. 3). Some of these patients have to undergo surgical intervention with an IOL exchange [3] (Fig. 4).

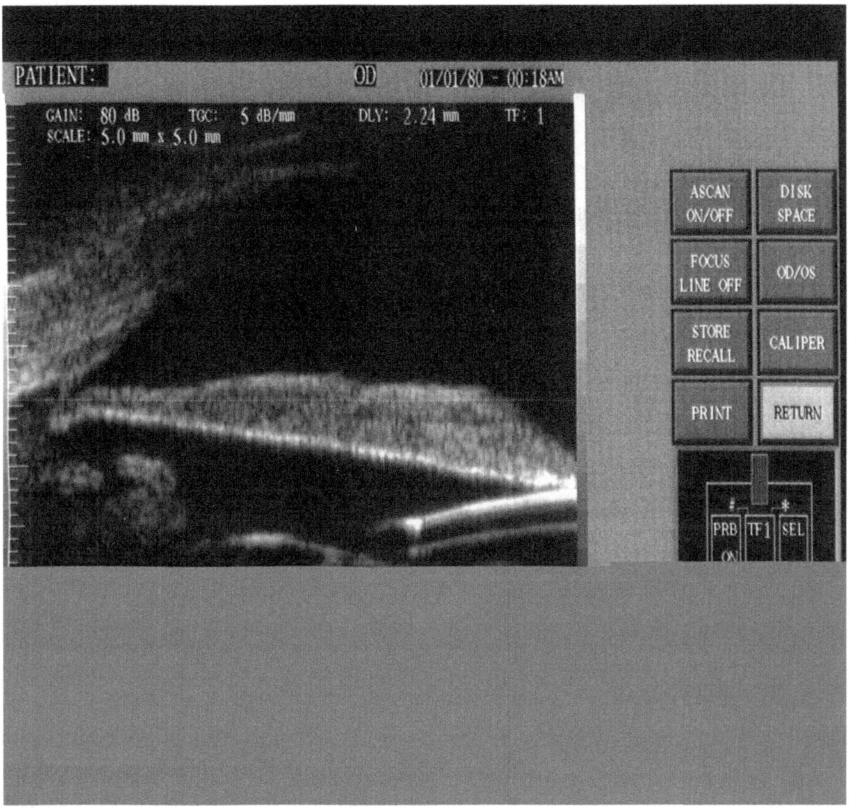

Fig. 1 UBM imaging of the anterior segment with visible contact of the iris with the anterior surface of a sulcus IOL

Conclusion

IOL implantation in the ciliary sulcus is a good alternative if anchoring in the capsular bag is not possible. The correct choice of IOL, precise knowledge of the anatomy of the ciliary sulcus and correct assessment of the surgical site, as well as a proper implantation technique, are the keys for a successful result.

Note: Any vitrectomy required should be performed while avoiding vitreoretinal traction and with complete removal of the lens material.

Useful hints for daily practice: In order to achieve a sufficient vitrectomy, marking of the prolapsed vitreous strands using triamcinolone acetate appears to be very helpful.

The symmetrical placement of an IOL suitable for the sulcus combined with the complete removal of the prolapsed vitreous are crucial for good results.

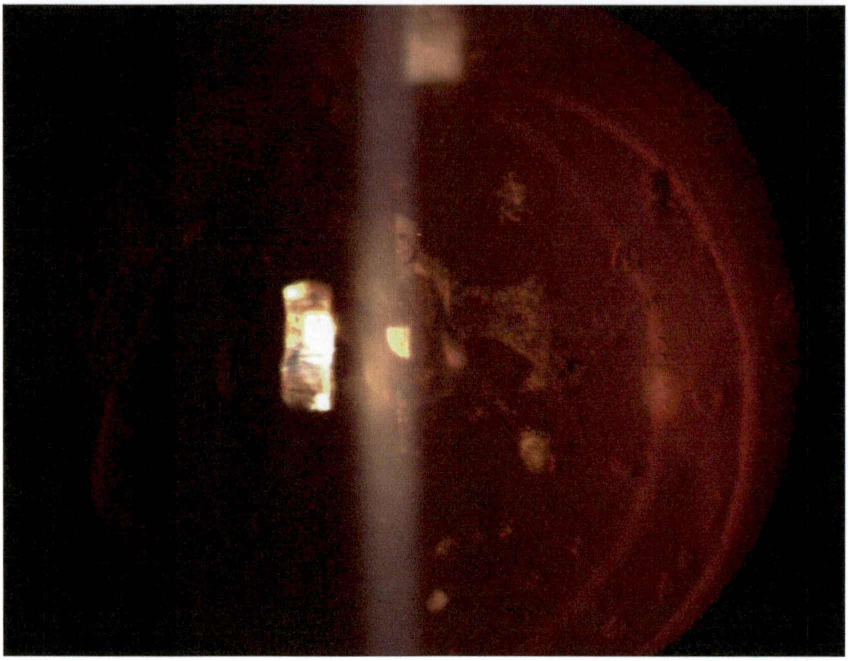

Fig. 2 Deposits of pigment and macrophages on the surface of a sulcus IOL

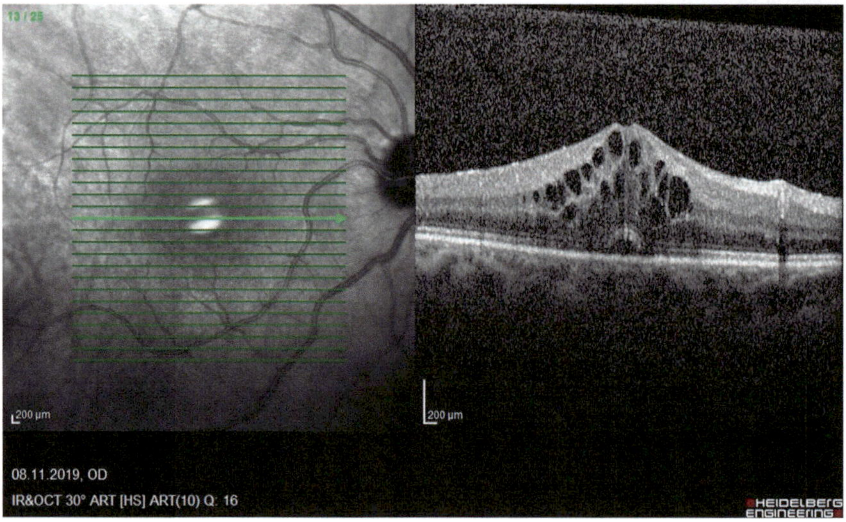

Fig. 3 Postoperative cystoid macular edema following implantation of a one-piece IOL in the ciliary sulcus

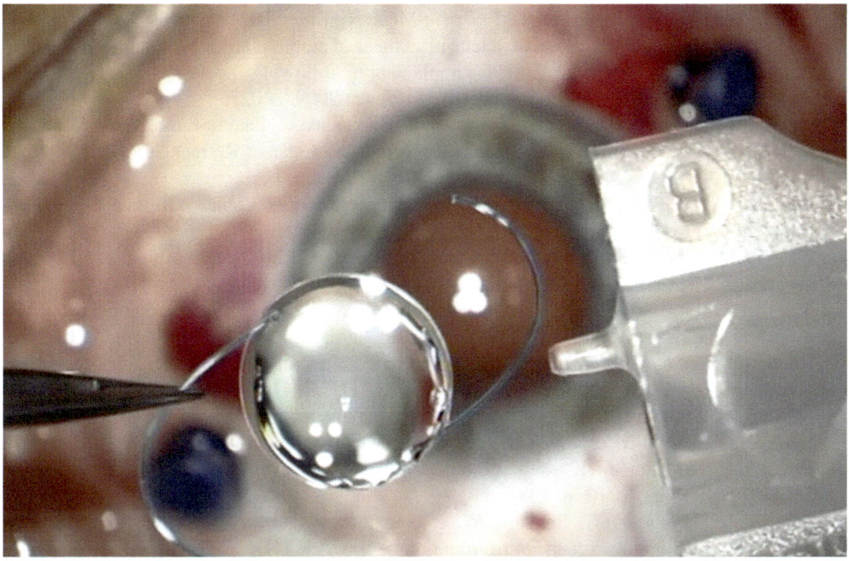

Fig. 4 (with Video) Implantation of a three-piece sulcus IOL with button-hole fixation after accidental intraoperative posterior capsular rupture during combined cataract surgery with pars-plana vitrectomy + membrane peeling

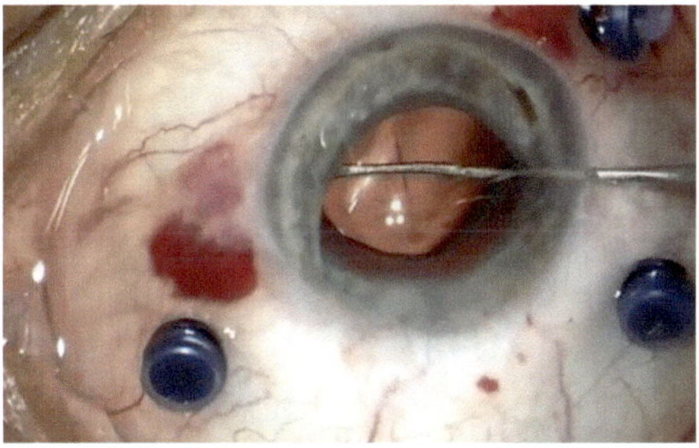

Video Implantation of a three-piece sulcus IOL with button-hole fixation after accidental intraoperative posterior capsular rupture during combined cataract surgery with pars-plana vitrectomy + membrane peeling (▶ https://doi.org/10.1007/000-8e3)

References

1. Abdelghany AA, Alio JL. Surgical options for correction of refractive error following cataract surgery. Eye Vis. 2014. https://doi.org/10.1186/s40662-014-0002-2.
2. Amon M, Wetzel B, Bernhart C, Kahraman G. Uveal and capsular biocompatibility of different IOLs for different indications. Spektrum Der Augenheilkunde. 2016. https://doi.org/10.1007/s00717-016-0305-x.

3. Chang DF, Masket S, Miller KM, Braga-Mele R, Little BC, Mamalis N, Oetting TA, Packer M. 2009. Complications of sulcus placement of single-piece acrylic intraocular lenses. Recommendations for backup IOL implantation following posterior capsule rupture. J Cataract Refract Surg. https://doi.org/10.1016/j.jcrs.2009.04.027.
4. Gimbel HV, Condon GP, Kohnen T, Olson RJ, Halkiadakis I. Late in-the-bag intraocular lens dislocation: incidence, prevention, and management. J Cataract Refract Surg. 2005. https://doi.org/10.1016/j.jcrs.2005.06.053.
5. Gimbel HV, DeBroff BM. Intraocular lens optic capture. J Cataract Refract Surg. 2004. https://doi.org/10.1016/j.jcrs.2003.11.035.
6. Kim T, DelMonte DW, Gupta PK, Chang DF, editors. Curbside consultation in cataract surgery. 2nd ed. NJ: Slack Incorporated; 2014. p. 153–67.
7. Masket S, Fram NR. Pseudophakic negative dysphotopsia: surgical management and new theory of etiology. J Cataract Refract Surg. 2011. https://doi.org/10.1016/j.jcrs.2011.02.022.
8. Mehta R, Aref AA. Intraocular lens implantation in the ciliary sulcus: challenges and risks. Clin Ophthalmol. 2019. https://doi.org/10.2147/OPTH.S205148.
9. Moshirfar M, Skanchy DF, Shah T. Intraoperative management of anterior capsular tear. Curr Opin Ophthalmol. 2017. https://doi.org/10.1097/ICU.0000000000000325.
10. Randleman JB, Ahmed IIK, editors. Intraocular lens surgery, vol. 10–18. New York: Thieme Medical Publishers; 2016. p. 138–78.
11. Schulze S, Bertelmann T, Sekundo W. Implantation von Intraokularlinsen in Den Sulcus Ciliaris. Ophthalmologe. 2014. https://doi.org/10.1007/s00347-013-2855-5.

Retropupillary Iris Claw Intraocular Lens Implantation for Aphakia Correction

Walter Sekundo

Introduction

Secondary aphakia correction, as well as the correction of aphakia within the scope of a very complicated cataract surgery (with an inadequate capsular bag apparatus) requires an anatomically satisfactory and less time-consuming alternative to suture- or haptic-fixed surgical techniques in the age of short operating times [1–3]. The technique of retropupillary implantation of iris claw IOLs (Artisan, Ophtec BV, Groningen, Netherlands, formerly known as Verisyse, distributed by AMO, Santa Ana, USA), which is described in the following, comes very close to this requirement.

Historical Information

The Artisan or Verisyse intraocular lens for the correction of aphakia is a rigid polymethyl methacrylate (PMMA) IOL with a total length of 8.5 mm and thickness of 1.04 mm. The lens has a 5 mm optic and was originally designed by the Dutch ophthalmologist Jan Worst, (Groningen, Netherlands), who first presented his "Iris-Claw Lens" back in 1971 [4]. His original design which was then modified as a convex-concave lens in 1986 was primarily intended for anterior implantation, i.e. on the anterior iris, in the anterior chamber. In 1980, Amar implanted the first iris-claw lenses in the retropupillary position in the convex-concave optical path [5]. This report, however, was basically an extended case report and discussed among other things, retropupillary implantation as part of a "triple procedure" (I.e. combined with penetrating keratoplasty) [6]. And so we have Mohr, Hengerer and

W. Sekundo (✉)
Marburg, Germany
e-mail: sekundo@med.uni-marburg.de

M. Shajari et al. (eds.), *Cataract and Lens Surgery*,
https://doi.org/10.1007/978-3-031-05394-8_61

Eckard to thank for their publication in 2002, who standardized the technique and reported outcomes on a larger number of eyes. In these cases, the lens was implanted in the opposite position than Amar, namely plano-convex. This was done with the aim of minimising the risk of iris pigment exfoliation chronic irritation, due to a small distance between the lens and the pigment epithelium. By using a 5° angled haptic, they also achieved a distance between the lens and the pigment epithelium that corresponds to that of a sulcus-fixed HVAC [7]. Pure anterior segment surgeons in particular hesitated in adopting Mohr's technique because they feared a loss of the IOL into the vitreous cavity during implantation. Sekundo countered these concerns by developing an instrument set in 2004 in cooperation with Braun (Feinwerkzeugmacher, Geuder GmbH), whose tweezers grasped the IOL from below like a support plate. As a result, this almost completely eliminated the risk of IOL loss into the vitreous cavity (see below) [8] (Fig. 1). Originally, the adoption of the retropupillary technique by the manufacturer, Ophtec BV, was also viewed very cautiously and was considered an "off-label" modification of the lens approved for the anterior chamber. Since then, however, retropupillary fixation of iris claw IOLs is being practiced worldwide and a considerable number of peer-reviewed publications that substantiate satisfactory results, which will be discussed below.

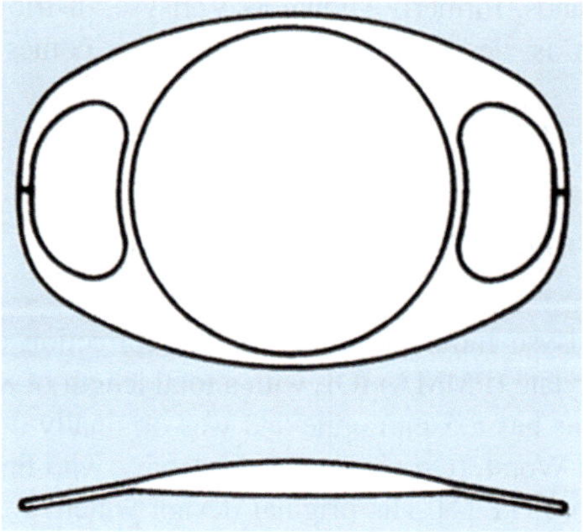

Fig. 1 Schematic drawing of the Artisan Aphakia IOL. Front view above and side view below

Surgical Procedures

Irrespective of which instruments are used, a careful anterior (or complete) vitrectomy should be performed before implantation. In any case, it must be ensured that the vitreous is also removed retropupillary in the area of the planned iris enclavation.

Practical tip Start
In order to avoid injury to the iris with the vitrector, a bimanual technique is recommended. We advised a continuous infusion either via a paracenthesis into the anterior chamber (anterior chamber maintainer) or via the pars plana. This frees the second hand, which then allows a Sinskey hook or a "push–pull" to be used to gently pull the iris over the vitrector peripherally and secure it. < Practical tip stop>.

The Technique Using Standard Instruments ("Artisan Tweezers")

Due to its rigidity and size, the implantation of an iris claw IOL requires a usually self-closing, "frown-incision" type sclero-corneal tunnel of 5.2–5.3 mm. If the incision is placed closer to the limbus or is purely corneal, the size of the incision can be reduced tof 5.1–5.2 mm, though this must always be sutured at the end of the operation [9]. If there is no history of glaucoma and the sclera is intact, we prefer a sclerocorneal tunnel, as this (1) is often self-closing and (2) has a limited effect on the astigmatism (in our hands approx. 0.75–1.0 dpt cyl against the rule for superior access). This incision is usually made at 12 o'clock and the IOL is fixed horizontally so the procedure is described here with this position in mind. There are certainly situations, however, where the IOL is inserted vertically (e.g. in the case of complicated phacoemulsification via a temporal incision, or in the case of iris lesions that do not allow perfect horizontal implantation). Another, but time-consuming modification is the preparation of a 5.2 mm temporal sclerocorneal tunnel (astigmatism induction of approx. 0.5–0.75 dpt with the rule) for the insertion of the IOL, followed by a 2 mm corneal incision for the lens forceps at 12 o'clock (astigmatism induction of approx. 0.3–0.5 dpt cyl against the rule). Since the two induced astigmatisms almost cancel each other out, the lens can be implanted horizontally in this technique almost astigmatism neutral and without sutures.

The lens is advanced into the anterior chamber with the concave side facing upwards using standard implantation tweezers under viscoelastic protection. The lens is initially inserted along it's the narrow axis in the direction of 6 o'clock and then rotated to the 3–9 o'clock position using any instrument or cannula. While the anterior chamber can be relatively stable with a sufficiently long sclero-corneal tunnel, a short corneal incision can be made with one loose continuous or two lateral single sutures, e.g. with 10.0 nylon thread, so that the anterior chamber does not collapse after insertion of the holding forceps. We additionally support the positive intraocular pressure during the implantation via the anterior chamber or pars plana infusion, which, however, is switched from "continuous" to foot switch operation during this step which helps avoid way the unintentional iris prolapse. The lens is grasped at the optic rim either with the "Artisan forceps" (Duckworth & Kent/GB) designed for anterior chamber implantation or the forceps developed by Mohr (ASICO/USA) or the one designed by Grehn (Geuder GmbH). By adding acethylcholine, the pupil can be slightly constricted while the IOL is brought into the retroiridal space. Threading of the mid-peripheral iris is done by gentle pressure between the haptic claws with a long spatula (Fig. 1c) or with the help of the enclavation needle. When using the spatula, a single horizontal paracentesis at 3 or 9 o'clock position is usually sufficient (depending on the dominant hand). When using the needle a technique analogous to prepupillary implantation is used—two downward paracenteses are applied at 10 and 2 o'clock. During needle enclavation, the forceps holding hand must also be changed intraoperatively, which is a technically more difficult and dangerous in retroiridal IOL position. Based on our experience, we believe that the latter technique is not recommended. If one has little experience and fears poor centration, similar to the prepupillary implantation of phakic Artisan®/Artiflex® IOLs, the iris can be marked preoperatively in the periphery using argon/diode lasers which works well with dark irises. However, the most common mistake is too enclavate the lens too centrally which leads to an oval pupil. Therefore, the iris should be enclaved as peripherally as possible.

Special Instruments to Facilitate Safe Implantation

The Sekundo forceps (Geuder GmbH, Fig. 1a, b) differ from conventional tweezers by using a different gripping principle. The lens is not held between the branches of the tweezers like a "sandwich", but nestles like a "tongue" on a supporting plate under the optics of the IOL. Thus, it acts simultaneously as a holding tweezers and a supporting plate and prevents the IOL from sliding into the vitreous space. The extendable support plate also has a notch that corresponds to the IOL centre, when the lens is anchored in the forceps. This makes it easy to locate the centre of the lens during enclavation, despite the retroiridal position of the IOL and the iris distortion. This is helpful in centring the lens. The individual steps are shown in Fig. 2. Figure 3 shows the final result of such an operation.

Author's recommendation

Make sure that the two haptic parts are not offset after enclavement, but opposite each other. You can feel this by touching the respective haptic parts with the spatula. If the two "claw parts" are offset, you will notice a step!

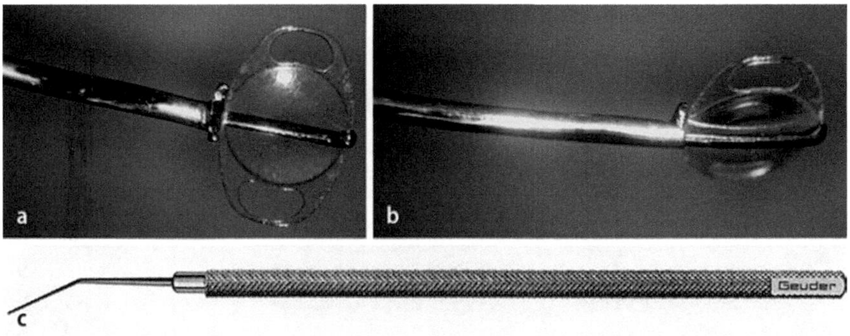

Fig. 2 Schematic representation of the implantation tweezers according to Sekundo. The branches of the tweezers are arranged in the vertical direction to avoid accidental opening during implantation. A support plate adapted to the curvature of the IOL with three small "hooks" ensures that the IOL is firmly anchored in the instrument. View from above (**a**) and below (**b**). **c** Special fine elongated spatula with an internal twist for one-handed iris claviculture into the proximal and distal haptics

Another modification (Schulze, Marburg, private communication) describes an alternative fixation technique when the Sekundo forceps have already been removed from the eye. Using a single lateral swivel movement, the IOL is brought behind the iris and is enclavated. There is no need to grasp the IOL with the tweezers inside the eye, though this modification requires a 7 mm sclerocorneal tunnel.

Lens calculation and position.

Due to the posterior localization, the A constant of the iris claw IOL changes compared to anterior chamber implantation (A = 115.0 for anterior).

Author's recommendation

We use the A constant of 116.8 for the SRK-T formula and IOL master (Carl Zeiss Meditec AG, Jena) [10].

This was calculated using postoperative data from our and other groups by W. Haigis at the University Eye Hospital Würzburg and is available at htttp://www.augenklinik.uni-wuerzburg.de/ulib/c1.htm. Other authors prefer higher values like 117.0 [11, 12] and 117.2 [13]. Galvis et al. used a personalized A constant of 117.5 and Haigis formula and thus achieve a rather high predictability of −0.62 ± 1.06 D around the target refraction [14, 15]. The heterogeneity of the refraction results is due to a reduced predictability of the effective lens position, which among other things, indicates a significant anterio-posterior movement with differing head positions. In one of our studies on this implant, the median change in anterior chamber depth compared to supine position/deep face was 155 μm [16], i.e. more than twice as high as in the iris claw design for phakic eyes [17]. This is explained by the lack of a real lens diaphragm and thus a larger iris IOL excursion. This fact

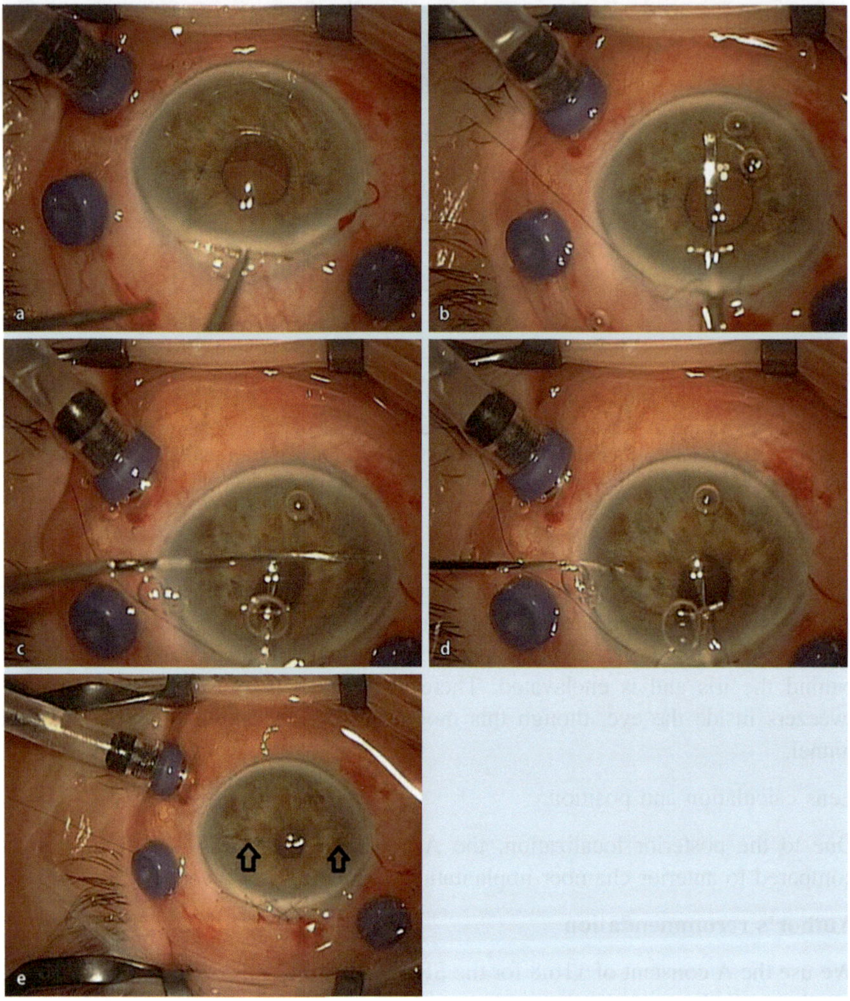

Fig. 3 Surgical steps. Aphakia after ppV, right eye, view under operating microscope. **a** After the creation of a self-closing 5.2 mm sclerocorneal tunnel, an anterior chamber infusion is inserted into the temporal lower limbus via a paracentesis. A further paracentesis is inserted at 3 o'clock. The inverted claw iris lens (IOL) is inserted into the anterior chamber under viscoelastic protection. **b** The IOL was rotated to the 3–9 o'clock position and the holding tweezers with the support plate were moved under the lens optic. **c** The IOL is firmly fixed between the holding hooks of the tweezers by a slight spatula pressure on the optic with simultaneous retraction of the supporting plate. **d** After the IOL has been brought retroiridally and centred using a central orientation notch, the pupil is narrowed by an injection of acetylcholine. The IOL is thus held in the forceps with the leading hand. A special fine spatula is then inserted through the lateral paracenthesis with the second hand and gradually presses iris tissue between the "claws" of the haptic. The pressure on the shaft of the forceps releases the now firmly encycled IOL from the forceps and removes the forceps from the eye. During removal, the infusion is interrupted to prevent iris prolapse. The bulb is then toned. Temporal and nasal. **e** The wound is closed. The pupil is round and the lens well centred [24]

can also be used clinically: when looking down, the patient reaches about half a diopter of pseudo accommodation. Of course, this does not apply to all eyes, because other factors, such as the nature of the iris, the location and amount of the encased iris tissue, and the vitreous status (partially and fully vitrectomised) can also contribute to a reduction in precision [10].

Complications

Potential complications in the immediate postoperative period include ocular hypo- and hypertension, IOL decentration, pupil opalization (which improves over time), cystoid macular edema, hypha or vitreous bleeding, uveitis, toxic anterior segment syndrome, retinal detachment and endophthalmitis [11, 12, 18, 19]. Apart from pupil ovalisation, the incidence of all other complications is well below 10%, the occurrence of which depends very much on experience and surgical technique. In our experience, one long-term postoperative complication is a de-enclavation of the IOL, which can occur in up to 8.7% of cases, but is almost always harmless, as both haptics almost never tear out at the same time. A repair via two small corneal accesses is usually easy [12]. This requires a 2.5 mm incision for the enclavation forceps and a paracentesis for the enclavation spatula (Fig. 1). The IOL is grasped and pulled up into the pupillary plane while the haptic is "fed" with new iris tissue. De-enclavation can be caused by tissue fatigue (tearing of the haptics), trauma or cyclophotocoagulation [20]. We consider an iridotomy unnecessary, provided that the retroiridal vitreous is extensively and completely removed. This is also important to minimise the risk of retinal detachment: In the case of incomplete vitrectomy and incarceration of the vitreous between the haptics, the risk of iatrogenic retinal detachment is high. Treatment of Irvin-Gass syndrome by injection of slow-release steroid implants (e.g. Ozurdex® or Illuvien®) is not recommended, as the implant can bypass the IOL and enter the anterior chamber, where it can irreversibly damage the endothelium.

Comparison with Other Implants and Implantation Techniques

In 2004, Mennel et al. compared the retropupillary iris claw IOL with a PMMA IOL fixated to a scleral suture and concluded that a faster and atraumatic implantation is possible, with the same visual acuity [3]. Seven years later, Hara et al. compared the iris claw lens with both the scleral suture-fixed PMMA lens and with a scleral suture-fixed foldable acrylic lens. The iris claw IOL had almost no complications, while the scleral suture-fixed IOL had some complications and with an operating time of almost 50 min, more than twice as long as for the iris claw IOL that took about 20 min [2].

In a comparative study of the modified haptic-fixation technique according to Scharioth, the retropupillary iris claw IOL performed only marginally better; however, the difference in operating time of 32 versus 50.5 min confirmed the experience of Mennel and Hara. Interestingly, there was also no significant difference in surgically induced astigmatism, despite the iris claw IOL requiring an incision of more than 5 mm, while a flexible IOL can be implanted through less than 3.0 mm. In the most recent publication, Toro and colleagues compared prepupillary and retropupillary implantation of an iris claw lens over a 5-year period. Apart for the number of pigment precipitates on the IOL (higher for anterior chamber implantation), the results and complication rate were almost identical. The low endothelial cell loss was also unexpectedly comparable in both groups [21].

Contraindications/Disadvantages

The implantation of an iris-fixed IOL naturally requires an intact iris diaphragm, although in the case of small iris defects these can be corrected by threading the IOL "between the claws" (Fig. 4). A 5 mm optic proves to be disadvantageous in vitreoretinal procedures. For this reason, a good rehabilitation of the posterior segment of the eye, and in particular the peripheral retina, is essential. As mentioned above, this includes a "clean" and generous anterior or pars plana vitrectomy. Glare is hardly ever reported, despite the small optics. On the one hand, this is due to the fact that older eyes have smaller pupils anyway, but at the same time

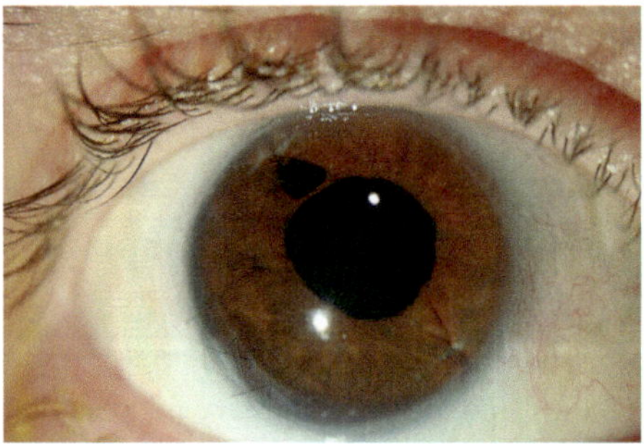

Fig. 4 Example of iris defect closure in the context of a secondary iris claw lens implantation. A giant iridectomy at 10:30 h from previous operations was significantly reduced by enclaving the peripheral iris adjacent to the defect between the haptics. No more diplopia. For this purpose, the incision was made temporally at the bottom (suture still visible) and the IOL was anchored in the 10:30–4:30 h position

there is certainly a similar pupil reduction effect as that described for the phakic Artisan® IOL [22].

Author's recommendation

Eyes with uveitis and/or ischaemic vitreoretinopathies (e.g. in diabetes or after vascular occlusion etc.) seem to us to be unsuitable for any kind of iris fixation.

On the other hand, the literature contains positive experiences in difficult initial situations such as Gilles de la Tourette's disease [23] or megalophthalmos [15]. A combination with keratoplasty is particularly advantageous because the "open sky" phase is short and the globe deformation is less severe than with scleral fixation [11].

Conclusion

- The retropupillary implantation of iris claw lenses is by far the fastest technique for anatomically correct rehabilitation of aphakic eyes without capsule structures
- Extensive anterior or pars plana vitrectomy is necessary for safe enclavation
- Special instruments facilitate the anchoring of the IOL and make it safer
- The complication rate is relatively low compared to other posterior segment IOL fixation techniques
- The technique is not suitable for eyes with defective iris diaphragm, ischemic vitreoretinal pathologies and uveitis.

Images
Figures 1, 2 and 3 please from the publication Sekundo et al. (2014) Technique of retropupillary iris claw intraocular lens implantation in aphakia. Ophthalmologe 111:315–319. There are Figs. 2, 3 and 4.

References

1. DeSilva SR, Arun K, Maghizh A, Glover N, Patel CK, Poznan P. Iris-claw intraocular lenses to correct aphakia in the absence of capsule support. J Cataract Refract Surg. 2012;37:1667–72.
2. Hara S, Borkenstein AF, Ehmer A, Ascension GU. Retropupillary fixation of iris-claw intraocular lens versus transscleral suturing fixation for aphakic eyes without capsular support. J Refract Surg. 2011;27:729–35.
3. Mennel S, Sekundo W, Schmidt JC, Meyer CH. Retropupillary fixation of an iris claw lens in aphakia. Is the scleral suture-fixed intraocular lens still state of the art? Spectr Ophthalmol. 2004;18:279–83.
4. Worst JG. Iris claw lens. J On Intraocul Implant Soc. 1980;6:166–7.

5. Amar L. Implant a pinces de chambre posterieure (type Amar) apres surgery intra-capsulaire de la cataracte. Bull Soc Ophthalmol Fr. 1982;82(6–7):847–50.
6. Rijneveld WJ, Beekhuis WH, Hassmann EF, Dellaert MM, Geerards AJ. Iris claw lens: anterior and posterior iris surface fixation in the absence of capsular support during penetrating keratoplasty. J Refract Corneal Surg. 1994;10:14–9.
7. Mohr A, Hengerer F, Eckardt C. Retropupillary fixation of the claw lens in aphakia. One-year results of a new implantation technique. Ophthalmol. 2002;99:580–3.
8. Secundo W. New forceps and spatula for easy retropullary implantation of iris-claw lenses in aphakia: experience in four years of use. Eur J Ophthalmol. 2008;18:442–44.
9. Baykara M, Ozcetin H, Yilmaz S, Timucin OB. Posterior iris fixation of the iris-claw intraoular lens implantation through a scleral tunnel incision. On J Ophthalmol. 2007;144:586–91.
10. Secundo W. Response to: position dependent accommodative shift of retropupillary fixed iris-claw lenses. Graefes Arch Clin Exp Ophthalmol. 2013;251:2485–6
11. Gonnermann J, Torun N, Klamann MK, et al. Visual outcomes and complications following posterior iris-claw aphakic intraocular lens implantation combined with penetrating keratoplasty. Graefes Arch Clin Exp Ophthalmol. 2013;251:1151–6.
12. Gonnermann J, Klamann MK, Maier AK, et al. Visual outcome and complications after posterior iris-claw aphakic intraocular lens implantation. J Cataract Refract Surg. 2012;38:2139–43.
13. Hsing YE, Lee GA. Retropupillary iris claw intraocular lens for aphakia. Clin Exp Ophthalmol. 2012;40:849–54.
14. Galvis V, Tello A, Carreño VI, Revelo ML. Apahakic retropupillary iris-claw intraocular lens (IOL) pseudophakic accommodation. Letter to the Editor. Graefes Arch Clin Exp Ophthalmol. 2013;251:2483–4.
15. Galvis V, Tello A, Miotto G, Rangel C. Artisan Aphakic Lens for cataract surgery in anterior megalophthalmos. Case Rep Ophthalmol. 2012;3:428–33.
16. Creator K, Berger A, Basket C, Stoffelns BM, Pfeiffer N, Sekundo W. Position dependent accommodative shift of retropupillary fixed iris-claw lenses. Graefes Arch Clin Exp Ophthalmol. 2012;250:1827–34.
17. Sekundo W, Tietjen A, Bißmann W. Behaviour of the phakic iris-claw intraocular lens (Artisan®/Verisyse®) during accommodation: an optical coherence biometry study. Eur J Ophthalmol. 2007;17:904–8.
18. Rüfer F, Saeger M, Nölle B, Roider J. Implantation of retropupillary iris claw lenses with and without combined penetrating keratoplasty. Graefes Arch Clin Exp Ophthalmol. 2007;247:457–62.
19. Saleh M, Heitz A, Bourcier T, et al. Sutureless intrascleral intraocular lens implantation after ocular trauma. J Cataract Refract Surg. 2013;39:81–6.
20. Kičová N, Sekundo W, Mennel S. Subluxation of a retropupillary fixed claw iris lens after cyclophotocoagulation. Ophthalmologe. 2011;108:167–9.
21. Toro MD, Longo A, Avitabile T, Nowomiejska K, Gagliano C, Tripodi S, Choragiewicz T, Kaminska A, Figus M, Posarelli C, Forlini M, Jünemann AGM, Reibaldi M, Reidak R. Five-year follow-up of secondary iris-claw intraocular lens implantation for the treatment of aphakia: anterior chamber versus retropupillary implantation. PLoS ONE. 2019;10(14): e0214140.
22. Dick HB, Aliyeva S, Tehrani M. Change in pupil size after implantation of an iris-fixated toric phakic intraocular lens. J Cataract Refract Surg. 2005;31:302–7.
23. Gaillard MC, Wolfensberger TJ. Automutilation with lens dislocation in Gilles de la Tourette's disease, treated with retropupillary iris claw lens. Clin Monatsbl Ophthalmol. 2004;221:435–7.
24. Besgen V, Sekundo W. Aphake Artisan®/Verisyse® intraocular lenses as retropupillary implants. Ophthalmologe. 2017;114:1038–1041.

Implantation of Scleral-Fixed Intraocular Lenses

Thomas C. Kreutzer and Sorcha Ní Dhubhghaill

The secondary implantation of scleral-fixated artificial lenses and the scleral refixation of sub- or completely luxated artificial lenses has increased significantly in recent years. Scleral fixation becomes necessary when the capsular bag complex (including the zonulae) is no longer able to guarantee a stable support of the artificial lens. In addition to secondary scleral fixation, the implantation of iris-fixated artificial lenses or the implantation of anterior chamber lenses can be considered as alternatives. When the artificial lens luxates in the eye and the surgeon wishes to refixate it without replacement, it is also possible to attach it to the iris as an alternative to scleral fixation.

Since iris problems can be more commonly associated with this and the scleral fixation of intraocular implants has made significant technical progress in recent years, the technique of iris suture fixation of artificial lenses is not currently recommended, in the opinion of the author, and not discussed in this chapter.

There are many different techniques and models of intraocular lens implants for the purposes of scleral fixation but to describe the myriad of different techniques could fill a whole book. In this chapter we will limit ourselves to current techniques for scleral fixation with a minimally invasive approach. In addition, these techniques can be carried out with many conventional lens models for capsular bag implantation, as found in most surgical units. Using minimally invasive techniques, it has become possible to implant intraocular lens (even in cases of secondary implantation) through corneal incisions of a maximum size of 3.0 mm and a minimum of 1.8 mm. This technical advance achieves more advantageous refrac-

Supplementary Information The online version contains supplementary material available at https://doi.org/10.1007/978-3-031-05394-8_62. The videos can be accessed individually by clicking the DOI link in the accompanying figure caption or by scanning this link with the SN More Media App.

T. C. Kreutzer (✉) · S. N. Dhubhghaill
München, Germany
e-mail: thomas.kreutzer@med.uni-muenchen.de

M. Shajari et al. (eds.), *Cataract and Lens Surgery*,
https://doi.org/10.1007/978-3-031-05394-8_62

tive results for the patient by specifically respecting and reducing corneal astigmatism. The authors of this chapter have already used the described techniques several times and will discuss the advantages and disadvantages of the techniques mentioned.

A prerequisite for successful scleral fixation and reduction of complications is the performance of a careful anterior vitrectomy. The surgeon should therefore master the technique of anterior vitrectomy and specifically, the removal of the anterior part of the vitreous, behind the iris as well. This can significantly reduce the risk of one of the most serious complications of scleral fixation, namely retinal detachment. In addition, it is advisable to remove any remaining capsular bag remnants as well, since in the event of preexisting fibrosis or fibrosis in the future, these can negatively influence the position of the scleral fixated intraocular implant by induction of tilt or decentration.

Scleral Pocket Fixation of 3-Piece IOLs

In 2010, Scharioth described the first minimally invasive approach for scleral fixation of an intraocular lens (Video 1) [1]. A key aspect of his approach was the creation of 180° offset intrascleral pockets. The haptics of a 3-piece artificial lens could then be inserted or retracted in these pockets through sclerotomies. A great advantage of this technique was the possibility of using foldable artificial lenses for secondary implantation as well as for the refixation of sub- or luxated 3-piece artificial lenses. One-piece lenses, however, were not appropriate for this technique.

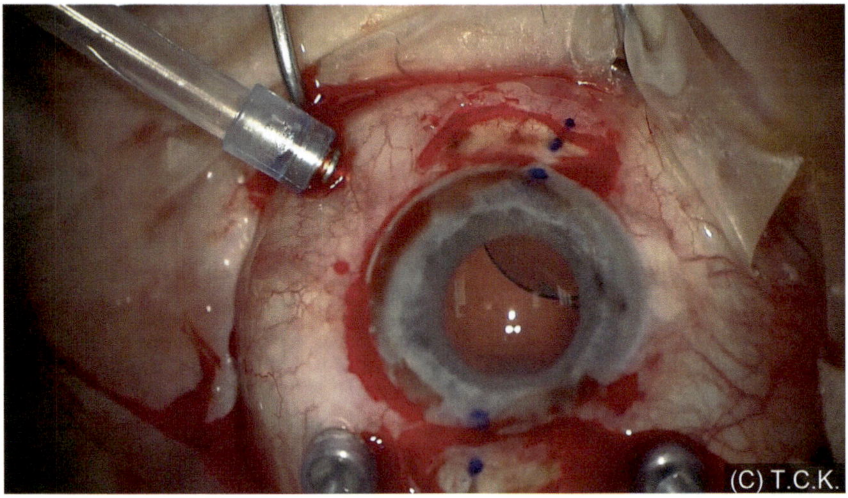

Video 1 Scleral fixation of a 3-piece intraocular lens with the technique according to Scharioth (▶ https://doi.org/10.1007/000-8e7)

When performing this technique, pars plana vitrectomy access, at least in the form of an infusion line is preferred, but an anterior chamber maintainer should always be used, for stability and endothelial protection. If a vitrectomy infusion is used, the sclerotomy knife can also be used to create the sclerotomies for haptic externalisation and trocar systems up to 27G can be used. The conjunctival pockets require a scleral tunnel preparation, are first prepared freely 180° apart, and two sclerotomy access points are marked 2 mm posterior to the limbus. After the infusion line has been placed to pressurize the eye, paracentheses are placed to allow optimal manipulation of the IOL haptics in the eye.

For the implantation of the three-piece intraocular lens with a total diameter of at least 13.5 mm, the corneal incision should be placed on the steep axis, if possible, in case of existing corneal astigmatism, otherwise it should be placed temporally. After filling the anterior chamber with viscoelastic, the artificial lens is implanted into the anterior chamber, leaving the trailing haptic outside the corneal incision for simplicity. Next the sclerotomies are created at the previously marked points using the sclerotomy knife. Intrascleral tunnels of 2 mm starting from the sclerotomy are created either with a 1.1 mm curved paracenthesis lance or with a 27 g needle, which is becoming more popular.

Now the leading haptic is grasped via the first sclerotomy with crocodile forceps corresponding to the access size at the haptic end and externalized via the sclerotomy. Gripping the haptic end is particularly important to prevent the haptic from bending during externalization. The same maneuver is now repeated with the following haptics via the second sclerotomy. Once both haptics have been externalized, they are inserted or pulled into the scleral tunnels using a 25G or 27G crocodile forceps or, if the needle technique is used, inserted into the needle which is then removed from the scleral pocket, leaving the haptic inside the sclera. Then the artificial lens is centered and fixated. Depending on the size of the sclerotomy, it may need to be sutured, and the conjunctiva is then closed.

When refixing luxated or subluxated 3-piece artificial lenses that had previously been implanted in the capsular bag, they must first be cut free of capsular bag residue using a vitrectomy cutter. Once the lens is cleaned and the haptics freed, these lenses can then be refixated in the same way. It is important to pay attention to the possibility of existing distortion of the haptics due to an extended period of implantation in the capsular bag or by surgical manipulation during the cleaning process. If there is any distortion, the artificial lens should be replaced, as good centering without tilting can no longer be guaranteed in the presence of haptic damage.

The advantages of this technique are that good centering is possible, that little additional surgical material is needed over that which is routinely available in an operating room, and that the patient's own luxated lens can be used (if it is a 3-piece). The disadvantages are the extensive number of incisions and the technically rather tricky insertion of the haptic ends into the scleral pockets.

Scleral Suture Fixation of 1-Piece IOLs

In 2010, Szurman (Video 2) described a technique of minimally invasive suture fixation of single-piece hydrophobic artificial lenses through a clear cornea incision [2]. This technique also allows a minimally invasive refixation of subluxated or luxated single-piece artificial lenses. Here too, the conjunctiva is opened at a 180° offset and the sclera is exposed over approx. 2 mm laterally and 5 mm posteriorly. Once again, two points 2 mm posterior to the limbus are marked, 180° apart. After a thorough anterior vitrectomy, a double-reinforced 9.0 or 10.0 prolene suture is inserted with a straight needle on one side and docked into a contralaterally inserted 27G needle. The prolene suture which now runs through the eye is externalized and cut via a clear cornea incision (CCI) of at least 2.2 mm, creating two suture ends which protrude from the CCI and run to each of the two scleral points with a straight needle at their ends.

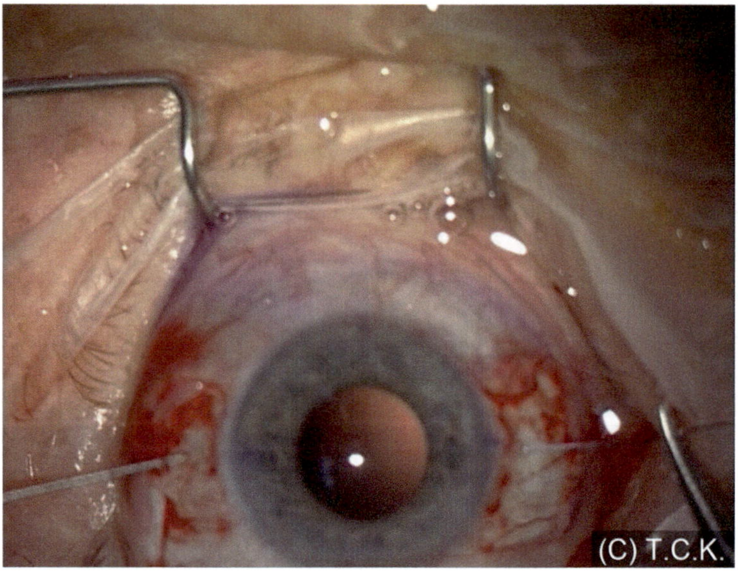

Video 2 Scleral fixation of a one-piece, hydrophobic artificial lens on the sclera using the technique according to Szurman (▶ https://doi.org/10.1007/000-8e5)

A one-piece hydrophobic artificial lens, ideally with slightly raised haptic ends, is now loaded into the injector in such a way that the leading haptic comes out of the cartridge straight when pushed forward. The artificial lens is now advanced so far that the leading haptic extends straight out of the cartridge. One half of the cut prolene thread is now knotted to the haptic end, and ideally the knot is guided to the outside of the haptic. The cartridge with the sutured haptic is now inserted into the incision and implanted into the anterior chamber but the trailing haptic should remain in the incision. The second half of the cut prolene thread is now knotted to it in the same way. Now the artificial lens can be fully inserted into the anterior chamber and then brought into position by pulling on the two ends of the prolene suture threads.

The prolene threads are then permanently fixed by winding intrascleral needle guidance within the sclera, with five stitches of approx. 3 mm in length guided intrasclerally. After the last intrascleral stitch, the thread is cut short at the end. This ensures a secure permanent fixation without the need for a knot at the end. The great advantage of this technique lies in the possibility of scleral fixation of single-piece hydrophobic artificial lenses, which are usually present in every surgical unit, the predominant manipulation in the anterior eye segment and the minimally invasive approach with possible small incision technique. The disadvantages are the technically somewhat more demanding knotting of the prolene thread at the haptic ends and the possibility of iris pigment loss if the artificial lens is fixed too loosely and thereby pushing against the posterior iris which can cause uveitis-glaucoma-hyphema (UGH) syndrome.

Modified Yamane Scleral Fixation of 3-Piece IOLs

In 2014, Yamane (Videos 3 and 4)described an elegant modification to the technique for the intrascleral fixation of three-piece artificial lenses [3]. The technique was further optimized in 2017 to be even more minimally invasive by a transconjunctival approach [4]. Ultimately, it is a technique that has been further minimized in its invasiveness, based on the procedure according to Scharioth and the “glued IOL technique” by Agarwall [5]. In Yamane’s case, three-piece artificial lenses are anchored intrasclerally by means of a hot cautery thickening at the haptic ends to create a bulb.

It is advantageous to use an artificial lens model with uncoated prolene haptics as these are most suitable for this maneuver. A good melt of the haptic ends can be problematic with coated prolene haptics. Yamane initially places a marking 1.5–2 mm posterior to the limbus on the conjunctiva at the 3- o’clock and 9 o’clock position, 180° apart. The conjunctiva does not need to be opened. After a thorough anterior vitrectomy, the three-piece artificial lens is implanted into the anterior chamber, the trailing haptic end can remain in the CCI for the time being. Again, an infusion line via a vitrectomy trocar at the pars plana is recommended. For the 3/9 h fixation, the haptics in the anterior chamber are rotated to the 6 and 12 h position. A 2 mm transconjunctival tunnel is now created by the intrascleral insertion of a 27G needle (or 30G needle with thin steel wall) at the conjunctival markings and then entering the vitreous cavity. The course of the needles should follow the haptic course of the artificial lens in the eye. The needles should be bent at an angle before the tunneling process, similar to bending a rhexis needle without manipulating the

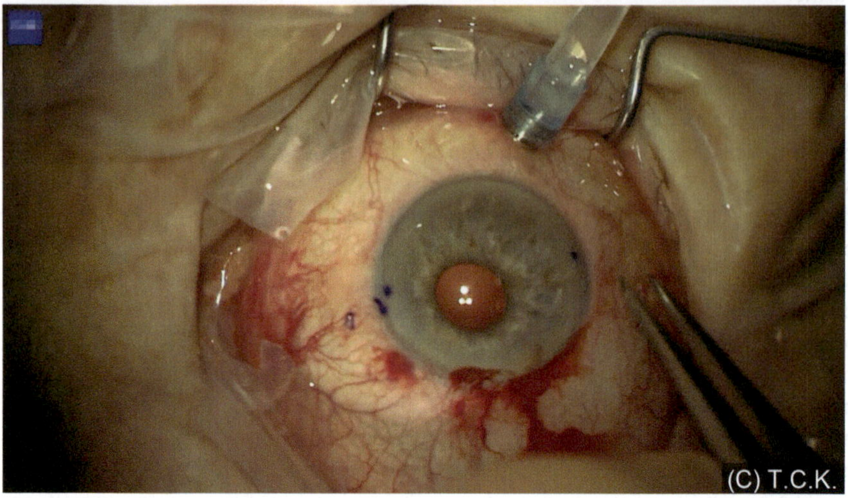

Video 3 Scleral fixation of a three-piece artificial lens using the Yamane technique (▶ https://doi.org/10.1007/000-8e6)

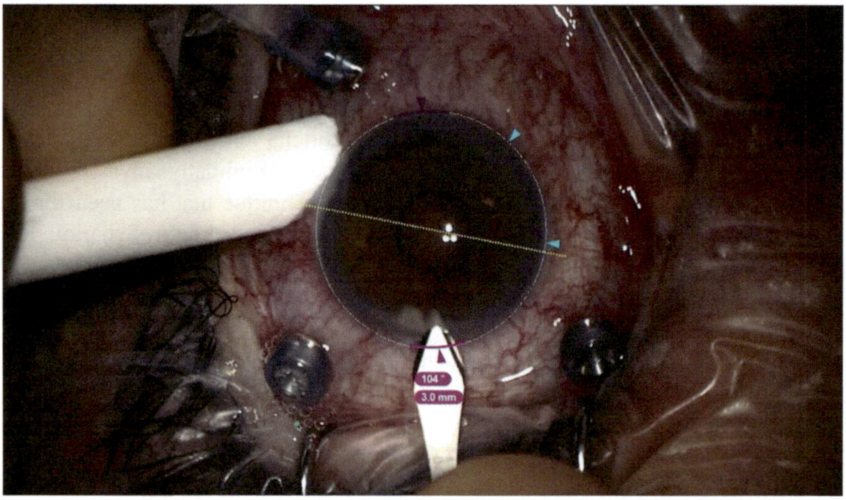

Video 4 Learning video of scleral fixation with the technique according to Yamane by M. Shajari (▶ https://doi.org/10.1007/000-8e4)

needle tip. It remains the preference of the surgeon whether they first insert both needles, puts them down and continues to advance or whether the second needle only pierces after the first haptic is externalized and fixated. The needles are then used to externalize the haptics.

The leading haptic at 6 h is then inserted into the left needle tip using an intraocular forceps. The author favors a curved 25 g crocodile forceps. Even with a reusable rhexis forceps, which can be inserted via a paracentesis, the haptics can be safely inserted into the needle end. The first haptic is now either externalized directly with the needle cannula following the course of the needle, grasped with a knotting forceps and melted with the cautery in order to fix it in place, or left in the needle after only partial retraction and the needle is discarded for the time being. The following haptic is now inserted into the second needle cannula. This is the more demanding maneuver. If the following haptic is located in the CCI, it can first be grasped there with the forceps and then, in a direct step, be introduced into the anterior chamber and inserted into the right needle. If it is already in the anterior chamber and therefore in the chamber angle, the artificial lens should first be manipulated either with a rotating hook or with the needle for insertion so the haptic end comes into the surgeon's field of vision.

The author strongly advises against "haptic fishing" with the forceps in the chamber angle without clear visualization of the haptic, as this can cause unpleasant iris bleeding and, in the worst-case, iris base defects. Now the second haptic can be externalized and cauterized, or both haptics can now be externalized and cauterized one after the other. They are then pushed back through the conjunctiva and into the scleral tunnels with tying forceps and should be fixed in place. The artificial lens should be centered unless the ends of the haptics are bent or the tunnels have not been applied properly.

The advantages of the Yamane technique are the highly minimally invasive approach, the possibility of CCI implantation on a steep corneal axis with a possible incision size of at least 2.6 mm and the sequence of surgical measures, which can be reproduced and standardized after an initial learning curve. The duration of the surgery is also usually very predictable. The disadvantages are the initial learning curve, an elevated technical demand especially with regard to the precise and uniform scleral tunnel preparation guiding the needles, in order to guarantee the most exact positioning of the artificial lens with the least possible tilt. Furthermore, long-term data are currently lacking with regard to position stability, the risk of infection (possible migration endophthalmitis) and the stability of the haptics.

Multi-point Scleral Fixation of IOLs

The disadvantage of a scleral fixation at two points is the susceptibility of the intraocular lens implant to tilt so additional points of fixation offer advantages. In 2014, Khan described the first scleral fixation of a one-piece hydrophilic lens with four loops using a Goretex® thread (Video 5) [6]. The conjunctiva is opened mainly nasally and temporally over 6 mm and the sclera exposed. The marking is made 180° offset 2 mm posterior to the limbus nasally and temporally. An alternative superior and inferior placement is also possible, but may jeopardize any glaucoma surgery measures that may be necessary later. Further markings are made 2 mm posterior to the limbus on both sides of the initial markings, offset by 1.5 mm. Sclerotomies are created to these 4 additional markings with a 25G scleral lance.

A double reinforced 6.0 Gore-Tex thread, which is used in neurosurgery and vascular surgery, is then cut in half and the end needles removed. Using a CCI for lens implantation, the end of the first thread is inserted into the anterior chamber and externalised with the aid of 25G crocodile tweezers via the lower left sclerotomy from the surgeon's perspective. The contralateral end of the thread is now passed from behind through the right haptic loop of the artificial lens and then back out of the left haptic loop. This thread end is then reintroduced into the anterior chamber via the CCI and externalised with crocodile forceps via the right upper sclerotomy. The artificial lens haptics are looped and the thread ends externalised with the 2nd half of the thread via the temporal sclerotomies. Once all the sutures have been secured, the artificial lens can be implanted with folding tweezers via a 3.2 mm CCI.

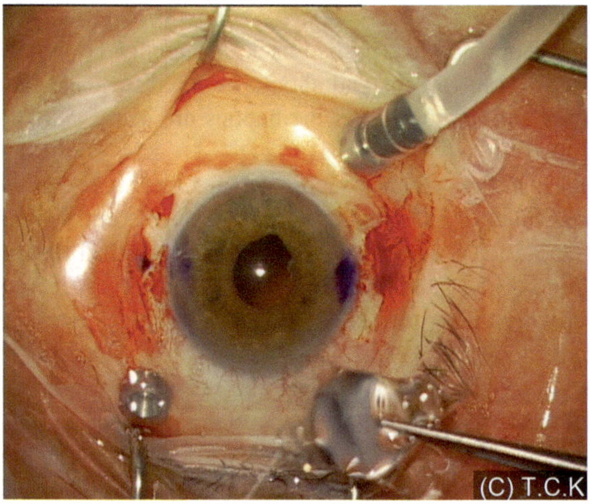

Video 5 Scleral fixation of a one-piece loop haptic artificial lens with Goretex® thread over a 3.2 mm CCI (▶ https://doi.org/10.1007/000-8e8)

The lens is positioned by pulling on the threads. The sutures are then knotted 3-1-1 on the sclera and the ends of the account are sunk through the respective contralateral inverted sclerotomy. The conjunctiva is closed and the sutures remain visible underneath. A modification by the author enables the implantation and fixation of the artificial lens through a 2.0 mm incision by looping the haptics in an implantation cartridge (video 6).

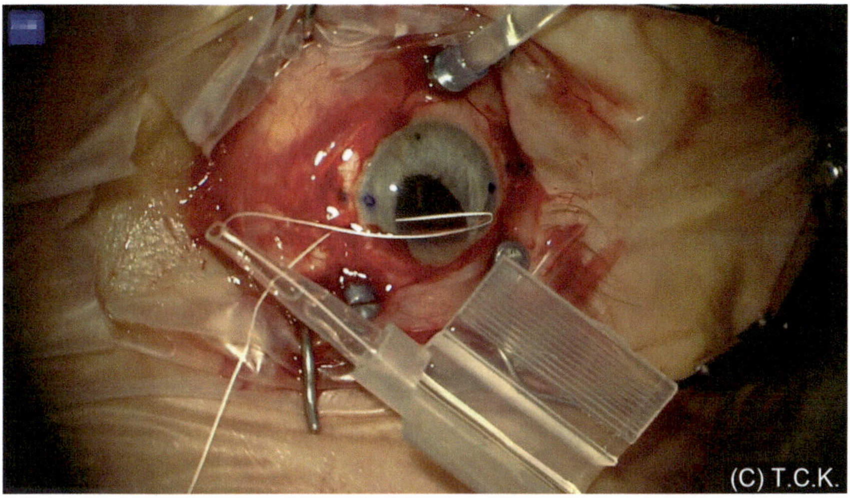

Video 6 Implantation of an artificial lens fixed with Goretex thread Sclera with loop haptics (▶ https://doi.org/10.1007/000-8e9)

The advantages of this technique are the very good rotation and tilt stability of the scleral fixation of a hydrophilic artificial lens via a micro incision. Disadvantages are the advanced technical demands with and learning curve, and steps that are not always reliably reproducible and thus reduced predictability of the duration of surgery (Video 7). The Goretex® thread used is not approved by the company for use in the eye.

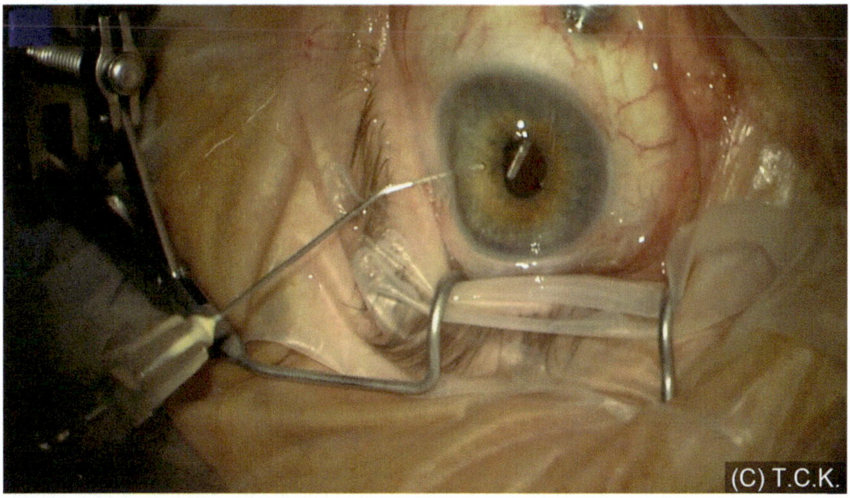

Video 7 Refixation of a luxated one-piece loop haptic artificial lens using Goretex® four-point fixation on the sclera (▶ https://doi.org/10.1007/000-8ea)

The Carlevale IOL

The Carlevale artificial lens is an intraocular lens specially designed and approved for scleral fixation. It can be implanted through a CCI between 2.4 and 3.0 mm, depending on the dioptric strength of the artificial lens [7]. The lens is made of a hydrophilic material and has a T-shaped fixation system for the sclera at both ends. The implant is also available as in a toric version for astigmatic correction but as usual, a thorough anterior vitrectomy must be performed first. First, after sectoral opening of the conjunctiva, two 3.5 × 3.5 mm scleral flaps are prepared offset by 180°. A sclerotomy is performed with a 25G needle 1.5 mm posterior limbus, under the lid. Now the artificial lens is implanted via a clear cornea incision (CCI). The leading haptic can be grasped over the sclerotomy with 25G forceps and then externalised. The following haptics remain either in the CCI or in the anterior chamber. Then, in a "handshake technique", the following haptics can be transferred to the 25G forceps with a pair of tweezers, which then externalises this haptic via the second sclerotomy. The T-feet are aligned parallel to the limbus and the scleral flaps are sutured over them. The conjunctiva is then closed. The Carlevale artificial lens enables a very standardized and reproducible procedure for scleral fixation. A disadvantage is the necessity of preparing the scleral flaps and conjunctival opening.

Summary

Scleral fixation of intraocular lenses is possible today using a variety of techniques. The fixation technique according to Yamane is becoming increasingly popular due to its reproducibility and stability. The Carlevale artificial lens also allows a very standardised procedure. Ideally, the advanced lens surgeon should have mastered several of these techniques to customize their approach to the patient. With the procedures described above, both three-piece and one-piece intraocular lenses can be fixated to the sclera.

Author's recommendation

A good command of anterior vitrectomy techniques is essential for scleral fixation of artificial lenses. The fixation techniques described by Szurman and the Carelvale artificial lens implantation offer good approaches for scleral fixation, especially for beginners. The Yamane technique and the Goretex 4-point fixation require much more bimanual skill and therefore have a somewhat more difficult learning curve.

References

1. Scharioth GB, Prasad S, Georgalas I, Tataru C, Pavlidis M. Intermediate results of sutureless intrascleral posterior chamber intraocular lens fixation. J Cataract Refract Surg. 2010;36(2):254–9. https://doi.org/10.1016/j.jcrs.2009.09.024.
2. Szurman P, Petermeier K, Aisenbrey S, Spitzer MS, Jaissle GB. Z-suture: a new knotless technique for transscleral suture fixation of intraocular implants. Br J Ophthalmol. 2010;94(2):167–9. https://doi.org/10.1136/bjo.2009.162180.

3. Yamane S, Inoue M, Arakawa A, Kadonosono K. Sutureless 27-gauge needle-guided intrascleral intraocular lens implantation with lamellar scleral dissection. Ophthalmology. (2014);121(1):61–6. https://doi.org/10.1016/j.ophtha.2013.08.043.
4. Yamane S, Sato S, Maruyama-Inoue M, Kadonosono K. Flanged intrascleral intraocular lens fixation with double-needle technique. Ophthalmology. 2017;124(8):1136–42. https://doi.org/10.1016/j.ophtha.2017.03.036.
5. Kumar DA, Agarwal A, Prakash G, Jacob S, Saravanan Y, Agarwal A. Glued posterior chamber IOL in eyes with deficient capsular support: a retrospective analysis of 1-year post-operative outcomes. Eye. 2010;24(7):1143–8. https://doi.org/10.1038/eye.2010.10.
6. Khan MA, Gerstenblith AT, Dollin ML, Gupta OP, Spirn MJ. Scleral fixation of posterior chamber intraocular lenses using gore-tex suture with concurrent 23-gauge pars plana vitrectomy. Retina. 2014;34(7):1477–80. https://doi.org/10.1097/IAE.0000000000000233.
7. Rossi T, Iannetta D, Romano V, Carlevale C, Forlini M, Telani S, Imburgia A, Mularoni A, Fontana L, Ripandelli G. A novel intraocular lens designed for sutureless scleral fixation: surgical series. Graefe's archive for clinical and experimental ophthalmology. Albrecht Graefe's Arch Clin Exp Ophthalmol. 2020. https://doi.org/10.1007/s00417-020-04789-3.

Cataract Surgery After Trauma

Armin Wolf and Ferenc Kuhn

Introduction

In general, functionality of the human crystalline lens can be damaged by trauma in various ways. Main manifestations of trauma on the lens are either the loss of transparency (Cataract) or the change in position in relation to the optical axis (luxation/subluxation of the lens). Both pathologies—opacification or (sub-)luxation can be caused by either direct mechanical exposure or secondary to a trauma, i.e. not mechanically, for example, induced by post-traumatic inflammatory reactions or accidents with electric current, radiation and chemicals.

The approach as well as the timing and planning of surgery for traumatic cataracts can differ greatly from standard cataract surgery. Timing in traumatic cataract surgery is important and it is therefore essential to choose the right timeline for surgery. Primary cataract surgery in a complex trauma needs to be considered and compared with secondary intervention during the course of the posttraumatic rehabilitation. The decision is not only based on the type of injury, but is also influenced by other trauma-related conditions and post-traumatic pathologies in the affected eye.

Supplementary Information The online version contains supplementary material available at https://doi.org/10.1007/978-3-031-05394-8_63. The videos can be accessed individually by clicking the DOI link in the accompanying figure caption or by scanning this link with the SN More Media App.

A. Wolf (✉)
Ulm, Germany
e-mail: armin.wolf@icloud.com

F. Kuhn
Birmingham, England
e-mail: fkuhn@mindspring.com

M. Shajari et al. (eds.), *Cataract and Lens Surgery*,
https://doi.org/10.1007/978-3-031-05394-8_63

The following is an overview of the numerous mechanisms of injury, the surgical options and factors determining the time of surgery for a trauma-related cataract. Only limited robust data exist on many aspects of traumatic cataract surgery due to the nature and intraindividual variance in ocular traumatology.

Injury Mechanisms

Half of the cases in the largest database of eye injuries (The United States Eye Injury Registry, with more than 17,000 entries), involve the lens. Traumatic cataract occurs mainly in people under 30 years of age, is common in children, and shows a marked predilection for male patients. In addition, approximately half of the eyes showed retinal, iris or corneal injuries and more than three-quarters of the eyes underwent surgery more than once. Only about 40% of the cases achieved a best-corrected visual acuity of 20/10 or better after completion of treatment [1].

There are different injury mechanisms to consider. For the nomenclature and for correct assessment it is best to follow the "Birmingham Eye Trauma Terminology" (BETT) system. Open-globe injuries (rupture, caused by a blunt object, versus laceration, caused by a sharp object, and within the latter category, penetrating, intraocular foreign body, perforating) are usually caused by impacts with higher kinetic energies. The causative objects may have high kinetic energy (knives, toys, glass, rubber bands, fishhooks, wire, pencils or fireworks). Closed globe injuries (contusion or lamellar laceration) are often caused by a fist punch, impacts from balls and rubber bands [2]. They occur most frequently at home. The second most frequent environment where injuries occur are in the workplace, followed by traffic accidents, sports and other circumstances. Safety glasses were worn at the time of injury in only 2% of cases [1].

Cataract in Open Globe Injuries

Open globe injuries (mostly penetrating injuries with or without IOFB) are responsible for about 70% of traumatic cataracts [1]. In penetrating injuries, the cataract may develop quickly after opening of the lens capsule by a foreign body or a sharp object. When the lens capsule is opened, the inner lens begins to hydrate and turns white by denaturing lens proteins [3].

However, in pediatric cases, a focal defect of the lens capsule may not necessarily lead to a hydration of the complete lens. In this instance the defect with the focal hydration may be monitored and, in some cases, a self-sealing circumscribed fibrosis occurs. In these cases, cataract surgery may be postponed to a later age.

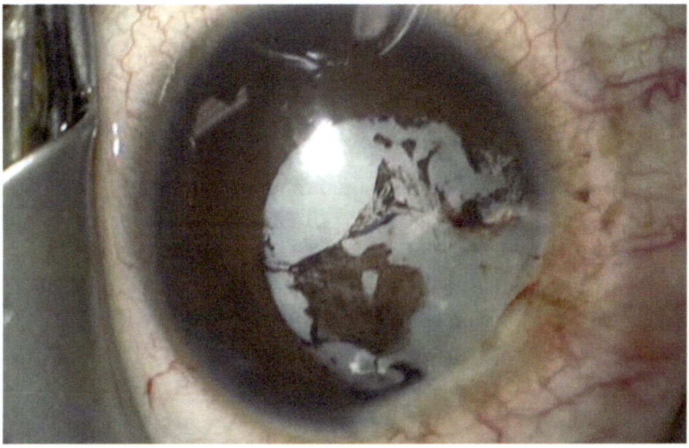

Video 1 Treatment of a traumatic cataract in a child with an iris defect
(▶ https://doi.org/10.1007/000-8eb)

Cataract in Closed Globe Trauma (Contusion)

Cataracts after contusion account for about 30% of all traumatic cataracts.

A mechanical trauma to the lens without rupturing the capsule can lead to a cataract that is initially subcapsular and often appears in a star-shaped pattern [4]. These injuries typically occur in young men. The identification of a potential role of trauma in cataract is essential. While in many cases the trauma is recent, in a large number of cases the trauma may have been many years previously and the patient may not be able to recall it. In addition, a history of repeated injury (for example martial arts in young men) might not have been perceived as trauma by the patient themselves. Traumatic cataract often leads to intraoperative complications as a result of zonular injury, such as zonulolysis, and complicated capsulorhexis or vitreous prolapse. Therefore, the potential diagnosis of a traumatic cataract is important even if the clinical history is negative for trauma or if there was no direct previous trauma reported. People working under hazardous conditions, such as welders and glassblowers or those working with high-voltage also may develop specific forms of cataracts [3].

Other lens changes caused by contusion of the globe include dislocation of the crystalline lens and—very infrequently—posterior rupture of the lens capsule.

Timing of Cataract Surgery

In the absence of comparative studies and in the face of the variety of post-traumatic conditions and accompanying pathologies, it is controversial whether the visual outcome is influenced by the timing of cataract extraction or IOL implantation [5]. Therefore, no overall recommendation should be given. There are various advantages and disadvantages of primary and secondary IOL-Implantation. The timing of secondary intervention is also not clearly defined in the available literature. One of the first decisions the surgeon has to make during the primary repair of a traumatized eye whether a primary or a secondary lens extraction is to be carried out. Similarly, the need for a primary or secondary lens implantation must be considered [5].

Advantages and Disadvantages of Primary Lens Extraction

Lens extraction during primary care refers to the removal of the lens during the initial treatment of the penetrating trauma. It has some advantages and is useful in certain situations. An examination of the posterior segment of the eye, which was not previously possible through the cloudy lens, can now be carried out and pathologies of the posterior segment of the eye can be detected. Therefore, one potential disadvantage of delayed cataract extraction is not being able to have detailed assessment of retinal pathologies which may have a better prognosis in an early intervention.

The visualization during pars plana vitrectomy, especially in case of intraocular foreign body or retinal detachment may make a primary lens removal necessary at that point. It is also useful in cases with dislocated fragments of the crystalline lens into the vitreous. Swelling caused by a capsule-breaching injury, might also indicate an earlier lens removal, especially if it leads to a pupil block. Special attention for this situation must be given in pediatric cases as such swelling is a significant risk in children. Faster visual rehabilitation may be another factor for early lens surgery.

The following conditions may be considered as indications for a timely lens removal:

(1) Discharge of lens material into the anterior chamber, especially with increase in pressure or increase in inflammatory intraocular reaction
(2) Large defect of the anterior or posterior lens capsule
(3) Lack of adequate assessment of the posterior segment of the eye due to lens opacification/lens hydration
(4) Acute secondary glaucoma

As stated above, traumatic cataract surgery may be accompanied by a large number of complicated situations. Therefore, we feel that the surgery should be performed by an experienced (trauma) surgeon so that these eyes are not treated as "routine, age-related" cases. Additionally, as mentioned above, some lens injuries may be observed and have better surgical options under more controlled circumstances at a later point of time. For example, biometry is more precise at a later point of time with a stable and reliable corneal surface and anterior chamber depth. The choice of the best IOL is dependent on other ocular conditions i.e. retinal detachment, epiretinal membrane and others, which may become less probable after a longer time post trauma. Many of these factors can influence the outcome of the lens surgery, which may be performed more optimally at a later time.

Author's Recommendation

Careful consideration is needed to indicate acute and primary lens surgery in pediatric cases, as opposed to delaying it in eyes with focal lens injuries, very hard lenses as well as "difficult-to-judge" situations caused by corneal concomitant injuries. Delayed surgery may be preferable in terms of surgical conditions.

In these cases, the immediate post-traumatic inflammatory reaction should be reduced by anti-inflammatory treatment and the operation should be performed after the intraocular inflammation has subsided.

Advantages and Disadvantages of Secondary Lens Extraction

The ideal time for secondary cataract surgery is not well established in the literature and usually varies between 2 weeks and 6 months. Ultimately, the decision of timing for secondary cataract surgery depends on individual factors, especially the pathologies of injury to other eye structures, such as the retina. A clearing-up of the cloudy cornea during follow-up may lead to better visibility during surgery and therefore allows a more controlled operation.

A more reliable keratometry at a time point after initial corneal wound healing also argues in favor of delayed correction of a traumatic aphakia: immediately after open globe trauma irregular astigmatism is increased due to sutures and corneal edema. Thus, the possible fitting of a toric lens correcting regular astigmatism may only be considered at a later stage, after the trauma.

Furthermore, a later correction of aphakia frequently allows for a better initial condition for reconstruction of other structures of the anterior and posterior segment.

At a later time-point, stabilization of the blood ocular barrier has re-established. This means that the postoperative inflammatory reaction is usually less severe after the post-traumatic inflammation has subsided [5].

Primary Aphakia and Secondary Implantation

In severely injured eyes, primary lens extraction may be beneficial for intraoperative management. However, this does not necessarily justify primary lens implantation. This is the case, for example, if posterior segment structures such as the retina are primarily affected or an intraocular foreign body needs to be removed [5]. If a pars plana vitrectomy is necessary, a cloudy lens decreases the visualization, thus lens extraction may be performed in primary surgery and the eye may be left aphakic for later IOL. It may be advisable in some of these cases to use pars plana lensectomy and vitrectomy as the primary procedure to reduce the risk of proliferative vitreoretinopathy [5]. Once the primary care is complete, the post-traumatic inflammation has subsided and corneal wound-healing has stabilized, the refractive power of the intraocular lens may be calculated more reliably and a secondary IOL may be implanted safely.

Surgical Technique Traumatic Cataract Extraction

The surgical technique for traumatic cataract usually differs significantly from the technique used in senile cataract extraction. Aggravating surgical conditions such as clouding of the cornea are often present, especially after acute trauma. It is also often accompanied by a rupture of the posterior capsule, which may be detected preoperatively by UBM or OCT in some cases [6].

In the case of a subluxated crystalline lens, a rhexis with smaller diameter may be beneficial to prevent total luxation. At a later point during surgery the rhexis may be widened with intraocular scissors for sufficient space to allow IOL implantation.

In the case of a central capsule defect, a controlled rhexis may be performed by widening the defect with intraocular scissors so that the rhexis can be guided away from the defect as a curvilinear rhexis. In the case of peripheral defects of the lens, it is recommended not to integrate the defect into the rhexis but perform a decentralized rhexis away from the opening.

The zonular apparatus is frequently affected in cases of ocular contusion and hyphema may be present. Particularly in these cases, hypotonic or hypertonic conditions may additionally complicate the surgery. If the zonules are only partially preserved, the implantation of a capsular tension ring or scleral fixation of the capsular bag with a Cionni ring may be possible [7]. However, in young patients especially, the extra mass of a CTR or similar may result in IOL luxation later in life. Intraoperatively, stabilization of the lens capsule with capsule hooks [8] or other devices can bring a certain degree of stabilization. Femtosecond laser-assisted cataract surgery [9] may ease the operation of a subluxated lens in selected cases but if there is too much damage to the lens supportive apparatus, extracapsular cataract extraction may be preferred. Other procedures such as pars plana lensectomy or lens retrieval from the vitreous need to be considered according to the scenario. In many traumatic cases, maintaining the capsular bag may not be possible or not advised, and the IOL needs to be fixated alternatively. In these cases, a variety of options for correcting aphakia exist. Scleral-fixated or iris-fixated lens [10] with or without sutures are the most common alternatives. An iris-clip lens is not always feasible due to iris defects. Additionally, anterior chamber lenses may increase the risk of further corneal decompensation and are not advised in young patients [11]. Overall, it is advisable to have a traumatic cataract treated by a surgeon experienced in both vitreoretinal as well as cataract surgery.

Postoperative Complications

In cases of traumatic cataract, especially in case of involvement of the iris base, the ciliary body and/or the lens zonules, intraocular pressure tends to be unstable postoperatively. Cases with increased or reduced intraocular pressure are often difficult to control. The risk of postoperative endophthalmitis after traumatic cataract surgery seems also to be increased [12]. Secondary intraocular lens dislocation is possible if the zonular apparatus is weak. Retinal detachment and postoperative macular edema are more common in traumatized eyes and therefore the follow-ups need to be conducted accordingly. This is further emphasized by the fact that more than three-quarters of the eyes are operated on more than once and the improvement of vision may take several years.

Traumatic Cataract in Children

In a US study, more than 60% of children undergoing surgery for traumatic cataract were able to achieve a vision of 0.5 or better [13]. Other studies usually show worse or even much worse results. As many cases of pediatric traumatic cataract are unilateral, age-adopted amblyopia treatment/prophylaxis, should be started as early as possible, and seems to be crucial for development of good visual acuity.

There is no consensus among experts on the most ideal rehabilitation methods for pediatric aphakic conditions. This is true for the type of correction as well as for the timing of secondary correction of aphakia [14]. There are various situations where primary cataract extraction with primary IOL implantation is preferred over a secondary procedure and/or secondary IOL implantation.

The situation cannot be compared to the already complex situation in adults: As in pediatric cases the eye is still in growth, many factors needed for adequate IOL calculation are not predictable. An empiric myopic shift which is usually incorporated into IOL calculation in pediatric cases may not be fully applicable to traumatized pediatric eyes.

Primary cataract extraction with primary IOL implantation is frequently performed in infants and children up to 10 years of age when timely visual rehabilitation is needed to prevent amblyopia in unilateral situations. In pediatric cases, "primary" does not necessarily indicate "immediate". In some situations, it is possible to wait a few weeks after the initial trauma to avoid postoperative complications due to the increased scarring tendency in wound healing in pediatric cases. A timely post-operative fitting of an aphakia correcting contact lens is one of the options to be considered, however contact lens intolerance may be found in some of the traumatic cases [15]. In the author's own experience contact lenses are frequently better tolerated by children than one would assume, especially if the parents are motivated.

Scleral or iris-fixated lenses in pediatric cases are also possible [16], but should be considered as a secondary option after careful consideration as revisions of sclera-fixated IOL may be challenging.

On the other hand, a multi-stage procedure with primary closure and several follow-up operations creates intervals during which irreversible amblyopia may develop [5, 14]. Postoperative monitoring including examination under anesthesia if necessary, should be rigorous.

Author's recommendation

In children at risk for amblyopia, even minimal opacity of the lens may require early surgery. This is especially true for centrally located opacifications. The recommendations for surgery for congenital cataract may also apply in these cases, even though the traumatized eye may bear an increased risk for complications.

Inflammatory reactions, macular edema and also secondary posterior capsule opacification are much more pronounced and more frequent in children after cataract surgery [9]. This secondary posterior capsule opacification may require repeated removal by vitrectomy [17]. A primary posterior capsulorhexis with extended anterior vitrectomy prevents this complication and ideally, this surgical step is performed with a vitrectomy probe. At this point, it has to be emphasized that in these pediatric cases it is of utmost importance to avoid any retinal damage —which can be induced by vitreo-retinal traction during anterior vitrectomy. The author's recommendation is therefore that this step should be performed by an experienced VR surgeon.

In cases with zone III involvement (posterior segment), removal of the complete capsular bag may be indicated to reduce the risk of anterior vitreoretinopathy and to avoid postoperative hypotony due to capsular contraction.

In young children sulcus-fixed lenses may cause more severe inflammation due to mechanical interactions of the IOL with the iris. In all of these cases, it should be kept in mind that complications in pediatric patients are more difficult to diagnose and may lead to amblyopia.

In children who are not at risk of amblyopia, it is advisable to delay the removal of the cataract and IOL implantation, until the eye is fully grown and there is a stable refraction. In the meantime, the correction may be carried out with a contact lens, which needs to be fitted repeatedly.

Summary

Traumatic cataracts have a significantly higher risk of complications than the age-related variant, and there should be a clear strategy for managing intraoperative complications prior to surgical treatment.

In general, there is a greater probability of an increased refractive error after cataract surgery. Given this background, if possible, the operation of traumatic cataract should be performed under planned conditions based upon a reliable, reproducible biometry.

References

1. May DR, Kuhn FP, Morris RE, Witherspoon CD, Danis R, Matthews G, et al. The epidemiology of serious eye injuries from the United States eye injury registry. Graefes Arch Clin Exp Ophthalmol. 2000;238(2):153–7.
2. Loncar VL, Petric I. Surgical treatment, clinical outcomes, and complications of traumatic cataract: retrospective study. Croat Med J. 2004;45(3):310–3.
3. Gupta VB, Rajagopala M, Ravishankar B. Etiopathogenesis of cataract: an appraisal. Indian J Ophthalmol. 2014;62(2):103–10.
4. Davidson M. Lens lesions in contusions: a medico-legal study. Am J Ophthalmol. 1940;23 (3):252–71.
5. Rumelt S, Rehany U. The influence of surgery and intraocular lens implantation timing on visual outcome in traumatic cataract. Graefes Arch Clin Exp Ophthalmol. 2010;248(9):1293–7.
6. Tabatabaei SA, Soleimani M, Etesali H, Naderan M. Accuracy of swept source optical coherence tomography and ultrasound biomicroscopy for evaluation of posterior lens capsule in traumatic cataract. Am J Ophthalmol. 2020.
7. Oudjani N, Renault D, Courrier E, Malek Y. Phacoemulsification and Zonular weakness: contribution of the capsular tension ring with a thread. Clin Ophthalmol. 2019;13:2301.
8. Masket S. Traumatic cataract with cyclodialysis and normal intraocular pressure: July consultation# 1st. J Cataract Refract Surg. 2018;44(7):917–8.
9. Trivedi RH, Wilson ME. Posterior capsule opacification in pediatric eyes with and without traumatic cataract. J Cataract Refract Surg. 2015;41(7):1461–4.
10. Kelkar A, Shah R, Vasavda V, Kelkar J, Kelkar S. Primary iris claw IOL retrofixation with intravitreal triamcinolone acetonides in cases of inadequate capsular support. Int Ophthalmol. 2018;38(1):111–7.
11. Veronese C, Maiolo C, Armstrong GW, Primavera L, Torrazza C, Della Mora L, et al. New surgical approach for sutureless scleral fixation. Eur J Ophthalmol. 2020;30(3):612–5.
12. Lemley CA, Han DP. Endophthalmitis: a review of current evaluation and management. Retina. 2007;27(6):662–80.
13. Yardley AM, Ali A, Najm-Tehrani N, Mireskandari K. Refractive and visual outcomes after surgery for pediatric traumatic cataract. J Cataract Refract Surg. 2018;44(1):85–90.
14. Vasavada AR, Vasavada V. Current Status of IOL implantation in pediatric eyes: an update. Expert Rev Med Devices. 2017:1–9.
15. Paryani M, Khandekar RB, Dole K, Dharmadhikari S, Rishikeshi N. Visual outcome and impact on quality of life after surgeries differ in children operated for unilateral and bilateral cataract (Pune study 2011). Oman J Ophthalmol. 2012;5(3):150–6.

16. Sen P, Kumar V, Bhende P, Rishi P, Rishi E, Rao C, et al. Surgical outcomes and complications of sutured scleral fixed intraocular lenses in pediatric eyes. Can J Ophthalmol. 2018;53(1):49–55.
17. Mohan A, Kumar A, Sen P, Shah C, Jain E, Sen A. Outcome of Surgical membranectomy with a vitrector via limbal approach for posterior capsular opacity in children. J Pediatric Ophthalmol Strabismus. 2020;57(1):33–8.

Paediatric Cataract Surgery

G. Darius Hildebrand

Introduction

The advances made in paediatric cataract surgery over the last decades have been remarkable. In 1957, Costenbader and Albert still felt compelled to conclude after having reviewed the literature that "cases of monocular congenital cataract surgery with production of satisfactory visual acuity have not come to our attention" and that "surgery for unilateral congenital cataract is strongly advised against" [1]. Even as recently as 1979, François remarked that "everyone knows the uselessness of operating on unilateral congenital cataracts, as the functional result is always very bad" ([2], Chap. 11). However, the apparent hopelessness of the situation reversed in 1981 when, in a landmark paper, Creig Hoyt and colleagues from San Francisco reported a series of outstanding long-term visual outcomes of 20/20–20/30 in five out of eight cases and none worse than 20/80 following surgery very early (41 days) to extremely early (7 h) after birth. With their report, Hoyt and colleagues provided evidence that "surgery during the neonatal period is not only justified but probably essential in any successful treatment of monocular congenital cataracts" [3].

Advances in microscopy, instrumentation, operating machines, OVDs, lens design, and a far better understanding of amblyopia and its effective management, including its early detection by screening and its correction through careful optical rehabilitation and patching, have resulted in unprecedented improvements in surgical and visual outcomes for children and especially infants since then. This

Supplementary Information The online version contains supplementary material available at https://doi.org/10.1007/978-3-031-05394-8_64. The videos can be accessed individually by clicking the DOI link in the accompanying figure caption or by scanning this link with the SN More Media App.

G. Darius Hildebrand (✉)
Oxford, United Kingdom
e-mail: dariushildebrand@yahoo.co.uk

M. Shajari et al. (eds.), *Cataract and Lens Surgery*,
https://doi.org/10.1007/978-3-031-05394-8_64

chapter describes the latest surgical techniques for children with cataracts, techniques that have reduced the complications of paediatric cataract surgery and that are bringing the prospect of a life with vision to more and more children and their families.

Immediate Versus Delayed Sequential Surgery

In cases of bilateral cataracts, same-day bilateral surgery is an option in some cases, as it has been shown to take less overall anesthetic time than sequential bilateral surgery on two separate days, only requires one general anesthetic and is sometimes logistically and medically the safest and most pragmatic option available. However, because of the risk of simultaneous bilateral complications, such as bacterial endophthalmitis and TASS, it is mandatory in these cases that meticulous precautions are taken and strictly adhered to, including that all instruments and solutions are changed and the machine cassettes replaced between cases, that each eye is cleaned and draped separately. The surgeons must rescrub and regown in order to reduce the risk to a minimum, if such an approach is taken.

Wound Construction

If no IOL implantation is planned, only one to two corneal stab paracentesis incisions with an MVR blade are required for coaxial or bimanual irrigation and lens aspiration. Traditionally, this is done at the 10 and 2 o'clock positions to allow the upper lid to cover the wounds for increased comfort and protection, however sometimes a temporal approach is more suitable to gain best access. The incision is directed towards the opposite limbus to create a self-sealing effect and reduce post-operative leakage. This and the routine use of corneal sutures will reliably prevent post-operative hypotony and shallowing of the anterior chamber in all young children, especially in babies. When IOL implantation is planned, the main wound is best placed superiorly for the reasons given by corneal, limbal or scleral tunnel incision. The scleral tunnel has a lower risk of wound leak, but causes conjunctival scarring that may make it more challenging to perform glaucoma surgery in those cases that need tit later (i.e. mostly in young infants).

Author's recommendation

Due to the different biomechanical properties of the paediatric cornea and globe, all surgical wounds should be sutured to reliably prevent post-operative hypotony. Unlike in adults, simple wound hydration alone is not recommended as this provides only a temporary sealing effect.

Pupil Dilation

In most children, pupil dilation is achievable simply by the preoperative application of mydriatic drops, such as a combination of phenylephrine 2.5% plus cyclopentolate 0.5% in infants, or phenylephrine 2.5% plus cyclopentolate 1% from one year of age. It is important to be aware of the greater risk of systemic side effects of topical mydriatics in younger children (and especially infants) and to use reduced concentrations of them. In the largest such study, Neffendorf et al. reported 1,246 eye examinations in premature infants with 2.5% and cyclopentolate 0.5% and showed 3 applications at least 5 min apart to be both safe and effective [4]. Phenylephrine 10% should **never** be used in children because of cardiovascular adverse reactions. Intracameral mydriatics, such as diluted adrenaline, phenylephrine or Mydrane® (a combination intracameral injection containing tropicamide 0.2 mg/ml (0.02%), phenylephrine 3.1 mg/ml (0.31%) and lidocaine 10 mg/ml (1%)) are very useful, especially if pupil constriction occurs during surgery. However, a word of caution: It is possible that the mydriatic gains venous access, for example when applied in the presence of bleeding conjunctival blood vessels immediately after wound construction, resulting in very high and sustained systemic hypertension and tachycardia. This can be prevented by avoiding cutting conjunctival and limbal vessels, applying cautery as necessary and not to use more solution than is recommended. Most anesthetists can advise on safe doses and will appreciate being informed in advance in order to recognise and respond to any cardiovascular effects early. Judicious application of HPMC to the cornea and the conjunctival sac can also further prevent systemic absorption by the venous or nasolacrimal routes.

Author's recommendation

It is important to discuss any use and the permissible dosages of adrenaline, phenylephrine, Mydrane® or any other similar solution with the paediatric anesthetist in case of any systemic adverse effects.

If pharmacological dilation and the use of the standard viscoelastics are not enough, the best mechanical pupil-dilating devices are iris hooks. In teenagers with nearly adult-sized eyes the Malyugin ring can be used as well. Fine pupil sphincterotomies (e.g. with VR scissors) can be quite effective, but will cause an irregular pupil. Pupil stretching with Kuglen hooks is best avoided in children, as it can cause significant uveitis, posterior synechiae and a distorted pupil. If the pupil is kept constricted by a fine pupillary membrane, the membrane can be carefully stripped and this may result in remarkable dilation with no other action required. In the case of marked pupil constriction or severe eccentration of the pupil, a permanent solution is to use the 23G vitrector to create a permanently larger and centralised pupil with a few judicious vitrector bites into the pupillary border. Bleeding is uncommon with this, presumably due to an often abnormal and atrophic iris (see Fig. 1).

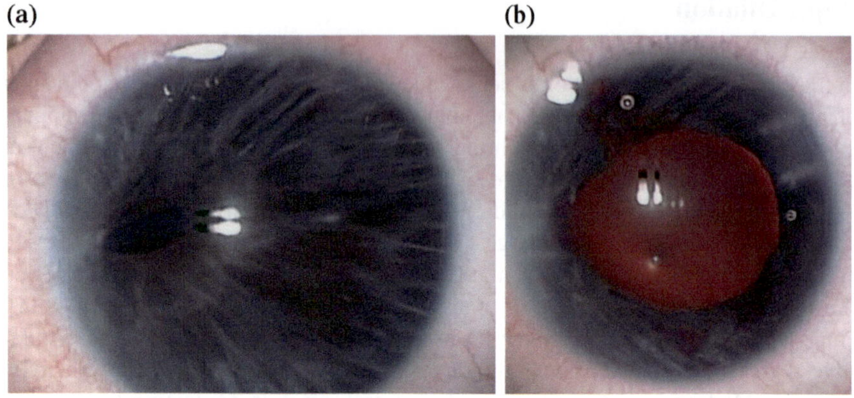

Fig. 1 **a** 23G vitrector pupiloplasty for extreme miosis and corectopia in a 1-year-old boy before treatment. **b** Adequately sized, round, central pupil after 23G vitrector pupiloplasty. No bleeding, iritis, glaucoma or photophobia during follow up

TIP (P), CCC, Vitrectorrhexis and Other Paediatric Anterior Capsulotomy Techniques

Making an intact anterior capsulotomy of the correct size, shape and centration is arguably the most challenging step in successful paediatric cataract surgery, especially in newborn and infant eyes. This is, in part because the younger the eye, the more elastic and stronger the capsule is. In addition, the anterior chamber of infants and especially neonates have a tendency to collapse, once opened, due to the greater scleral elasticity of the children eyes compared to the relative scleral rigidity seen in adults. As mentioned already, both the anterior and posterior capsules of neonates and children are much stronger and far more elastic compared to adults. Overall tensile strength falls by a factor of five and extensibility by at least a factor of two from birth to late adulthood ([5], Chap. 17).

These factors all combine to make the capsulotomy technically much more difficult in very young children and especially in neonates. For this reason, a number of special methods have been developed for anterior capsulotomy in children, the most important of which are the classic manual continuous curvilinear capsulorhexis (CCC), vitrectorrhexis and two-incision push-pull capsulorhexis (TIPP), which will be described in more detail together with a modification the author has used for over 10 years, namely two-incision push capsulorhexis (TIP).

Author's recommendation

Making a correctly sized, round and central intact anterior capsulotomy is the most difficult part of paediatric cataract surgery. Different techniques have been developed to achieve this, including manual continuous curvilinear capsulorhexis, vitrectorrhexis, two-incision push-pull capsulorhexis (TIPP), and two-incision push capsulorhexis (TIP).

Author's recommendation

It is helpful to use the Purkinje images 1 (corneal reflex) and 4 (posterior surface of the crystalline lens) to align the visual axis optimally to create a central capsulotomy.

Continuous Curvilinear Capsulorhexis (CCC)

This classic technique was independently described by Neuhann and Gimbel in adults and later applied to children with important modifications. While free-hand CCC gives a strong and smooth rhexis, it is technically much harder to complete successfully, centrally and of the desirable size in infants and toddlers.

The paediatric capsule, especially the neonatal capsule, has a constant tendency to 'run out' due to its greater inherent capsular elasticity. In addition, the sclera of young children and especially infants is much less rigid and when the eye is opened the anterior chamber has an immediate tendency to collapse, resulting in a forward displacement of the lens and a centrifugal and posterior pull on the anterior capsule due to increased radial zonular tension.

A high molecular weight ophthalmic viscosurgical device (OVD) such as healon GV or healon 5 is of vital importance to maintain the anterior chamber, push back the lens, flatten the anterior capsule and create laxity of the radial zonules, all of which help to prevent the rhexis running out. Reloading with viscoelastic is often necessary to maintain optimal working conditions, especially if non-VR small diameter forceps are used. A good gauge for how much viscolelastic to use is to look for a small concave indent in the anterior capsule. In newborn babies, the cornea becomes slightly hazy with high pressure caused by overfilling of the anterior chamber. Simply releasing some of the viscoelastic until the cornea is clear will immediately clear the cornea again. Using a high viscosity OVD not just to flatten, but to create a slight concave impression in the anterior capsule is another simple way to avoid the rhexis running out, effectively causing a slope up rather than a slope down effect.

Once the anterior chamber is filled with viscoelastic and the anterior lens capsule flattened or rendered slightly concave, the handling of the capsular flap is of paramount importance. Unlike in standard capsulotomy, the capsule flap needs to be pulled constantly towards the center while also slightly anteriorly to counteract the simultaneously centrifugal and slightly posterior pull by the radial zonules. It is best to start the CCC rhexis centrally and gradually spiral out with frequent regrasping of the capsular flap with vitreoretinal or similar small incision forceps close to the rhexis edge to maintain maximum control over the direction and size of the CCC at all times. Frequent refilling of the anterior chamber is recommended with larger forceps that can cause escape of viscoelastic through the wound. Finer VR forceps introduced through a small stab incision prevents this problem.

Trypan blue staining of the capsule has greatly facilitated the visualisation of the elastic anterior capsule and has been shown to reduce the elasticity of the paediatric capsule. Trypan blue is a godsend in most young children and infants, especially in the presence of a white cataract, and should be used routinely in most paediatric cases.

Author's recommendation

Anterior chamber filling with sufficient OVD and careful handling of the capsule flap with constant central and slightly anterior pull are vital to prevent a run-out rhexis, especially in infants. The use of trypan blue capsule stain is recommended for most paediatric cataract cases.

Vitrectorrhexis

Because of the greater technical difficulties with manual CCC in very young children, some surgeons prefer vitrector-cut anterior capsulotomy (vitrector-'rhexis') in very young children under 2 years and manual CCC in older ones. Vitrectorrhexis is generally not advised for children above 6–8 years as manual CCC is quite straightforward and more predictable at that age and gives a stronger rhexis for IOL implantation.

Vitrectorrhexis is more correctly termed a capsulectomy rather than a capsulotomy or rhexis. Two corneal stab incisions for the vitrector handpiece and the irrigation cannula are made. Ideally, the two incisions should be of a similar diameter to allow swapping instruments between both hands during surgery with minimum leakage and maximum anterior chamber stability. The vitrector handpiece is placed with the cutter facing down to the anterior capsule. The recommended machine settings are a slow cutting rate (e.g. 150 cuts/min) and high infusion rate ([6], Chap. 17). A Venturi pump is best for this technique. With the vitrector cutter facing the anterior capsule, a central opening is made and gradually enlarged in a spiral manner. The aim is to create a rounded capsulotomy and to avoid right-angled edges that are more prone to radial tears. Though a very useful technique, experimental work has shown that the capsulotomy strength by vitrectorrhexis is less than that of a manual capsulorhexis and less resistant to manipulation during irrigation and aspiration, IOL implantation and manipulation ([6], Chap. 17).

Author's recommendation

Because the edge of the vitrectorrhexis is less resistant to tearing out, it is wise to avoid capsular stretching manoeuvres with this technique, such as for optic capture or the BIL techniques.

Two-Incision Push-Pull Capsulorhexis (TIPP) and Two-Incision Push Capsulorhexis (TIP)

Building on earlier work by Auffarth and colleagues in the albino rabbit model [7], Nischal described an ingenious and simple method to create an anterior (and posterior) capsulotomy in 2002 that has proven extremely safe, reliable and consistent in infants and young children [8]. It combines the maximum rhexis strength of a manual CCC technique with safety and reliable precision in children in the first few years of life. They published their five-year experience in children as young as 4 weeks and reported 100% completion rates and no tear-out during anterior capsulotomy in all 84 paediatric cataract operations, including 12 cases carried out by the trainee. Furthermore, it was possible to create a precise target anterior opening diameter of 4–4.5 mm in all cases [9].

Two stab incisions are made in the capsule with the microvitreoretinal (MVR) blade, both proximally and distally. This determines the overall diameter and location of the anterior capsulotomy. The distance can be measured with caliper marking on the cornea or along the limbus or with an intraocular ring caliper made by Morcher. Alternatively, some newer microscope manufacturers can project any capsulotomy ring size into the operating field view. The diameter needs to be less than the diameter of the IOL optic. Because of capsular elasticity, the final CCC will be slightly larger than measured. In the case of a 6 mm optic diameter, one would aim for 4–4.5 mm leading to a 4.5–5 mm rhexis for a 6 mm IOL optic with a 0.5 mm anterior capsular overlap around the IOL optic.

Because of the inherent capsular elasticity in very young children, the initial capsular slit immediately changes shape to a horizontal ellipse in a toddler and even a small circle in a newborn. The degree of this immediate expansion of the original slit is useful to gauge the likely amount of anterior capsular elasticity during the capsulotomy (the more expansion of the slit the more elastic the capsule). Forceps are used to first grasp one end of the proximal stab incision to push the capsule towards the centre to create a quarter circle. This pushing manoeuvre is then repeated for the other end of the proximal capsule edge to create a proximal capsular half circle (see Fig. 2a). Then, the proximal edge of the distal stab is pulled, one end at the time, towards the centre to create the second half circle before connecting the two into a full circle capsulotomy. The combination of push and pull using two stabs gives rise to the name two-incision push–pull (TIPP) technique.

For more than 10 years, I have simplified the classic TIPP technique to a two-incision push capsulorhexis (TIP) to complete the entire rhexis by pushing away from the proximal stab all the way towards the distal second stab, completing one side and then the other (see Fig. 2a and Video 1) with great safety.

The reason TIP(P) is so safe is because the tearing vector at all times is directed centripedally. The reason for their reliability and accuracy is that by making the two initial stab incisions in the anterior capsule the surgeon controls the exact diameter and location of the manual capsulorhexis. Because TIP(P) is a rhexis method, the capsular edge is very strong like with CCC.

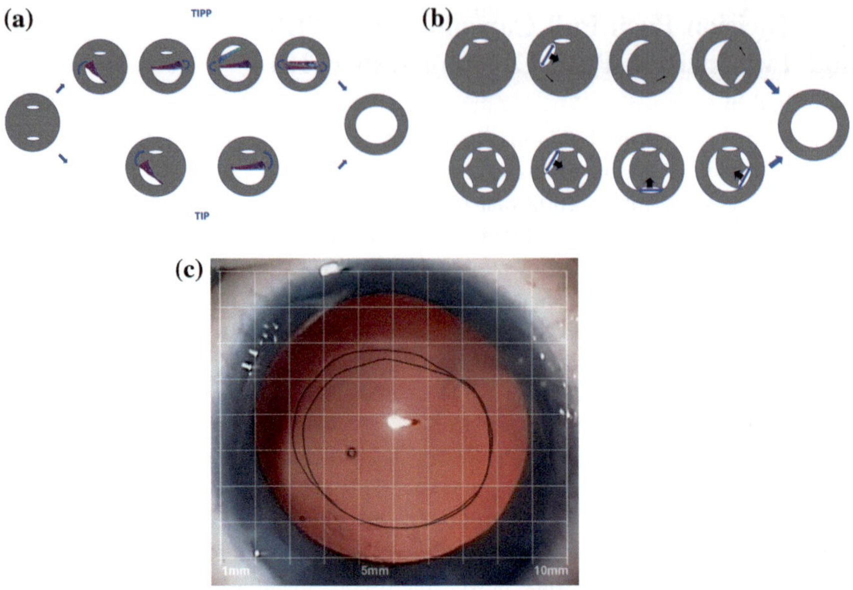

Fig. 2 **a** Two-incisional push-pull capsulotomy (TIPP) after Nischal and modified two incision push capsulotomy (TIP) after Hildebrand. Both are extremely safe and versatile in newborns, infants and toddlers. **b** Circumferential posterior incisional capsulotomy (CPIC, after Hildebrand). Unlike the can-opener technique in adults, the CPIC results in a continuous and strong posterior capsule edge. **c** Precision of congruent shape, centration and size within 1mm accuracy between ACCC and PCCC is shown for the comnination of TIP(P) for ACCC and CPIC for PCCC in an infant, allowing for reliable optic capture as early as the newborn age

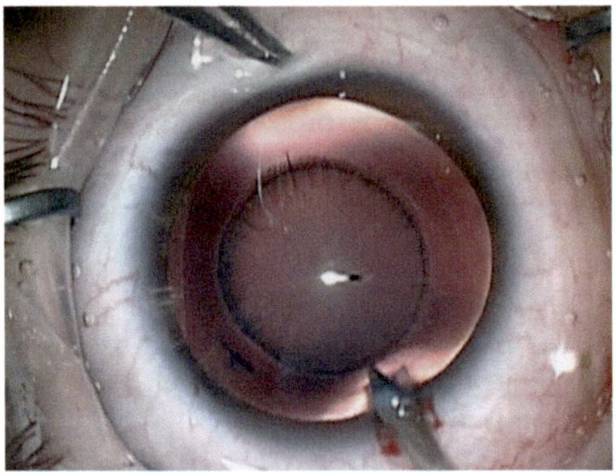

Video 1 Two-incisional push (TIP) capsulotomy technique (modification after Hildebrand) (▶ https://doi.org/10.1007/000-8ee)

Author's recommendation

TIPP and TIP are very safe techniques to achieve a secure, predictably precise and very strong anterior capsulotomy with little risk of running out, especially in infants and very young children.

Author's recommendation

If you are not sure whether to choose a classic manual CCC or TIP(P) in a child a few years old, use the MVR blade to make an initial central stab in the anterior capsule and observe whether the opening becomes elliptical. If it does, the capsule is significantly elastic and proceed with the usual TIP(P) technique. If there is minimal ovalisation of the thin MVR slit, this indicates the capsule is no longer significantly elastic and a classic manual CCC will be the better option.

Other Anterior Capsulotomy Techniques

Less commonly used methods include the Fugo blade that employs plasma technology and radiofrequency diathermy developed by Kloti. More recently, femto-laser assisted capsulotomies have also been used in children.

Special Case of Intumescent White Cataracts

Intumescent white cataracts in children are very high-risk cases for causing a run-out rhexis and a so-called 'Argentinian flag sign'. The reasons for this are severalfold. In addition to the elasticity of the capsule the presence of one or more high intralenticular high-pressure compartments may cause uncontrolled expansion of the anterior capsule after initial opening. Intraoperative high-resolution OCT reveals the internal complexity of these cataracts in children with multicompartments and fine attachments between these and the inner aspect of the capsule (see Video 2).

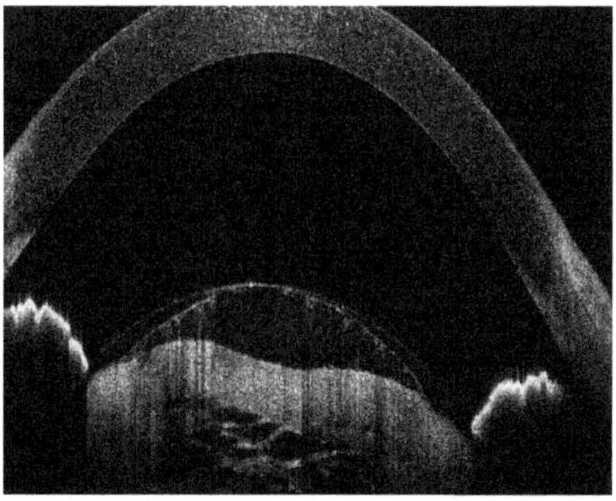

Video 2 Intraoperative OCT of intumescent white cataract in 9-year-old with rapid vision loss over 3 weeks due to insulin-dependent diabetes mellitus revealing detailed complex internal subcompartments and capsular adhesions.png (▶ https://doi.org/10.1007/000-8ed)

If the anterior chamber pressure is lower than the intralenticular pressure, it is easy to see how capsular rupture may immediately ensue. It is therefore important to use high molecular weight OVD during all steps of the capsulotomy to avoid capsular rupture whichever capsulotomy technique is used. A simple way to determine whether the OVD has created enough anterior chamber pressure is to look for the beginning of a concave impression of the anterior capsule, indicating the anterior chamber pressure is now greater than the intralenticular pressure and the capsulotomy can be attempted. A common technique is to then make a small initial central opening or even an initially very small wound rhexis and to release ('milky smoke sign') or aspirate some of intralenticular fluid with a fine cannula to decompress the intralenticular pressure (see Video 1). Once this has been achieved, the situation is much safer and manual CCC (spiralling technique), vitrectorrhexis or the TIP(P) technique can be used to complete the full anterior capsulotomy.

Hydrodissection and Hydrodelineation

While cortical cleaving hydrodissection is mandatory in older adults, hydrodissection in children and teenagers is generally not necessary and even contraindicated where the anterior or posterior capsule is not intact or suspected to be particularly weak (e.g. posterior lenticonus). Complications include iris prolapse, nucleus prolapse into the anterior chamber, rupture of the anterior and posterior capsules and posterior dislocation of the lens. Similarly, gentle hydrodelineation is not generally required for the same reasons, but may be employed in selected cases.

Lens Aspiration and Lensectomy

Strictly speaking, lensectomy is the total removal of the entire lens protein and capsule. Such a radical approach was more common in the past, but is nowadays typically reserved for cases of advanced subluxation. In most paediatric cataract cases, the intent is to carry out lens aspiration to remove the cataractous lens matter and the central anterior and posterior capsules, but to leave the peripheral capsular bag behind for immediate or future IOL implantation. To remove the lens matter, the cortex is engaged with the aspiration instrument and gently stripped away from the inner capsule surface in a systematic fashion. It is advisable to first free the peripheral 360 degrees of cortex in this manner, leaving the posterior cortex till the end in case of a present posterior capsular defect. A wide choice of irrigation and aspiration instruments are available, including bimanual, coaxial and vitrector I&A. Direct cortex removal or stripping by bimanual or coaxial aspiration is usually straightforward in paediatric cataract surgery.

It is important to remove all visible lens material as much as possible and to polish the capsule in an effort to minimise postoperative lens epithelial proliferation and visual axis opacification, the most frequent post-operative complication of cataract surgery.

Author's recommendation

A thorough aspiration of all visible lens material and capsular polishing are advised in an attempt to minimise postoperative lens epithelial proliferation and visual axis obscuration.

Posterior Capsulotomy

If the paediatric posterior capsule is left intact at the end of surgery, it will inevitably opacify over time and interfere with optical quality and visual development in children. To prevent this, standard practice is to perform a primary posterior capsulotomy (PPC) in all young children up to the age when subsequent waking cooperation with Nd-YAG laser capsulotomy is anticipated to be possible. While some children are outstandingly cooperative and can be lasered as young as 7–8 years, some older teenagers with learning difficulties may not be able to tolerate laser treatment awake and therefore should have a primary posterior capsulotomy even as teenagers or adults. Significant nystagmus in a child may be another reason to carry out a PCC. If in doubt, it is safer to perform a PCC in children.

The surgical approach can be anterior or posterior by pars plana or pars plicata. With a posterior approach, transpupillary illumination in the dark helps to demarcate the true location of the anatomic ciliary body. The techniques for PPC are the same as for anterior capsulotomy, i.e. CCC, vitrectorrhexis or TIP(P). Another very reliable and safe technique developed by the author in infants and very young children is using the MVR blade to create sequential stab incisions at the desired location in the posterior capsule, each time followed by a centripedal and circumferential push to extend and connect neighbouring capsulotomy stabs to create a continuous extension until the 360 degree circle is completed (circumferential posterior incisional capsulotomy (CPIC), see Fig. 2b and Video 3). Unlike the can-opener technique in adults, CPIC results in a continuous and strong posterior capsule opening. With this method it is possible to create a PCC of exact shape and size routinely less than 1 mm exact overlap between the anterior and posterior capsules (see Fig. 2c and Video 3).

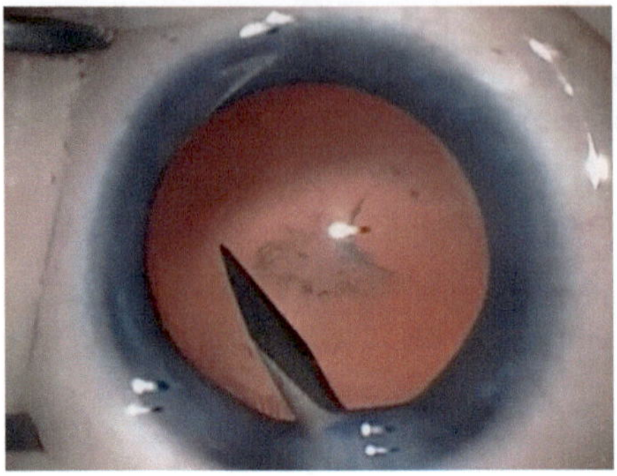

Video 3 The Circumferential posterior incisional capsulotomy technique (CPIC after Hildebrand) (▶ https://doi.org/10.1007/000-8ec)

A special case is persistent fetal vasculature (PFV) in which posterior plaques may be so thick as to require VR scissors to cut out a posterior opening often in combination with endocautery to coagulate perfused posterior tunica vasculosa lentis blood vessels. Supine Nd-YAG laser capsulotomy was popular for primary or secondary PCC, but is much less used nowadays with the availability of more effective surgical techniques and reduced availability of instruments. If necessary, a standard capsulotomy laser machine can be brought to theatre and the patient be lasered in the supine position with the head flexed towards the side of the laser positioned right next to the bed.

Anterior Core Vitrectomy

Because of the real risk of anterior vitreous face opacification, it is widespread practice to combine PCC with an anterior core vitrectomy in preschool children (0–5 years). This was popularised by Taylor and Parks, though other authors have achieved also very good results without routine anterior vitrectomy using for example Robert Stegmann's optic capture technique [10] or Marie-José Tassignon's pioneering bag-in-the-lens (BIL) technique [11]. The vitrectomy can be carried out either by limbal or posterior approaches depending on age, anatomic findings and surgeon's preference.

Aphakia or Pseudophakia?

Primary IOL implantation is accepted standard of care in older children, but there is a debate as to whether there should be a young age cut-off and if so, when? There are reports against as well as in favour of early IOL implantation.

The Infant Aphakia Treatment Study (IATS, prospective randomised, 114 infants under 7 months with unilateral cataracts only) reported no different visual outcomes at 5 years or difference in glaucoma at 10 years, but more reoperations in the pseudophakic group at one year. Because of the increase in reoperations in the pseudophakic group, the IATS group recommended that "babies aged younger than 7 months with unilateral cataract typically be left aphakic after cataract surgery" [12].

The IOLunder2 study (non-randomized prospective observational study, 158 children aged 2 years or younger, with uni- and bilateral cataracts) reported at 5 years no better vision and no protection from secondary glaucoma in bilateral cases, but a 5 times increased rate of reoperation for visual axis obscuration in bilateral cataracts and a 20 times increased risk in unilateral cases. The authors did not recommend IOL implantation under 2 years [13].

On the other hand, a large meta-analysis of 470 children and 659 cataracts (median surgical age of 3 months) found that primary IOL implantation was significantly protective against secondary glaucoma compared with aphakia (hazard ratio 0.1, 95% CI 0.01–0.76, $p = 0.03$) [14].

In addition, recalculation of the IOLunder2 data appeared to demonstrate a significant 3.5 times greater rate of glaucoma in the aphakes (14/70) compared with pseudophakes (5/88; $p = 0.005$) in the IOLunder2 study [15].

Furthermore, the only randomized controlled study of bilateral cataract surgery in children younger than 2 years reported similar low rates of VAO requiring surgery (8% aphakic vs. 10% pseudophakic groups, $p = 0.76$) and the authors stated that "primary in-the-bag IOL implantation … has an acceptable complication rate and offers immediate visual benefit in children up to 2 years of age with bilateral cataracts" [16].

The high reoperation rate in the IATS pseudophakic group has caused observers to scrutinise their surgical protocols and one important criticism has been that infants in the aphakic group underwent only a lensectomy and anterior vitrectomy by the limbal route, while in the pseudophakic group the vitrectomy and posterior capsulotomy were routinely carried out not limbally, but by additional pars plana/plicata surgery, unless a pre-existing opening was noted in the posterior capsule or a rent developed intraoperatively, or in some eyes with persistent fetal vasculature in which only a limbal approach was used.

This means that in the IATS Study most pseudophakic infants had both anterior and posterior segment surgery (anterior lens aspiration and PPV) compared to just an anterior lens aspiration with anterior vitrectomy in the aphakic group**.** This is in contrast to the already cited only randomized controlled study of bilateral cataract surgery by Vasavada et al., whose surgical protocol prescribed identical surgical procedures (only difference implantation or not) all by the same surgeon [16].

Moreover, IOLunder2 was an observational study with only 18 unilateral aphakes, requiring caution in generalising their findings from this small cohort.

Moreover, IATS and IOLunder2 reported VAO as the main complication of primary implantation. In fact, of the 36 infants who needed additional intraocular surgery in the first year in the pseudophakic group in the IATS Study, 34 needed this to treat VAO and 42 out of 50 patients in the 10-year assessment, showing that traditional lens-in-the-bag or lens-in-the-sulcus placements are associated with a high risk of VAO [12]. Therefore, neither IATS nor IOLunder2 studies used the optic capture or the bag-in-the-lens (BIL) techniques. Importantly, it is the BIL and the optic capture techniques that have been shown to have very low VAO and reoperation rates (see below), removing this reason for not implanting a primary IOL in otherwise suitable eyes of infants.

Aphakia

If the surgical aim is to leave the child aphakic, an anterior capsulotomy, lens aspiration, posterior capsulotomy and an anterior core vitrectomy are carried out as described above to clear the visual axis and to prevent secondary VAO. Leaving a capsule ring remnant provides support for future IOL implantation. A common mistake is to make the capsulotomies too small, especially if the pupil was not well dilated during surgery, leading to later phimosis or even complete closure and the need for reoperation within months.

Author's recommendation

The risk of capsular phimosis is reduced by making large capsulotomies. The phimosis risk is further reduced by making a number of small perpendicular sphincterotomy cuts into the capsulotomies with VR scissors at the end of the case to prevent delayed phimosis.

The anterior and posterior capsulotomies should be 5–6 mm and congruent to maximise overlap and sealing of the anterior and posterior capsules to reduce the growth and escape of Elschnig pearls and LEC migration from the capsular equator into the visual axis (see Fig. 3a).

Some surgeons prefer a small prophylactic vitrector peripheral iridectomy as a precaution against secondary pupil block that can rarely be caused by protruding vitreus later. However, a good core vitrectomy in the first place can usually obviate this complication. In addition, a PI can cause hyphema and vitreous hemorrhage in a hypotonic vitrectomised eye overnight that may then require surgical removal, if severe enough to be amblyogenic.

Based on the biometry and refraction, many surgeons place an aphakic contact lens at the end of surgery for two reasons: It makes the eye more comfortable after surgery and provides immediate optical rehabilitation. It is certainly much easier to place a contact lens in an anesthetised than an awake child!

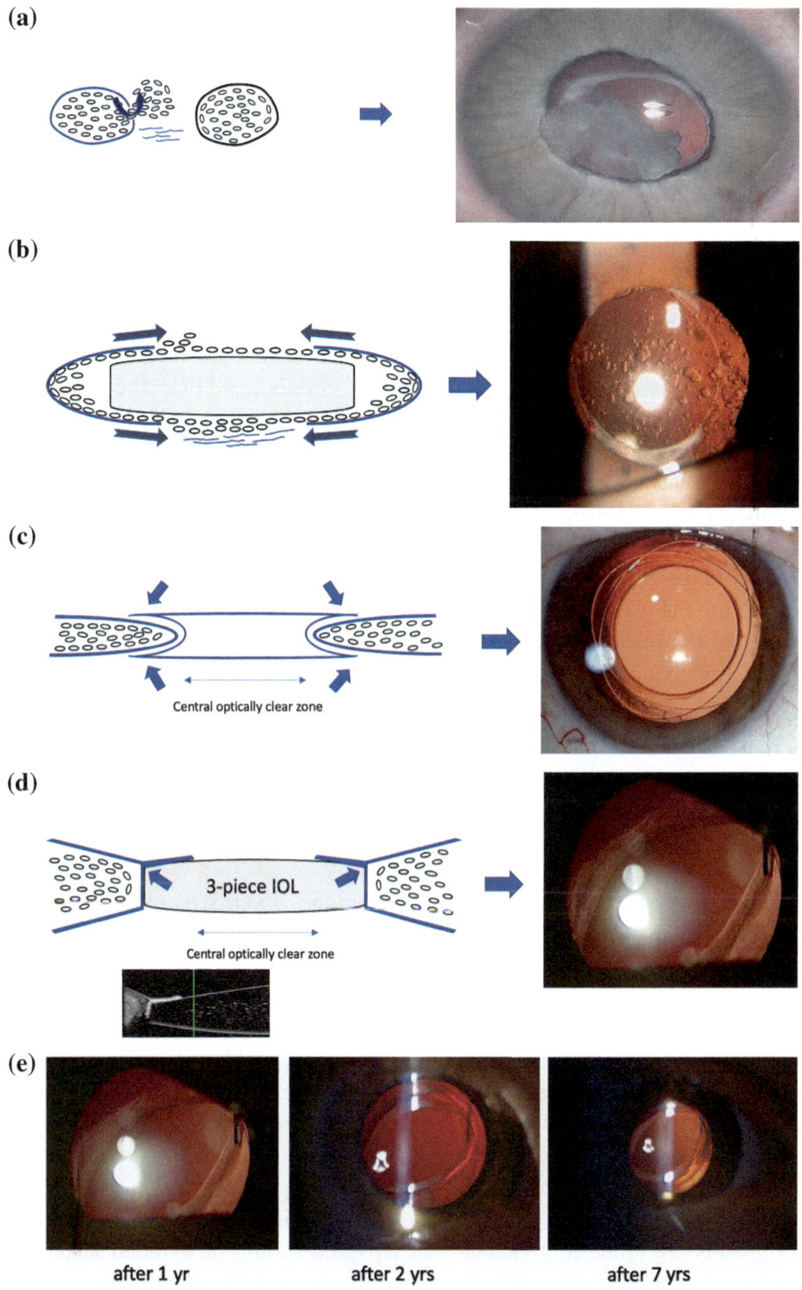

Fig. 3 **a** Aphakia. Escape of LECs outside the bag with Elschnig pearls and VAO formation in aphakia (Fig. 3a) and conventional uncaptured IOL-in-bag (Fig. 3b) techniques. **b** Conventional IOL in bag. **c** Bag-in-the-lens technique (with kind permission of Prof. M-J Tassignon Antwerpen Belgium. **d** Optic capture technique of IOL. **e** Optic capture IOL stays clear after 1, 2 and 7 years in same toddler

Author's recommendation

Placing an aphakic contact lens at the end of the case is practical and provides immediate optical correction and comfort post-operatively.

Lens Power

If an IOL is chosen, the lens power is generally chosen to undercorrect to aim for hypermetropia in anticipation of the future physiological myopic shift, especially in the first two years of life. A number of useful tables are available that make recommendations for target refractions by the child's age [17]. The resultant hyperopia and any significant astigmatism must also be corrected with glasses or contact lenses as early as possible. As discussed for aphakic cases above, it is advisable to place a contact lens at the end of the operation based on the biometry calculation for IOL power or intraoperative refraction in order to provide immediate refractive correction to stimulate visual development immediately post-operatively and to avoid the avoidable challenge of attempting the insertion of a contact lens in a struggling baby or child in the days after eye surgery. In trauma cases, the biometry of the opposite eye can be used to calculate lens power, if both eyes had similar refractions previously.

Traditional IOL Implantation Technique Associated with High VAO and Reoperation Rate in Young Children

The most widely used IOL implantation technique is still IOL placement into the bag or sulcus. This technique works very well in adults who have a less pronounced healing response and a mature visual system. However, as the IATS and IOLu2 studies have clearly shown, the problem with this technique in infants and children under two years is the high rate of visual axis obscuration, leading to a high reoperation rate. Even the use of anterior vitrectomy and high-quality single piece IOLs with square edge designs are not enough to prevent visually significant VAO in too many cases with this approach which is ineffective in providing an effective barrier to the escape of LECs into the visual axis (see Fig. 3b).

Because conventional IOL implantation in the bag or the sulcus is still the most common IOL technique in children, the complications with this technique have unfortunately led some to conclude that all IOLs should be avoided in the under 2-year and especially the under 7-month-old children. However, this would do injustice to better surgical techniques in children that have been well established for decades and that have been shown to have a very low VAO and reoperation rate, while offering the advantages of primary IOL implantation. These will be discussed next.

Optic Capture and BIL Technique to Reduce Reoperations Due to VAO

As already mentioned, the main surgical complication of paediatric cataract surgery is visual axis obscuration and LEC overgrowth requiring reoperations. The traditional technique of IOL placement into the bag provides little protection against VAO as shown (see Fig. 3b). However, prevention of VAO can successfully be achieved by the bag-in-the-lens (BIL) and optic capture techniques (see Fig. 3c, d) with long-term visual axis clarity (Fig. 3e).

The pioneering BIL lens (Morcher) was designed by Prof Marie-José Tassignon and is made of hydrophilic acrylic biomaterial [18]. It measures 7.5 mm in overall diameter with a biconvex optic of 5 mm. A 360 degree circumferential sulcus surrounds the optic into which the anterior and posterior capsulotomies are placed together to achieve a secure fit. Subsequent fusion between the anterior and posterior capsule very effectively seal off the capsule bag and prevent any LEC migration into the visual axis. Of 50 children under 2 years at BIL implantation, only 5 (10%) developed VAO at a median follow-up of 35 months [19]. When correctly executed, the BIL technique is associated with a very low VAO and reoperation rate and is now considered the standard of care for paediatric cataract surgery in Sweden, including in infancy.

For surgeons who prefer a traditional IOL or when the BIL is not available, optic capture is an invaluable alternative first used by Stegmann [10] and Gimbel [20, 21]. A three-piece IOL is introduced into the eye either by injection or by folding. There are two main variations of the optic capture technique depending on the position of the haptics. The haptics can be placed into the bag in which case the optic is pushed with a Sinskey hook through the posterior capsulotomy only. The advantage is having the haptic in the bag, but it is only the posterior capsule that buttonholes the optic and there is less overlap between anterior and posterior capsule to form a seal. The second technique involves placing the haptic into the ciliary sulcus and pushing the optic through both the anterior and posterior capsulotomies. This gives extra stability and added security and provides for maximum apposition of the anterior and posterior capsulotomies. The optic capture technique is shown (see Video 4). Once the IOL is captured, it is important to lower the bottle height to a minimum before removing the viscoelastic to avoid excessive posterior pressure and dislocation of the lens.

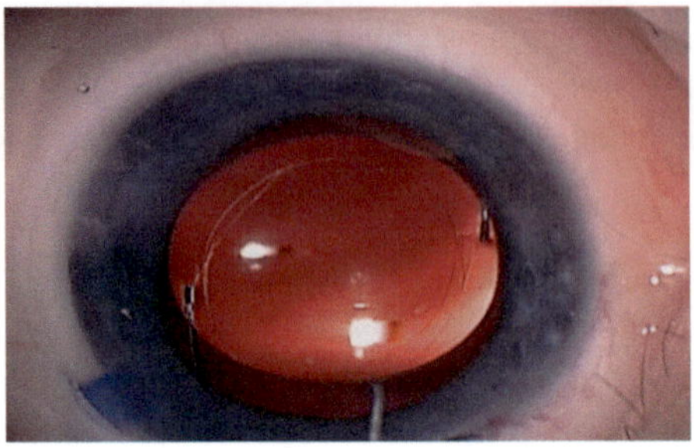

Video 4 Optic capture technique in a 2-year-old boy. Placement of haptic in bag or sulcus. The optic is then pushed through the posterior rhexis (with haptic in bag) or through both anterior and posterior rhexes (with haptic in sulcus) (▶ https://doi.org/10.1007/000-8ef)

The optic capture technique takes less than a minute to perform (see Video 4) and offers long-term centration, stabilization, preventing pupil capture, providing an effective vitreous barrier, counteracting capsular phimosis and inhibiting posterior capsular opacification. A recent review of reports of optic capture in children showed an absence of posterior capsular opacification in 18 of the 20 reports of optic capture listed [22]. This is confirmed by a recent meta-analysis which found that optic capture significantly reduced VAO (RR 0.12, 95% CI: 0.02–0.85; p = 0.03) and decentration (RR 0.09; 95% CI: 0.02 to 0.46; p = 0.004) [23].

All these advantages are achieved by spending less than a minute extra operating time on capturing the optic with no need for any special instrumentation.

The main requirements for successful optic capture are the achievement of an accurately sized, shaped and centred anterior and posterior capsulotomy. The capsulotomy techniques described above, especially the TIP(P) and CPIC techniques (see Fig. 2a–c and Videos 1 and 2), achieve this and give very predictable results in my experience. The final capsulotomy sizes should be 0.5–1 mm smaller than the optic size, i.e. 5–5.5 mm for a 6 mm optic.

Surgical Correction of Aphakia

If a child is left aphakic, it will require optical rehabilitation with aphakic contact lenses or glasses. Most patients and their families will want a permanent correction sooner or later and will therefore require further surgery.

With good capsular support, options include open the peripheral capsular ring, wash out the Soemmering ring and lens epithelial cells and try to insert an IOL into the bag remnant. Attempting this is not without risks, however. If there is enough

(a) (b)

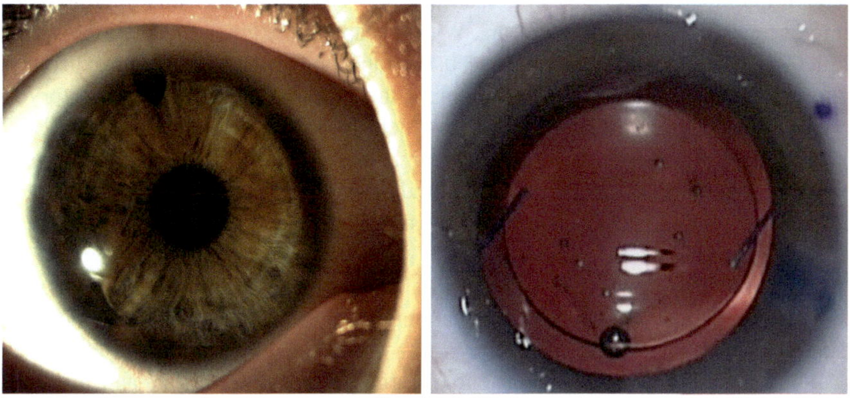

Fig. 4 **a** Secondary IOL with retropupillary Artisan iris claw lens 6 years after surgery at age 2 years with excellent BCVA 2020 for distance and N5 for near. **b** Secondary IOL with Yamane technique in 3-year-old boy

space in the ciliary sulcus as determined by pre-operative UBM assessment or exploration intraoperatively, a very reasonable and safer alternative is to implant a three-piece IOL into the ciliary sulcus with or without optic capture ([5], Chap. 31).

If there is not enough capsular support for bag or sulcus implantation, surgical options include an iris claw lens with anterior or posterior fixation, or a trans- or intrascleral fixation technique (see Figs. 4a, b) ([24], [25], Chap. 32). An anterior chamber IOL is another option in older teenagers, but not in younger or very active children.

Completing the Operation

The anterior chamber of young children and especially infants tend to collapse once opened and therefore all incisions must be closed to avoid wound leakage, hypotony, the risk of endophthalmitis and anterior chamber flattening, resulting in increased post-operative glaucoma.

Nylon is less inflammatory than vicryl sutures, but requires a general anesthetic in a child to remove electively or emergently later on. Many surgeons therefore prefer interrupted self-absorbable 10–0 vicryl sutures in children. If any focal inflammation or a sterile abscess is noticed, this can be controlled with more preservative-free topical steroids and antibiotics and review.

Children have a stronger inflammatory response and therefore adequate steroid management is important. In addition to topical application (preservative-free, especially if contact lens is used), steroids can be given by the intracameral, peri-ocular, and systemic route. I don't use routine intracameral steroids, but give subconjunctival and orbital floor injections in all infants and children to prevent early inflammation and have not seen post-op hypopyon with this approach and only one case of fibrin over the years. With this approach, I usually add unpreserved topical steroids (e.g. Dexamethasone 0.1%) and antibiotics (e.g. levofloxacine or chloramphenicol) four times a day, unless there is iris microtrauma, a history of uveitis or other predisposing factors in which the steroid regime is increased and prolonged. It is important to give enough steroids early to prevent longterm problems, but these should be reviewed and tapered as soon as possible because of the real risk of secondary adrenal suppression in young children even with topical steroids alone [26].

The use of intracameral antibiotics in all infants and children (same dose as in adults) at the end of surgery and topical antibiotics post-operatively is standard in most units now.

Povidone iodine 5% drops at the end of surgery is useful for further antisepsis and to check the wounds are Seidel sign. To prevent post-operative pressure spikes, intravenous acetazolamide at the end of the operation and twice afterwards at 8–12-h intervals can be given, especially if some of the viscoelastic has been left behind.

A short- and long-acting anesthetic drop (e.g. proxymethacaine and bupivacaine) and sometimes a small subconjunctival injection of the latter at the end of surgery can be very helpful to control post-operative pain. Finally, a clear shield should be applied to prevent the child rubbing the operated eye.

Importance of Data Bases for Progress

At an incidence of about 2/10,000 in the first year of life and 4/10,000 in the first 5 years of life [27], it is important to collect and share clinical experience as much as possible in clinical registries. The future **European Registry for Childhood Cataract Surgery** (EuReCCa) will be launched by the ESCRS in 2021, allowing surgeons to contribute their results to this large international data registry. EuReCCa aims to advance the understanding of paediatric cataract surgery by collecting large data sets to an extent that could not be gained individually or nationally alone. Building and contributing to such an international registry will help further progress and answer current questions about timing and method of IOL implantation and how to futher improve outcomes for children and their families.

Summary

Cataract surgery in children is very different from adults and requires special techniques and approaches. Children's eyes have different physiological and tissue properties, pathologies and healing responses, superimposed on an immature and developing visual system and children are much more difficult to examine and treat.

Kenneth Wright summed up the surgeon's task: "Not all children treated aggressively will obtain that lofty goal of good visual acuity and binocular vision, but it is guaranteed that without aggressive treatment virtually all children with a visually significant cataract at birth will end up with a blind eye and strabismus...". ([2], Chap. 11).

The purpose of this section was to present the latest specialist techniques in paediatric cataract surgery that are reducing the rate of complications in children and offering new chances for a life with vision for the children and their families. Early detection and rapid access to effective, modern surgery are of paramount importance to prevent irreversible amblyopia. The main complication of IOL implantation in very young children is VAO which is largely preventable with the bag-in-the-lens and optic capture techniques. TIP, TIPP and other techniques described in this chapter are very safe and create reliable capsulotomies for these newer implantation techniques.

The development of paediatric cataract surgery shows how the thoughtful application of research and innovative surgical thinking can transform a once incurable disease into a treatable condition with good or even near normal vision in many cases, affirming as Hermann Hesse put it:

> Damit das Mögliche entsteht, muss immer wieder das Unmögliche versucht werden!
>
> In order for the possible to arise, the impossible must be attempted again and again.

References

1. Costenbader FD, Albert DG. Conservatism in the management of congenital cataract. AMA Arch Ophthalmol. 1957;58:426–30.
2. Trivedi RH, Wilson ME. Historical overview (chapter 11). In: Wilson ME, Trivedi RH, editors. Pediatric cataract surgery. Techniques, complications and management. Wolters Kuwer: Philadelphia; 2014. p. 77–83.
3. Beller R, Hoyt CS, Marg E, Odom JV. Good visual function after neonatal surgery for congenital monocular cataracts. Am J Ophthalmol. 1981;91:559–65.
4. Neffendorf JE, Mota PM, Xue K, Hildebrand GD. Efficacy and safety of phenylephrine 2.5% with cyclopentolate 0.5% for retinopathy of prematurity screening in 1246 eye examinations. Eur J Ophthalmol. 2015; 25: 249–53.
5. Trivedi RH, Wilson ME. Epidemiology of pediatric cataracts and associated blindness (chapter 3). In: Wilson ME, Trivedi RH, editors. Pediatric cataract surgery. Techniques, complications and management. Wolters Kuwer: Philadelphia; 2014. p. 22–25.
6. Wilson ME, Trivedi RH. Anterior capsule management. In: Wilson ME, Trivedi RH, editors. Pediatric cataract surgery. Techniques, complications and management. Wolters Kuwer: Philadelphia; 2014. p. 112–120.
7. Auffarth GU, Wesendahl TA, Newland TJ, Apple DJ. Capsulorhexis in the rabbit eye as a model for pediatric capsulectomy. J Cataract Refract Surg. 1994;20:188–91.
8. Nischal KK. Two-incision push-pull capsulorhexis for pediatric cataract surgery. J Cataract Refract Surg. 2002;28:593–5.

9. Hamada S, Low S, Walters BC, Nischal KK. Five-year experience of the 2-incision push-pull technique for anterior and posterior capsulorrhexis in pediatric cataract surgery. Ophthalmol. 2006;113:1309–14.
10. Grieshaber MC, Pienaar A, Stegmann R. Posterior vertical capsulotomy with optic entrapment of the intraocular lens in congenital cataracts—prevention of capsule opacification. J Cataract Refract Surg. 2005;31:886–94.
11. Tassignon M-J, De Veuster I, Godts D, Kosec D, Van den Dooren K, Gobin L. Bag-in-the-lens intraocular lens implantation in the pediatric eye. J Cataract Refract Surg. 2007;33:611–7.
12. Plager DA, Bothun ED, Freedman SF, Wilson ME and Lambert SR. Complications at 10 years of follow-up in the Infant Aphakia Treatment Study. Ophthalmology. 2020 (in press).
13. Solebo AL, Cumberland P, Rahi JS. British Isles Congenital Cataract Interest Group. 5-year outcomes after primary intraocular lens implantation in children aged 2 years or young with congenital or infantile cataract: findings from the IoLunder2 prospective inception cohort study. Lancet Child Adolesc Health. 2018; 2:863–71.
14. Mataftsi A, Haidich AB, Kokkali S, Rabiah PK, Stager DR, et al. Postoperative glaucoma following infantile cataract surgery. An indivisual patient data meta-analysis. JAMA Ophthalmol. 2014;132:1059–1067.
15. Hildebrand GD, Tasignon MJ, Vasavada AR, Nischal KK, Nyström A. Intraocular lens implantation in children with cataract. Lancet Child Adolesc Health. 2019;3:e6-7.
16. Vasavada AR, Vasavada, Shah SK, et al. Five-year postoperative outcomes of bilateral aphakia and pseudophakia in children up to 2 years of age: a randomized clinical trial. Am J Ophthalmol 2018; 193:33–4.
17. Weil NC, Lambert SR. Primary intraocular lens implantation (chapter 13). In: Kraus CL, editors. Pediatric cataract surgery and IOL implantation. A case-based guide. Springer Nature: Switzerland AG; 2020. p. 137–4.
18. Tassignon M-J. Bag-in-the-lens. Pediatric Cataract Surgery. In: Wilson ME, Trivedi RH, editors. Techniques, complications and management. Wolters Kuwer: Philadelphia; 2014. p. 178–7.
19. Nyström A, Almarzouki N, Magnusson G, Zetterberg M. Phaocoemulsification and primary implantation with bag-in-the-lens intraocular lens in children with unilateral and bilateral cataract. Acta Ophthalmol. 2018;96:364–70.
20. Gimbel HV, DeBroff BM. Posterior capsulorhexis with optic capture: maintening a clear visual axis after pediatric cataract surgery. J Cataract Refract Surg. 1994;20:658–64.
21. Gimbel HV. Posterior continuous curvilinear capsulorhexis and optic capture of the intraocular lens to prevent secondary opacification in pediatric cataract surgery. J Cataract Refract Surg. 1997;23:652–6.
22. Xie YB, Ren MY, Wang Q, Wang LH. Intraocular lens optic capture in pediatric cataract surgery. Int J Ophthalmol. 2018;11:1403–10.
23. Zhou HW, Zhou F. A meta-analysis on the clinical efficacy and safety of optic capture in pediatric cataract surgery. Int J Ophthalmol. 2016;9:590–6.
24. Wilson ME, Ramappa M, Trivedi RH. Intraocular lens implantation in the absence of capsular support. In: Wilson ME, Trivedi RH, editors. Pediatric cataract surgery. Techniques, complications and management. Wolters Kuwer: Philadelphia; 2014. p. 211–9.
25. Hildebrand GD, Xue K. Experience of early implantation of retropupillary iris-claw intraocular lens in childhood. Graefes Arch Clin Exp Ophthalmol. 2016;254:1655–8.
26. Bangsgaard R, Main KM, Boberg-Ans G, la Cour M, et al. Adrenal suppression in infants treated with topical ocular glucocorticoids. Ophthalmology. 2018;125:1638–43.
27. Solebo AL and Rahi JS. Epidemiology of congenital cataract (chapter 2). In: Lloyd IC, Lambert SR. editors. Congenital cataract. A concise guide to diagnosis and management. Springer; 2017. pp. 15–25.

Cataract Surgery for Corneal Pathologies

Loay Daas, Elias Flockerzi, Shady Suffo, and Berthold Seitz

When should we perform a triple procedure? Lens first or cornea first?

Penetrating keratoplasty (PKP) still accounts for 40% of all corneal transplants in Germany—even in the "lamellar age" [1, 2]. The classic triple procedure (PKP and cataract extraction (CE) as well as implantation of a posterior chamber lens (PCIOL) was introduced in the mid-seventies [3, 4]. In the classic, simultaneous (one-stage) triple procedure, the cataract extraction and the PCIOL implantation are performed via the open sky technique during PKP. The title "triple" is an anachronism as, at that time in the 1970s, removal of the cataract and implantation of the lens were considered two steps and the PKP was the third part of the triple procedure. Nowadays, the triple procedure title refers to combined corneal transplantation (PKP or lamellar) with cataract surgery. If the cornea is still sufficiently transparent, the cataract surgery can be performed immediately before the PKP by means of phacoemulsification via a separate incision. A sequential (two-stage)

Supplementary Information The online version contains supplementary material available at https://doi.org/10.1007/978-3-031-05394-8_65. The videos can be accessed individually by clicking the DOI link in the accompanying figure caption or by scanning this link with the SN More Media App.

L. Daas (✉) · E. Flockerzi · S. Suffo · B. Seitz
Homburg, Germany
e-mail: loay.daas@uks.eu

E. Flockerzi
e-mail: veit.flockerzi@uks.eu

S. Suffo
e-mail: shady.suffo@uks.eu

B. Seitz
e-mail: Berthold.Seitz@uks.eu

M. Shajari et al. (eds.), *Cataract and Lens Surgery*,
https://doi.org/10.1007/978-3-031-05394-8_65

procedure means performing the cataract surgery with PCIOL implantation either after PKP or—rarely—before PKP.

The classic triple procedure is basically the method of choice in elderly patients with lens and corneal opacities as a necessary simultaneous procedure [5], as elderly patients tend to have a rapid progression of their nuclear opacities after pure PKP [6, 7]. In 2019, 19 (5%) of the 378excimer laser-assisted perforating KPs were performed as triple procedures in Homburg (Video 1).

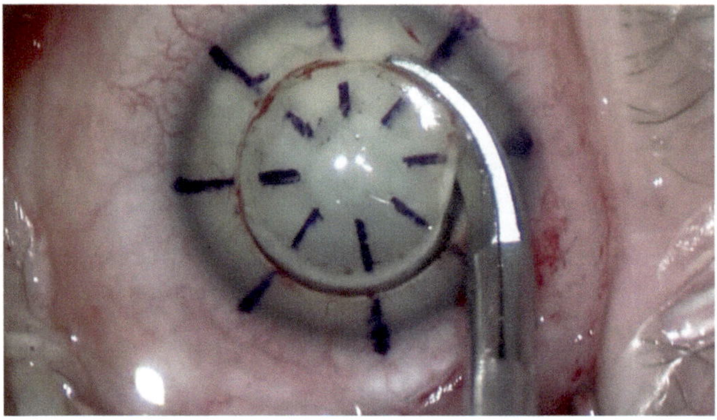

Video 1 Performing a triple procedure (▶ https://doi.org/10.1007/000-8ej)

The triple procedure allows for faster visual rehabilitation and a second procedure to open the globe can be avoided. Furthermore, there is no significant difference in the amount of astigmatism in the course after triple procedure and PKP alone [1, 5]. The refractive deviations after a triple procedure can be reduced by using multiple regression analysis for the PCIOL calculation [8]. Disadvantages include the increased risk of capsular rupture, vitreous prolapse, increased risk of capsulorhexis run out, expulsive haemorrhage and artificial lens decentration if the PCIOL is (partially) located in the sulcus. The fibrin reaction after the triple procedure appears to occur more frequently than with a pure PKP, likely due to the breakdown of the blood-chamber water barrier in the early phase [3, 9]. To combat this, a more intensive topical steroid therapy should be applied postoperatively in the triple procedure than in pure PKP.

Author's recommendation

We routinely prescribe prednisolone acetate eye drops (8 × a day) after triple procedure from the first postoperative day onwards, even in the presence of a corneal epithelial defect.

In younger patients with incipient cataract, the two-stage procedure (cataract surgery after PKP) is the therapy of choice. However, sequential (two-stage) cataract surgery should only be performed when the curvature of the cornea is stable, i.e. $\geq$6 weeks after suture removal (typically >18 months) after PKP [10]. This allows the intraocular lens to be calculated more accurately as well as offering the advantage of possibly reducing postoperative astigmatism.—The prerequisite for this approach, however, is a good endothelial cell count. Potential disadvantages are the theoretically increased risk of immune reaction, the increased risk of infections due to the need for two procedures, the increased risk of herpes reactivation and endothelial cell loss after phacoemulsification. In PKP in cases with a known history of proven herpes (e.g. PCR positive) sequential cataract surgery under topical and systemic aciclovir protection is recommended [3].

For regular astigmatism in young patients after keratoplasty who have a clear crystalline lens, it is possible to implant a phakic intraocular lens if the anterior chamber depth is sufficient (>3 mm) and the endothelium is good. After triple procedure, high astigmatism and/or high anisometropia can also be corrected after suture removal using a toric add-on IOL via corneal small incision technique.

Cataract surgery prior to PKP is relatively rare in practice. This procedure is used, for example, in keratoconus patients with cataracta complicata in the context of systemic steroid therapy, neurodermatitis or diabetes mellitus. The target refraction is based on the refraction of the contralateral eye and the potential need for a subsequent PKP.

Author's recommendation

Rule of thumb for artificial lens determination: Haigis formula, assumed keratometry of 43 diopters, target refraction −1.5 diopters. Check that no hyperopia is achieved with the calculated artificial lens even with an assumed postoperative refractive power of the graft of 41 diopters.

What can the a pinhole lens do?

The pinhole lens, or small-aperture IOL "IC-8™-IOL" (AcuFocus Inc., Irvine, CA) belongs to the group of extended-depth-of-focus (EDOF) intraocular lenses [11–13] providing more depth of field at all ranges, but especially at near and intermediate range. The IC-8™ IOL is actually intended for presbyopia correction but it is also used for severe corneal irregularities to increase subjective visual perception and reduce high-order aberrations and coma. The IC-8™ can has been particularly useful in patients with pellucid marginal degeneration (PMD), patients with irregular astigmatism, and after refractive surgery e.g. after decentrated PRK/LASIK ablation or radial keratotomies (Fig. 65.1). However, calculating the IOL for central astigmatism (3 mm zone) of more than 8 diopters is challenging, as with advanced stages of keratoconus [14]. However, a residual refraction—slight hyperopic shift—is well tolerated by most patients. Furthermore, patients can tolerate a residual

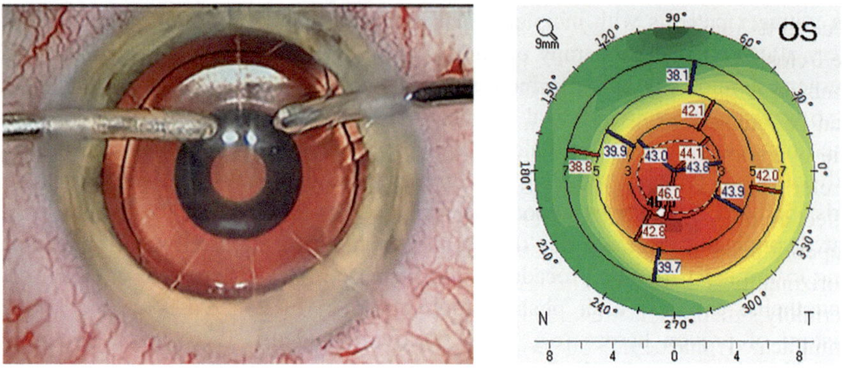

Fig. 65.1 a and b with video: **a** IC-8™ IOL implantation in a patient with post-radiotherapy keratotomies (external), **b** IC-8™ IOL implantation in a patient with a condition following decentrated ablation in the context of hyperopic photorefractive keratotomies (external)

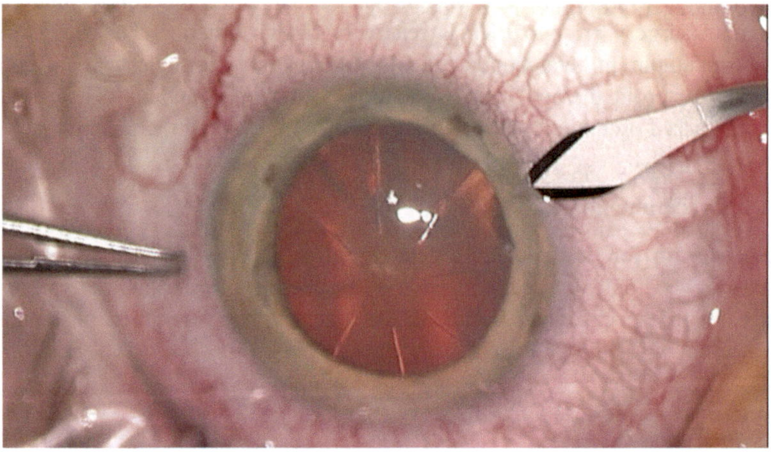

Video 2 IC8 Implantation (▶ https://doi.org/10.1007/000-8eh)

astigmatism of up to 1.5 diopters with the IC-8™ IOL. Optical phenomena such as glare, halos, visual fluctuations and reduced night vision may occur but are typically within an acceptable range [15].

Note: Before implantation of an IC-8 IOL, every patient must be informed about a restricted visual field, especially 90° visual field, as well as a restricted funduscopic view of the retina!

What about cases of MDFD? Or of Salzmann?

The corneas of both eyes must always be examined before any cataract operation and, if possible, after mydriasis and with retro illumination.

Author's recommendation

In principle, we operate on eyes from "outside to inside", i.e. we optimize the eyelids first, then the corneal surface, and only then the lens.

Map dot fingerprint dystrophy (MDFD, Fig. 65.2a) is an epithelial basement membrane dystrophy (EBMD) and belongs to the epithelial and subepithelial group of dystrophies [16]. It is the most common form of anterior corneal dystrophy. The prevalence varies widely and has been reported between 2 and 42% [17]. MDFD is a superficial corneal dystrophy and can be treated with excimer laser assisted phototherapeutic keratectomy (**excimer PTK**) with good results [17, 18]. PTK in MDFD with an optical zone of 10 mm and an ablation depth of 15 μm (after epithelial removal leaving Bowman's membrane intact) can be classified as minimally invasive. Because it is so superficial, no special IOL calculation is necessary as would be needed after treatment of deeper corneal pathologies. However, a postoperative interval of at least 6 weeks until cataract surgery should be planned [17].

The situation is different in cases of pre-existing Salzmann nodular corneal degeneration [19] (Fig. 65.2b). Here, (mid-) peripherally located elevations can also lead to asymmetric tear film pooling with asymmetric "optical cornea plana" [19, 20].

Note: Salzmann nodules always requires a pannectomy and excimer PTK beforehand to enable a valid artificial lens calculation. Cataract surgery should not be planned until at least 6 weeks after PTK at the earliest.

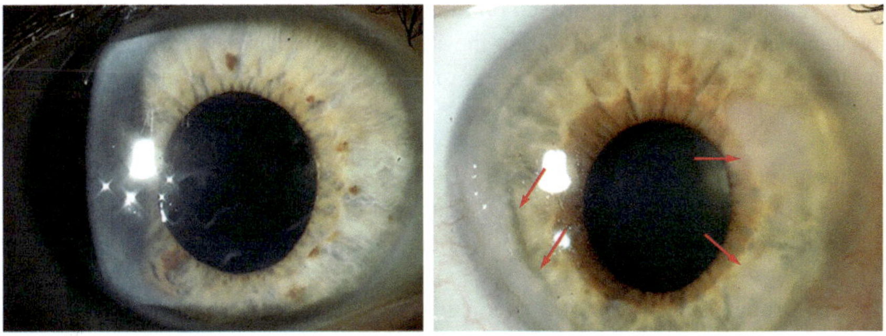

Fig. 65.2 **a** Classical maps in the context of map dot fingerprint dystrophy (epithelial basement membrane dystrophy). **b** Salzmann's nodular corneal degeneration **(arrows)** with asymmetric **"tear film pooling" and "optic cornea plana"**

How for keratoconus? When toric IOL?

Intraocular lens (IOL) calculation in keratoconus is challenging, as it is after past keratorefractive surgery. There are a variety of reasons that can lead to inaccurate results with postoperative hyperopia ("refractive surprise") [21, 22]. The keratometric index with (n = 1.3375, IOL master) overestimates corneal refractive power in keratoconus and leads to underestimation of IOL power [23]. Keratometers and corneal topography may give incorrect values due to the asymmetry of corneal curvature in keratoconus. IOL formulas have been developed for healthy eyes, however keratoconus typically has steeper corneal curvature and greater anterior chamber depth which limits the precision of the predicted effective lens position in any formula. Postoperative "refractive surprise" also depends on the stage of keratoconus. Great caution is required with K values above 48 diopters. In the early stages of keratoconus, the artificial lens calculation is quite predictable using the SRK/T formula. In the intermediate to advanced stage, the predictability of artificial lens calculation decreases [21]. As other formulas have a tendency to hyperopic due to underestimation of IOL power, the SRK/T formula is a good choice as it includes overestimation of IOL power. In any case, we compare the results with those of the Haigis formula.

In cases of incipient to mild keratoconus and cataract, clear central optical axis, stable refraction and topography for at least 6 months, patients usually benefit from implantation of a toric intraocular lens. Some authors suggest that outcomes may be better in pellucid marginal degeneration (PMD) than in keratoconus because the astigmatism is central and, unlike keratoconus, more often regular [23]. Toric phakic IOLs (e.g. ICL) have also been successfully implanted in PMD [24].

Note: The target refraction is based on the refraction of the contralateral eye and the potential need for sequential PKP. In the stable keratoconus of the older patient, we target −1.5 to −3.0 diopters depending on the refraction of the contralateral eye.

Author's recommendation

We recommend contact lens abstinence for 4 weeks for form-stable, for 2 weeks for soft contact lenses before any IOL calculation in keratoconus patients, though compliance with these recommendations can be difficult to enforce.

How to proceed in case of severe corneal irregularities?

In very severe irregularities, especially after a previous penetrating keratoplasty (Fig. 65.3, external), the first option (provided that the patient has a clear lens) is a repeat excimer laser-assisted keratoplasty (Re-PKP) with a larger diameter—typically 8.5 mm diameter [25].

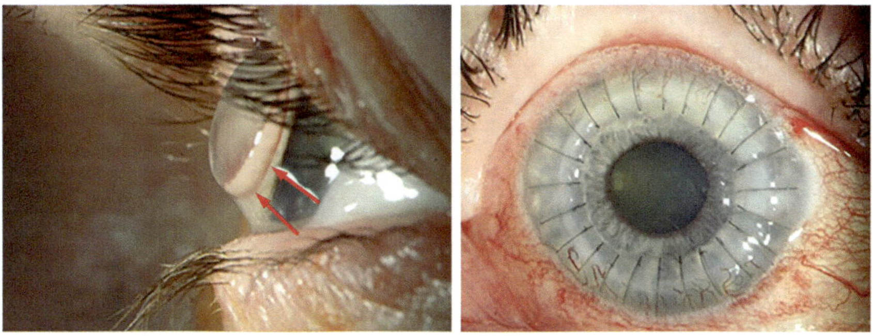

Fig. 65.3 a with video and b. **a** Pronounced step formation (arrows) in condition after penetrating keratoplasty (L:1996, external) for keratotorus. **b** 4 days after excimer laser-assisted re-keratoplasty (8.5/8.6 mm) with 24 single knot sutures

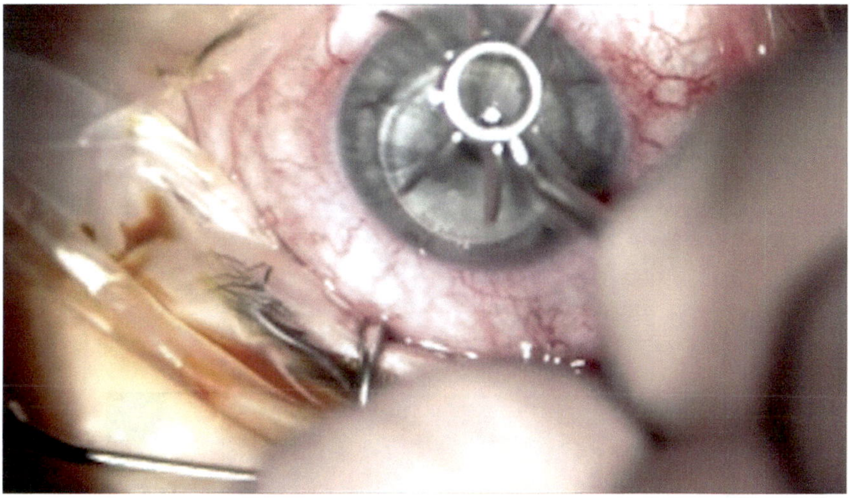

Video 3 Re KPL (▶ https://doi.org/10.1007/000-8eg)

Note: In case of centred re-keratoplasty due to high irregular astigmatism, the old graft should be removed completely, if possible, depending on the corneal size and graft decentration.

Six weeks after the last suture removal (typically >18 months) after PKP, cataract surgery can be performed if lens opacity is present. In case of high regular astigmatism, cataract surgery with implantation of a toric IOL or implantation of a phakic toric IOL (ICL) can be performed.

Alternatively, in the case of high regular astigmatism after PKP, limbus-parallel keratotomies with compression sutures (Fig. 65.4) can first be performed to reduce

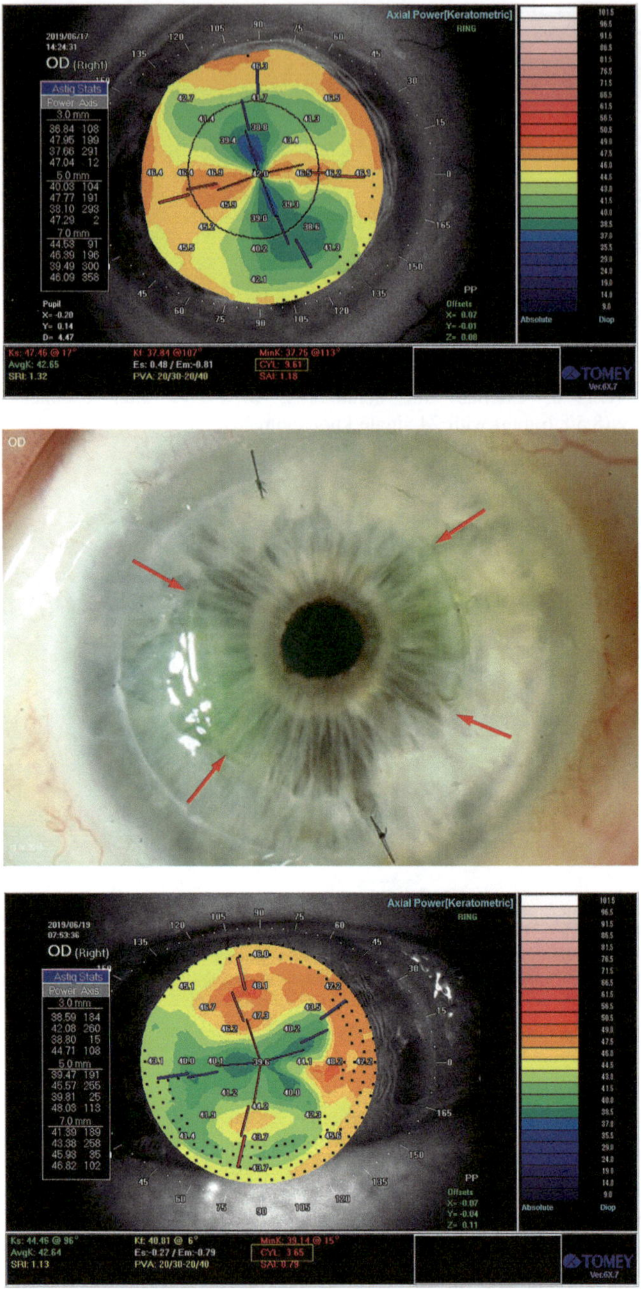

Fig. 65.4 a, b with video, and c. **a** Illustration of topographic images (Tomey TMS-5) after keratoplasty before limbus-parallel keratotomies (arrows) with compression sutures **b** Slit lamp biomicroscopic image after limbus-parallel keratotomies with compression sutures. **c** Topographic image (Tomey TMS-5) taken early after limbus-parallel keratotomies with compression sutures. The height of the astigmatism is clearly reduced, the axis is rotated by approx. 90° (initial "overcorrection")

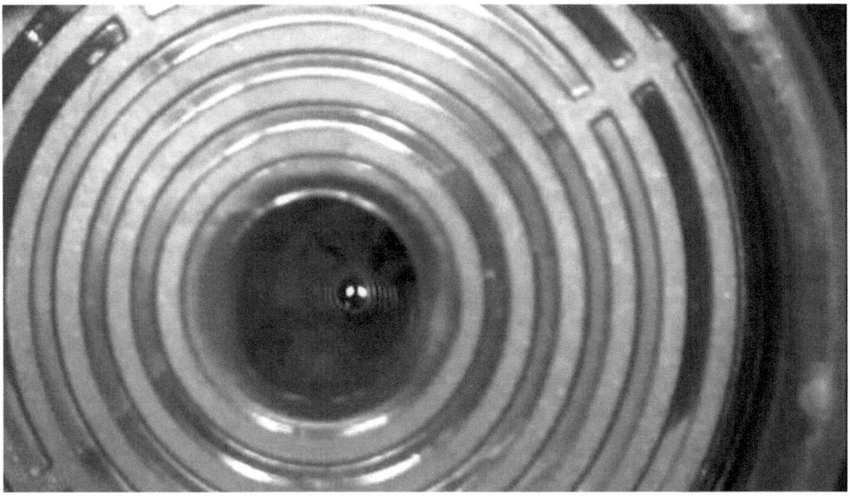

Video 4 (Limbusparallele Kompre.-Nähte) _xvid (▶ https://doi.org/10.1007/000-8ek)

astigmatism. This is particularly recommended if the astigmatism is very high or if toric artificial lens implantation is not an option for the patient as a self-payer [26, 27].

A prerequisite for toric IOL implantation after PKP is a sufficient endothelial cell count to avoid potential postoperative corneal endothelial epithelial decompensation (HEED). The risk of immune reaction and/or herpes reactivation may be increased after phacoemulsification. If there is a positive ocular history of herpes, cataract surgery should be performed under topical and systemic aciclovir protection.

References

1. Seitz B, Langenbucher A, Kus MM, Küchle M, Naumann GOH. Nonmechanical corneal trephination with the excimer laser improves outcome after penetrating keratoplasty. Ophthalmology. 1999;106:1156–65. https://doi.org/10.1016/S0161-6420(99)90265-8.
2. Seitz B, Daas L, Milioti G, Szentmàry N, Langenbucher A, Suffo S. Excimer laser-assisted penetrating keratoplasty-On 01.07.2019, penetrating excimer laser keratoplasty celebrated its 30th birthday. Video Article Ophthalmologe. 2019;116:1221–30. https://doi.org/10.1007/s00347-019-00990-w.
3. Seitz B, Langenbucher A, Viestenz A, Dietrich T, Küchle M, Naumann GOH. Cataract and keratoplasty—simultaneous or sequential surgery? Klin Monatsbl Augenheilkd. 2003;220:326–9. https://doi.org/10.1055/s-2003-39429.
4. Taylor DM. Keratoplasty and intraocular lenses. Ophthalmic Surg. 1976;7:31–42. https://doi.org/10.3928/1542-8877-19760401-06.

5. Das S, Langenbucher A, Jacobi C, Nguyen NX, Kruse FE, Naumann GO, Seitz B. Long-term refractive and visual outcome after penetrating keratoplasty only versus the triple procedure in Fuchs' dystrophy. Graefes Arch Clin Exp Ophthalmol. 2006;244:1089–95. https://doi.org/10.1007/s00417-005-0156-7.
6. Rathi VM, Krishnamachary M, Gupta S. Cataract formation after penetrating keratoplasty. J Cataract Refract Surg. 1997;23:562–4. https://doi.org/10.1016/s0886-3350(97)80214-3.
7. Martin TP, Reed JW, Legault C, Oberfeld SM, Jacoby BG, Yu DD, Dickens A, Johnson HP. Cataract formation and cataract extraction after penetrating keratoplasty. Ophthalmology. 1994;101:113–9. https://doi.org/10.1016/S0161-6420(13)31252-4.
8. Davis EA, Azar DT, Jakobs FM, Stark WJ. Refractive and keratometric results after the triple procedure. Experiences with early and late suture removal. Ophthalmology. 1998;105:624–30. https://doi.org/10.1016/S0161-6420(98)94015-5.
9. Nguyen NX, Langenbucher A, Seitz B, Graupner M, Cursiefen C, Küchle M, Naumann GOH. Blood-aqueous barrier breakdown after penetrating keratoplasty with simultaneous extracapsular cataract extraction and posterior chamber lens implantation. Graefe's Arch Clin Exp Ophthalmol. 2001;239:114–7. https://doi.org/10.1007/s004170000244.
10. Dietrich T, Viestenz A, Langenbucher A, Naumann GOH, Seitz B. Accuracy of artificial lens calculation in cataract surgery after penetrating keratoplasty - retrospective study in 72 eyes. Klin Monatsbl Augenheilkd. 2011;228:698–703. https://doi.org/10.1055/s-0029-1245640.
11. Dick HB, Piovella M, Vukich J, Vilupuru S, Lin L. Prospective multicenter trial of a small-aperture intraocular lens in cataract surgery. J Cataract Refract Surg. 2017;43:956–68. https://doi.org/10.1016/j.jcrs.2017.04.038.
12. Grabner G, Ang RE, Vilupuru S. The small-aperture IC-8 intraocular lens: a new concept for added depth of focus in cataract patients. Am J Ophthalmol. 2015;160:1176–84. https://doi.org/10.1016/j.ajo.2015.08.017.
13. Schojai M, Tim Schultz, Corinna Jerke, Jörg Böcker DI, Dick HB. Prospective Randomized comparative trial: visual performance comparison of two enhanced depth of focus IOLs—symphony and IC-8. J Cataract Refract Surg. 2020. https://doi.org/10.1097/j.jcrs.0000000000000068. Epub ahead of print. PMID: 32050214.
14. Shajari M, Mackert MJ, Langer J, Kreutzer TC, Wolf A, Kohnen T, Priglinger S, Mayer WJ. Safety and efficacy of a small-aperture capsular bag-fixated intraocular lens in eyes with severe corneal irregularities. J Cataract Refract Surg. 2020;46:188–92. https://doi.org/10.1097/j.jcrs.0000000000000045.
15. Agarwal S, Thornell EM. Cataract surgery with a small-aperture intraocular lens after previous corneal refractive surgery: visual outcomes and spectacle independence. J Cataract Refract Surg. 2018;44:1150–4. https://doi.org/10.1016/j.jcrs.2018.06.028.
16. Seitz B, Lisch W, Weiss J. The revised latest IC3D classification of corneal dystrophies. Klin Monbl Augenheilkd. 2015;232:283–94. https://doi.org/10.1055/s-0041-100774.
17. Pogorelov P, Langenbucher A, Kruse F, Seitz B. Long-term results of phototherapeutic keratectomy for corneal map-dot-fingerprint dystrophy (Cogan-Guerry). Cornea. 2006;25:774–7. https://doi.org/10.1097/01.ico.0000214801.02195.d4.
18. Seitz B, Flockerzi E, Daas L. Significance of imaging pathological non-inflammatory findings of the corneal surface for phototherapeutic keratectomy. Z Prakt Ophthalmolog. 2020;41(125):134.
19. Das S, Link B, Seitz B. Salzmann's nodular degeneration of the cornea: a review and case series. Cornea. 2005;24:772–7. https://doi.org/10.1097/01.ico.0000153100.74033.ef.
20. Viestenz A, Bischoff-Jung M, Langenbucher A, Eppig T, Seitz B. Phototherapeutic keratectomy in salzmann nodular degeneration with "optical cornea plana." Cornea. 2016;35:843–6. https://doi.org/10.1097/ICO.0000000000000816.
21. Savini G, Abbate R, Hoffer KJ, Mularoni A, Imburgia A, Avoni L, D'Eliseo D, Schiano Lomoriello D. Intraocular lens power calculation in eyes with keratoconus. J Cataract Refract Surg. 2019;45:576–81. https://doi.org/10.1016/j.jcrs.2018.11.029.

22. Seitz B, Langenbucher A, Nguyen NX, Kus MM, Küchle M. Underestimation of intraocular lens power for cataract surgery after myopic photorefractive keratectomy. Ophthalmology. 1999;106:693–702. https://doi.org/10.1016/S0161-6420(99)90153-7.
23. Alió JL, Peña-García P, Abdulla Guliyeva F, Soria FA, Zein G, Abu-Mustafa SK. MICS with toric intraocular lenses in keratoconus: outcomes and predictability analysis of postoperative refraction. Br J Ophthalmol. 2014; 98:365–370. https://doi.org/10.1136/bjophthalmol-2013-303765.
24. Kamiya K, Shimizu K, Kobashi H, Igarashi A, Komatsu M. Three-year follow-up of posterior chamber toric phakic intraocular lens implantation for moderate to high myopic astigmatism. Br J Ophthalmol. 2015;99:177–83. https://doi.org/10.1136/bjophthalmol-2014-305612.
25. Szentmáry N, Seitz B, Langenbucher A, Naumann GO. Repeat keratoplasty for correction of high or irregular postkeratoplasty astigmatism in clear corneal grafts. Am J Ophthalmol. 2005;139:826–30. https://doi.org/10.1016/j.ajo.2004.12.008.
26. Seitz B, Naumann GOH. Limbus-parallel keratotomies and compression sutures in excessive astigmatism after penetrating keratoplasty. Ger J Ophthalmol. 1993;2:42–50.
27. Vilchis E, Seitz B, Langenbucher A, Küchle M, Kus MM, Naumann GO. Limbus-parallel keratotomies with compression sutures for the treatment of high astigmatism after perforating keratoplasty: a vector-analytical and topographical study. Klin Monatsbl Augenheilkd. 1997;211:151–8. https://doi.org/10.1055/s-2008-1035115.

Cataract Surgery Strategies for Iris Pathologies

Peter Szurman

Combined or two-step treatment?

If these iris defects are not treated at the time of cataract surgery, an otherwise successful cataract extraction will fail, leaving the patient dissatisfied. This is because pupillary or iris defects impair vision, increase glare sensitivity and halos, and reduce contrast vision. Cataract surgery alone with implantation of a conventional intraocular lens may exacerbate these symptoms and generate additional photic phenomena of the exposed IOL edge, particularly double vision, polyopsia, and photophobia.

Mnemonic
The cosmetic aspect of the surgery should not be underestimated either, as patients (most of whom are young) can suffer from a significantly reduced quality of life.

The question about comorbidities

This question is of course relevant to ask before any cataract operation, but it is particularly important in the case of combined iris pathology. This is because iris defects, depending on their cause, almost always have accompanying ocular comorbidities that can make cataract surgery considerably more difficult. Causes can be traumatic, developmental, or iatrogenic.

Traumatic partial or complete aniridia usually have multiple pathologies and often show zonular insufficiency, primary capsular defects, vitreous prolapse, and

---

Supplementary Information The online version contains supplementary material available at https://doi.org/10.1007/978-3-031-05394-8_66. The videos can be accessed individually by clicking the DOI link in the accompanying figure caption or by scanning this link with the SN More Media App.

P. Szurman (✉)
Sulzbach, Germany
e-mail: Peter.Szurman@kksaar.de

M. Shajari et al. (eds.), *Cataract and Lens Surgery*,
https://doi.org/10.1007/978-3-031-05394-8_66

compromised corneal endothelium. Postoperative complications such as retinal detachment, pressure spikes, and especially corneal decompensation are common [1].

Congenital and developmental iris defects occur in a variety of conditions including congenital aniridia, coloboma, ICE syndrome, and Axenfeld–Rieger syndrome. Many of these patients have simultaneous zonular and capsular anomalies. Especially in congenital aniridia, the capsule may be thin and rigid. Congenital iris colobomas may be associated with colobomas of the ciliary body and partial zonular defects (pseudo-lens coloboma), complicating cataract surgery.

Iatrogenic iris injuries during cataract surgery, on the other hand, are often due to difficult conditions, especially IFIS and vitreous pressure (see chapter "General cataract surgery"). In these cases, iris reconstruction should only be performed in the irritation-free interval under controlled conditions (e.g., under general anaesthesia).

Mnemonic
Iris defects are not only technically challenging, but they also increase the risk of complications for the cataract surgery itself.

Strategic considerations for iris reconstruction

The second important question concerns the type of iris defect. The highly variable iris pathology requires highly individualized surgical strategies. Accordingly, the multitude of iris reconstructive approaches and available techniques seem confusing at first glance. However, in actuality, it is much simpler. It is very helpful to understand that all iris defects can be divided into four categories in which defined strategic approaches are applicable:

- Iris coloboma (sector defect)
- Iris dialysis
- Persistent mydriasis
- Subtotal or total aniridia

The first three types of injury can often be treated with special suturing techniques, which are presented in detail below. However, it should be noted that only small-to-moderate defects can be reconstructed by primary suturing. As elastic as the iris tissue appears during pupillary movement, the iris stroma allows only a surprisingly limited amount of gathering and stretching to bridge larger iris defects. Such sutures under tension are often seen to "migrate" through the iris stroma over the years. Accordingly, only a moderate extent of traumatic mydriasis can be adequately gathered with a tobacco pouch suture. Artificial iris implants are used for larger defects [8].

Mnemonic
Sutured iris tissue never grows together. The closed defect must be held in place for life by the iris sutures.

Traumatic coloboma (sector defect)

Not every iris defect needs to be sutured; some patients feel little disturbance. Superior defects are covered well by the upper eyelid, and congenital iris colobomas usually cause no discomfort despite their typical inferonasal location. On the other hand, the lacrimal meniscus contributes a prismatic effect that can make even small iridotomies symptomatic. As always, asking the patient about their symptoms and expectations helps.

If the decision is made to reconstruct the iris, the guiding principle is to proceed as cautiously and as simply as possible. Sector defects can usually be treated well with one of the following suture techniques:

The McCannel suture is the simplest variant of the primary iris suture. It is suitable for small-to-medium sector defects. Historically, this ab externo method has often been used as a pupil suture for the closure of a preceding radial pupillotomy, performed to facilitate ICCE in small pupils [5]. Today, it involves passing a 10-0 polypropylene suture through two paracenteses created perpendicular to the iris defect. The suture needle will grab both iris edges. A third paracentesis is then created above the defect. A hook is used to externalize loops of both sutures through the paracentesis, where they are cut and the ends are tied externally, and the knot is allowed to slide back into the anterior chamber (see Fig. 1a). Typically, this

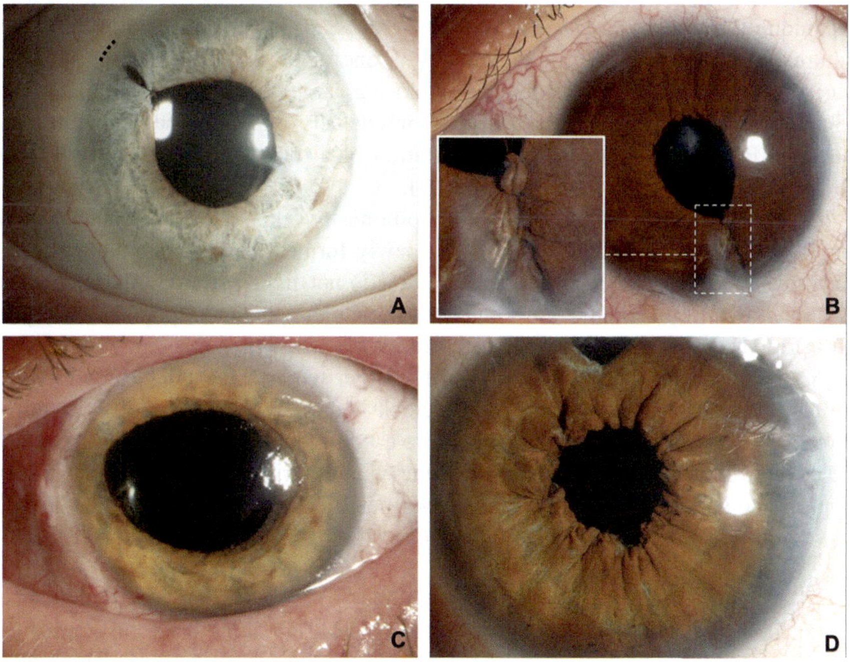

Fig. 1 Slit-lamp photography of primary iris sutures: **a** McCannel suture after traumatic iris coloboma, shown here together with a scleral fixed IOL. **b** Pupilloplasty with opaque suture spacing. **c** Iris base refixation with oval pupil. **d** Iris cerclage with a slightly serrated aspect of the pupillary margin

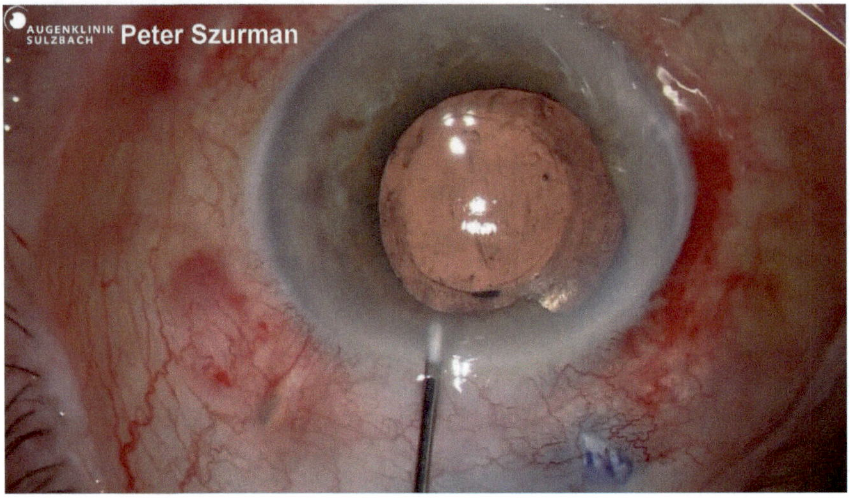

Video 1 Pupilloplasty with an Engels sliding knot (▶ https://doi.org/10.1007/000-8ep)

technique involves only a single pupillary suture and leaves a triangular peripheral iridectomy. Therefore, this method is limited to superior defects.

The sliding knot according to Engels, on the other hand, is an ab interno technique that can be used very specifically to adapt larger defects with multiple sutures (see Video 1) [2]. This technique is one of the multiple Siepser slipknot variations and is perfectly suitable for closing larger traumatic colobomas (see Fig. 1b), iridectomies that are too large, or iris defects (e.g., after the removal of iris tumors). Pupilloplasty, that is, the restoration of a round pupil, can also be performed with the Engels suture (see Fig. 2).

Corectopia can also be treated with pupilloplasty. This involves closing the old pupil with Engels sutures and creating a newly formed, centred one with the vitrectomy cutter. However, this artificial pupil is not light reactive. Therefore, the treatment decision should always be based on whether sufficient pupil reactivity is still present or whether it seems worth preserving (see Fig. 3).

Sector iris implants are an alternative for larger sector defects that can no longer be closed with primary iris sutures (>2 clock hours). Whereas rigid poly (methyl methacrylate) (PMMA) segment rings were used in the past, these defects can now be covered more effectively and gently with flexible iris prostheses tailored to the appropriate size and shape (Customflex ArtificialIRIS®, HumanOptics, Erlangen). A very good cosmetic result can be achieved through the custom colour design.

Author's recommendation

Sector defects can be treated well with iris sutures, but some basic rules must be observed:

- Only healthy iris stroma can be sutured; in atrophic stroma the sutures will migrate through. Here, assessment in the regressive light of the slit lamp is helpful.

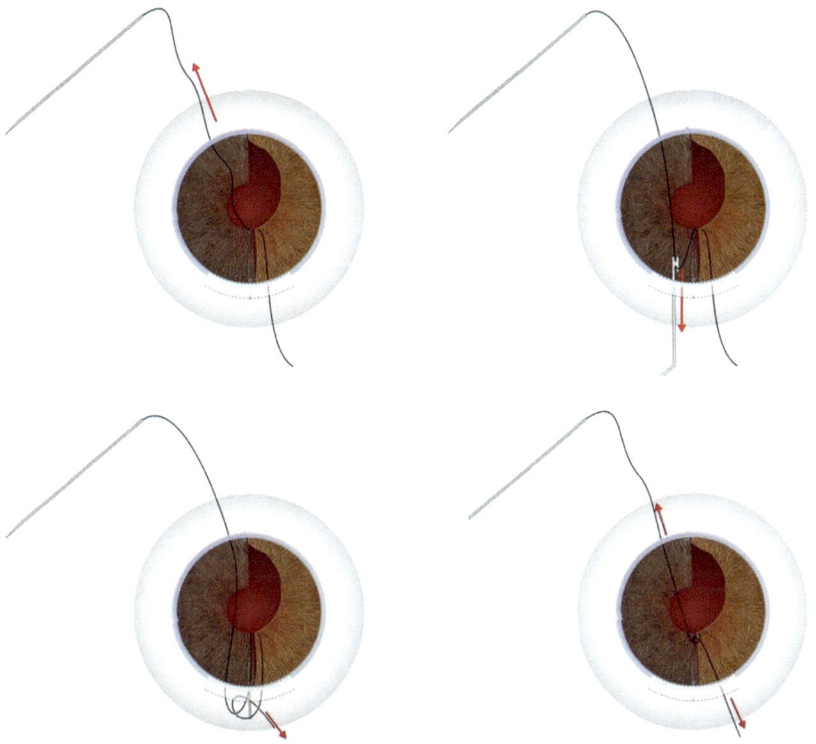

Fig. 2 Schematic instructions for pupilloplasty with an Engels sliding knot. A single-armed Prolene 10-0 suture is inserted via a paracentesis, pierced through both iris edges, and then passed out again on the other side through a paracentesis. A loop of the posterior suture is pulled out with a push–pull hook in order to create a single suture and loop for knotting. The single thread is pulled through the loop from below and rethreaded through the newly formed loop from above

- Iris tissue has only limited elasticity. Therefore, only small-to-medium defects up to a maximum of 2 clock hours can be primarily adapted.
- Opaque sutures must be used. If the suture distance is too wide, the resulting polycoria leads to very disturbing double or multiple images (Fig. 1b).

Traumatic iris dialysis

Iris dialysis, in which the iris root is torn off by the scleral spur (not to be confused with cyclodialysis), most commonly occurs due to trauma. Surgically induced iris base avulsion is also quite common, either as a result of marked iris prolapse or accidental entanglement with a surgical instrument. Typically, this occurs during frustrated insertion of the phaco tip through a tunnel that is too narrow, which, after overcoming resistance, suddenly and uncontrollably penetrates the iris and tears off the iris base.

Iris base refixation can be achieved quite easily with transscleral mattress sutures (U-sutures) (see Video 2). Both needles of a double-armed Prolene 10-0 suture are

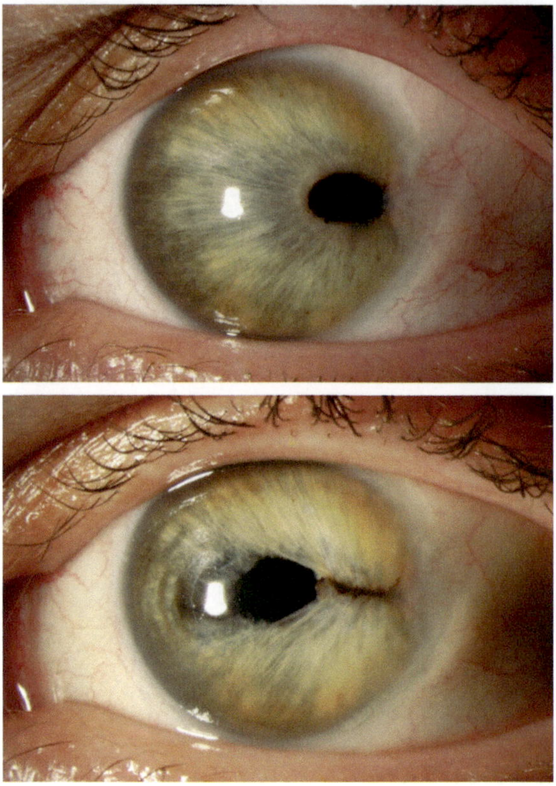

Fig. 3 Slit-lamp photograph of a corectopia due to an old iris prolapse into the temporal tunnel incision after childhood cataract surgery: before (top) and after (bottom) pupilloplasty with a newly formed pupil

inserted sequentially over an opposite paracentesis, pierced through the iris base about 1 clock hour apart, and then passed out through the sclera from the inside. The needles are cut, the two ends of the suture are knotted, and the knot is buried into the sclera by rotating the U-suture (see Fig. 4).

Author's recommendation

The surgeon must be aware that the iris base will be shortened by the sutures, pulling the pupil toward the iridodialysis. To avoid an oval-distorted pupil, the sutures should only be loosely tightened. Regardless, the iris base does not grow together with the sclera and is held for life only by the mattress suture. Even if this rule is followed, these eyes often show oval-mydriatic pupils postoperatively because the iris base tear leads to permanent denervation in this sector (Fig. 1c).

Traumatic mydriasis

Chronic mydriasis is a consequence of an atonic pupil (i.e., permanent failure of the iris sphincter). The causes are manifold; it is most commonly due to blunt trauma (traumatic mydriasis), acute glaucoma, or uveitis, but it also occurs after surgical

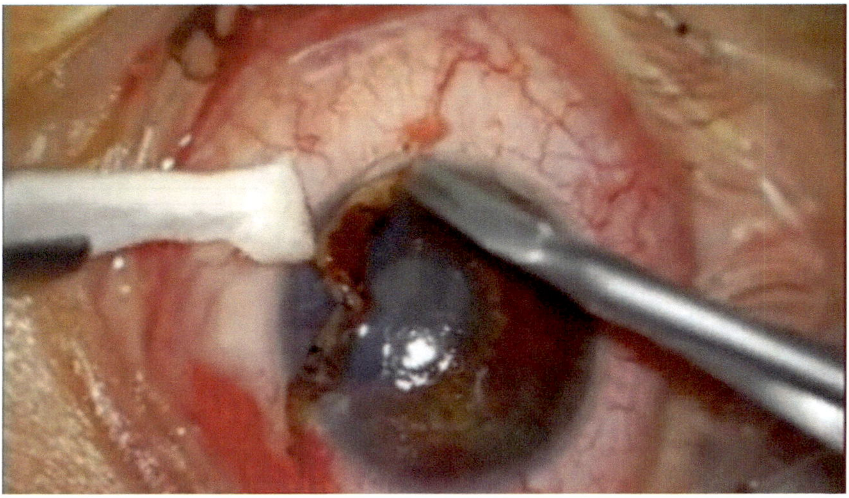

Video 2 Iris base refixation in traumatic iris base avulsion (▶ https://doi.org/10.1007/000-8en)

dilatation of narrow pupils (via iris stretching, iris retractors, or pupil expanders; see chapter "General Cataract Surgery").

Iris cerclage is the treatment of choice. This is a tobacco-pouch suture, in which small bites are taken around the pupillary circumference, and the annular suture is then pulled together and knotted (see Video 3). In total, three paracenteses at 120° intervals are created. A single-armed 10-0 polypropylene thread with a 13 mm straight needle is inserted and repetitively pierced through the pupillary margin at short intervals. The pupil should be threaded with approximately 5–6 bites per 120°. The ends of the sutures are knotted outside the tunnel, and the knot is slid into the eye with a push–pull hook. The pupil size can be dosed well by the thread tension. Note that the pupillary rim must be grasped with the suture sufficiently often (approximately 15 punctures) to prevent the pupil from acquiring an angular configuration and to avoid cheese wiring (Fig. 1d).

If mydriasis is too pronounced or the iris stroma is atrophic, iris cerclage is no longer feasible. Alternatively, a flexible iris prosthesis (fiber-free) can be implanted behind the iris remnant. Often the iris prosthesis does not need to be sutured transsclerally because it is held in place by the remaining iris base in the sulcus. For the implantation technique, see details below. Both techniques can be combined well with cataract surgery.

Author's recommendation

Anterior PVR can also pull the iris into the chamber angle (up to pseudo-aniridia). These PVR membranes can be peeled in a similar way to retinal surgery, allowing the iris to be remobilized.

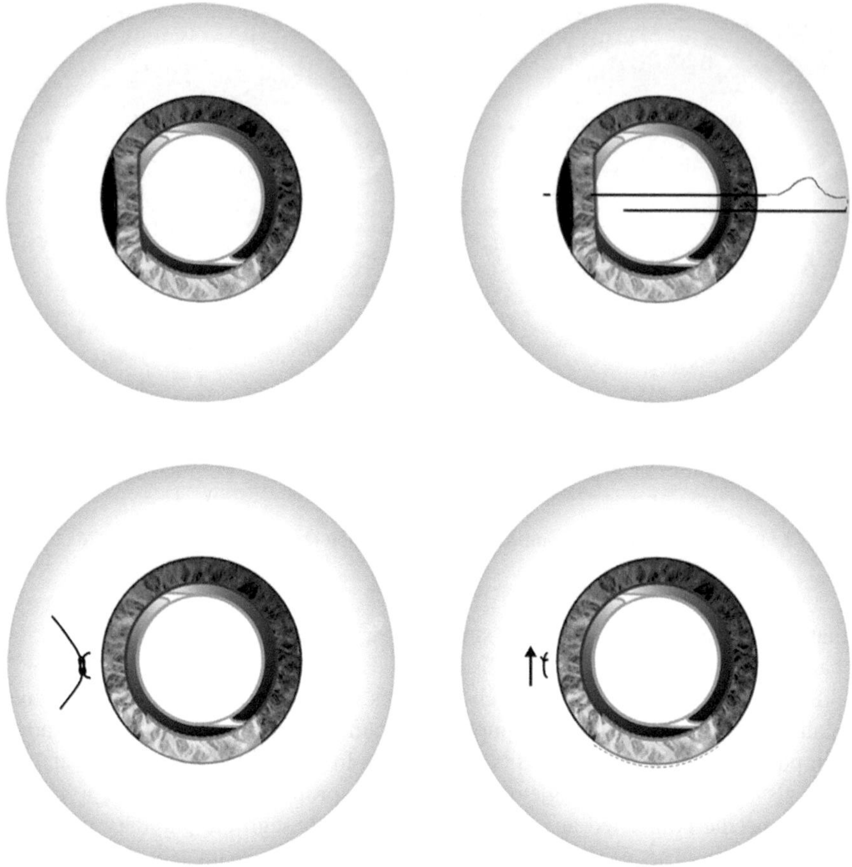

Fig. 4 Schematic instructions for iris base refixation; see text

Partial or complete aniridia

If not enough vital iris tissue is available, iris prosthetic systems must be used [4]. The trend here is clearly moving away from rigid implants made of PMMA and towards flexible iris prostheses that can be cut to size and customized in color.

Aniridia intraocular lenses (Morcher, Stuttgart) have been available since 1991 and contain a 10 mm, black PMMA diaphragm with a central opening, thereby providing an aperture function. They are implanted into the capsular bag or sutured transclerally into the ciliary sulcus in eyes without sufficient capsular bag support. The PMMA lenses require a sclerocorneal tunnel incision of up to 14 mm [10]. For several years, these lenses have also been available with a color-printed diaphragm (type 308) instead of the black one, which improves the cosmetic aspect.

Morcher 50-C ring segments (Rosenthal–Rasch) consist of two overlapping, implanted aniridia rings and are available in three pupil sizes (3.5, 4, and 6 mm). It

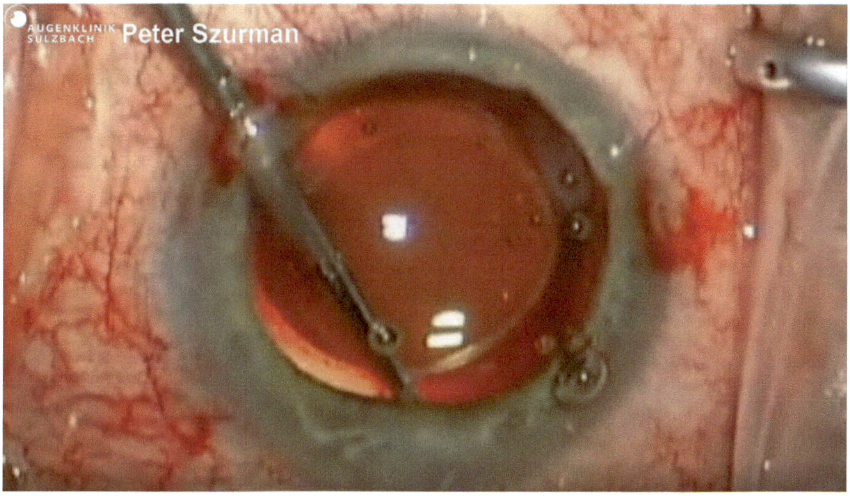

Video 3 Iris cerclage for traumatic mydriasis (▶ https://doi.org/10.1007/000-8em)

should be noted that the black PMMA material breaks very easily, and the pupil size stated by the manufacturer is usually optimistically small. In practice, this results in pupil sizes that are too large. The implants are also available as partial implants for sector defects (see Fig. 5a).

The Iris Prosthetic System (IPS®) according to Hermeking is a modular system from Ophtec (Groningen, NL) with different implants that are inserted individually into the anterior chamber and "plugged together" there. A very common complication seems to be endothelial decompensation (see Fig. 5b).

The Customflex ArtificialIRIS® according to Koch (HumanOptics, Erlangen) is the first foldable iris implant with an individually made iris drawing. The multilayered implant consists of a silicone carrier matrix with an integrated color pigment. The iris is designed individually for each patient according to a slit-lamp image of the fellow eye and provides excellent cosmetic results. The implant has a diameter of 12.8 mm and pupil size of 3.35 mm and is available with or without an embedded fiber mesh as a design variant.

The iris prosthesis is intended for implantation into the sulcus and is only recommended for pseudophakic or aphakic eyes. The prosthesis is foldable and can be implanted via a 3.5 mm tunnel incision, either as a full prosthesis (see Video 4) or an individually tailored, partial prosthesis (see Video 5). Detailed step-by-step instructions can be found in Szurman and Jaissle [8].

Full prostheses can be implanted directly into the sulcus without transsceral sutures if sufficient supporting iris residual tissue is available. If not, fixation is performed with up to three transscleral Prolene sutures with knot-free external Z-suture fixation [9]. Fiber-free implants are suitable for full prostheses. These are more flexible and thinner than those including a fiber mesh, can be easily folded and punched to the correct diameter, and adapt well to the sulcus' anatomy

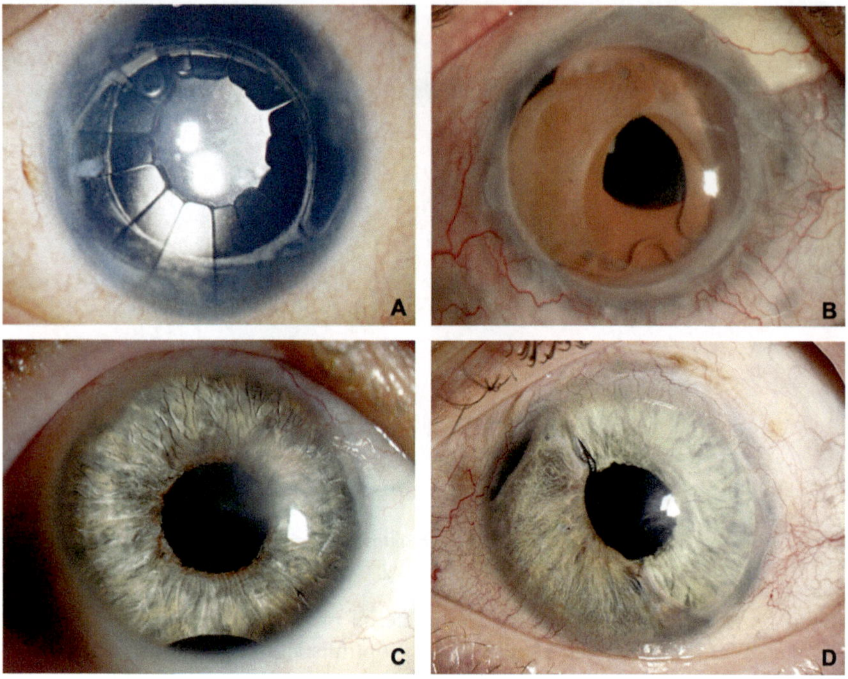

Fig. 5 Slit-lamp photography of different iris prosthetic systems: **a** Rosenthal–Rasch segmental rings. **b** Mounted IPS® implants. **c** Flexible, full prosthesis without tissue and an Ando iridectomy created with silicone oil. **d** Flexible, partial prosthesis with side-to-side anastomoses

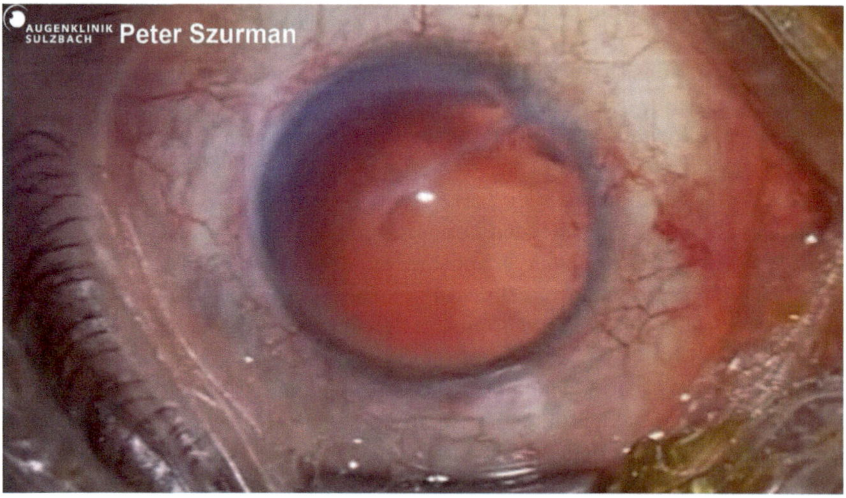

Video 4 Iris prosthesis as full prosthesis in complete aniridia (▶ https://doi.org/10.1007/000-8eq)

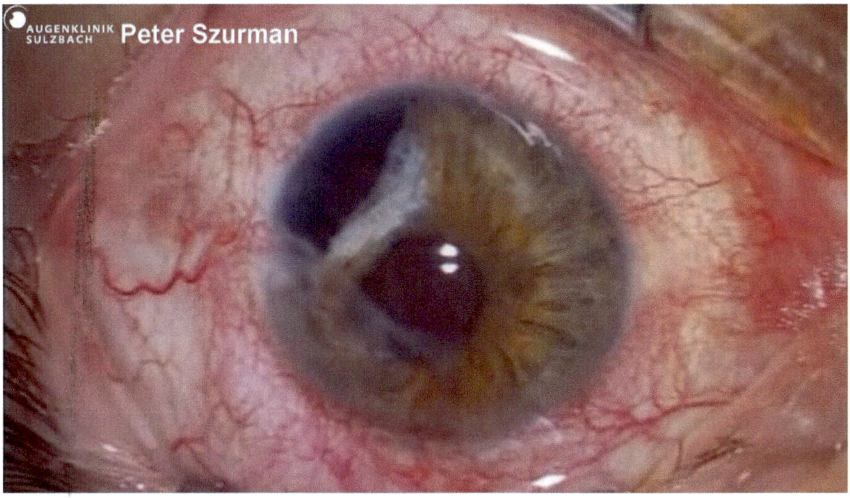

Video 5 Iris prosthesis as partial prosthesis in partial aniridia (▶ https://doi.org/10.1007/000-8er)

(Fig. 5c). In addition, they can be combined well with cataract surgery, although in practice it is noticeable that these severely ill eyes are almost all aphakic [6]. However, the full prosthesis can also be combined well with scleral-fixated intraocular lenses [7].

Partial prostheses are suitable for the treatment of partial aniridia (larger sector defects). Implantation is considerably more complex than with full prostheses, as stable side-to-side connections are required in addition to transscleral sulcus sutures (Fig. 5d). Therefore, implants with fibers are preferred because they ensure greater stiffness and suture holdability. However, the primarily cast-in fibers are exposed during punching and cutting and have been shown to cause a high rate of glaucoma [3] and chronic anterior chamber irritation.

In addition to the usual complications such as CME, hemorrhaging, endothelial decompensation, and hypotony, we identified two aspects in particular in a long-term study over 7 years [6]. First, the increased glaucoma rate can be significantly reduced by using prostheses without polymer fibers. Second, a darkening of the residual iris is observed in the long-term course, which leads to a cosmetically worse outcome; this is preventable by the use of a fiber-free material.

Author's recommendation

- Whenever possible, full prostheses (fiber-free) should be used instead of partial prostheses (containing fibers), even if larger iris remnants are still present. Full prostheses are much gentler on the tissue and shorten the surgical time, which are especially important considerations for severely diseased eyes. Simply sliding the full prosthesis behind the iris remnants is recommended.
- When punching the correct prosthesis diameter, the manufacturer's recommendation (according to vertical white-to-white distance) is very inaccurate and

often results in implants that are too large, bulging up in the eye and putting pressure on the chamber angle. Deviating from this recommendation, we recommend following a simple rule that has been proven in a large case series: in all normal-sized eyes (90% of cases), an 11 mm diameter iris is perfect. A 12 mm iris should be chosen only for very large eyes and a 10 mm iris for very small eyes.

Conclusion

Cataract surgery can be combined well with iris reconstruction, considering the increased complication rate of cataract surgery. Although the initial situation is always complex and unique, almost every initial situation can be solved satisfactorily with the suture techniques and individually adapted prostheses presented here. Due to the vulnerability of the pre-damaged eyes, the guiding principle is to proceed as cautiously and as simply as possible. The iris reconstructive challenges may be great, but so is the resulting satisfaction of both surgeon and patient. The combined treatment not only improves visual quality with reduced glare sensitivity but also has a favorable cosmetic effect. Both improve the quality of life of these patients, most of whom are young.

References

1. Burk SE, Da Mata AP, Snyder ME, et al. Prosthetic iris implantation for congenital, traumatic, or functional iris deficiencies. J Cataract Refract Surg. 2001;27:1732–40.
2. Engels T. Irisnähte in der geschlossenen Vorderkammer. Ophthalmo-Chirurgie. 1998;10:21–8.
3. Jonsson NJ, Sahlmüller MC, Ruokonen PC, et al. Komplikationen nach kosmetischer Irisimplantation. Ophthalmologe. 2011;108:455–8.
4. Mavrikakis I, Mavrikakis E, Syam PP, et al. Surgical management of iris defects with prosthetic iris devices. Eye (Lond). 2005;19:205–9.
5. McCannel MA. A retrievable suture idea for anterior uveal problems. Ophthalmic Surg. 1976;7:98–103.
6. Rickmann A, Szurman P, Januschowski K, Waizel M, Spitzer MS, Boden KT, Szurman GB. Long-term results after artificial iris implantation in patients with aniridia. Graefes Arch Clin Exp Ophthalmol. 2016;254:1419–24.
7. Spitzer MS, Yoeruek E, Leitritz MA, et al. A new technique for treating posttraumatic aniridia with aphakia: first results of haptic fixation of a foldable intraocular lens on a foldable and custom-tailored iris prosthesis. Arch Ophthalmol. 2012;130:771–5.
8. Szurman P, Jaissle G. Künstliche Iris. Ophthalmologe. 2011;108:720–7.
9. Szurman P, Petermeier K, Aisenbrey S, et al. Z-suture—a new knotless technique for transscleral suture fixation of intraocular implants. Br J Ophthalmol. 2010;94:167–9.
10. Thompson CG, Fawzy K, Bryce IG, Noble BA. Implantation of a block diaphragm intraocular lens for traumatic aniridia. J Cataract Refract Surg. 1999;25:808–13.

Cataract Surgery in Special Circumstances—PEX and Zonular Weakness

Michael Müller, Boris Malyugin, and Mehdi Shajari

The zonular apparatus can either be weak initially before the operation (e.g., in pseudoexfoliation (PEX), after trauma or previous ocular surgery) or damaged during the surgical procedure. Depending on the degree of damage, various techniques and auxiliary instruments can help the surgeon to perform the procedure successfully. When dealing with complicated and challenging cases, it is important to have a structured approach allowing to compensate for the difficulties of the situation.

How does the procedure differ compared to standard cataract surgery?

In principle, every cataract operation should be performed in such a way that the intraoperative stress on the eye structures and especially on the fragile zonular apparatus is kept as low as possible. It is therefore important to consider the most important strains during cataract surgery:

- Light exposure of the retina
- Changes in the intraocular pressure
- Hydrodynamic forces and fluid currents in the anterior chamber
- Ultrasonic energy

Supplementary Information The online version contains supplementary material available at https://doi.org/10.1007/978-3-031-05394-8_67. The videos can be accessed individually by clicking the DOI link in the accompanying figure caption or by scanning this link with the SN More Media App.

M. Müller (✉)
Frankfurt, Germany
e-mail: michael.mueller@kgu.de

B. Malyugin
Moscow, Russia

M. Shajari
München, Deutschland

M. Shajari et al. (eds.), *Cataract and Lens Surgery*,
https://doi.org/10.1007/978-3-031-05394-8_67

- Mechanical stress on the lens zonular apparatus caused by the movements of the vibrating phaco tip or other surgical instruments
- The stress on the capsular bag and zonular fibers during lens fragmentation and rotation

In general, it is recommended that every surgery is performed under the lowest possible microscope light, lowest infusion pressure and fluidic parameters, with minimal amount of mechanical stress, rotational movements and pressure with the phaco and IA tips and other instruments. These principles are even more important when operating eyes with weak zonular apparatus.

What distinguishes a PEX eye from a non-PEX eye?

The eyes with PEX are having several characteristic features including poor pupil dilation, weak zonular apparatus, unstable intraocular pressure (IOP) and disruption of blood-aqueous barrier. Moreover, PEX is a progressive condition, thus all the above mentioned will definitely worsen with time [1].

The surgeon should be prepared for the following technical challenges complicating cataract surgery in an eye having PEX:

- Reduced pupil response to mydratic eye drops and, as a result, a narrower pupil
- Lower strength of the zonular fibers
- In advanced PEX, the possibility of phacodonesis
- Reduced thickness of the lens capsule making it more prone to mechanical damage
- Higher risk of the capsule rupture and vitreous loss

How can the surgeon avoid or reduce the stress on a (PEX) eye during cataract surgery?

- with the choice of the "right" anesthesia when preparing for the operation:
  - Topical plus intracameral anesthesia in a cooperative patient
  - Peribulbar anesthesia in a complicated case with synechiae, very narrow pupil, hard lens, marked phacodonesis and the increased possibility of capsular rupture potentially leading to vitrectomy
  - General anesthesia in an uncooperative and/or very anxious patient.
- with oculocompression, especially in short, hyperopic eyes, to reduce IOP intraoperatively (Honnan ballon).
- with the lowest possible intraoperative infusion pressure, vacuum and flow to minimize the stress on the zonular fibers
- with the lowest possible microscope light setting to minimize light exposure to the retina
- with very careful and complete hydrodissection and hydrodelineation

Author's recommendation

Cataract surgery in an eye with PEX should, if possible, be performed earlier. Lower lens hardness will help to avoid the excessive stress on the zonular apparatus.

In eyes with PEX, surgery should never be performed by a novice surgeon.

An experienced cataract surgeon should be aware that it is a PEX eye and take appropriate care.

Preoperative considerations

Proper diagnostics may help to diagnose zonular weakness and dehiscence and to build the proper surgical plan. Unusually shallow or excessively deep anterior chamber when compared to the healthy eye, may help the surgeon to anticipate zonular pathology. Ultrasonic biomicroscopy (or UBM) allows for direct visualization of the lens zonular apparatus. Typical findings in PEX are the broken and over-extended zonular fibers and PEX material attached to the zonules.

Various medications are used for pupil dilation. The most common topical protocol consists of the combination of cycloplegic and adrenergic receptor agonists. The use of nonsteroidal anti-inflammatory drugs (NSAIDs) preoperatively has also been shown to support mydriasis and/or prevent miosis [2]. Preoperative administration of NSAIDs decreases the chance of pupil constriction during the surgical procedure by reducing the number of prostaglandins released into the aqueous humor.

Incisions and OVD

If the phacodonesis is pronounced, it makes sense to perform the phacoemulsification from the superior position. This makes it easier to change to an ECCE/ICCE or, in the case of a capsular defect with vitreous prolapse, to extend it to a pars plana vitrectomy.

We recommend to perform the paracentesis only (not the main incision) at the beginning of the procedure and, after filling the anterior chamber with viscoelastic substance, testing the strength of the zonular system by gentile pressure on the center of the anterior capsule with the spatula or other blunt instrument. If the zonular system is too weak and the cataract is very dense switching directly to ECCE/ICCE is the best choice.

In these challenging cases the main incision should not be a clear corneal incision but rather a sclero-corneal tunnel which can be widened, if necessary, at a later stage.

During surgery a cohesive viscoelastic should be used to keep the anterior chamber stable. Again, it is also very critical not to overfill the eye and cause additional stress on the zonular fibers.

Pupil management strategies

Small pupil is a factor significantly affecting the ability of the surgeon to visualize the surgical field and getting the access to the lens capsule and lens capsular bag content. Small pupil is a risk factor associated with numerous complications during cataract surgery. One of the most significant is vitreous loss. In patients whose pupils failed to dilate the risk increases two-fold [3, 4].

The intracameral use of mydriatic agents to augment the preoperative mydriatic instillations is currently gaining popularity. Two main options are available: bolus injection of pharmacological agent or its constant irrigation during the phacoemulsification procedure. The former is aimed to expand the pupil, while the latter is mostly preventing the pupil from constriction.

If the pupil is not sufficiently dilated, mechanical pupil dilation may be necessary. There are several surgical maneuvers to be considered when the pupil is not sufficiently dilated. They are: synechiolysis, pupil stretching, iris cutting and the use of mechanical pupil expanders [5].

Pupil stretching is performed with two iris hooks introduced through the opposite incisions (Video 1). However, it is important to know that this forceful maneuver is mostly effective in breaking the fibrotic pupils. Excessive and repeated iris tissue touch can lead to a pupillary constriction by reflex. After synechiolysis or pupil stretching, highly cohesive viscoelastic (e.g., Healon GV or Healon 5) should be used to stabilize the iris.

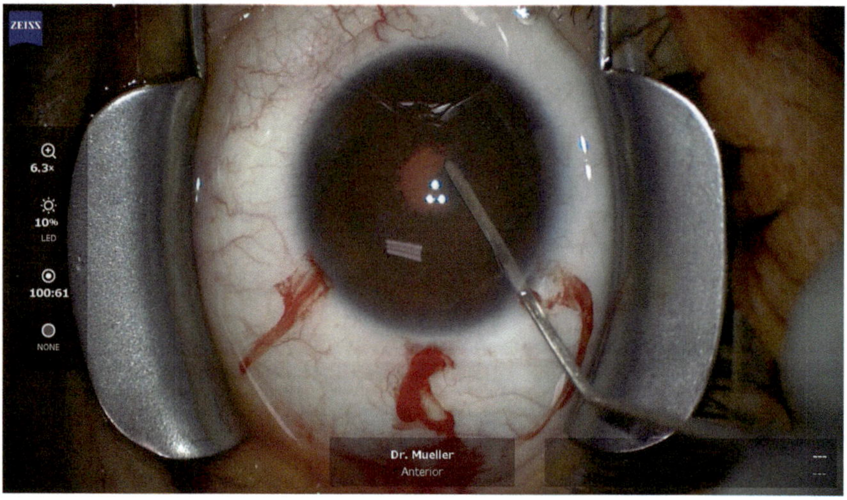

Video 1 Releasing a posterior synechiae and pupil stretching (▶ https://doi.org/10.1007/000-8et)

Nowadays, many surgeons prefer a stable pupillary dilation with a ring device (e.g., Malyugin ring) or iris hooks. Iris hooks since the early days of their introduction into the clinical practice gained wide popularity all over the world [6]. Usually, four evenly spaced paracentesis are performed and the hooks are introduced catching the iris edge. The sleeve of each hook is adjusted in order to expand the pupil to the desired size. Advantages of this technique include ease of manipulations and wide availability of the hooks manufactured in different sizes, materials, and designs. The drawbacks of this technique include iris sphincter tears and risk of bleeding.

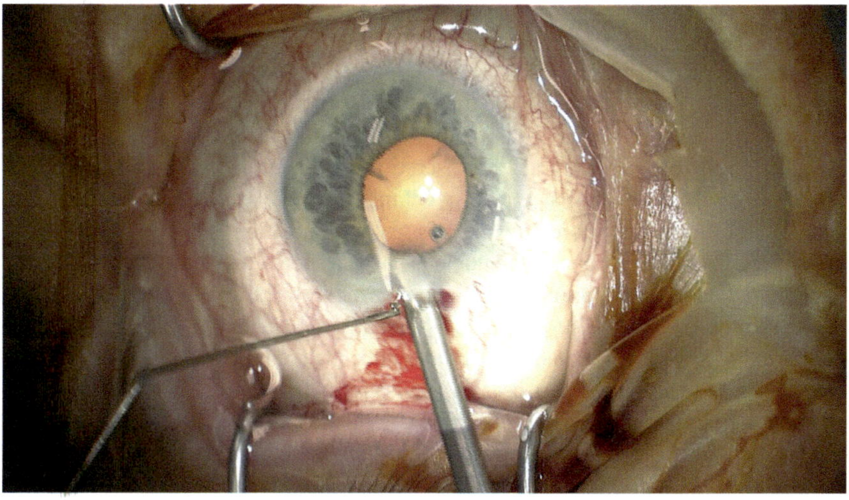

Video 2 Implantation and explantation of Malyugin Ring in patient with IFIS (▶ https://doi.org/10.1007/000-8es)

Currently one of the most popular pupil expansion devices is the Malyugin ring (MicroSurgical Technology Inc.). It is a square foldable instrument made of 4-0 or 5-0 polypropylene. The one-piece planar design features four circular curls located at equidistant points on the ring [7, 8]. The profile of the ring is thin, making it very easy and safe to manipulate inside the eye. The device is injected into the anterior chamber and removed from the eye with the injection system (Video 2).

The Maluygin Ring is providing pupil dilation and iris tissue stabilization by effectively preventing the iris billowing which is very important especially in patients with floppy irises [9].

Following the success of the Malyugin ring several manufacturers introduced pupil expansion devices of various designs. They are differing with materials, pupillary margin fixation mechanisms, and easiness of manipulations during implantation and removal.

Capsulorhexis techniques

There are several characteristic signs of zonular weakness the surgeon may find during anterior capsulotomy. Lack of countertraction from zonules make the anterior capsule more flaccid. That is why after applying pressure on the center of the anterior lens capsule, radial capsular folds can be seen. The second sign is the excessive mobility of the lens during tearing of the anterior capsule and creating CCC.

Opening the anterior capsule with femtosecond laser is one of the good options helping the surgeon to create the round and well-centered capsulorhexis. It also reduces the stress on the zonular apparatus during capsulotomy. Laser application to the anterior lens capsule may be challenging in cases with insufficient mydriasis.

Lens fragmentation strategies

The question of which technique should be used for lens fragmentation (e.g., divide and conquer or phaco chop) is a matter of the surgeon's preference. The common knowledge is that the forces on the zonular apparatus are less with the phaco chop technique. But it is basically on the discretion of the surgeon to choose the technique he/she is most familiar with. Switching from the customary fragmentation technique could be the source of unnecessary complication.

One of the options is to use lens nucleus pre-fragmentation. That can be achieved either with mechanical instrument (pre-chopper) or with femtosecond laser. The latter helps to soften the lens prior to removal by creating radial, circular or cubical patterns of laser energy. Pre-fragmentation helps to reduce the amount of US energy as well as the number of manipulations necessary to disassemble and remove the nucleus.

The other important thing to consider is adjusting the parameters of the phaco system. Lowering the infusion pressure by adjusting the bottle height or limiting the amount of irrigation entering the anterior chamber (with pressure-controlled systems) is very helpful in preventing excessive zonular stress. The other recommendation is to increase the US power (up to 10–30%) above the regular levels. This helps to fragment the lens more effectively, causing less stress to the capsule.

Cortex aspiration

Residual cortical material can be aspirated with coaxial or bi-manual systems. The latter is preferrable as it increases the accessibility of the cortex to the whole circumference of the capsular bag equator.

During cortex aspiration the surgeon can sometimes witness the lens particles located behind the posterior capsule. This was first described by Maloney in 1993 and called "infusion misdirection syndrome" (IMS) [10] during phacoemulsification in patients with intact posterior capsule (PC), when the fluid passes through the lax or even sometimes seemingly intact zonules into the retrolenticular space. The exact mechanism of that complication resulting from Wieger's ligament rupture and detachment of anterior vitreous hyaloid was described in our publication utilizing the intraoperative visualization of the posterior lens capsule and retrolenticular space with intraoperative OCT [11].

Lens particles in in the Berger's space is a sign of the anterior vitreous detachment and zonular laxity. IMS is characteristic for patients having zonulopathy and increased permeability of the zonular apparatus. It is leading to increased mobility of the posterior lens capsule making it prone to aspiration during cortical material removal. It is an additional risk factor predisposing to the PC rupture in patients with weak zonules.

Zonule-supporting and replacement strategies

Capsular tension rings (CTR) are to be considered in cases with severe zonulopathy. They reduces the stress on the zonules by replacing the zonular defect (if it is not exceeding 2–3 clock hours), by stretching the equator of the bag and by distributing centripetal forces to the bag (Video 3).

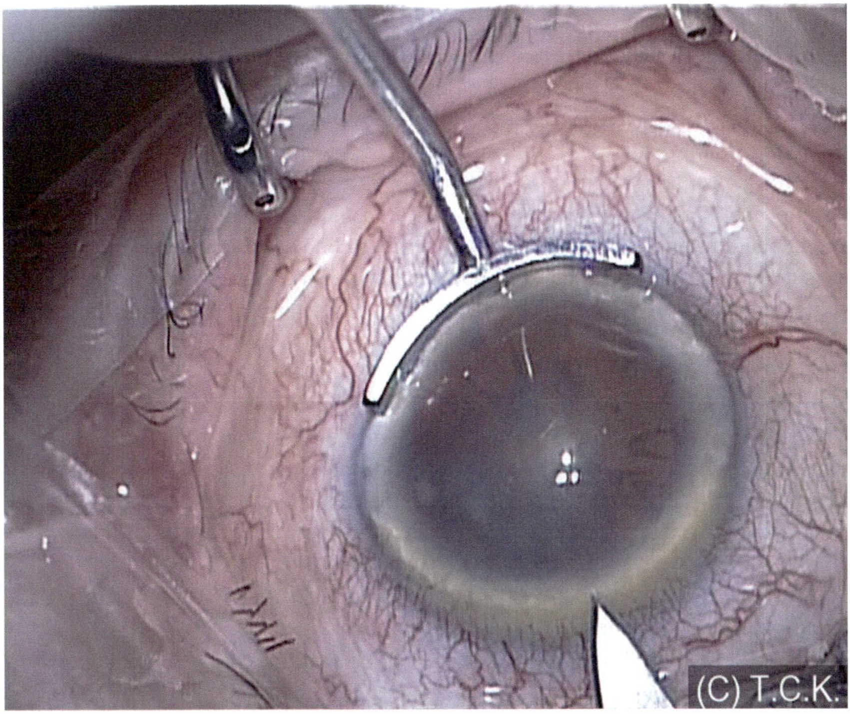

Video 3 Implantation of a conventional capsular tension ring (▶ https://doi.org/10.1007/000-8ev)

Conventional CTR can be used for cases with generalized zonular weakness and/or zonular defects not exceeding 2 clock hours. It is a good idea to get familiarized with several CTR insertion techniques (forceps, injector, Sinskey hook-assisted, safety suture-assisted, fishtail).

Conventional CTRs do not prevent progressive zonular disease characteristic to PEX in the long-term period after cataract surgery. However, they help the surgeon to complete the surgery successfully, to save the capsular bag and to ensure capsular IOL fixation.

In cases of zonulolysis exceeding 3 clock hours and even more, modified capsular tension rings (Cionni or Malyugin) should be implanted. These devices are having special fixation elements with eyelets designed for CTR suturing to the sclera [5, 12]. It is important to ensure that the ring is injected in the direction of the zonular defect to cause little stress on the remaining zonular apparatus.

The other option is to augment the conventional CTR with the Ahmed capsular tension segment – CTS.

It is important to mention that polypropylene (neither 10-0 nor 9-0) should not be used for CTR and CTS. Gore-Tex suture or flanged Polypropylene suture (5-0 or 6-0) are the current options to be considered.

IOL options

In mild zonular weakness there is no need to change the IOL design and to abandon in-the-bag fixation. In more severe cases one of the options is to place the 3-piece IOL haptics in the ciliary sulcus and prolapse its optic into the capsular bag, achieving double (sulcus-capsular) fixation.

If the capsular system is extremely loose, it can be assumed that a capsular tension ring is no longer of any benefit (the capsule is unstable and very deformed), and depending on the experience of the surgeon, one should consider removing the capsule completely and fixate the IOL to the Iris (iris claw) or to the sclera. It is sometimes necessary to perform an adequate anterior vitrectomy in these situations.

Postoperative management

Significant variations in the ocular and systemic co-morbidity may require the whole spectrum of pharmacological tools. As the eyes with PEX are having disrupted blood-aqueous barrier, it is a good idea to treat these patients more aggressively with prolonged steroid and NSAIDs regimes. Frequent IOP checks postop are also mandatory as well as examining the macula (with OCT).

Summary

Minor zonular weakness:

With minor zonular weakness, no lens movement induced by the rhexis can be detected. The surgeon should keep the stress on the eye **low** by adjusting the phaco power and fluidics. Minor phacodonesis, if present, does not require any changes in the usual surgical procedure.

Moderate zonular weakness:

In the case of **moderate** zonular weakness, i.e. moderate phacodonesis with forced eye movements or lens movement during rhexis, the surgical procedure should be adapted accordingly:

- Repeated injections of OVD in the anterior chamber to achieve good mechanical stabilization of the lens position. It is however important not to "overfill" the anterior chamber as this also causes stress on the zonular fibers.
- Careful irrigation of the eye during hydrodissection in order to protect the lens capsule from excessive pressure. Hydrodissection should be thorough and complete to ensure a freely rotating lens.
- Adjust the US power according to the hardness of the lens in order to ensure that the lens is not excessively pushed by the phaco tip during phacoemulsification and thus generating unnecessary zonular stress.
- Careful removal of the cortex with low suction, using tangential (oblique) peeling movements and removal of only small pieces to minimize stress on the capsule and zonules during the I/A phase.

Severe zonular weakness:

In the case of **severe** zonular weakness, which is indicated preoperatively by strong phacodonesis even without forced eye movements at the slit lamp. Cataract surgery is a challenge even for an experienced surgeon. Alternative methods of cataract removal (ECCE, ICCE) and IOL fixation (iris, sclera) should be considered.

References

1. Liu Y-C, Wilkins M, Kim T, Malyugin B, Mehta J. Cataracts. Lancet Semin. 2017. http://dx.doi.org/https://doi.org/10.1016/PII.
2. Grob SR, Gonzalez-Gonzalez LA, Daly MK. Management of mydriasis and pain in cataract and intraocular lens surgery: review of current medications and future directions. Clin Ophthalmol. 2014; 8:1281–9.
3. Bartlett JD, Miller KM. Phacoemulsification techniques for patients with small pupils. Compr Ophthalmol Update. 2003; 4:171–6.
4. Asaria RH, Galloway P, Sparrow JM. The cataract national dataset electronic multicentre audit of 55 567 operations: risk stratification for posterior capsule rupture and vitreous loss. Eye. 2009; 23:31–7.
5. Malyugin B. The results of cataract surgery in patients with Marfan's syndrome with the new CTR. Zdrav Vestn Suppl. Slov Med J. 2012; 61–66.
6. De Juan E, Jr, Hickingbotham, D. Flexible iris retractor [letter]. Am J Ophthalmol. 1991; 110:776–7.
7. Malyugin B. Cataract surgery in small pupils. Indian J Ophthalmol. 2017; 65(12):1323–1328. https://doi.org/10.4103/ijo.IJO_800_17
8. Malyugin B. Recent advances in small pupil cataract surgery. Curr Opin Ophthalmol. 2018; 29(1):40–7.
9. Lockington D, Wang Z, Nan Qi, Malyugin B, et al. Modelling floppy iris syndrome and the impact of pupil size and ring devices on iris displacement. Eye (Basingstoke). 2020. https://doi.org/10.1038/s41433-020-0782-7.
10. Mackool RJ. Infusion misdirection syndrome. J Cataract Refract Surg. 1993; 19(5):671–2.
11. Anisimova N, Arbisser L, Shilova N, Melnik M, Belodedova A, Knyazer B, Malyugin B. Anterior vitreous detachment: risk factor for intraoperative complications during phacoemulsification. J Cataract Refract Surg. 2020. https://doi.org/10.1016/j.jcrs.2019.08.005.
12. Cionni R, Osher R. Endocapsular ring approach to the subluxated cataractous lens. J Cataract Refract Surg.1995; 21(3):245–249.

Cataract Surgery for Retinal Diseases

Nicolas Feltgen

Preoperative assessment of the vitreous and retina is an essential diagnostic component, when planning a lens operation as pathological changes can have an immediate effect intraoperatively. Here, increased mobility of the zonular apparatus in the absence of a vitreous body should always be kept in mind, as well as the compromised or absent red reflex in the case of vitreous or retinal hemorrhages. Even minor pathological changes can lead to serious complications. If such special circumstances are recognized when planning the operation, intraoperative difficulties can in many cases be avoided or at least mitigated.

In the first section, we discuss the intraoperative peculiarities associated with lens surgery in these cases, and the second section deals with postoperative complications.

1. Special intraoperative features of cataract surgery in retinal diseases

a. Reduced red reflex

The presence of a good red reflex cannot be overstated in cataract surgery. Although an absent or reduced red reflex can be compensated for with the help of dyes which can be used for staining the anterior lens capsule, visibility is still unsatisfactory in some cases. When the red reflex is reduced by bleeding, the contrast is reduced until it disappears entirely. The most common cause of a reduced red reflex in this context is vitreous hemorrhage, but extensive subretinal hemorrhage, such as in the case of mass hemorrhaging due to choroidal neovas-

N. Feltgen (✉)
Göttingen, Germany
e-mail: nicolas.feltgen@med.uni-goettingen.de; nfeltgen@gmx.de

M. Shajari et al. (eds.), *Cataract and Lens Surgery*,
https://doi.org/10.1007/978-3-031-05394-8_68

cularisation, can also considerably reduce the red reflex. Extensive retinal detachment can also alter the red reflex noticeably in some cases, which must be taken into account when planning combined surgical approaches. Finally, another (frequently overlooked) cause of an altered red reflex is a defect or atrophic region in the macular retinal pigment epithelium (RPE). This tends to whiten the red reflex and is typically seen in high myopia with focal points of retinal stretching. In these cases, the image is often obscured and the rhexis edges of the anterior capsule are less visible due to reduced contrast. Dyes for staining the lens capsule should be used generously in the cases. If the reduced red reflex is only discovered perioperatively after the initial opening of the anterior capsule, the use of these dyes, especially if the anterior chamber has been filled with viscoelastic material, is not only technically more difficult, but results in a lower staining intensity. When planning the operation, it is advisable to assess the lens with the help of retro illumination and to estimate whether the fundal red reflex is likely to sufficiently rich in contrast.

Author's recommendation

If there is a suspicion when planning the operation that the intraoperative contrast might be reduced for a reliable assessment of the rhexis, staining of the anterior lens capsule with dye should be considered. When in doubt, stain early.

b. **Cataract surgery for injured posterior capsule**

During vitreoretinal surgery, contact with the posterior capsule of the lens is always a possibility. This can happen during a pars plana vitrectomy as well as during a supposedly simple intravitreal injection. This complication occurs more frequently in patients with high myopia or retinal detachment. In high myopia, the capsular-lens complex may be displaced slightly backwards, which is why the standard intravitreal injection limbus distance of 3.5 mm is too short in individual cases. In a vitrectomy to treat a retinal detachment, the peripheral vitreous body must be carefully removed as far as possible. This brings the vitrector very close to the posterior capsule so a lens touch may occur, especially in older people with a thicker lens. For this reason, some surgeons also remove relatively clear lenses in the same procedure, especially in the case of retinal detachment, but this cannot be considered a standard procedure and there is some debate in the field.

It is recommended that the lens should always be assessed preoperatively in retro illumination light, because defects of the posterior capsule can be visualised better (Fig. 1).

Author's recommendation

In cataract patients with high myopia and a history of previous intravitreal injection and in patients with previous vitrectomy for retinal detachment, the possibility of iatrogenic cataract due to lens contact should be considered.

Lens surgery following lens touch may be associated with a tear of the posterior capsule and the chance of dropping the entire lens into the vitreous is higher. In

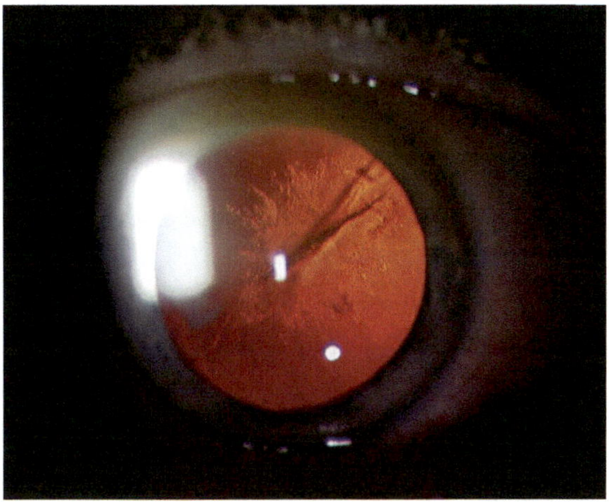

Fig. 1 Lens touch after intravitreal injection from temporal above. The defect is mainly visible on retro illumination, in addition to the contact surface, a diffuse opacity of the posterior subcapsular parts around the canaliculus is also visible

some cases, this is unavoidable, but it is nevertheless advisable to try to work with as little pressure as possible throughout the entire operation. A particularly careful hydrodissection is essential because the added pressure in the bag can propagate a small, subtle, posterior capsular tear to create a large split. If the posterior capsule defect is seen preoperatively, hydrodissection should be avoided completely and only hydrodelineation should be carried out to separate the cortex and lens core. This leaves a protective epinuclear shell which provides added protection during the lens nuclear removal. During phacoemulsification and also during subsequent capsule polishing, particularly low intraocular pressure should be used. At every point during the surgery, care must be taken to ensure that vitreous does not luxate through the posterior capsule. It is helpful here to observe the configuration of the posterior capsule defect, which—if not peripherally extended—can often be widened to a round shape with a capsular microforceps, forming a safe posterior capsulorhexis. In any case, a combined cassette for phacoemulsification and vitrectomy should be chosen, and the possibility of complete lens loss into the vitreous cavity should be considered in the surgical planning.

It is also advisable not to create too large of a rhexis. Firstly, the stability of the capsule apparatus is improved even in the case of a posterior capsule rupture, and secondly, in an emergency, the artificial lens can still be inserted into the ciliary sulcus with the option of optic capture.

c. **Increased mobility of the zonulae and capsule**

Excessive mobility of the zonulae can cause difficulties during cataract surgery. and the rhexis of the lens capsule and phacoemulsification can be particularly surprising. This mobility can be caused by high myopia, a previous trauma, pseudoexfoliation syndrome or a previous vitrectomy, so that either the lens suspension is too loose or defective, or the stabilizing attachment of the anterior vitreous is missing. During anterior capsular rhexis, a vertical shift posteriorly together with the iris is typically observed during surgery. Here, a little more stability can be provided with highly viscous viscoelastic material, occasionally a mechanical pupil dilatation must also be used.

During phacoemulsification, this posterior shift of the lens-iris complex can be particularly problematic and the risk of posterior capsule damage is increased. In addition, the patient can often perceive this shift as a painful sensation. It is helpful to plan a little more time for the entire procedure and to work with less suction. Above all, however, the preoperative assessment is important so that one can adapt to the particular situation.

Author's recommendation

The vertical mobility of the zonula apparatus is increased in cases of high myopia and prior vitreous surgery and should be taken into account when planning the operation. Lifting the iris with a second instrument before introducing the infusion into the anterior chamber can help distribute the pressure and avoid the sudden deepening.

d. **Cataract surgery for oil-filled eyes**

This special constellation is rare outside of the retinal clinics, because phacoemulsification is usually combined with oil removal. Nevertheless, this special situation is worth mentioning. A cataract operation in an oil-filled eye is more complicated because the increased pressure from the vitreous chamber caused by the rising oil leads to a more unstable anterior chamber. Figure 2 shows how the posterior capsule reflexes change when the anterior chamber flattens. However, the danger of anterior chamber flattening can usually be well controlled with highly

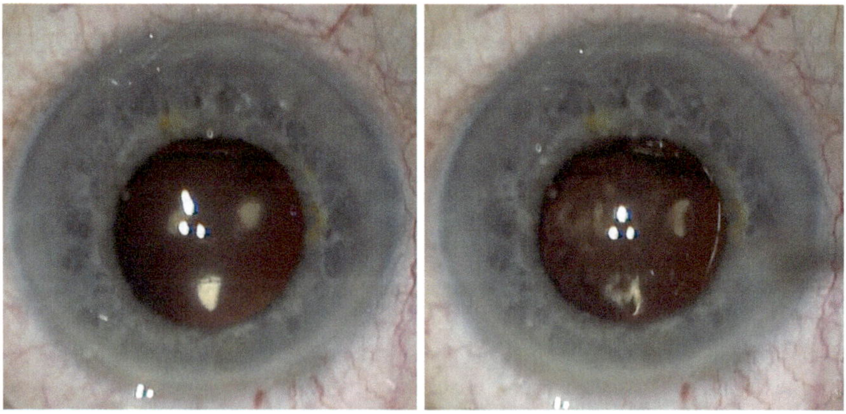

Fig. 2 Dynamics of the posterior capsule after removal of the handles for irrigation/aspiration. In the left picture the anterior chamber is still stable, the rear capsule oil reflex shows a smooth rear capsule. In the right picture a few seconds later the anterior chamber is flattened by the pressure of the oil and the posterior capsule is wrinkled

viscous viscoelasticum. In patients with already increased intraocular pressure (posterior pressure) it may be advisable to perform the procedure under general anesthesia in order to generate as little additional pressure as possible. In any case a cohesive viscoelastic should be used.

Conversely, the operation can actually be somewhat easier because the posterior capsule is much more stable and less fluttery due to the oil tamponade. The risk of a rupture of the posterior capsule during polishing is reduced in most cases.

2. Postoperative complications after cataract surgery

Postoperative complications include retinal detachment and endophthalmitis, but also cystoid macular edema, alteration of a pre-existing macular disease and lens dislocation due to the simultaneous use of an intraocular tamponade in combined surgery. The topics of endophthalmitis and postoperative cystoid macular edema are covered in other chapters, so they will not be discussed here.

a. **Pseudophakic retinal detachment**

Even a cataract operation without no complications is associated with an increased risk of retinal detachment in the years afterward. In a recent analysis, the rate for primary rhegmatogenous retinal detachment in Europe is 13/100,000 inhabitants [1]. This rate appears to be rising, which has attributed to the increased number of cataract surgeries and surgeries in younger patients [2]. There are different data in the literature regarding the frequency of a pseudophakic retinal detachment. The incidence varies in large meta-analyses and database analyses between 0.21 and 2.9%, but on average, there is a 10-fold increased risk that can be attributed to lens surgery [3–8]. The timing of retinal detachment after cataract surgery has also been well studied and it is important to note that detachment does not occur immediately after lens surgery. It takes between 6 and 23 months to diagnose retinal detachment [4, 5]. As a result, patients should be informed and reminded of the symptoms of a retinal detachment and regular check-ups take place within the first 2 years.

Detachment after a capsular rupture is typically seen more quickly. In these cases, the retinal detachment occurs, after 44 days on average, which means that patients with a complicated cataract operation have to be closely examined and informed of the symptoms within the first 2 months [4]. The risk of a retinal detachment after complicated cataract surgery is also increased. The literature describes a 10–40-fold increase in risk, compared to the normal population [3, 9]. It is particularly worth mentioning that the rate of retinal complications is high in young myopic patients. Here there is an up to 20-fold increased risk of a pseudophakic retinal detachment. As a rule, retinal detachment is observed after about 45 months [9–11]. These data clearly advise against ‘clear-lens extraction’ in myopic patients.

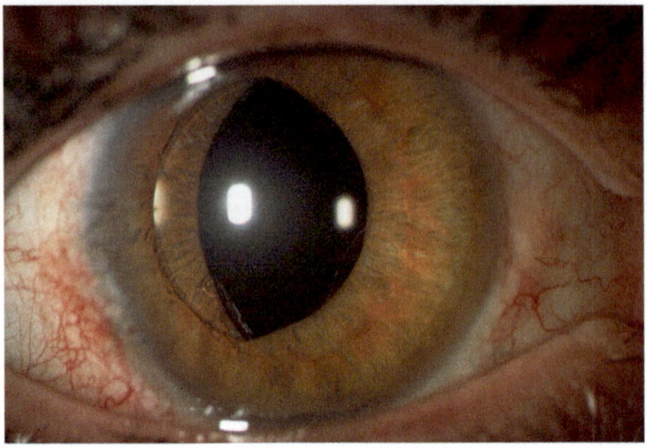

Fig. 3 Iris capture after combined surgery with gas tamponade

Author's recommendation

A retinal detachment after cataract surgery is, unfortunately, not rare and patients should be informed about the symptoms. Check-ups are recommended up to 2 years after lens surgery.

b. **Tamponade-related lens dislocation**

A less dramatic complication is the dislocation of the artificial lens by an intraocular tamponade such as gas or oil. Postoperative lens dislocation can occur, especially in complicated anterior segment procedures with vitrectomy, where the artificial lens was implanted into the sulcus (Fig. 3). Even the intraoperative use of pupil-constricting medication is of limited help. If possible, an attempt should be made to avoid maximum gas filling during the retinal surgery. However, this is not always possible, which is why the complication of iris capture is repeatedly observed. Lens reduction is usually only useful once the tamponade has been absorbed (gas) or removed again (oil). Due to the lens prolapse, the iris may remain slightly overstretched and even after successful reduction, the artificial lens often dislocates again. That being said, lens dislocations are easily manageable complications that rarely cause permanent damage.

References

1. Li JQ, Welchowski T, Schmid M, Holz FG, Finger RP. Incidence of rhegmatogenous retinal detachment in Europe—a systematic review and meta-analysis. Ophthalmol J Int Ophtalmol Int J Ophthalmol Z Augenheilkd. 2019;242:81–6.
2. Nielsen BR, Alberti M, Bjerrum SS, la Cour M. The incidence of rhegmatogenous retinal detachment is increasing. Acta Ophthalmol (Copenh). 2020. (online).
3. Bechrakis NE, Dimmer A. Rhegmatogenous retinal detachment: epidemiology and risk factors]. Ophthalmol Z Dtsch Ophthalmol Ges. 2018;115:163–78.

4. Day AC, Donachie PHJ, Sparrow JM, Johnston RL. Royal College of ophthalmologists' national ophthalmology database: united kingdom national ophthalmology database study of cataract surgery: Report 3: Pseudophakic retinal detachment. Ophthalmology 2016; 23:1711–1715.
5. Kassem R, Greenwald Y, Achiron A, Hecht I, Man V, Ben Haim L, Bukelman A. Peak occurrence of retinal detachment following cataract surgery: a systematic review and pooled analysis with internal validation. J Ophthalmol. 2018;2018:9206418.
6. Mitry D, Charteris DG, Fleck BW, Campbell H, Singh J. The epidemiology of rhegmatogenous retinal detachment: geographical variation and clinical associations. Br J Ophthalmol. 2010;94:678–84.
7. Sheu S-J, Ger L-P, Ho W-L. Late increased risk of retinal detachment after cataract extraction. At J Ophthalmol. 2010;149:113–9.
8. Qureshi MH, Steel DHW. Retinal detachment following cataract phacoemulsification-a review of the literature. Eye Lond Engl. 2020;34:616–31.
9. Kim J, Ryu SY, Hong JH, Chung EJ. Incidence and risk factors for retinal detachment after cataract surgery in Korea: a nationwide population-based study from 2011 to 2015. Graefes Arch Clin Exp Ophthalmol Albrecht Von Graefes Arch Klin Exp Ophthalmol. 2019;257:2193–202.
10. Laube T, Brockmann C, Lehmann N, Bornfeld N. Pseudophakic retinal detachment in young-aged patients. PLoS ONE. 2017;12: e0184187.
11. Lin JY, Ho WL, Ger LP, Sheu SJ. Analysis of factors correlated with the development of pseudophakic retinal detachment—a long-term study in a single medical center. Graefes Arch Clin Exp Ophthalmol. 2013; 251(2):459–65. https://doi.org/10.1007/s00417-012-2043-3. Epub 2012 May 5. PMID: 22555898.

Cataract and Glaucoma

Marc J. Mackert

Glaucoma is the second most common cause of blindness worldwide with a prevalence of 3.5% [1] while cataract is the leading cause of blindness worldwide. Both conditions increase with age, and comorbidity is high, with a reported prevalence of 19.1% in the literature [2].

Cataract surgery in general has a low complication rate of 0.1–5% [3] and may have an additional benefit in lowering intraocular pressure (IOP) in glaucoma patients. IOP reduction is currently the only medically treatable factor to prevent the progression of glaucoma [4]. In this context different treatment modalities and plans can be distinguished. These options include cataract surgery as a stand-alone procedure, cataract surgery after previous glaucoma surgery, and combined procedures such as minimally invasive glaucoma surgery (MIGS) with cataract surgery.

Preoperative considerations:

From the moment the cataract is diagnosed in a patient with glaucoma, the question arises as to how high the potential IOP reduction alone through cataract surgery can be. In the Ocular Hypertension Treatment Study, a large prospective randomized study regarding ocular hypertension, the average IOP reduction after cataract surgery was 16.5% and 39.7% of eyes achieved >20% IOP reduction, which is about half the IOP reducing effect of prostaglandin analogues [5]. In 2015 a report from

Supplementary Information The online version contains supplementary material available at https://doi.org/10.1007/978-3-031-05394-8_69. The videos can be accessed individually by clicking the DOI link in the accompanying figure caption or by scanning this link with the SN More Media App.

M. J. Mackert (✉)
Munich, Germany
e-mail: marc.mackert@med.uni-muenchen.de

M. Shajari et al. (eds.), *Cataract and Lens Surgery*,
https://doi.org/10.1007/978-3-031-05394-8_69

the American Academy of Ophthalmology further investigated the effect of phacoemulsification on IOP of glaucoma patients. In primary open angle glaucoma (POAG), the IOP reduction was 13% and the reduction of glaucoma medication was 12%. In pseudoexfoliation (PEX) glaucoma, the IOP reduction was as high as 20% and the reduction of medication was 35%.

In acute angle-closure glaucoma, cataract surgery is often the most important causal therapy and can in fact lead to a cure of the disease. When cataract surgery is performed in the acute stage, an IOP reduction of 71% can be achieved and hardly any long-term medication maybe needed. In chronic angle-closure glaucoma the IOP lowering effect is still 30% and the medication reduction 58%. However, advanced stages of the disease and poorly regulated glaucoma patients were not taken into account [6]. Other studies also report a beneficial effect in advanced glaucoma, and the IOP lowering effect seems to depend on the baseline pressure (the higher the baseline IOP, the higher the IOP reduction). However, it is not clear how long this effect lasts. In summary cataract surgery alone results in a reduction of IOP. This effect is highest in angle-closure glaucoma, followed by PEX glaucoma, POAG and ocular hypertension.

But what is the benefit of cataract surgery for people with a glaucomatous, damaged optic nerve? In cases of advanced cataract and in the absence of fundus view, the swinging flashlight test is essential to rule out a positive relative pupil defect (RAPD). For follow-up of glaucoma in patients with significant cataract, "pattern standard deviation" (PSD) is most useful in perimetry, as localized scotomas are less affected by cataract [7]. Cataract does not produce deep scotomas in static perimetry, but relative scotomas may obscure glaucomatous defects. Cataract also affects the overall sensitivity of the visual field which is represented by the "mean deviation" (MD). In general, if there is a deep central scotoma in two or less meridians, the patient is likely to achieve a significant improvement in visual acuity with cataract surgery [8]. Quality of life also increases significantly, even in advanced glaucoma [9]. Follow up of glaucoma patients with perimetry improves also after cataract surgery and is therefore more conclusive.

Older patients in particular can benefit from a combined procedure of cataract surgery and minimally invasive glaucoma surgery (MIGS). The combined approach avoids the need for a second surgery and compliance can be improved in these patients. The main indications for MIGS are intolerance of IOP-lowering eye drops, reduced compliance in administration of eye drops and difficulties with eye drop application. While a reduction in the number of eye drops can be achieved, a combined procedure can also be useful in cases of significant cataract and uncontrolled glaucoma. It should be noted however that a longer operation time and the increased invasiveness leads to an increased inflammatory reaction. With the injection of two minimally invasive trabecular implants, the iStent inject (Glaucos Co., CA, USA), the IOP lowering effect of cataract surgery can be further improved in mild to moderate open angle glaucoma (including pseudoexfoliation glaucoma). This is currently the smallest known approved medical device for implantation in humans (Fig. 1).

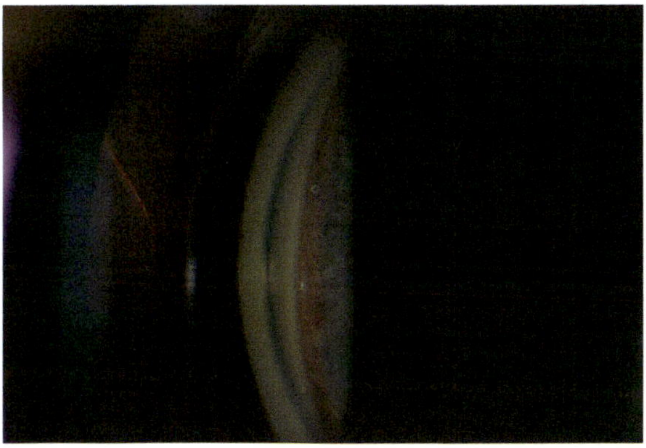

Fig. 1 Gonioscopy: iStent inject implanted in the trabecular meshwork

In a prospective randomized study of cataract surgery alone versus combined cataract surgery with the iStent inject, the results showed a $\geq 20\%$ reduction of IOP after 24 months in 61.9% versus 75.8% (in the combined group) with excellent safety [10]. If cataract is the primary concern in mild/moderate glaucoma, the combination of cataract surgery with a trabecular bypass system (iStent inject) can be performed to reduce glaucoma medication. In moderate to severe open angle glaucoma, cataract surgery can be combined with minimally invasive filtrating glaucoma surgery such as the XEN GEL Stent (Allergan Inc., CA, USA) or the PRESERFLO MicroShunt (Santen Pharmaceutical Co., Ltd., Osaka, Japan) with the goal of avoiding more invasive surgery. IOP reduction in these subconjunctival filtrating procedures (Xen Gel Stent, Preserflo MicroShunt) is effective and achieves IOP reduction similar to trabeculectomy (TET). Therefore, these procedures can be used in uncontrolled and/or progressive glaucoma. Unlike the gold standard of the classic TET there is no disadvantage in combining these procedures with cataract surgery. The Xen Gel Stent is implanted ab interno with an outflow from the anterior chamber into the subconjunctival space (Fig. 2).

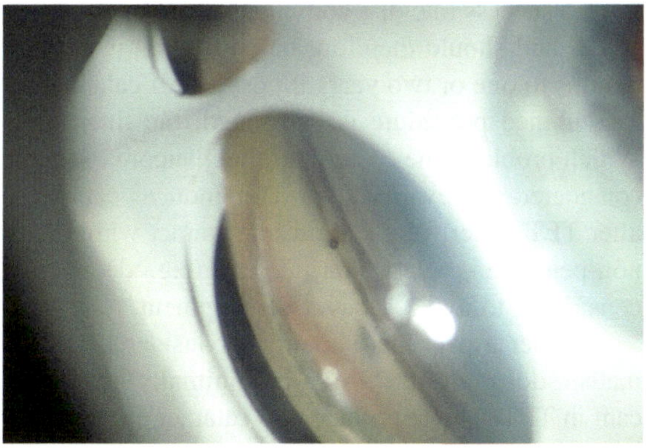

Fig. 2 Gonioscopy: XEN gel stent in the anterior chamber angle

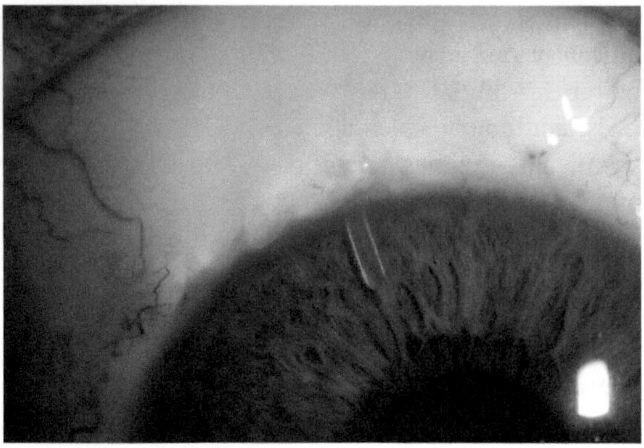

Fig. 3 Slit lamp photo: preserflo microShunt in the anterior chamber

In a prospective study an IOP reduction from 21.4 to 15.2 mmHg was achieved after two years, and 44.7% of eyes were still without IOP-lowering medication after two years. Comparison of combined surgery with XEN Gel Stent implantation alone showed no significant difference [11]. The Preserflo MicroShunt is a procedure ab externo with filtration from the anterior chamber under the conjunctiva (Fig. 3).

In a prospective study IOP was reduced from 23.8 mmHg at baseline to 10.7 mmHg (55% reduction) after three years. The number of glaucoma medications was reduced from 2.4 to 0.7 after three years and there was no significant difference between the combined procedure and MicroShunt implantation alone [12].

In combined subconjunctival filtration procedures, the eye should be prepared ten days before surgery, because the prolonged use of anti-glaucomatous medication, especially prostaglandin analogues, lead to conjunctival injection and inflammation. Local anti-glaucomatous therapy should be discontinued and temporarily replaced by oral acetazolamide (e.g. 250 mg tablets two to three times a day). A preservative free topical corticosteroid (dexamethasone) should be administered three times a day to achieve an optimal surgical site without inflammation, for these combined operations.

The success rate of a combined TET operation is usually lower than a combined MIGS and should therefore be performed in two steps with an interval of several months to one or two years if possible. If cataract surgery is performed too early or a combined procedure is performed, the filtering function of the TET is at risk. Which problem, the cataract or the glaucoma, is a question that should be carefully considered and evaluated. A TET induces cataract formation. Half of the patients after TET suffer from significant cataract within five years [13]. In young patients, non-penetrating glaucoma surgery (e.g. deep sclerectomy) should therefore be considered to avoid cataract development.

Another aspect that should be considered is corneal astigmatism. While astigmatism does not play a role in minimally invasive glaucoma surgery, it is significant in TET. The advantage of a cataract operation in the second step is that if there is any astigmatism induced by TET, this can be corrected with a toric lens implant during cataract surgery. In order to counteract scarring of the bleb after subconjunctival filtrating procedures, 5-fluorouracil should be injected subconjunctivally during cataract surgery. Unlike valve surgery, cataract surgery may impair the IOP control in eyes after filtrating procedures. Cataract development is also induced after valve surgery (for example Baerveldt or Ahmed Valve) and implantation of valves is easier in pseudophakia. Therefore, if possible, cataract surgery should be performed before implantation of a valve.

The intraocular lens design is another aspect that should be considered preoperatively before cataract surgery. Multifocal lenses are a contraindication for glaucoma patients, as they further impair contrast vision, which is already reduced due to the optic nerve damage. Aspherical lenses, on the other hand, are the lens of choice because they increase contrast vision and depth of field. In cases of significant corneal astigmatism (especially after TET) toric lenses are an option, as mentioned previously. However, toric lenses are contraindicated in cases of pseudoexfoliation (PEX) or unstable zonula and are also unsuitable for combined procedures with cases of unpredictable astigmatism. Hydrophobic acrylates have less capsular shrinkage, posterior capsule opacification and a slow controlled unfolding of the IOL intraoperatively, which can be useful in existing zonula defects, especially with PEX. PEX can also present additional surgical problems such as a narrow pupil, so iris hooks or a Malyugin ring should be considered. If the zonula is unstable, a capsular tension ring should be considered, or in the case of zonulolysis a sulcus fixated IOL is a viable and reliable alternative.

Intraoperative considerations:

The most common drug family used to reduce IOP are the prostaglandin analogues, which have side effects such as eyelash growth and blepharitis. Thorough disinfection with povidone iodine is mandatory (as usual) but particular care should be taken to ensure that the long eyelashes are well taped by the sterile draping. Glaucoma patients often have deep-set eyes due to atrophy of the orbital fatty tissue, which is also a side effect of prostaglandin analogues. Not every eyelid speculum is suitable. The open Barraquer speculum or an adjustable eyelid speculum such as the Bangerter can be good options here. If the deep-set eye is still a problem, a retrobulbar injection of Balanced Salt Solution (BSS) or Mepivacain to increase the orbital volume and to allow the eye to bulge out of the orbit can be helpful. The positioning of the corneal incision may also need to be adapted for the glaucoma patient. If the anterior chamber is shallow, for example in the case of angle-closure glaucoma, the incision should be placed further in the clear cornea, more centrally, and not at the limbus to avoid iris prolapse through the corneal wound. In the case of a bleb, the incision should be made at a different location, for example temporally, in order to avoid damage to the bleb. Furthermore, corneal wound healing in the area of the bleb may be impaired by the application of antimetabolites.

In a combined TET, the incision can be made in the sclera via the prepared scleral flap or temporally in the clear cornea, away from the superior TET. After cataract surgery, the incision should be sutured with a single nylon suture for safety reasons. Cohesive ophthalmic viscoelastic device (OVD) causes fewer IOP spikes postoperatively than dispersive OVD, as these can be better removed completely at the end of the operation [14, 15]. At the end of the operation, all residual OVD should be thoroughly rinsed out of the anterior chamber angle with BSS. In patients with more shallow anterior chambers, the endothelial cells can be more prone to damage during the cataract surgery. In these cases, a combination of dispersive and cohesive OVD should be used (soft-shell technique). During the capsulorhexis, you should also be aware that PEX changes the nature of the capsule, making it more brittle. In order to avoid damaging the zonula fibers in PEX when manipulating the cataract, the largest possible rhexis opening should be performed (that can still safely hold the IOL). If the rhexis is too small, postoperative anterior capsular contraction syndrome can develop which can pull on the zonula fibers. These patients are also prone to smaller pupils so intracameral epinephrine is recommended. In combined procedures, however, a slightly smaller rhexis opening may be advantageous, as the IOL is firmly seated in the capsular bag and does not luxate out of the capsular bag during the following glaucoma surgery. After valve surgery (for example Ahmed Valve), care should be taken to ensure that the anterior chamber is stable, as the intracameral part of the tube can injure the capsular bag.

During phacoemulsification in glaucoma patients, a low bottle height is preferred, to protect the retinal ganglion cells. A low bottle height is also useful in the case of an existing bleb, as an excessive outflow with a large forming bleb should be avoided. When irrigating/aspirating cortex material, it is important to ensure that the cortex material is removed thoroughly, so that an increased inflammatory reaction does not occur postoperatively. In PEX, tangential suction of the cortex material has proven to be effective in order to protect the zonula fibers (hurricane aspiration). At the end of the operation, any PEX material still present in the area of the anterior chamber angle can also be aspirated. In case of partial zonulolysis, the insertion of a capsular tension ring or a sulcus-fixed IOL may be useful and should be considered. In cataract surgery after filtrating procedures, 5-fluorouracil should be injected subconjunctivally in the area of the bleb to prevent fibrosis, and the eye should be rinsed with plenty of BSS due to the toxicity of 5-Flurouracil for the cornea [16]. If the filtration is not working properly then a needling procedure with a 27-gauge needle can be performed in the area of the bleb at the end of the operation (Video 1).

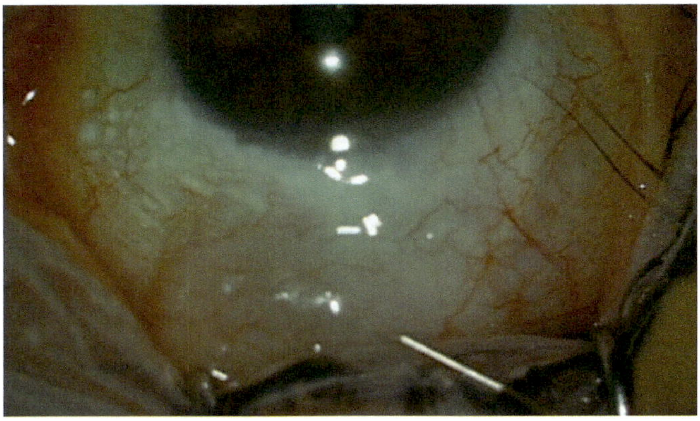

Video 1 Needling procedure with 5-fluorouracil (▶ https://doi.org/10.1007/000-8ey)

A few selected procedures for combined cataract and glaucoma surgery are described below, as all combined procedures are beyond the scope of this chapter.

iStent inject:

After cataract surgery, the pupil is constricted with acetylcholine and a cohesive OVD of high viscosity, (e.g. Healon GV or Eyefill SC), is injected into the anterior chamber (Video 2). The microscope is then tilted 35 degrees towards the surgeon and the patient's head is turned 35 degrees away from the surgeon. Using a gonioscope, (e.g. a single use gonio lens, Swan-Jacobs or Vold gonio lens), the nasal anterior chamber angle can be displayed under a 10–12 × magnification. After cataract surgery, you can often see so-called *reflux bleeding* in the trabecular meshwork, which indicates the localization for the correct implantation site (Fig. 4).

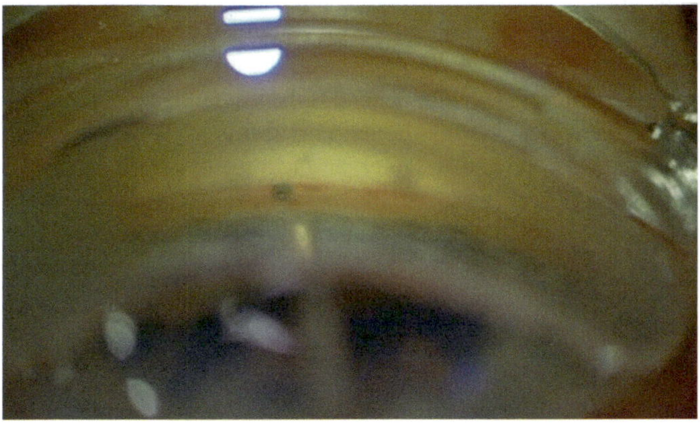

Video 2 iStent inject implantation (▶ https://doi.org/10.1007/000-8ex)

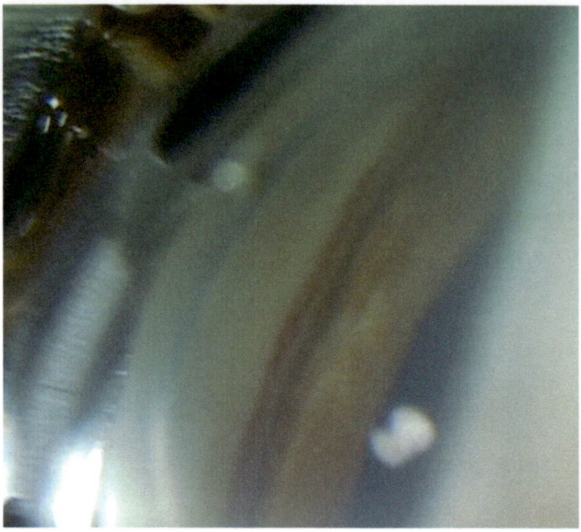

Fig. 4 Gonioscopy: reflux bleeding in Schlemm's canal intraoperatively after cataract surgery

The clear cornea incision can be used for implantation if a cataract surgery with temporal approach was performed, otherwise with superior approach the paracentesis can be enlarged to 1.5 mm at the temporal side. The injector is inserted to the middle of the anterior chamber and the protective cover of the injector is retracted. While localizing the trabecular meshwork with the gonio lens, the injector is brought to the target site and the meshwork is indented so that a "V-shape" is seen. The first implant is positioned by pressing the release button. The release button should remain pressed until the injector is removed from the implant. If a reflux of blood is seen entering the anterior chamber, the implant is positioned in the right place. The same technique is used to implant the second iStent about 60–90 degrees away. In order to achieve the best possible outflow, the prominent episcleral veins at the limbus should be inspected before implantation, as these are usually larger collector vessels, especially inferior-nasal. Should the implant luxate out of the trabecular meshwork, it can be picked up with the injector or an intraocular forceps and re-implanted. Attention should be paid if the implantation is too peripheral from the incision, as there is a risk that the guiding needle in the injector will be bent or displaced in such a way that a faulty or incomplete injection can occur. After implantation, the OVD material should be removed thoroughly, preferably with irrigation/aspiration, and the anterior chamber pressurized with BSS. It is recommended to pressurize the eye to the higher side of normal to avoid further anterior chamber bleeding and an upright position immediately after the operation is also advisable.

XEN:

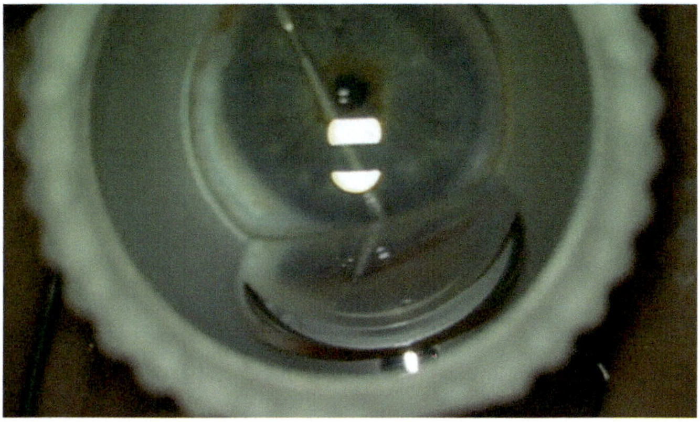

Video 3 Xen gel stent implantation (▶ https://doi.org/10.1007/000-8ew)

In XEN implantation, the pupil is constricted after cataract surgery and the anterior chamber is filled with a cohesive OVD (Video 3). An Ahmed gonio lens is used to check the implantation site, above the trabecular meshwork in the nasal superior quadrant. Position the mirror of the gonio lens on the opposite side. The conjunctiva at the implantation site in the nasal superior quadrant is marked with a marking pen, 3 mm from the limbus. Then 0.1 ml of mitomycin C (0.2 mg/ml) is injected with a 30-gauge needle in this area under the Tenon's capsule. A 1.8 mm keratome is used to create a clear corneal incision inferotemporally. A preexisting paracentesis in this area can also be widened, or the clear cornea incision of a cataract surgery (if it was temporal) can be used. The preloaded 27-gauge injector is then inserted into the anterior chamber and the XEN is implanted superonasally using a gonio lens. One millimeter of the implant should be in the anterior chamber, two millimeter in the scleral canal and three millimeter in the subconjunctival space. A modified needling procedure in the subconjunctival area of the implant tip can be carried out so that the implant is free and mobile. After removal of the OVD, 4 mg of dexamethasone is injected peribulbar.

MicroShunt:

After cataract surgery, the clear cornea incision is temporarily stitched with a single 10.0 nylon knot, and the pupil is constricted (Video 4). A corneal traction suture is applied superior with silk 6.0 and the eye is pulled down. A fornix based subconjunctival/subtenon flap is created superonasal or superotemporal over two to three clock hours and undermined. Small sponges soaked with mitomycin (0.2 mg/ml) are placed under the flap for two minutes, as peripherally as possible and thoroughly rinsed with BSS after removal. The episcleral tissue is removed with a hockey knife and any bleeding vessels are cauterized. The implantation site is

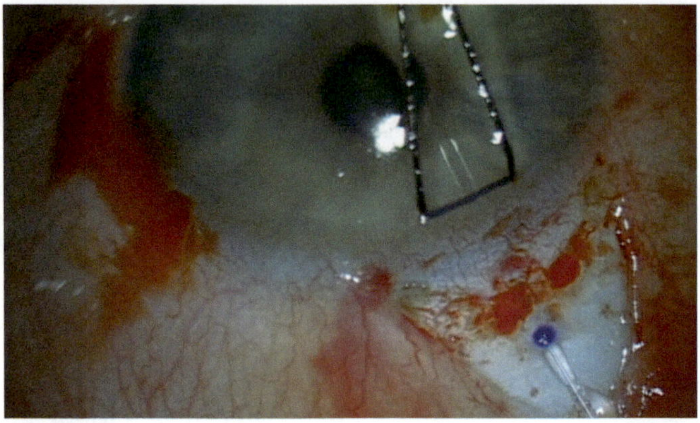

Video 4 Preserflo MicroShunt implantation (▶ https://doi.org/10.1007/000-8ez)

marked 3 mm away from the limbus. A 1 mm lance is used to create a scleral pocket at this site, in order to fixate the wings of the implant intrascleral without any sutures later. Using this pocket, a bent 25-gauge needle is used to penetrate the anterior chamber in such a way that the implant can be placed between the iris and the cornea. It is important to ensure that the beveled side of the implant points upwards. The pressure in the eye is then increased with BSS via a paracentesis, and the flow through the implant is checked. If no sufficient flow is visible, the implant can be flushed from the outside. An important step is that the tenon´s membrane and conjunctiva are placed over the implant and fixed watertight to the limbus with Vicryl 9.0 single interrupted sutures. The traction suture and the nylon suture are removed and 4 mg dexamethasone injected peribulbar.

In case of neovascularization glaucoma, an anti-vascular endothelial growth factor drug can be injected intravitreal at the end of the operation.

Postoperative notes:

The risk of intraocular pressure peaks after cataract surgery in glaucoma patients is increased and the already damaged optic nerve is particularly vulnerable to further nerve fiber loss. Increased risk is associated with long axial length, status post trabeculectomy or laser trabeculoplasty and high numbers of glaucoma medications [17]. Three to seven hours after cataract surgery almost half (46.4%) of the patients with glaucoma have an IOP increase to more than 28 mmHg [18]. Even well controlled glaucoma patients, especially those with pseudoexfoliation, have a significant increase in IOP in the first 24 h [19]. It is therefore advisable to measure the IOP in these patients on the same day and to treat if necessary. Useful drugs, which can also be given prophylactically, preferably one hour before surgery, are fast-acting topical alpha-2 agonists or oral carbonic anhydrase inhibitors [20]. The risk of postoperative IOP spikes with certain OVDs has also been reported.

In order to avoid failure of an already existing bleb after cataract surgery, it is recommended that corticosteroids should be used intensively in the beginning and to inject 5-fluorouracil subconjunctival in the first two weeks if necessary. Glaucoma patients have an increased risk for a steroid response and almost 90% of patients with POAG have an IOP increase after steroid therapy so this should be monitored carefully [21]. In most cases IOP increases after two to six weeks of steroid therapy and the increase in IOP depends on the potency of the steroids. Due to the lower penetration, hydrocortisone 0.5% has a lower IOP increase than prednisolone 1% and especially dexamethasone 0.1% [22].

Topical prostaglandin analogues pre- and postoperatively increase the risk of cystoid macular edema after cataract surgery [23]. Inflammation (flare) in the anterior chamber is also increased postoperatively in these patients [24]. However, the discontinuation of prostaglandins pre- or postoperatively is controversial due to the lack of evidence-based data. It seems reasonable to discontinue prostaglandin analogues postoperatively for four weeks in patients who have another risk factor for the development of cystoid macular edema, such as diabetic retinopathy, retinal vein occlusion or uveitis. A combination of topical steroids and non-steroidal anti-inflammatory drugs (NSAIDs) should also be considered prophylactically in these patients [25].

References

1. Pascolini D, Mariotti SP. Global estimates of visual impairment: 2010. Br J Ophthalmol. 2012;96(5):614–8.
2. Tseng VL, Yu F, Lum F, Coleman AL. Risk of fractures following cataract surgery in medicare beneficiaries. JAMA. 2012;308(5):493–501.
3. Linebarger EJ, Hardten DR, Shah GK, Lindstrom RL. Phacoemulsification and modern cataract surgery. Surv Ophthalmol. 1999;44(2):123–47.
4. Kass MA, Heuer DK, Higginbotham EJ, Johnson CA, Keltner JL, Miller JP, et al. The ocular hypertension treatment study: a randomised trial determines that topical ocular hypotensive medication delays or prevents the onset of primary open-angle glaucoma. Arch Ophthalmol. 2002;120(6):701–13; discussion 829–30.
5. Mansberger SL, Gordon MO, Jampel H, Bhorade A, Brandt JD, Wilson B, et al. Reduction in intraocular pressure after cataract extraction: the ocular hypertension treatment study. Ophthalmology. 2012;119(9):1826–31.
6. Chen PP, Lin SC, Junk AK, Radhakrishnan S, Singh K, Chen TC. The effect of phacoemulsification on intraocular pressure in glaucoma patients: a report by the American academy of ophthalmology. Ophthalmology. 2015;122(7):1294–307.
7. Guthauser U, Flammer J. Quantifying visual field damage caused by cataract. Am J Ophthalmol. 1988;106(4):480–4.
8. Hayashi K, Hayashi H, Nakao F, Hayashi F. Influence of cataract surgery on automated perimetry in patients with glaucoma. Am J Ophthalmol. 2001;132(1):41–6.
9. Xu X, Sun Q, Ma YY, Zou HD. Vision-related quality of life outcomes of cataract surgery in advanced glaucoma patients. J Glaucoma. 2016;25(1):e5-11.

10. Samuelson TW, Sarkisian SR Jr, Lubeck DM, Stiles MC, Duh YJ, Romo EA, et al. Prospective, randomized, controlled pivotal trial of an ab interno implanted trabecular micro-bypass in primary open-angle glaucoma and cataract: two-year results. Ophthalmology. 2019;126(6):811–21.
11. Reitsamer H, Sng C, Vera V, Lenzhofer M, Barton K, Stalmans I, et al. Two-year results of a multicenter study of the ab interno gelatin implant in medically uncontrolled primary open-angle glaucoma. Graefes Arch Clin Exp Ophthalmol. 2019;257(5):983–96.
12. Batlle JF, Fantes F, Riss I, Pinchuk L, Alburquerque R, Kato YP, et al. Three-year follow-up of a novel aqueous humour microshunt. J Glaucoma. 2016;25(2):e58-65.
13. Patel HY, Danesh-Meyer HV. Incidence and management of cataract after glaucoma surgery. Curr Opin Ophthalmol. 2013;24(1):15–20.
14. Rainer G, Stifter E, Luksch A, Menapace R. Comparison of the effect of Viscoat and DuoVisc on postoperative intraocular pressure after small-incision cataract surgery. J Cataract Refract Surg. 2008;34(2):253–7.
15. Rainer G, Menapace R, Findl O, Georgopoulos M, Kiss B, Petternel V. Intraocular pressure after small incision cataract surgery with Healon5 and Viscoat. J Cataract Refract Surg. 2000;26(2):271–6.
16. Sharma TK, Arora S, Corridan PG. Phacoemulsification in patients with previous trabeculectomy: role of 5-fluorouracil. Eye (Lond). 2007;21(6):780–3.
17. Slabaugh MA, Bojikian KD, Moore DB, Chen PP. Risk factors for acute postoperative intraocular pressure elevation after phacoemulsification in glaucoma patients. J Cataract Refract Surg. 2014;40(4):538–44.
18. Ahmed II, Kranemann C, Chipman M, Malam F. Revisiting early postoperative follow-up after phacoemulsification. J Cataract Refract Surg. 2002;28(1):100–8.
19. Levkovitch compound H, Habot-Wilner Z, Burla N, Melamed S, Goldenfeld M, Bar-Sela SM, et al. Intraocular pressure elevation within the first 24 hours after cataract surgery in patients with glaucoma or exfoliation syndrome. Ophthalmology. 2008;115(1):104–8.
20. Hayashi K, Yoshida M, Manabe SI, Yoshimura K. Prophylactic effect of oral acetazolamide against intraocular pressure elevation after cataract surgery in eyes with glaucoma. Ophthalmology. 2017;124(5):701–8.
21. Armaly MF. Effect of corticosteroids on intraocular pressure and fluid dynamics. II. The effect of dexamethasone in the glaucomatous eye. Arch Ophthalmol. 1963;70:492–9.
22. Jones R 3rd, Rhee DJ. Corticosteroid-induced ocular hypertension and glaucoma: a brief review and update of the literature. Curr Opin Ophthalmol. 2006;17(2):163–7.
23. Miyake K, Ibaraki N, Goto Y, Oogiya S, Ishigaki J, Ota I, et al. ESCRS Binkhorst lecture 2002: Pseudophakic preservative maculopathy. J Cataract Refract Surg. 2003;29(9):1800–10.
24. Arcieri ES, Santana A, Rocha FN, Guapo GL, Costa VP. Blood-aqueous barrier changes after the use of prostaglandin analogues in patients with pseudophakia and aphakia: a 6-month randomised trial. Arch Ophthalmol. 2005;123(2):186–92.
25. Hollo G, Aung T, Cantor LB, Aihara M. Cystoid macular edema related to cataract surgery and topical prostaglandin analogues: mechanism, diagnosis, and management. Surv Ophthalmol. 2020;65(5):496–512.

Cataract Surgery in Patients with Radiation-Induced Cataract

Raffael G. Liegl and Nikolaos E. Bechrakis

The most common entity that associated with radiation-induced cataract is choroidal melanoma, (including ciliary body and iris melanomas) which is associated with the frequency of radiotherapy used in intraocular tumours. A basic rule of thumb is that tumors located more anteriorly are associated with a higher and earlier risk of cataract development, as they are usually accompanied by a higher radiation dose to the lens. However, cataract development can also occur associated with cancers in other areas of the head, when radiation is applied to the lens. In this chapter, the special features of these cataracts and the optimal timing of treatment will be discussed, taking into account both the literature and our own experience.

Fundamentals of Radiobiology

The lens belongs to the kind of body tissues that are particularly vulnerable to radiation. The main determinants that have an impact on tissue alteration due to radiotherapy are the cumulative dose, the single dose per fraction when applying

---

Supplementary Information The online version contains supplementary material available at https://doi.org/10.1007/978-3-031-05394-8_70. The videos can be accessed individually by clicking the DOI link in the accompanying figure caption or by scanning this link with the SN More Media App.

R. G. Liegl (✉)
Bonn, Germany
e-mail: Raffael.Liegl@ukbonn.de

N. E. Bechrakis
Essen, Germany
e-mail: nikolaos.bechrakis@uk-essen.de

M. Shajari et al. (eds.), *Cataract and Lens Surgery*,
https://doi.org/10.1007/978-3-031-05394-8_70

several fractions of radiotherapy, as for example in case of proton beam radiation, the time interval between the fractions, as well as the overall time of radiotherapy.

There are differences in the time between radiation exposure and tissue reaction, with some displaying an early reaction and others manifesting with a late tissue reaction. These differences are associated with the proliferation capability. Body tissues with a high proliferation rate show an earlier reaction in comparison to those with a lower rate. The *International Commission for Radiological Protection (IRCP)* estimates that the lens belongs to the group of body tissues that shows a late tissue reaction. Thus, even small doses can affect the lens and it is assumed that 0.5 Grey are sufficient to cause an incidence of cataract development of 1% [1]. Conversely, radiation-induced cataracts occur with a distinct latency after radiotherapy.

The most common forms of radiotherapy for intraocular tumors are brachytherapy and teletherapy, mostly using proton beam therapy. Radiosurgery using gamma- or cyberknife or other options of conventional convergence irradiation can also be considered as possible treatment options. The dose of radiation that is applied to the tumor has a great variety depending on the form of radiotherapy and the profile of radiation that comes along with it. Thus, it is difficult to conduct a comparison between the dose that is applied between the different forms of radiation.

Frequency of Cataract Development After Radiotherapy of the Eye

The incidence of developing a cataract further along the course of treatment following irradiation seems to be quite comparable among the different treatment modalities. It is commonly assumed that up to 50% of patients develop a radiation-induced cataract within five years after irradiation with the need of surgical intervention depending on the treatment plan and the amount of radiation applied to the lens. The radiation can hit the posteriorly localized tumor from anterior, depending on the form of radiotherapy that is being used. Proton beam therapy can serve as an example for that, since 20% of the patients develop a cataract when only 10% of the lens is localized in the field of radiation that is applied.

Form of Cataract After Radiotherapy

Typically, radiation-induced cataracts show a posterior subcapsular cataract formation. Nevertheless, the development of cataracts can occur in any manner. Since uveal melanomas are detected at a higher age, age-related cataract forms can be found in any case. From our own experience a clear opacity of the cortex can dissemble an intumescent cataract, whereby the nucleus can still be quite soft. Thus, less energy of phacoemulsification is needed than initially assumed.

Keypoint

Radiation-induced cataracts occur commonly as a subcapsular cataract. They can give the impression of a hard lens, although, the nucleus is oftentimes rather soft. Therefore, an aggressive approach regarding effective phaco time and CDE is not necessary in many cases.

Rationales for Performing Cataract Surgery

Multiple studies have shown that surgery of radiation-induced cataracts can result in an improvement of visual acuity [2, 3]. On the other hand, older studies have reported no significant advantages with regard to improvement of sight [4]. However, the techniques of cataract surgery as well as the sources of radiation used in those days are not directly comparable with the techniques that are used nowadays [4]. Other than the improvement of visual acuity for the patient, cataract surgery also allows to better assess the tumor through a clear lens. Further, its visualization facilitates the option to perform adjuvant therapy, such as laser coagulation, transpupillary thermotherapy or even intravitreal injections of various substances with higher safety (Videos 1 and 2).

Dissemination of Tumor Cells Due to Cataract Surgery

Even though there are case reports of disseminated tumor cells after cataract and filtering glaucoma surgeries, the probability of this dissemination is very low. In the case of a malign entity, one should perform cataract surgery only when a robust statement regarding local tumor control is possible in order to minimize the hypothetical risk of dissemination however.

Timing of Cataract Surgery

Even though recurrence can occur decades later, from our own experience, in most cases tumor control can be determined within the first two years after treatment. Since radiation-induced cataract usually develops at a later stage, depending on the dose of radiation that is applied to the lens, the choice of timing for cataract surgery seems unproblematic. Rarely, the opacity of the lens can have progressed so far that the tumor cannot be assessed clinically and ultrasonography. When medical imaging via MRI may substantiate the suspicion of a recurrence, we would first plan treatment of the tumor and perform cataract surgery at a later stage.

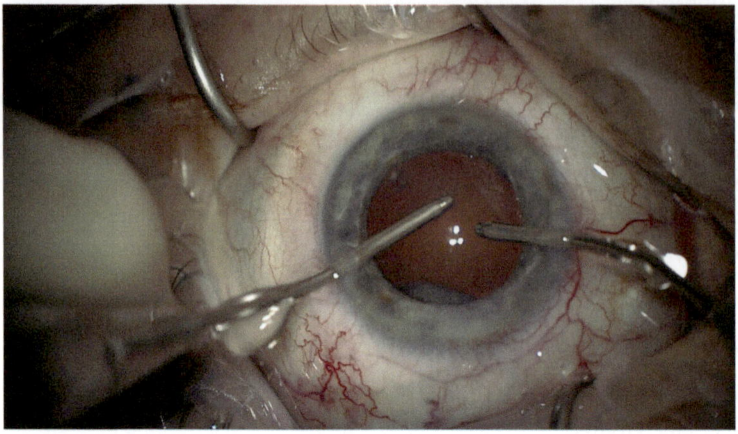

Video 1 Cataract surgery for an intraocular tumour may be accompanied by changes in the anterior segment (such as displacement of the iris, synechiae, etc.).
(▶ https://doi.org/10.1007/000-8f1)

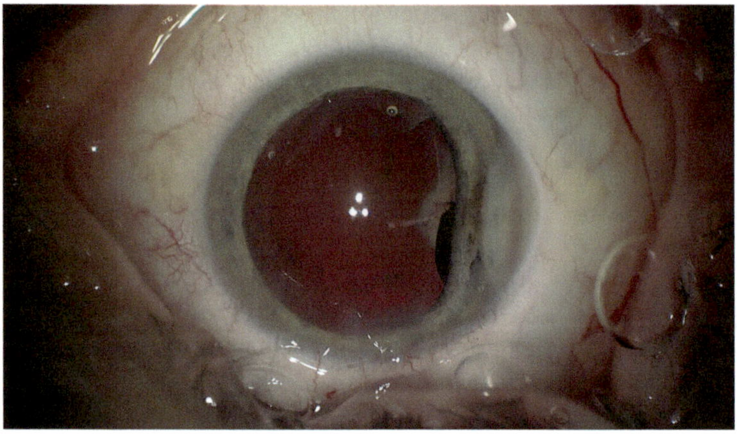

Video 2 Successful lens implantation is nevertheless possible in most eyes
(▶ https://doi.org/10.1007/000-8f0)

Author's recommendation

"Cataract surgery should only be performed at a time when a robust statement regarding the local control of the intraocular tumor that has been treated can be made. When tumor recurrence occurs, this is often appreciated within the first years after radiation. In case of benign tumors, the time point of cataract surgery should be scheduled according to the usual criteria of standard cataract surgery."

Reflection on Cataract Surgery

Cataract surgery itself is performed as a standard cataract procedure. Neither cryo-coagulation of the incision site nor any other particular precaution is necessary. It should be taken into account however that the complication rate concerning posterior capsular rupture is higher in the literature [5]. Furthermore, it has to be considered that especially tumors that are located anteriorly can weigh or push on the lens or the capsule and its apparatus. Thus, the operative approach can be challenging. In addition, for any astigmatism noted a verification of its origin should be pursued using corneal imaging technologies in order to avoid surprises when the tumor is becoming smaller. Further, the red reflex can be reduced drastically in patients that have an exudative retinal detachment.

Cataract surgery can be especially challenging in cases of entire iris/anterior segment proton beam Irradiation for diffuse iris melanomas. These patients will all eventually develop a complicated form of cataract that will usually be associated with secondary glaucoma and severe dry eye syndrome. The cataracts in these cases are usually intumescent with a swollen cortex. Special precautions have to be taken to avoid the "Argentinian flag phenomenon" during the initiation of a capsulorhexis after having injected a capsular dye in the anterior chamber for better visualization of the lens capsule.

Generally, eyes that have undergone cataract surgery after any kind of ocular irradiation have a much higher propensity for dry eye related problems.

Keypoint

In case of patients with an exceptionally high and asymmetric astigmatism that have a known or unknown intraocular tumor, it should always be ruled out that a tumor is located in the very anterior part of the eye.

Contraindications for Cataract Surgery

A permanent deterioration of sight in patients, that have received radiotherapy, is usually not caused by alterations of the lens, but due to radiation retinopathy and maculopathy or optic neuropathy. Furthermore, synechia and/or rubeosis iridis, that can present with anterior chamber hemorrhage should be anticipated. These changes do not constitute a contraindication for cataract surgery and can be handled in the same way as in patients with proliferative diabetic retinopathy. Similar to diabetic patients, postoperative inflammation can be increased and can fully deploy on the second or third day after operation. This situation can be managed well by using an intensified, local steroid therapy. From our point of view, a solitary cataract surgery without prior treatment of the uveal melanoma should be omitted, whenever possible.

References

1. ICRP ICRP Publication 127. Annals of the ICRP. Radiol Prot Ion Beam Radiother. 2014.
2. Gragoudas ES, Egan KM, Arrigg PG, Seddon JM, Glynn RJ, Munzenrider JE. Cataract extraction after proton beam irradiation for malignant melanoma of the eye. Arch Ophthalmol. 1992;110(4):475–9. https://doi.org/10.1001/archopht.1992.01080160053029.
3. Seibel I, Cordini D, Hager A, Riechardt AI, Rehak M, Böker A, et al. Cataract development in patients treated with proton beam therapy for uveal melanoma. Graefes Arch Clin Exp Ophthalmol. 2016;254(8):1625–30. https://doi.org/10.1007/s00417-016-3356-4.
4. Augsburger JJ, Shields JA. Cataract surgery following cobalt-60 plaque radiotherapy for posterior uveal malignant melanoma. Ophthalmology. 1985;92(6):815–22. https://doi.org/10.1016/s0161-6420(85)33955-6.
5. Wachtlin J, Bechrakis NE, Schueler AO, Helbig H, Bornfeld N, Foerster MH. Phacoemulsification following treatment of choroidal melanoma. Graefes Arch Clin Exp Ophthalmol. 2000;238(12):942–8. https://doi.org/10.1007/s004170000208.

Systematic Overview

Cataract Surgery in Eyes with Uveitis

Vita Dingerkus, Matthias Becker, and Stephan Thurau

Introduction

Cataract surgery in patients with uveitis is challenging with regard to both the indication and the timing of surgery. The preoperative initial situation and the prognosis of visual acuity in uveitis eyes can be complicated by the associated risks of band-keratopathy, endothelial cell loss especially in anterior uveitis, posterior synechiae, pre- or retrolental fibrosis, vitreous opacities, optic atrophies and retinal changes such as atrophies, fibrosis or macular edema.

The risk of postoperative complications is also significantly increased and includes posterior synechiae with the intraocular lens implant, the lens capsule, the anterior vitreal membrane, inflammatory deposits on the IOL (Fig. 2), retrolental fibrosis with traction on the ciliary body, hypotension, and cystoid macular edema. Thus, the postoperative prognosis for visual acuity can be highly variable and significantly reduced [1].

Depending on the uveitis entity, up to 2/3 of the eyes develop cataract [2–4] (Fig. 1). Up to 1.2% of all cataract surgeries are performed in eyes with a history of

---

Supplementary Information The online version contains supplementary material available at https://doi.org/10.1007/978-3-031-05394-8_71. The videos can be accessed individually by clicking the DOI link in the accompanying figure caption or by scanning this link with the SN More Media App.

V. Dingerkus · M. Becker
Cityhospital Zurich Triemli, Birmensdorferstr. 497, 8063 Zurich, Switzerland
e-mail: Vita.Dingerkus@triemli.zuerich.ch

M. Becker
e-mail: Matthias.Becker@triemli.zuerich.ch

S. Thurau (✉)
Munich, Germany
e-mail: Stephan.Thurau@med.uni-muenchen.de

M. Shajari et al. (eds.), *Cataract and Lens Surgery*,
https://doi.org/10.1007/978-3-031-05394-8_71

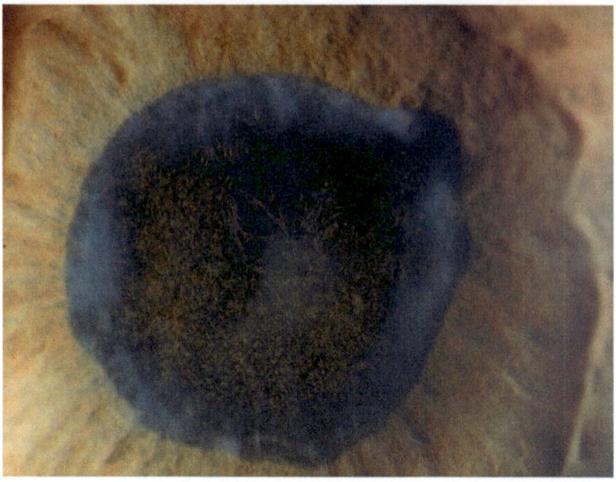

Fig. 1 Secondary cataract with circular posterior synechiae and pigment cells on the anterior surface of the lens

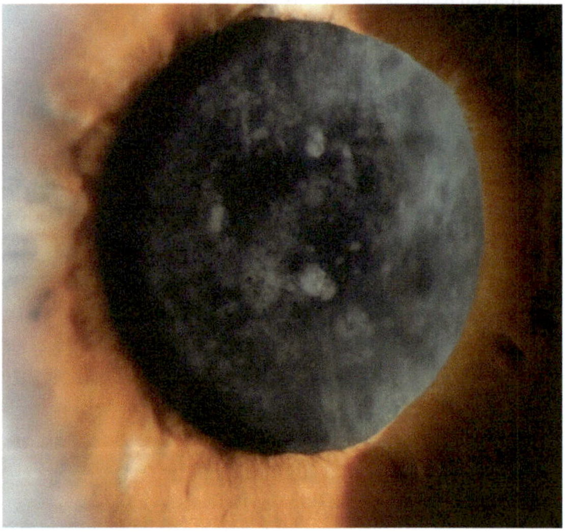

Fig. 2 IOL implant with granuloma-like inflammatory deposits on the anterior and posterior surface of the lens. Removal with the Nd:YAG laser should be avoided as it carries the risk of an increased inflammatory response. Intraocular steroids are the therapy of choice

uveitis because both intraocular inflammation and therapy with local or systemic steroids can induce cataract [5, 6].

Preoperative Goals

Control of inflammation preoperatively is particularly important. Quiescence for at least 3 months prior to surgery is recommended, though may not always be possible [7, 8]. Systemic therapies with disease modifying anti-rheumatic drugs (DMARDs) and/or topical steroids continue to be the first-line treatments to achieve this goal. In the case of autoimmune uveitis, interdisciplinary cooperation with a rheumatologist or pediatric rheumatologist is highly advised and usually required. In cases of an infectious aetiology, an appropriate antibiotic or antiviral therapy must be initiated and time provided to recover from the episode [9, 10]. Intravitreal steroid therapy with dexamethasone (0.7 mg) or fluocinolone (0.19 mg) implants can reduce intraocular inflammation quickly and safely [11, 12]. With these implants, a quiescent eye can be achieved much better than with topical therapy. However, the risk of developing steroid induced glaucoma needs to be considered as it limits the treatment with intraocular steroids. The goal is a to achieve a maximum anterior chamber cell count of 0.5 + (according to SUN assessment criteria), which corresponds to 1–5 cells in a 1 × 1 mm light beam of the slit lamp [13]. Anterior chamber flare (intensity of Tyndall's effect) is not considered here.

In general, anterior uveitis is associated with a higher incidence of postoperative flare-ups than intermediate or posterior uveitis. With respect to inflammation, cataract surgery in Fuchs uveitis has a better prognosis than in patients with juvenile idiopathic arthritis (JIA)- or HLA-B27-associated iritis [3, 14]. In contrast, posterior uveitis has a worse prognosis for visual acuity, not because of the risk of postoperative inflammation, but because of pre-existing damage to the posterior pole (macular edema, epiretinal gliosis, atrophy) that limits the maximum potential visual outcome. Preoperative control of inflammation is particularly important in children. If quiescence to the extent defined above can be achieved, the prognosis can be relatively favourable.

In children especially, a pre-lenticular membrane can simulate a dense media opacity, while the lens behind may, in fact be relatively clear. In this case, if the membrane is delicately and meticulously peeled, the lens itself may be clear and left in situ.

Surgical Procedure

In principle, a primary IOL implantation can be planned if the inflammation is well controlled. The capsulorhexis should be kept to the smaller side to reduce the risk of posterior synechiae. In cases of more severe uveitis entities such as JIA, the posterior capsule should be opened and an anterior vitrectomy with removal of the anterior vitreal membrane should be performed. While this is more complex than a standard cataract operation, the aim here is to reduce the risk of cyclic membranes with secondary lens decentration, ciliary body traction and hypotension [3, 15]. Nevertheless, Kulik et al. reported membrane formation in almost half of the eyes with posterior capsulorhexis and combined anterior vitrectomy in eyes with JIA-associated uveitis [16]. Phacoemulsification is associated with less postoperative inflammation and complications (such as synechiae, capsular fibrosis, epiretinal membranes or macular edema) than extracapsular extraction (Video 1) [17].

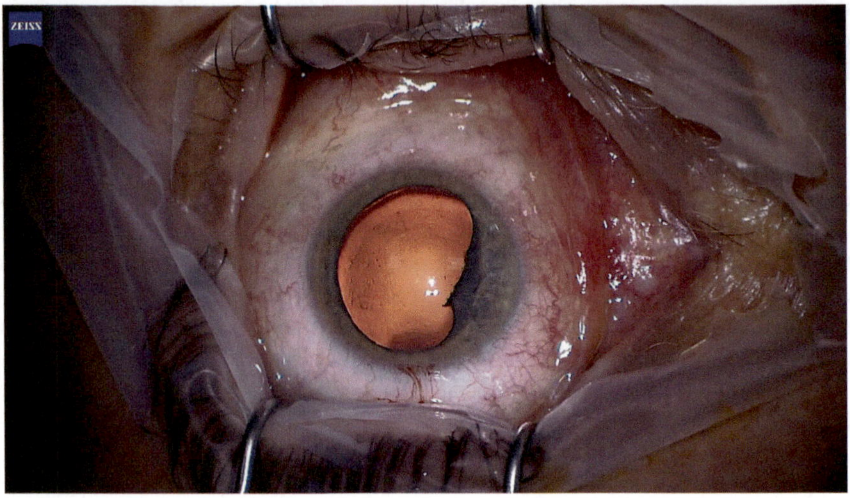

Video 1 Solution of a rear synechia (▶ https://doi.org/10.1007/000-8f2)

Type of Intraocular Lens

In general, acrylate lenses or heparin surface-modified polymethylmethacrylate (PMMA) lenses are much better tolerated (with regard to inflammation) than uncoated PMMA or silicone lenses [18–20]. It is not clear whether there are major differences in outcome between PMMA lenses and hydrophobic acrylic lenses [16]. The risk of posterior capsule opacity is also reduced in uveitis eyes by a square edge IOL [15]. Primary aphakia should be considered when the inflammatory activity in the anterior segment of the eye cannot be reduced to the required 0.5 + cells. If the eye is aphakic, an optimal contact lens fitting must be provided during follow-up, and, in children, an intensive amblyopia therapy and patching must be carried out. Under those conditions very good visual acuity can be achieved in aphakic eyes. Secondary IOL implantations are rarely performed.

Postoperative Care

The most common postoperative complication, if surgical opening of the posterior capsule has not been performed, is secondary cataract (or posterior capsular opacification), which can easily be treated with the Nd-YAG laser in a quiescent interval [21]. Macular edema is a consequence of the breakdown of the blood-eye barrier. Postoperatively, effective inflammation control with local steroidal and non-steroidal anti-inflammatory eyedrops is required, which must be adapted to the inflammatory activity [22]. In addition, oral steroids (up tp 1 mg/kg prednisolone) are often given one to two weeks preoperatively with postoperative tapering over the following weeks. Intraoperative pulse-dose steroids (e.g. 15 mg/kg methylprednisone) can also be considered. Depending on the postoperative inflammatory reaction oral prednisone can be given and tapered accordingly. Intravitreal steroid implants are an effective alternative especially in unilateral cases, if steroid-induced glaucoma is not a contraindication [23, 24]. If necessary, interferon-α2a can also be administered subcutaneously, but systemic side effects must be considered (fever-like symptoms, depression, induction of autoimmune diseases) [25].

Author's recommendation

Pre-operative control of the inflammation is an indispensable prerequisite for a high-quality long-term result. The appropriate therapy depends on whether the uveitis is infectious or autoimmune. Intravitreal steroid implants are an important addition to pre- and post-operative inflammation therapy where necessary. In anterior uveitis, implantation of an IOL is associated with an increased risk of postoperative inflammation and complications, while in posterior uveitis the prognosis of visual acuity may be reduced due to structural damage to the posterior segment of the eye. If a quiet eye cannot be achieved preoperatively, IOL implantation should be avoided. After surgery, the eye must be closely monitored for an extended time in order to adapt the therapy to the course of the inflammation.

References

1. Sharief L, Lightman S, Baltinas J, Tomkins-Netzer O. Long-term effect of cataract phacoemulsification on the inflammation control and clinical outcome in uveitis patients. Clin Exp Ophthalmol. 2018;46(9):1048–1054.
2. Hooper PL, Rao NA, Smith RE (1990) Cataract extraction in uveitis patients. Survey Ophthalmol. 1990;35(2):120–44.
3. Grajewski RS, Zurek-Imhoff B, Roesel M, Heinz C, Heiligenhaus A. Favourable outcome after cataract surgery with IOL implantation in uveitis associated with juvenile idiopathic arthritis. Acta Ophthalmol. 2012;90(7):657–62.
4. Chu CJ, Dick AD, Johnston RL, Yang YC, Denniston AK, Group UKPMES. Cataract surgery in uveitis: a multicentre database study. Br J Ophthalmol 2017;101(8):1132–1137
5. Thorne JE, Woreta FA, Dunn JP, Jabs DA. Risk of cataract development among children with juvenile idiopathic arthritis-related uveitis treated with topical corticosteroids. Ophthalmology 2010;117(7):1436–41.
6. Sijssens KM, Rothova A, Van De Vijver DA, Stilma JS, De Boer JH. Risk factors for the development of cataract requiring surgery in uveitis associated with juvenile idiopathic arthritis. Am J Ophthalmol. 2007;144(4):574–9.
7. Chan NS, Ti SE, Chee SP. Decision-making and management of uveitic cataract. Indian J Ophthalmol. 2017;65(12):1329–39.
8. Behndig A, Cochener-Lamard B, Guell J, Kodjikian L, Mencucci R, Nuijts R, et al. Surgical, antiseptic, and antibiotic practice in cataract surgery: Results from the European Observatory in 2013. J Cataract Refract Surg. 2015;41(12):2635–43.
9. Lu LM, McGhee CNJ, Sims JL, Niederer RL. High rate of recurrence of herpes zoster-related ocular disease after phacoemulsification cataract surgery. J Cataract Refract Surg. 2019;45 (6):810–5.

10. Moshirfar M, Somani AN, Motlagh MN, Ronquillo YC. Management of cataract in the setting of uveitis: a review of the current literature. Curr Opin Ophthalmol. 2020;31(1):3–9.
11. Sen HN, Abreu FM, Louis TA, Sugar EA, Altaweel MM, Elner SG, et al. Cataract surgery outcomes in uveitis: the multicenter uveitis steroid treatment trial. Ophthalmology. 2016;123 (1):183–90.
12. Jinagal J, Gupta G, Agarwal A, Aggarwal K, Akella M, Gupta V, et al. Safety and efficacy of dexamethasone implant along with phacoemulsification and intraocular lens implantation in children with juvenile idiopathic arthritis associated uveitis. Indian J Ophthalmol. 2019;67 (1):69–74.
13. Jabs DA, Nussenblatt RB, Rosenbaum, J. T. (2005). Standardization of uveitis nomenclature for reporting clinical data. Results of the First International Workshop. Am J Ophthalmol, 140 (3), 509–16.
14. Ji Y, Hu K, Li C, Li P, Kijlstra A, Eghrari AO, et al. Outcome and Prognostic Factors of Phacoemulsification Cataract Surgery in Vogt-Koyanagi-Harada Uveitis. Am J Ophthalmol. 2018;196:121–8.
15. Heiligenhaus A, Walscheid K, Pleyer U. Cataracts in Uveitis. Klin Monbl Augenheilkd. 2018;235(5):568–75.
16. Kulik U, Wiklund A, Kugelberg M, Lundvall A. Long-term results after primary intraocular lens implantation in children with juvenile idiopathic arthritis–associated uveitis. Eur J Ophthalmol. 2019;29(5):494–8.
17. Foster, R. E., Lowder, C. Y., Meisler, D. M., & Zakov, Z. N. (1992). Extracapsular cataract extraction and posterior chamber intraocular lens implantation in uveitis patients. Ophthalmology, 99(8), 1234–41 Issn: 0161–6420.
18. Chen JL, Bhat P, Lobo-Chan A-M. Perioperative Management of Uveitic Cataracts. Advances in Ophthalmology and Optometry. 2019;4:325–39.
19. Alio JL, Chipont E, BenEzra D, Fakhry MA. Comparative performance of intraocular lenses in eyes with cataract and uveitis. J Cataract Refract Surg. 2002;28(12):2096–108.
20. Abela-Formanek C, Amon M, Schauersberger J, Kruger A, Nepp J, Schild G. Results of hydrophilic acrylic, hydrophobic acrylic, and silicone intraocular lenses in uveitic eyes with cataract: comparison to a control group. J Cataract Refract Surg. 2002;28(7):1141–52.
21. Chiu H, Dang H, Cheung C, Khosla D, Arjmand P, Rabinovitch T, et al. Ten-year retrospective review of outcomes following phacoemulsification with intraocular lens implantation in patients with pre-existing uveitis. Can J Ophthalmol. 2017;52(2):175–80.
22. Cerqueira PMG, Silva F, Carricondo PC, Olivalves E, Hirata CE, Yamamoto JH. Outcomes of phacoemulsification in patients with uveitis at a tertiary center in Sao Paulo, Brazil: a review of cases from 2007 to 2012. Arq Bras Oftalmol. 2017;80(2):104–7.
23. Gupta G, Ram J, Gupta V, Singh R, Bansal R, Gupta PC, et al. Efficacy of Intravitreal Dexamethasone Implant in Patients of Uveitis Undergoing Cataract Surgery. Ocul Immunol Inflamm. 2019;27(8):1330–8.
24. Thorne JE, Sugar EA, Holbrook JT, Burke AE, Altaweel MM, Vitale AT et al (2019) Periocular Triamcinolone vs. Intravitreal Triamcinolone vs. Intravitreal Dexamethasone Implant for the Treatment of Uveitic Macular Edema: The PeriOcular vs. INTravitreal corticosteroids for uveitic macular edema (POINT) Trial. Ophthalmology, 126(2), 283–95.
25. Fardeau C, Simon A, Rodde B, Viscogliosi F, Labalette P, Looten V, et al. Interferon-alpha2a and Systemic Corticosteroid in Monotherapy in Chronic Uveitis: Results of the Randomized Controlled BIRDFERON Study. Am J Ophthalmol. 2017;177(5):182–94.

Systematic Overview of Cataract Surgery

Carolin Kolb-Wetterau and Mehdi Shajari

Visual Results

Surgical treatment of cataracts is one of the most frequently performed medical interventions. It leads to both an improved quality of life as well as a reduction in mortality [10]. The majority of interventions are carried out as standard micro-incision cataract surgery, i.e. without the use of a femtosecond laser and with implantation of a standard or "monofocal" lens. Although special lenses with complex optics offer some advantages for particular patients, monofocal posterior chamber lenses remain the most popular choice and are considered as the standard. Since most patients prefer optimal distance vision, the focus of these intraocular lenses (IOL) is usually in the distance.

Based on randomised controlled trial data, the mean corrected distance visual acuity (CDVA) is about 0.0 logMAR six months after implantation of a monofocal lens while the mean uncorrected intermediate visual acuity at a distance of 60 cm is 0.4 logMAR. This distance is particularly relevant for computer work, while the uncorrected near visual acuity is 0.65 logMAR [13]. Although the data on post-operative uncorrected distance visual acuity (UDVA) vary widely in the literature, it can be assumed that, in the absence of comorbidities and complications, a majority of patients achieve visual acuity of 0.3 logMAR or better and thus satisfactory distance vision.

While evaluating scores to assess the performance of certain tasks, it was found, unsurprisingly, that patients with monofocal lenses and target for the distance find it hard to work in the near distance without additional visual aids. Only about 5% of patients do not need visual aids for near vision tasks [13]. Other data suggest that about 17% of patients are spectacle-free after six months [3].

C. Kolb-Wetterau (✉) · M. Shajari
Goethe-Universität Frankfurt am Main, Frankfurt am Main, Germany
e-mail: carolin.kolb@kgu.de

M. Shajari et al. (eds.), *Cataract and Lens Surgery*,
https://doi.org/10.1007/978-3-031-05394-8_72

Keypoint
A standard micro-incision cataract surgery with implantation of a monofocal lens is a good option for patients who wish to have good uncorrected distance vision. In case of plano target refraction, an additional visual aid is usually required for near or computer vision.

However, visual results of randomised controlled trials are difficult to apply generally to the overall population. They are not typically representative because strict inclusion and exclusion criteria are set for participation. When looking to "real-world" results, often registry studies which include patients with comorbidities and complications provide better data as these aspects have a great influence on postoperative visual acuity [11]. The following information from large data collections refers to cataract surgery in general, without differentiating between different types of IOL.

The median postoperative UDVA is 0.2 logMAR, including only data from patients with a predicted postoperative spherical equivalent of ±0.5 dpt. Figure 1 shows the distribution of UDVA. Three quarters of patients have an UDVA of 0.3 logMAR or better after four months and about 25% of patients achieve an UDVA of at least 0.0 logMAR [7]. Even after mature cataract surgery, mean visual acuity of 0.2 logMAR or better can be obtained after three months [4].

The median of the best measured distance visual acuity improves from 0.5 logMAR preoperatively to 0.1 logMAR. Patients without additional ocular comorbidities have a postoperative median value of 0.0 logMAR. A best measured distance visual acuity of 0.3 logMAR or better is achieved by 90%. This value decreases to 80% if an ocular comorbidity is present, and that applies to about a quarter of patients, and increases to 95% in the absence of comorbidities [7].

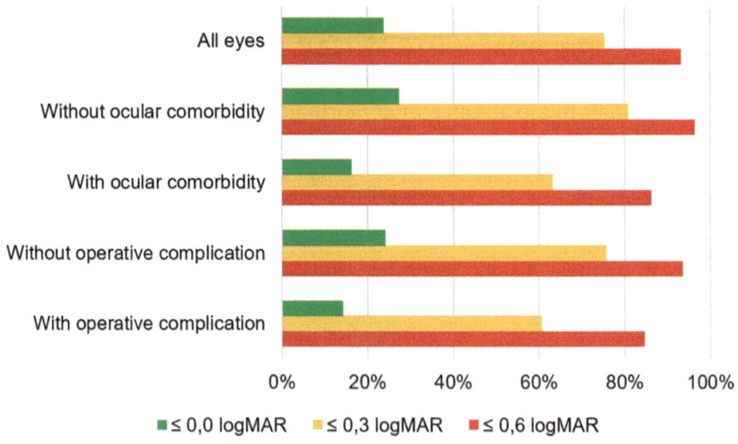

Fig. 1 Distribution of uncorrected distance visual acuity of patients with a predicted spherical equivalent of ±0.5 dpt

A CDVA of 0.0 logMAR or better is achieved after two months in more than 60% of all cases. Differentiating the results according to the presence and absence of ocular comorbidities gives values of 70% and 36% [11]. Even after mature cataract surgery, CDVA is about 0.1 logMAR after three months [4].

The most frequent comorbidities of cataract patients are age-related macular degeneration (10%), glaucoma (8%), and diabetic retinopathy (5%) [8]. The major risk factors for a poor outcome are amblyopia and macular degeneration. Nevertheless, cataract surgery can lead to a relevant improvement in visual acuity in these patients, especially if their preoperative visual acuity is poor, and should not be withheld.

In 93% of all cases, visual acuity improves as a result of the intervention but in 1.7% it worsens. Intraoperative complications increase the risk of the latter, especially dropped nucleus, vitreous loss, or capsule rupture. Furthermore, the better is the preoperative visual acuity, the higher is the risk, suggesting that "clear lens extraction" may not be worth it. Patients with ocular comorbidities but good preoperative CDVA need to be informed about the possibility of decreased postoperative visual acuity in 20–30% of cases [11].

Long-term observations illustrate the stability of treatment success. After 10 and 15 years, the median CDVA is 0.02 and 0.1 logMAR, respectively. About 87% and 81% of patients have a CDVA of 0.3 logMAR or better at the 10- and 15-year time points respectively. Compared to CDVA directly after surgery, visual acuity deteriorates by at least 0.1 logMAR in 40% of all cases after 15 years. About 10% have a worse CDVA at this point in time than before surgery. This finding can be explained by the occurrence of ocular comorbidities over time [14].

The mean absolute prediction error (PE), i.e. the difference between the achieved postoperative spherical equivalent (SE) and the predicted SE, is 0.42 dpt. Almost 75% of patients achieve a PE of $\pm$ 0.5 dpt after two months. However, there are wide variations depending on the institution where the procedure is performed. There are just as many patients more myopic than intended as hyperopic but more than 90% reach a PE within $\pm$ 1.0 dpt. In the absence of comorbidities and intraoperative complications, the mean absolute PE is 0.39 dpt. With a comorbidity, it is 0.52 dpt, with a complication 1.10 dpt, and with both this becomes 1.47 dpt. The most important comorbidities or complications for refractive errors are glaucoma and amblyopia or capsule rupture and vitreous loss. In addition, a below average preoperative CDVA and a history of previous corneal intervention may lead to a higher PE due to problems with preoperative biometry [12]. A further improvement in refractive results can be expected in the future by optimising biometric diagnostics and the lens power calculation.

Postoperative dysphotopsias are the main reason for patients' dissatisfaction after uncomplicated cataract surgery [10]. Halos or starbursts occur in about 40% of patients though less than 5% report strong optical phenomena [13]. According to one review, the rate of glares and halos is below 10% but it is not specified how much the patients are affected [3]. Overall, it can be stated that these phenomena are rarely perceived as very distracting despite being relatively often present with monofocal lenses.

Intraoperative Complications

Today, cataract surgery is one of the most frequently performed procedures as well as one of the safest. With the exception of long-term lens luxations, a steady decline in complication rates has been observed, due to the improvement and innovations in surgical techniques over the past decades.

The occurrence of intraoperative complications depends on several factors. In general, patients with ocular pathologies in addition to cataract have a higher risk and the rate of complications is about 4%. The most frequent incident is, by far, posterior lens capsule rupture (PCR) with or without vitreous loss, followed by iris trauma or prolapse and damage of the zonular fibres. Injury to the corneal epithelium or endothelium or the Descemet membrane may also occur, though this is less frequent. Figure 2 shows the most common intraoperative complications according to data by Day et al. [7].

PCR occurs in 2% of all interventions but the risk is doubled for inexperienced surgeons. In the case of a PCR, only about 75% of patients achieve a best measured distance visual acuity of 0.3 logMAR or better, and UDVA is 0.3 logMAR or better in 55% [7]. Possible consequences of a PCR are retained lens material in the anterior chamber or vitreous, cystoid macular edema (CME), vitreous prolapse, retinal detachment, endophthalmitis, or increased intraocular pressure (IOP) [10]. An axial length of less than 20 mm or greater than 26 mm significantly increases the probability of a PCR [8]. Patients with short eyes are more frequently associated with comorbidities, such as glaucoma or synechia, and an increased risk of intra-operative complications. Lens power calculation is more difficult in these eyes. Therefore, it is particularly important to provide appropriate preoperative counselling regarding these aspects. A mature cataract complicates the capsulorhexis

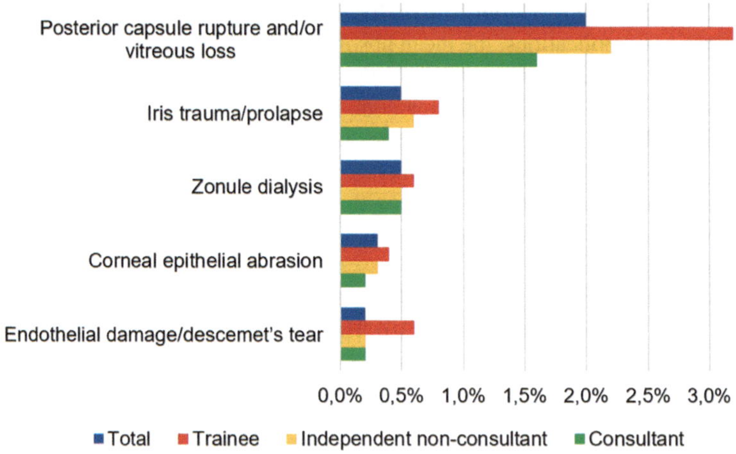

Fig. 2 Intraoperative complications depending on the surgeon's experience

and thus increases the risk of lens capsule rupture or vitreous loss. Furthermore, since more energy is required for phacoemulsification, endothelial cell loss or corneal oedema may occur more often.

Author's recommendation

In the discussion prior to a possible cataract surgery, the individual situation of the patient must be considered. Attention should be drawn to comorbidities or other factors that increase the risk of complications. In addition, the predictability of the postoperative refractive outcome must be addressed and expectations kept in line with reality.

Postoperative Complications

Early postoperative complications include transiently increased IOP (up to 18% of cases), corneal oedema, bleeding, and toxic anterior segment syndrome (which is an acute sterile inflammatory response). Corneal oedema is more common but is usually self-limiting after two to four weeks. In case of impaired corneal endothelium there is an increased risk for corneal oedema. In the worst cases, irreversible damage of the endothelium during surgery or due to prolonged inflammation or increased IOP postoperatively can lead to bullous keratopathy [10].

Endophthalmitis is a rare but very serious postoperative complication. Overall, the probability is about 0.03% within the first three months [7]. Posterior capsule rupture, possibly with vitreous loss, results in a six-fold increase in risk. Other risk factors include further intraoperative complications and a clear corneal incision [2]. A more frequent rate of endophthalmitis was found after combined procedures, such as combined glaucoma or corneal surgeries. Less than 50% of the affected patients achieve a final visual acuity of 0.3 logMAR or better. Preoperative disinfection of the skin and conjunctiva with povidone-iodine is therefore of particular importance, as is a tight closure of the corneal incision. The risk can be significantly reduced by intracameral injection of cefuroxime [10].

In addition to endophthalmitis, the following long-term complications should also be mentioned: development of posterior capsule opacification in up to 30% of patients, followed by CME, bullous keratopathy, capsular fibrosis, chronic uveitis, and retinal detachment [10].

The probability of clinically detectable CME is less than 2% within 90 days. In patients with diabetes, however, it is four times higher, especially in the presence of diabetic retinopathy. Other risk factors are epiretinal membranes, venous occlusion, previous retinal surgery, uveitis, and PCR. CME leads to a noticeable worse visual outcome [5].

Cataract surgery also significantly increases the risk for rhegmatogenous retinal detachment (RRD) compared to the overall population [16]. A posterior vitreous detachment occurs in 80% postoperatively, and its development is promoted by PCR [9]. This explains the increased risk of RRD in patients with a PCR compared to patients without this intraoperative complication [7]. Furthermore, intraoperative vitreous prolapse and loss leads to a higher probability of RRD. The total incidence of RRD after cataract surgery is 0.1–0.2% per year [16]. Hence, the risk increases with the duration of pseudophakia, except for in patients with PCR. In the latter case, one third of the detachments occur within one month [9]. Other risk factors for RRD are a long eye, young age, and ocular trauma. Only about 50% of the patients achieve visual acuity of at least 0.3 logMAR after RRD [16].

Keypoint
Since the risk for a retinal detachment after a posterior lens capsule rupture is increased especially in the first weeks, close dilated fundoscopic follow-up should be carried out in these patients. An explanation of symptoms of vitreous and retinal detachment can help to detect these complications early on.

Lens replacement or explantation is rarely necessary. The annual incidence is estimated at about 2.5/10,000. The most common causes are in the bag subluxation, out of the bag subluxation, and patient's dissatisfaction due to disturbing optical phenomena. The latter is particularly relevant for multifocal lenses and less frequently for monofocal lenses [1].

In most cases, the main reason for an in the bag dislocation is weakness and resulting rupture of the zonula fibres. Patients with a pseudoexfoliation syndrome, having an additional probability of fibrotic capsular shrinkage, are especially at risk. They account for about 1% of all surgical patients. Other causes are uveitis, trauma, or a long axis. Information on the frequency of in the bag subluxation varies in the literature and depends, among other things, on the prevalence of pseudoexfoliation syndrome. Observations over a period of 20 years show that less than 1% of all patients experience lens dislocation with required secondary surgery. The risk for subluxation increases with the duration of the pseudophakia [6]. Therefore, the number of required secondary interventions is likely to increase in the future.

Finally, another long-term postoperative complication is the decentration or tilting of the IOL. Decentration of more than 2 mm occurs in about 5% of patients within 20 years [15]. Decentration or tilt is particularly important because aspheric IOL correcting spherical aberrations are increasingly used. In these cases, the visual outcome depends crucially on the correct lens position.

References

1. Abdalla Elsayed MEA, Ahmad K, Al-Abdullah AA, et al. Incidence of intraocular lens exchange after cataract surgery. Sci Rep. 2019;9:12877. https://doi.org/10.1038/s41598-019-49030-2.
2. Cao H, Zhang L, Li L, Lo S. Risk factors for acute endophthalmitis following cataract surgery: a systematic review and meta-analysis. PLoS ONE. 2013;8: e71731. https://doi.org/10.1371/journal.pone.0071731.
3. Cao K, Friedman DS, Jin S, et al. Multifocal versus monofocal intraocular lenses for age-related cataract patients: a system review and meta-analysis based on randomized

controlled trials. Surv Ophthalmol. 2019;64:647–58. https://doi.org/10.1016/j.survophthal.2019.02.012.
4. Chen X, Yu Y, Song X, et al. Clinical outcomes of femtosecond laser-assisted cataract surgery versus conventional phacoemulsification surgery for hard nuclear cataracts. J Cataract Refract Surg. 2017;43:486–91. https://doi.org/10.1016/j.jcrs.2017.01.010.
5. Chu CJ, Johnston RL, Buscombe C, et al. Risk factors and incidence of macular edema after cataract surgery: a database study of 81984 eyes. Ophthalmology. 2016;123:316–23. https://doi.org/10.1016/j.ophtha.2015.10.001.
6. Dabrowska-Kloda K, Kloda T, Boudiaf S, et al. Incidence and risk factors of late in-the-bag intraocular lens dislocation: evaluation of 140 eyes between 1992 and 2012. J Cataract Refract Surg. 2015;41:1376–82. https://doi.org/10.1016/j.jcrs.2014.10.040.
7. Day AC, Donachie PHJ, Sparrow JM, et al. The royal college of ophthalmologists' national ophthalmology database study of cataract surgery: report 1, visual outcomes and complications. Eye (Lond). 2015a;29:552–60. https://doi.org/10.1038/eye.2015.3.
8. Day AC, Donachie PHJ, Sparrow JM, et al. The royal college of ophthalmologists' national ophthalmology database study of cataract surgery: report 2, relationships of axial length with ocular copathology, preoperative visual acuity, and posterior capsule rupture. Eye (Lond). 2015b;29:1528–37. https://doi.org/10.1038/eye.2015.198.
9. Day AC, Donachie PHJ, Sparrow JM, et al. United Kingdom national ophthalmology database study of cataract surgery: report 3: pseudophakic retinal detachment. Ophthalmology. 2016;123:1711–5. https://doi.org/10.1016/j.ophtha.2016.04.002.
10. Liu Y-C, Wilkins M, Kim T, et al. Cataracts. Lancet. 2017;390:600–12. https://doi.org/10.1016/S0140-6736(17)30544-5.
11. Lundström M, Barry P, Henry Y, et al. Visual outcome of cataract surgery; study from the European registry of quality outcomes for cataract and refractive surgery. J Cataract Refract Surg. 2013;39:673–9. https://doi.org/10.1016/j.jcrs.2012.11.026.
12. Lundström M, Dickman M, Henry Y, et al. Risk factors for refractive error after cataract surgery: Analysis of 282 811 cataract extractions reported to the European Registry of Quality Outcomes for cataract and refractive surgery. J Cataract Refract Surg. 2018;44:447–52. https://doi.org/10.1016/j.jcrs.2018.01.031.
13. Maxwell A, Holland E, Cibik L, et al. Clinical and patient-reported outcomes of bilateral implantation of a +2.5 diopter multifocal intraocular lens. J Cataract Refract Surg. 2017;43:29–41. https://doi.org/10.1016/j.jcrs.2016.10.026.
14. Mönestam E. Long-term outcomes of cataract surgery: 15-year results of a prospective study. J Cataract Refract Surg. 2016;42:19–26. https://doi.org/10.1016/j.jcrs.2015.07.040.
15. Mönestam E. Frequency of intraocular lens dislocation and pseudophacodonesis, 20 years after cataract surgery - a prospective study. Am J Ophthalmol. 2019;198:215–22. https://doi.org/10.1016/j.ajo.2018.10.020.
16. Qureshi MH, Steel DHW. Retinal detachment following cataract phacoemulsification-a review of the literature. Eye (Lond). 2020;34:616–31. https://doi.org/10.1038/s41433-019-0575-z.

Aspheric Intraocular Lenses

Zaid Shalchi and Mayank A. Nanavaty

Introduction

All optical systems have aberrations that can affect the image reaching the retina and hence the quality of vision patients obtain after cataract surgery. Although myopia, hyperopia and astigmatism account for the majority of image quality, higher order aberrations (HOAs) account for some 10% of the remainder and include spherical aberration (SA), coma and trefoil. Aspheric intraocular lenses (IOLs) are designed to reduce spherical aberration in the eye.

Spherical aberration occurs when light rays are refracted differently at different points on a lens or optical system. This spherical aberration can be positive or negative (Figs. 1 and 2). This occurs in the eye, where the average spherical aberration of the anterior corneal surface is positive (approximately + 0.27 μm), and typically remains stable throughout life. The young crystalline lens compensates for this positive sphericity, inducing a negative spherical aberration of –0.20 μm. However, as the lens ages, its spherical aberration shifts from negative to positive [1]. This positive spherical aberration adds to the positive spherical aberration of the cornea, potentially impairing visual quality.

Implanting a spherical IOL during cataract surgery means the positive spherical aberration of the cornea remains uncorrected. Furthermore, the spherical IOL will add further spherical aberration, leading to poor focus of an image onto the retina. This is particularly problematic in mesopic (reduced light) conditions when the pupil is large.

Z. Shalchi (✉)
Prince Charles Eye Unit, King Edward VII Hospital, Royal Berkshire NHS Foundation Trust, St Leonard's Road, Windsor SL4 3DP, UK
e-mail: zshalchi@gmail.com

M. A. Nanavaty
Sussex Eye Hospital, University Hospitals Sussex NHS Foundation Trust, Eastern Road, Brighton BN2 5BF, England
e-mail: mayank.nanavaty@nhs.net

M. Shajari et al. (eds.), *Cataract and Lens Surgery*,
https://doi.org/10.1007/978-3-031-05394-8_73

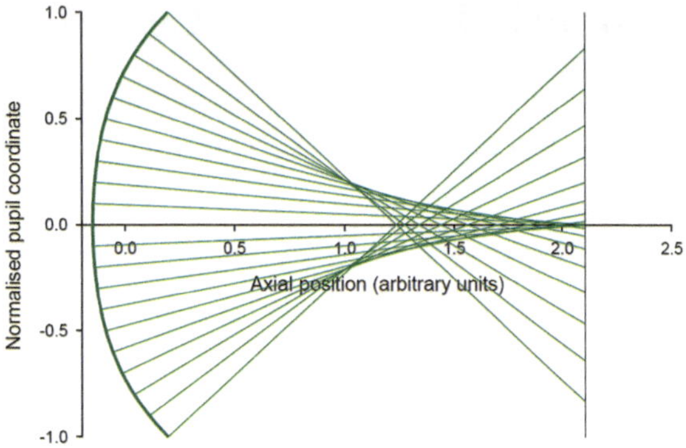

Fig. 1 Positive spherical aberration. Light rays refracted by the periphery of the lens converge greater than those passing through more centrally. (Reproduced from Nanavaty (2019). Aspheric intraocular lens in cataract surgery. https://openaccess.city.ac.uk/id/eprint/23663/)

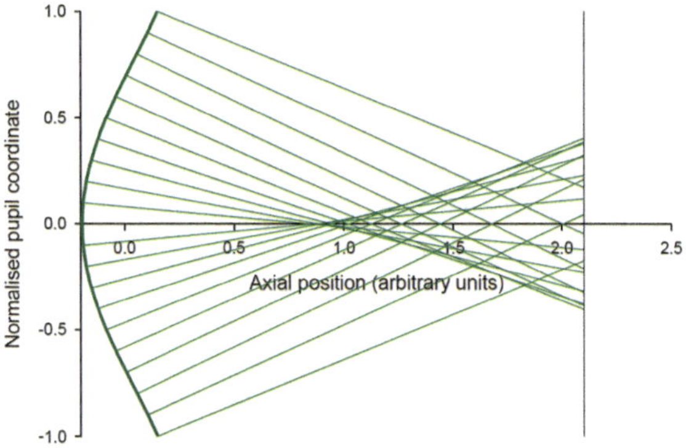

Fig. 2 Negative spherical aberration. Light rays refracted by the periphery of the lens converge less than those passing through more centrally. (Reproduced from Nanavaty (2019). Aspheric intraocular lens in cataract surgery. https://openaccess.city.ac.uk/id/eprint/23663/)

Aspheric IOL Design

Intraocular lenses can be classified as spherical, spherically neutral or aspheric. Spherical IOLs have positive spherical aberration and, therefore, add to the positive corneal spherical aberration. Spherically neutral IOLs are designed to have zero spherical aberration. Aspheric IOLs have negative spherical aberration designed to partially or fully compensate for the positive spherical aberration of the cornea. The Table 1 gives the asphericity of some commonly used IOLs.

Efficacy of Aspheric IOLs

Many investigators have performed randomised controlled trials (RCTs) comparing spherical and aspheric IOLs in cataract surgery. Schuster and colleagues performed a comprehensive Cochrane-style meta-analysis to compare the two IOL designs [2, 3]. This encompassed 43 studies and a total of 4,110 eyes.

Table 1 Asphericity of common intraocular lenses with mean residual ocular spherical aberration based on corneal spherical aberration of +0.27 μm

Intraocular lens	IOL asphericity (μm)	Residual spherical aberration (μm)
Acrysof MA60 (Alcon Laboratories, USA)	+0.20 (spherical)	+0.47
Sofport AO (Bausch & Lomb, USA)	0 (spherically neutral)	+0.27
Akreos (Bausch & Lomb, USA)	0 (spherically neutral)	+0.27
Softec HD (Lenstec, USA)	0 (spherically neutral)	+0.27
enVista (Bausch & Lomb, USA)	0 (spherically neutral)	+0.27
EyeCee One (Bausch & Lomb, USA)	−0.13 (negatively aspheric)	+0.14
Acrysof IQ (Alcon Laboratories, USA)	−0.20 (negatively aspheric)	+0.07
Tecnis 1 (Johnson & Johnson, USA)	−0.27 (negatively aspheric)	0.00

Best-corrected visual acuity (BCVA): This was reported in 38 studies (1,890 eyes with an aspheric IOL and 1,910 eyes with a spherical IOL). The mean difference in post-operative BCVA was −0.01 logMAR favouring aspheric IOLs, but the 95% confidence interval (−0.02 to 0.00) included zero, it was judged that aspheric IOLs do not improve BCVA.

Contrast sensitivity is an important indicator of the quality of vision and is quantified across various spatial frequencies (measured in cycles per degree). The meta-analysis considered contrast sensitivity in photopic and mesopic conditions. Twenty-nine studies reported contrast sensitivity in photopic conditions, typically at spatial frequencies of 1.5, 3, 6, 12 and 18 cycles per degree. This revealed no difference between eyes implanted with spherical and aspheric IOLs. Nevertheless, 25 studies reported contrast sensitivities under mesopic conditions across the 5 spatial frequencies listed above. For all spatial frequencies, contrast sensitivity was significantly better in eyes implanted with aspheric than spherical IOLs, with the highest effect observed at the 18 cpd spatial frequency. This effect is understandable, given pupils dilate under mesopic conditions thus increasing spherical aberration.

Patient-reported quality of vision was tested in 6 RCTs and based on the National Eye Institute VFQ-25 questionnaire, Visual Function Index (VF-14) or Activities of Daily Vision Scale (ADVS). This failed to show a significant difference between the two IOL groups but may be related to a ceiling effect as the questionnaires are designed to assess quality of life in patients with ocular disease. Nevertheless, 1 study utilising VF-14 showed a statistically significant benefit in favour of the aspheric IOL group [4], whilst another study using the ADVS also showed a benefit in favour of the aspheric IOL group [5].

Wavefront aberrometry was used in 32 studies to investigate residual spherical aberration in both IOL groups. Eyes receiving aspheric IOLs had significantly lower spherical aberration than those receiving spherical IOLs at 4, 5 and 6 mm pupil sizes. Aspheric lenses, however, had no effect on residual coma (14 studies) or trefoil (9 studies) in comparison to spherical IOLs [3].

Drawbacks of Aspheric IOLs

Due to their design, aspheric IOLs are less tolerant of tilt and decentration than spherical IOLs. For example, tolerance levels for the Tecnis aspheric lens require that it be decentred less than 0.4 mm and tilted less than 7 degrees in order to provide optical performance superior to that of a spherical lens [6]. Later studies have shown that the above values applied to monochromatic light only. In a real-world situation where polychromatic light is present, the above values nearly double, with about 0.8 mm of decentration and more than 10 degrees of tilt being tolerated [7]. A number of published studies over the past decade or more have shown that with a continuous curvilinear capsulorhexis and in-the-bag IOL implantation, modern cataract surgery results in average tilt and decentration that is typically well within such tolerance limits [8–10].

Benefits of Spherical Aberration

Some studies suggest that it is not necessary to correct spherical aberration completely, and in fact it is recommended to leave a slightly positive residual (+0.10 μm). A study performed on pilots of the American Air Force suggests that positive spherical aberration can be correlated with visual acuities of 20/15 or better [11].

Some investigators [12–14] have argued that an advantage of positive spherical aberration in the ageing eye is an increased depth-of-focus. Improving distance vision by correcting spherical aberration with an aspheric IOL might worsen near and intermediate vision. In fact, modern aspheric extended depth-of-focus (EDOF) IOLs make use of targeted spherical aberration to improve patient intermediate unaided acuity without compromising distance unaided vision. IOLs such as Eyhance, LuxSmart, MiniWell, and Vivity have some kind of central refractive zones which induce more spherical aberration, without the glare and halos associated with diffractive IOLs. A study comparing the Eyhance (comprising a central zone of positive spherical aberration) with the spherically neutral RayOne found improved intermediate acuity of 1.0 line with a broader defocus curve from −0.5D to −3.0D (Fig. 3) (data submitted for publication).

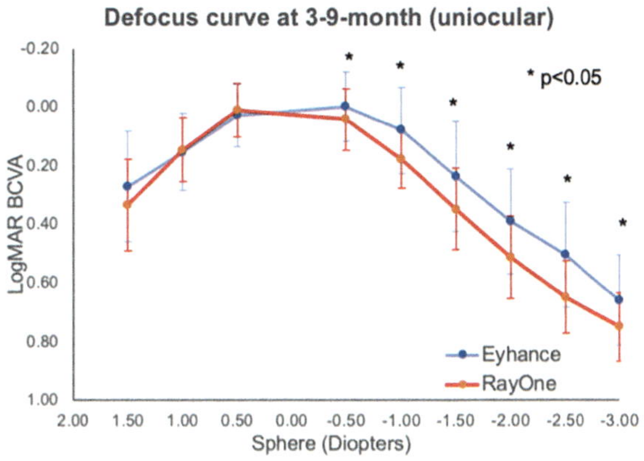

Fig. 3 Uniocular defocus curve comparing the Eyhance IOL with positive spherical aberration and RayOne spherically neutral IOL. The broader Eyhance curve shows patients enjoy better intermediate vision between −0.5 and −3.0D

Selecting the Correct IOL for the Patient

Several authors have proposed IOL selection according to the degree of corneal spherical aberration [15–17]. Ocular spherical aberrations can be corrected in a manner that is tailored to each individual. Yamaguchi and colleagues found that if a patient's pupil under mesopic conditions is smaller than 3.0 mm, an aspheric IOL will not reduce ocular spherical aberration. In eyes with a larger pupil under mesopic conditions, the IOL's impact on spherical aberration will increase [18]. This observation highlights the importance of pupil size in the selection of a particular IOL for an individual.

A patient who drives a lot at night may benefit from an aspheric IOL, which improves mesopic contrast sensitivity. A person who is an occupational reader or a computer worker may receive more benefit from a conventional spherical IOL. This highlights the importance of good history-taking for clinical decision-making.

Summary

Aspheric IOLs correct corneal spherical aberration, ensuring better focus of images on to the retina. They have been shown to improve mesopic contrast sensitivity. Modern aspheric extended depth-of-focus IOLs make use of targeted spherical aberration to improve patient intermediate unaided acuity without compromising distance unaided vision.

References

1. Glasser A, Campbell MC. Presbyopia and the optical changes in the human crystalline lens with age. Vision Res. 1998;38(2):209–29.
2. Schuster AK, Tesarz J, Vossmerbaeumer U. The impact on vision of aspheric to spherical monofocal intraocular lenses in cataract surgery: a systematic review with meta-analysis. Ophthalmology. 2013;120(11):2166–75.
3. Schuster AK, Tesarz J, Vossmerbaeumer U. Ocular wavefront analysis of aspheric compared with spherical monofocal intraocular lenses in cataract surgery: systematic review with metaanalysis. J Cataract Refract Surg. 2015;41(5):1088–97.
4. Luo M, Ji J, Zhao C, Fan X. Clinical study of Acrysof IQ aspheric intraocular lenses. Clin Exp Ophthalmol. 2010;38(4):358–62.
5. Denoyer A, Halfon J, Majzoub S, Pisella PJ. Visual function after cataract surgery in patients with an aspherical lens without spherical aberration. J Fr Ophtalmol. 2007;30(6):578–84.
6. Holladay JT, Piers PA, Koranyi G, van der Mooren M, Norrby NE. A new intraocular lens design to reduce spherical aberration of pseudophakic eyes. J Refract Surg. 2002;18(6):683–91.
7. Piers PA, Weeber HA, Artal P, Norrby S. Theoretical comparison of aberration-correcting customized and aspheric intraocular lenses. J Refract Surg. 2007;23(4):374–84.
8. Akkin C, Ozler SA, Mentes J. Tilt and decentration of bag-fixated intraocular lenses: a comparative study between capsulorhexis and envelope techniques. Doc Ophthalmol. 1994;87(3):199–209.
9. Hayashi K, Harada M, Hayashi H, Nakao F, Hayashi F. Decentration and tilt of polymethyl methacrylate, silicone, and acrylic soft intraocular lenses. Ophthalmology. 1997;104(5):793–8.
10. Mutlu FM, Bilge AH, Altinsoy HI, Yumusak E. The role of capsulotomy and intraocular lens type on tilt and decentration of polymethylmethacrylate and foldable acrylic lenses. Ophthalmologica. 1998;212(6):359–63.
11. Grimson JM, Schallhorn SC, Kaupp SE. Contrast sensitivity: establishing normative data for use in screening prospective naval pilots. Aviat Space Environ Med. 2002;73(1):28–35.
12. Nanavaty MA, Spalton DJ, Boyce J, Saha S, Marshall J. Wavefront aberrations, depth of focus, and contrast sensitivity with aspheric and spherical intraocular lenses: fellow-eye study. J Cataract Refract Surg. 2009;35(4):663–71.
13. Nishi T, Nawa Y, Ueda T, Masuda K, Taketani F, Hara Y. Effect of total higher-order aberrations on accommodation in pseudophakic eyes. J Cataract Refract Surg. 2006;32(10):1643–9.
14. Koch DD, Wang L. Custom optimization of intraocular lens asphericity. Trans Am Ophthalmol Soc. 2007;105:36–41; discussion 2
15. Packer M, Fine IH, Hoffman RS. Aspheric intraocular lens selection based on corneal wavefront. J Refract Surg. 2009;25(1):12–20.
16. Packer M, Fine IH, Hoffman RS. Aspheric intraocular lens selection: the evolution of refractive cataract surgery. Curr Opin Ophthalmol. 2008;19(1):1–4.
17. Solomon JD. Outcomes of corneal spherical aberration-guided cataract surgery measured by the OPD-scan. J Refract Surg. 2010;26(11):863–9.
18. Yamaguchi T, Negishi K, Ono T, Torii H, Dogru M, Yamaguchi K, et al. Feasibility of spherical aberration correction with aspheric intraocular lenses in cataract surgery based on individual pupil diameter. J Cataract Refract Surg. 2009;35(10):1725–33.

Systematic Overview of Toric Intraocular Lenses

Stefan Palkovits

Introduction

Toric intraocular lenses (IOL) are used to correct the cylindrical component of the refractive error. These IOLs, which are widely used today, are implanted into the capsular bag during cataract surgery . In addition to these lenses designed for the capsular bag, phakic toric IOLs are available, which can be used in refractive surgery. In both cases, the exact spherical and cylindrical power of the toric IOL, as well as the target axis must be accurately determined by the biometric data collected preoperatively. Nowadays, the accuracy of the biometry is an important cornerstone of lens surgery, as patients' expectations after surgery have increased enormously with the success of intraocular lens implantation in recent decades. About 47% of all patients undergoing cataract surgery have an astigmatism higher than 1D [3, 37] and about 20% of patients have an astigmatism higher than 1.5D [7, 12, 18, 23, 37, 39]. It has been shown, that, in the presence of astigmatism between 1 and 1.5D, reading ability is impaired as well as the ability to steer a vehicle at night [61, 62]. Therefore, this group of patients requires not only spherical correction but also correction of astigmatism in order to achieve a satisfactory, spectacle-free results after cataract surgery. In the case of implantation of multifocal IOL (mIOL), lower astigmatism values should also be corrected, since the function of the mIOL decreases drastically even with low residual astigmatism values [16].

In general, there are different methods available to reduce corneal astigmatism during cataract surgery [34]. These include reducing astigmatism by choosing the location of the main incision [2, 17, 45], laser surgery (such as LASIK or PRK), corneal incisions or limbal relaxing incisions [47] or toric IOLs. The latter are currently considered to be the most effective for correcting regular astigmatism

S. Palkovits (✉)
Department of Ophthalmology, Hanusch Hospital, Vienna, Austria
e-mail: office@palkovits.at

M. Shajari et al. (eds.), *Cataract and Lens Surgery*,
https://doi.org/10.1007/978-3-031-05394-8_74

during cataract surgery [21, 48]. Incisions and manual procedures, such as limbal and corneal incisions are more difficult to plan and may reduce corneal stability. Furthermore, the effect varies between patients and there may also be a prone to regression with time. Femtosecond lasers have been used to perform keratotomies for astigmatism correction [49] and the accuracy of astigmatism correction is higher, compared to manual, limbal relaxing incisions [46].

In the case of laser surgical procedures (such as LASIK or PRK), a second procedure—the treatment of the cornea is necessary in addition to cataract surgery. For the patient, this means a higher burden by two sperate operations.

Toric IOLs-Intracapsular

Schimizu et al. published the first case series with 47 patients who received a toric IOL during cataract surgery back in 1994 [53]. Unfortunately, the three-piece toric PMMA lens used rotated postoperatively more than 10° in 50% of cases and more than 30° in 20%. Nevertheless, these first results were very promising and since then there has been a rapid development in this field. In a meta-analysis published in 2016, Kessel et al. investigated the advantages, disadvantages and effectiveness of implanting a toric lens during cataract surgery in patients with regular astigmatism. In that study, 13 randomized controlled trials with a total of 707 eyes (toric IOL) and 706 eyes (monofocal IOL) were included. Uncorrected postoperative visual acuity was significantly higher in the group receiving a toric IOL (2–5 letters). The benefit of implanting a toric IOL was even more clearly seen in the proportion of patients with visual acuity of 0.1 logMAR or worse. This proportion was 35.2% in the group with a toric IOL while it was 60.4% in the group without a toric IOL. The dependence on glasses also differed significantly (toric IOL: 29.7%; spherical IOL: 53.2%). On the other hand, no significant difference in the rates of complications or side effects were found postoperatively. Thus, the superiority of toric lenses over non-toric lenses could be demonstrated in patients with regular corneal astigmatism [22].

Visser et al. summarized the results of 33 prospective controlled trials in 2014 and nearly all patients achieved uncorrected visual acuity of 0.5 (20/40) or better after implantation of a toric IOL. In 20–80% of cases, uncorrected visual acuity of 0.8 (20/25) was achieved. Independence of distance vision correction after bilateral implantation of a toric IOL (different models) was achieved in 70 to 100% of the eyes in the analyzed studies [58]. The review by Agresta et al. summarizes the data of uncorrected distant visual acuity (UDVA) and glasses independence from a total of 11 studies of patients, who underwent cataract surgery using toric IOLs [1]. These data show a significant increase in UDVA and a reduction in spectacle dependence postoperatively. However, the comparison with a monofocal control group is missing in this analysis.

In a Cochrane review, the effectiveness of toric lenses was compared with that of limbal relaxing incisions (LRI). 10 relevant studies were included in this review

[25]. The results showed a difference of 0.04 logMAR (2 letters on the logMAR chart) in favor of the toric IOL. The authors concluded that both methods contribute to reducing astigmatism, but with slightly better results using the toric IOL. On the other hand, the costs of treatment with toric lenses are much higher compared to LRI. The decision on which treatment method to use must therefore be made on an individual basis. It was pointed out that further studies are necessary for the long-term observation of LRI. Toric IOLs also showed a better efficacy compared to opposite clear corneal incisions in the correction of astigmatism [31].

A meta-analysis has recently compared the effect of toric lenses with that of incisional procedures (limbal relaxing incisions, corneal incisions and keratotomies). A total of 12 randomized controlled trials were included in the analysis and the results indicate the superiority of toric IOLs compared to other procedures [54].

Nagpal et al. compared the effectiveness of toric IOLs with that of implantation of a monofocal IOL followed by photorefractive keratectomy (PRK) [35]. The residual astigmatism in the group with toric IOL was higher than in the group with monofocal IOL + PRK (−0.5D vs. 0D). On the other hand, postoperative pain, higher order aberrations and glare phenomena were more frequent in the monofocal IOL + PRK group. A further disadvantage of the IOL + PRK method is the need for two separate interventions.

In general, implantation of a toric IOL is only recommended in the presence of regular astigmatism. However, in special cases of astigmatism, such as previous corneal surgery [27, 51, 60], keratoconus [20], or other corneal ectasias and degenerations [4, 19], good results with toric lenses were shown. However, the use of toric lenses in these special cases must be decided individually.

Positioning of the Toric IOL

A major cause for unsatisfactory postoperative findings after cataract surgery with toric lenses is the incorrect alignment of the toric IOL or its postoperative rotation [21]. The final axial position is mainly influenced by two factors: the intraoperative alignment of the IOL and the postoperative rotation.

A deviation of one degree of the final from the planned axis leads to a reduction of about 3% of the IOL's corrective power. A deviation of 10° reduces corrective power by approximately one third and if the deviation exceeds 45° the effect is completely lost, and the residual astigmatism may even be increased [29, 36, 44, 57].

Marking of the Target Axis

Nowadays, different methods are used for preoperative marking of the axis position [21]. A distinction should be made between manual and automated, computer-assisted methods [21, 63]. Numerous studies describe more accurate positioning of the toric IOL using automated methods but there are also contradictory data. In a meta-analysis by Zhou et al. the superiority of automated methods could be shown [63]. Five studies with a total of 257 eyes were used for this analysis and the results showed a lower axis deviation, lower postoperative astigmatism and smaller deviation of the resulting vector. However, no significant difference in postoperative uncorrected visual acuity was found.

Manual Marking Techniques

Manual marking of the axis position is usually performed in three steps: [59] (1) preoperative marking of the reference axis (0 and 180° or 90° and 270°), (2) intraoperative marking of the target axis using an angle measurement device based on the reference marking and (3) alignment of the axis of the toric IOL based on the target axis. Pre-operative marking in the upright position is necessary because a change of position from the upright to the lying position can cause cyclotorsion of the eye and twisting of the axis. The mean absolute cyclotorsion due

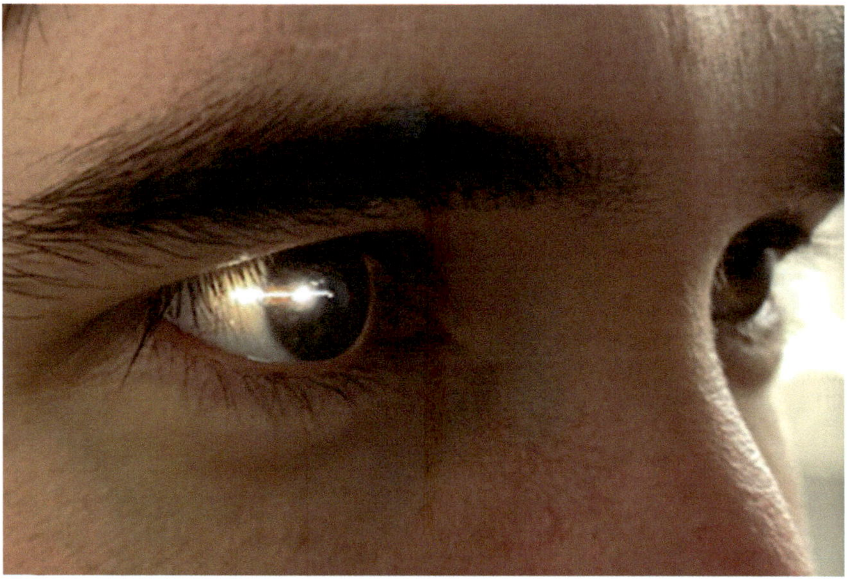

Fig. 1 Horizontal marking with the slit lamp

to a change of position is usually about 4° [56]. In some patients however, cyclotorsion can be much higher (up to 12°). In these cases, an exact alignment is not possible without a reference mark in the upright position.

Preoperative marking of the reference axis can be performed with different methods: Freehand marking, horizontal marking using the slit lamp, pendulum markers or the Nuijts/Lane bubble marker (Figs. 1 and 2, horizontal marking with the slit lamp).

In addition to the above-mentioned marking methods, it is also possible to mark the target axis directly. The Gueder tonometer marker, Neuhann one-step toric bubble marker or the Gueder-Geren pendulum marking system are available for this purpose.

Both the Nuijts/Lane bubble marker and the pendulum marker show very good results with a postoperative deviation of about 3° in both groups [9]. The highest accuracy was shown using the pendulum marker (Mean absolute error, MAE, 1.8° ± 2.2), followed by the slit lamp marker (MAE 2.3° ± 1.8), the Nuijts/Lane bubble marker (MAE 2.9° ± 1.9) and the tonometer marker (MAE 4.7° ± 2.9) [41].

The total deviation of the 3-step manual marking technique is about 5° [59]. These systems therefore represent a cost-efficient and accurate way of axis marking.

Applications developed for mobile phones represent a further marking aid to improve the results. First, two markings are applied to the cornea 180° from each other. Using the mobile phone, the cornea and the markings are photographed and

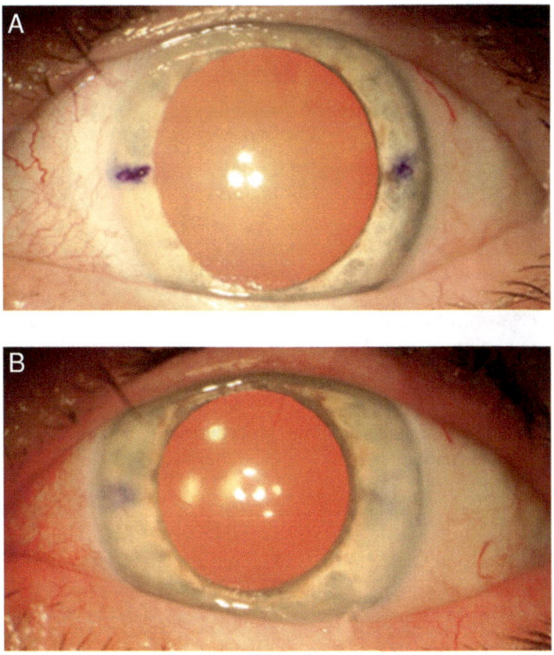

Fig. 2 **A** Preoperative marking of the reference axis at 0°; **B** Immediately postoperative toric IOL in position aligned with the target axis

the software measures the axis of the reference mark. The intraoperative steps are then performed as described above. A recent study could show that manual marking procedures can be improved with these apps [24].

Digital-Assisted Marking Techniques

Digital-assisted marking systems are based on a reference image of the anterior segment of the eye. Prominent reference points such as the iris configuration or limbal blood vessels are used for alignment and measurement. The target axis is then superimposed on the surgical microscope view using the reference image. This enables the surgeon to precisely align the toric IOL without the need for an additional marking instrument. (Fig. 3).

Different systems are available for electronic marking. The most widely used are CALLISTO Eye and Z align (Carl Zeiss Meditec AG), VERION image-guided system (Alcon) and TrueVision 3D Surgical System (Leica Microsystems).

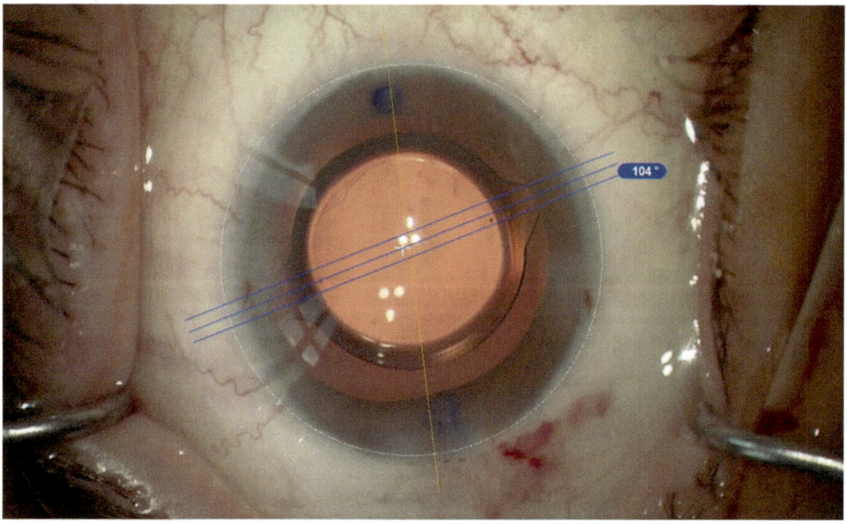

Fig. 3 In digital marking procedures, the surgeon aligns the lens according to the displayed markings

Intraoperative Alignment

In essence, the technique of cataract surgery using toric IOL differs very little from that of a standard monofocal IOL. The additional steps include the marking of the reference and target axis (as outlined before) and intraoperative orientation of the IOLs axis with the target axis.

As the axis of toric IOLs are by definition marked in the flat meridian (axis of the plus cylinder), it has to be superimposed to the steep axis of the cornea. After IOL implantation, it is recommended to rotate the lens close to target axis (within 10°). Then the viscoelastic behind the IOL should be removed completely and the IOL is brought into its final position. The aim of this maneuver is to avoid leaving residues of viscoelastic between haptic and capsule, which was shown to be a risk factor for early postoperative IOL rotation. However, these are recommendations of individual surgeons and depend on surgical preference [13].

Residual Astigmatism and Postoperative Rotation

Residual postoperative astigmatism is a common problem and a common cause of patient dissatisfaction. If an unexpected refraction occurs after surgery ("refractive surprise") after implantation of a toric IOL, the correct alignment of the IOL axis and the IOL calculation of must be checked. Rare causes such as mislabeling are described in the literature and must be considered in each individual case.

Postoperative rotation of the toric lens occurs frequently within the first hour after surgery and most rotations occur within 10 days [21, 33]. Incomplete removal of OVD from the capsular bag is a major cause of early lens rotation, whereas later rotation depends on the stability of the IOL in the capsular bag. This, in turn, depends on the lens design and material of the IOL as well as the anatomy of the eye. If an IOL is implanted into the capsular bag, the capsular bag collapses after only a few days. In the following weeks the capsular bag fibroses, causing the IOL to stick within it. In that regard, the material of the IOL is very relevant as it seems that hydrophobic acrylic IOLs show the strongest adhesion, followed by hydrophilic acrylic IOLs, PMMA and silicone IOLs [8, 28, 58]. Once both anterior and posterior capsule are fused, the IOL is basically firmly anchored. Despite this, rotations at this stage can still occur as a result of capsule shrinkage. In a randomized controlled trial, a reduction of postoperative rotation with simultaneous implantation of a capsule tension ring was shown ($1.85 \pm 1.72°$ vs. $4.02 \pm 2.04°$) [44]. In a second recent study, however, no difference (capsule tension ring vs. no capsule tension ring) could be found [14].

Numerous studies of the past years have investigated the rotational stability of different toric IOLs. The results were summarized in reviews in 2013 and 2017 [21, 58]. In general, toric lenses show good rotational stability with rotation values of up to 5° in the median [21, 26, 33]. However, in individual cases this rotation can be much higher and become clinically relevant. It is however, difficult to identify these patients preoperatively.

Risk factors for rotation include the retention of viscoelastic in the capsular bag [33], longer axial length [26, 52, 64] and lager capsulorhexis diameter [26, 33]. On the other hand, increased opacity of the anterior lens capsule counteracts the likelihood of IOL rotation [64].

Previous studies have found a reduced rotational stability of plate-haptic lenses compared to open-loop haptic lenses, especially in the early postoperative phase, but a higher rotational stability later after surgery [40]. In a later study, however, a good rotational stability was shown for both lens designs [43]. The diameter of the capsular bag was also discussed as a possible risk factor [50]. A larger haptic diameter showed slightly better rotational stability values (13 mm vs 12 mm). However, this difference was not significant [15].

At present there are no general recommendations when a misaligned toric IOL should be rotated. Felipe et al. recommend a rotation if misalignment is higher than 10°, since the effect on postoperative refraction is usually small (0.5D) with smaller deviations (<10°) [10]. Furthermore, the imaging quality is only slightly impaired in smaller deviations [57]. Patient satisfaction and amount of residual astigmatism are important factors in that regard. If a postoperative IOL rotation is required, various tools such as an online calculator (astimatismfix.org, Ocular Surgical Data LLC, Sioux Falls, SD, USA) are available for planning the further procedure. The data of the implanted lens, the information about the current subjective refraction as well as the initial calculated lens axis are taken into account and a decision is made between IOL rotation or lens exchange. In 2016, 12,000 data entries within this platform were analyzed [42]. In less than 1% of the entries the axis deviation was greater than 5°.

The incidence of postoperative IOL rotation is reported as 0.65–3.3% [5, 6, 21, 33]. This depends very much on the type of lens, the lens material, the measurement method and especially on the time of measurement or the comparison period of the individual study. In a large retrospective analysis of more than 6400 eyes a re-rotation was necessary in 0.65% of the cases [38]. The deviation could be reduced from 32.9° ± 15.7° to 8.8° ± 9.7° by the follow-up intervention. The earlier rotation (within 6 days) showed slightly worse results compared to the rotation after 7 days or later.

Additives IOLs and Special Lenses

Additive IOLs can be used to augment both natural or artificial lenses. In the first case, these treatment are in the field of refractive surgery, i.e. to reduce an existing high refractive error. In the second case, implantation is usually used to correct a deviation in the target refraction or to introduce additional features such as multifocality.

The toric versions of these lenses are based on two types of lenses: irisfixed IOLs and sulcus-supported IOLs. Overall, less data is available for these two lens types compared to the intracapsular versions. The orientation with respect to preoperative marking or intraoperative steps of both lens types does not differ from an intracapsular toric IOL. In the case of an irisfixed toric IOL there is usually very little room for rotation due to the fixation. Exact intraoperative alignment plays a decisive role in order to reduce misalignment and to prevent postoperative residual astigmatism [55, 59].

In a small study, a rotation of 3.0° ± 2.5° of a sulcus-supported toric IOL (Sulcoflex Toric 653 T) could be shown [11]. Higher rotation values were also published by McLintock (mean value: 8.23° the day after surgery,maximum rotation 17.63° in the post-observation period). About two thirds of the IOLs had to be re-rotated [30]. Higher rotation values were also found in a case series of patients with myopia and keratoconus [32].

Summary

The correction of corneal astigmatism is essential in many cases to achieve the best possible uncorrected refractive results. Toric IOLs, in the capsular bag as well as add-on lenses can be used very effectively for this purpose. Complication rates are similar to those of a monofocal IOL and the rotational stability of modern toric IOLs is very good.

To achieve a good uncorrected refractive result after cataract surgery, adequate correction of astigmatism is necessary. The implantation of a toric IOL is a cornerstone in this respect and should be offered to patients after appropriate indication, preparation and education.

References

1. Agresta B, Knorz MC, Donatti C, Jackson D. Visual acuity improvements after implantation of toric intraocular lenses in cataract patients with astigmatism: 2 systematic review. BMC Ophthalmol. 2012. https://doi.org/10.1186/1471-2415-12-41.
2. Altan-Yaycioglu R, Akova YA, Akca S, Gur S, Oktem C. Effect on astigmatism of the location of clear corneal incision in phacoemulsification of cataract. J Refract Surg. 2007. https://doi.org/10.3928/1081-597x-20070501-16.
3. Anderson DF, Dhariwal M, Bouchet C, Keith MS. Global prevalence and economic and humanistic burden of astigmatism in cataract patients: A systematic literature review. Clin Ophthalmol. 2018. https://doi.org/10.2147/OPTH.S146829.
4. Balestrazzi A, Baiocchi S, Balestrazzi A, Cartocci G, Tosi GM, Martone G, Michieletto P. Mini-incision cataract surgery and toric lens implantation for the reduction of high myopic astigmatism in patients with marginal pellucid degeneration. Eye (basingstoke). 2015. https://doi.org/10.1038/eye.2015.13.

5. Chang DF. Comparative rotational stability of single-piece open-loop acrylic and plate-haptic silicone toric intraocular lenses. J Cataract Refract Surg. 2008;34(11):1842–7. https://doi.org/10.1016/j.jcrs.2008.07.012.
6. Chang DF. Reduction technique and rate for toric intraocular lenses. J Cataract Refract Surg. 2009. https://doi.org/10.1016/j.jcrs.2009.02.035.
7. Day AC, Dhariwal M, Keith MS, Ender F, Perez VivesC, Miglio C, et al. Distribution of preoperative and postoperative astigmatism in a large population of patients undergoing cataract surgery in the UK. Br J Ophthalmol. 2019. https://doi.org/10.1136/bjophthalmol-2018-312025.
8. Draschl P, Hirnschall N, Luft N, Schuschitz S, Wiesinger J, Rigal K, Findl O. Rotational stability of 2 intraocular lenses with an identical design and different materials. J Cataract Refract Surg. 2017. https://doi.org/10.1016/j.jcrs.2016.12.011.
9. Farooqui JH, Koul A, Dutta R, Shroff NM. Comparison of two different methods of preoperative marking for toric intraocular lens implantation: bubble marker versus pendulum marker. Int J Ophthalmol. 2016. https://doi.org/10.18240/ijo.2016.05.11.
10. Felipe A, Artigas JM, Díez-Ajenjo A, García-Domene C, Alcocer P. Residual astigmatism produced by toric intraocular lens rotation. J Cataract Refract Surg. 2011. https://doi.org/10.1016/j.jcrs.2011.04.036.
11. Ferreira TB, Pinheiro J. Clinical results with a supplementary toric intraocular lens for the correction of astigmatism in pseudophakic patients. Eur J Ophthalmol. 2015;25(4):302–8. https://doi.org/10.5301/ejo.5000564.
12. Ferrer-BlascoT, Montés-Micó R, Peixoto SC, González-Méijome JM, Cerviño A. Prevalence of corneal astigmatism before cataract surgery. J Cataract Refract Surg. 2009. https://doi.org/10.1016/j.jcrs.2008.09.027.
13. Graether JM. Simplified system of marking the cornea for a toric intraocular lens. J Cataract Refract Surg. 2009. https://doi.org/10.1016/j.jcrs.2009.04.033.
14. Hahn U, Krummenauer F, Schmickler S, Koch J. Rotation of a toric intraocular lens with and without capsular tension ring: data from a multicenter non-inferiority randomized clinical trial (RCT). BMC Ophthalmol. 2019;19(1):143. https://doi.org/10.1186/s12886-019-1147-5.
15. Harrer A, Hirnschall N, Maedel S, Findl O. Influence of the overall intraocular lens diameter on rotational stability. Ophthalmic Res. 2015. https://doi.org/10.1159/000368658.
16. Hayashi K, Manabe SI, Yoshida M, Hayashi H. Effect of astigmatism on visual acuity in eyes with a diffractive multifocal intraocular lens. J Cataract Refract Surg. 2010. https://doi.org/10.1016/j.jcrs.2010.02.016.
17. Hey W, Zhu X, Du Y, Yang J, Lu Y. Clinical efficacy of implantation of toric intraocular lenses with different incision positions: a comparative study of steep-axis incision and non-steep-axis incision. BMC Ophthalmol. 2017. https://doi.org/10.1186/s12886-017-0528-x.
18. Hoffmann PC, Hütz WW. Analysis of biometry and prevalence data for corneal astigmatism in 23 239 eyes. J Cataract Refract Surg. 2010. https://doi.org/10.1016/j.jcrs.2010.02.025.
19. Kamiya K, Shimizu K, Hikita F, Komatsu M. Posterior chamber toric phakic intraocular lens implantation for high myopic astigmatism in eyes with pellucid marginal degeneration. J Cataract Refract Surg. 2010. https://doi.org/10.1016/j.jcrs.2009.08.021.
20. Kamiya K, Shimizu K, Miyake T. Changes in astigmatism and corneal higher-order aberrations after phacoemulsification with toric intraocular lens implantation for mild keratoconus with cataract. Jpn J Ophthalmol. 2016. https://doi.org/10.1007/s10384-016-0449-x.
21. Kaur M, Shaikh F, Falera R, Titiyal J. Optimizing outcomes with toric intraocular lenses. Indian J Ophthalmol. 2017. https://doi.org/10.4103/ijo.IJO_810_17.
22. Kessel L, Andresen J, Tendal B, Erngaard D, Flesner P, Hjortdal J. Toric intraocular lenses in the correction of astigmatism during cataract surgery a systematic review and meta-analysis. Ophthalmology. 2016. https://doi.org/10.1016/j.ophtha.2015.10.002.
23. Khan MI, Muhtaseb M. Prevalence of corneal astigmatism in patients having routine cataract surgery at a teaching hospital in the United Kingdom. J Cataract Refract Surg. 2011. https://doi.org/10.1016/j.jcrs.2011.04.026.

24. Khatib ZI, Haldipurkar SS, Shetty V. Verion digital marking versus smartphone-assisted manual marking and isolated manual marking in toric intraocular lens implantation. Indian J Ophthalmol. 2020. https://doi.org/10.4103/ijo.IJO_987_19.
25. Lake JC, Victor G, Clare G, Porfírio GJ, Kernohan A, Evans JR. Toric intraocular lens versus limbal relaxing incisions for corneal astigmatism after phacoemulsification. Cochrane Database Syst Rev. 2019. https://doi.org/10.1002/14651858.CD012801.pub2.
26. Li S, Li X, He S, Zheng Q, Chen X, Wu X, Xu W. Early postoperative rotational stability and its related factors of a single-piece acrylic toric intraocular lens. Eye (Lond). 2020;34 (3):474–9. https://doi.org/10.1038/s41433-019-0521-0.
27. Lockington D, Wang EF, Patel DV, Moore SP, McGhee CNJ. Effectiveness of cataract phacoemulsification with toric intraocular lenses in addressing astigmatism after keratoplasty. J Cataract Refract Surg. 2014. https://doi.org/10.1016/j.jcrs.2014.03.025.
28. Lombardo M, Carbone G, Lombardo G, De Santo MP, Barberi R. Analysis of intraocular lens surface adhesiveness by atomic force microscopy. J Cataract Refract Surg. 2009. https://doi.org/10.1016/j.jcrs.2009.02.029.
29. Ma JJK, Tseng SS. Simple method for accurate alignment in toric phakic and aphakic intraocular lens implantation. J Cataract Refract Surg. 2008;34(10):1631–6. https://doi.org/10.1016/j.jcrs.2008.04.041.
30. McLintock CA, McKelvie J, Gatzioufas Z, Wilson JJ, Stephensen DC, Apel AJG. Outcomes of toric supplementary intraocular lenses for residual astigmatic refractive error in pseudophakic eyes. Int Ophthalmol. 2019;39(9):1965–72. https://doi.org/10.1007/s10792-018-1027-7.
31. Mendicute J, Irigoyen C, Ruiz M, Illarramendi I, Ferrer-Blasco T, Montés-Micó R. Toric intraocular lens versus opposite clear corneal incisions to correct astigmatism in eyes having cataract surgery. J Cataract Refract Surg. 2009. https://doi.org/10.1016/j.jcrs.2008.11.043.
32. Meyer JJ, Kim BZ, Ziaei M, McGhee CNJ. Postoperative rotation of supplementary sulcus-supported toric intraocular lenses. J Cataract Refract Surg. 2017;43(2):285–8. https://doi.org/10.1016/j.jcrs.2016.12.014.
33. Miyake T, Kamiya K, Amano R, Iida Y, Tsunehiro S, Shimizu K. Rotational stability of a toric intraocular lens: Influence of axial length and alignment in the capsular bag. J Cataract Refract Surg. 2014. https://doi.org/10.1016/j.jcrs.2014.01.044.
34. Mozayan E, Lee JK. Update on astigmatism management. Curr Opin Ophthalmol. 2014. https://doi.org/10.1097/ICU.0000000000000068.
35. Nagpal R, Sharma N, Vasavada V, Maharana PK, Titiyal JS, Sinha R, et al. Toric intraocular lens versus monofocal intraocular lens implantation and photorefractive keratectomy: a randomised controlled trial. Am J Ophthalmol. 2015. https://doi.org/10.1016/j.ajo.2015.06.007.
36. Novis C. Astigmatism and toric intraocular lenses. Curr Opin Ophthalmol. 2000. https://doi.org/10.1097/00055735-200002000-00007.
37. Núñez MX, Henriquez MA, Escaf LJ, Ventura BV, Srur M, Newball L, et al. Consensus on the management of astigmatism in cataract surgery. Clin Ophthalmol. 2019. https://doi.org/10.2147/OPTH.S178277.
38. Oshika T, Inamura M, Inoue Y, Ohashi T, Sugita T, Fujita Y, et al. Incidence and outcomes of repositioning surgery to correct misalignment of toric intraocular lenses. Ophthalmology. 2018. https://doi.org/10.1016/j.ophtha.2017.07.004.
39. Ostri C, Falck L, Boberg-Ans G, Kessel L. The need for toric intra-ocular lens implantation in public ophthalmology departments. Acta Ophthalmol. 2015. https://doi.org/10.1111/aos.12584.
40. Patel CK, Ormonde S, Rosen PH, Bron AJ. Postoperative intraocular lens rotation: a randomised comparison of plate and loop haptic implants. Ophthalmology. 1999;106 (11):2190–5; discussion 2196. https://doi.org/10.1016/S0161-6420(99)90504-3
41. Popp N, Hirnschall N, Maedel S, Findl O. Evaluation of 4 corneal astigmatic marking methods. J Cataract Refract Surg. 2012. https://doi.org/10.1016/j.jcrs.2012.07.039.
42. Potvin R, Kramer BA, Hardten DR, Berdahl JP. Toric intraocular lens orientation and residual refractive astigmatism: An analysis. Clin Ophthalmol. 2016. https://doi.org/10.2147/OPTH.S114118
.

43. Prinz A, Neumayer T, Buehl W, Vock L, Menapace R, Findl O, Georgopoulos M. Rotational stability and posterior capsule opacification of a plate-haptic and an open-loop-haptic intraocular lens. J Cataract Refract Surg. 2011;37(2):251–7. https://doi.org/10.1016/j.jcrs.2010.08.049.
44. Rastogi A, Khanam S, Goel Y, Thacker P, Kumar P. Comparative evaluation of rotational stability and visual outcome of toric intraocular lenses with and without a capsular tension ring. Indian J Ophthalmol. 2018;66(3):411–5. https://doi.org/10.4103/ijo.IJO_875_17.
45. Rho CR, Joo CK. Effects of steep meridian incision on corneal astigmatism in phacoemulsification cataract surgery. J Cataract Refract Surg. 2012. https://doi.org/10.1016/j.jcrs.2011.11.031.
46. Roberts HW, Wagh VK, Sullivan DL, Archer TJ, O'Brart DPS. Refractive outcomes after limbal relaxing incisions or femtosecond laser arcuate keratotomy to manage corneal astigmatism at the time of cataract surgery. J Cataract Refract Surg. 2018. https://doi.org/10.1016/j.jcrs.2018.05.027.
47. Rubenstein JB, Raciti M. Management of astigmatism: LRIs. Int Ophthalmol Clin. 2012. https://doi.org/10.1097/IIO.0b013e31824b8786.
48. Rubenstein JB, Raciti M. Approaches to corneal astigmatism in cataract surgery. Curr Opin Ophthalmol. 2013. https://doi.org/10.1097/ICU.0b013e32835ac853.
49. Rückl T, Dexl AK, Bachernegg A, Reischl V, Riha W, Ruckhofer J, et al. Femtosecond laser-assisted intrastromal arcuate keratotomy to reduce corneal astigmatism. J Cataract Refract Surg. 2013. https://doi.org/10.1016/j.jcrs.2012.10.043.
50. Ruhswurm I, Scholz U, Zehetmayer M, Hanselmayer G, Vass C, Skorpik C. Astigmatism correction with a foldable toric intraocular lens in cataract patients. J Cataract Refract Surg. 2000. https://doi.org/10.1016/S0886-3350(00)00317-5.
51. Schiano Lomoriello D, Savini G, Naeser K, Colabelli-Gisoldi RM, Bono V, Pocobelli A. Customized toric intraocular lens implantation in eyes with cataract and corneal astigmatism after deep anterior lamellar keratoplasty: a prospective study. J Ophthalmol. 2018. https://doi.org/10.1155/2018/1649576.
52. Shah GD, Praveen MR, Vasavada AR, Vasavada VA, Rampal G, Shastry LR. Rotational stability of a toric intraocular lens: Influence of axial length and alignment in the capsular bag. J Cataract Refract Surg. 2012. https://doi.org/10.1016/j.jcrs.2011.08.028.
53. Shimizu K, Misawa A, Suzuki Y. Toric intraocular lenses: Correcting astigmatism while controlling axis shift. J Cataract Refract Surg. 1994. https://doi.org/10.1016/S0886-3350(13)80232-5.
54. Tan QQ, Liao X, Lan CJ, Lin J, Tian J. Comparison of Toric intraocular lenses and corneal incisional procedures for correction of low and moderate astigmatism during cataract surgery: a meta-analysis. Zhonghua yan ke za zhi] Chinese J Ophthalmol. 2019. https://doi.org/10.3760/cma.j.issn.0412-4081.2019.07.009.
55. Tehrani M, Dick HB, Schwenn O, Blom E, Schmidt AH, Koch H-R. Postoperative astigmatism and rotational stability after artisan toric phakic intraocular lens implantation. J Cataract Refract Surg. 2003;29(9):1761–6. https://doi.org/10.1016/s0886-3350(03)00014-2.
56. Terauchi R, Horiguchi H, Ogawa T, Shiba T, Tsuneoka H, Nakano T. Posture-related ocular cyclotorsion during cataract surgery with an ocular registration system. Sci Rep. 2020. https://doi.org/10.1038/s41598-020-59118-9.
57. Tognetto D, Perrotta AA, Bauci F, Rinaldi S, Antonuccio M, Pellegrino FA, et al. Quality of images with toric intraocular lenses. J Cataract Refract Surg. 2018. https://doi.org/10.1016/j.jcrs.2017.10.053.
58. Visser N, Bauer NJC, Nuijts RMMA. Toric intraocular lenses: Historical overview, patient selection, IOL calculation, surgical techniques, clinical outcomes, and complications. J Cataract Refract Surg. 2013. https://doi.org/10.1016/j.jcrs.2013.02.020.
59. Visser N, Berendschot TTJM, Bauer NJC, Jurich J, Kersting O, Nuijts RMMA. Accuracy of toric intraocular lens implantation in cataract and refractive surgery. J Cataract Refract Surg. 2011. https://doi.org/10.1016/j.jcrs.2011.02.024.
60. Wade M, Steinert RF, Garg S, Farid M, Gaster R. Results of toric intraocular lenses for post-penetrating keratoplasty astigmatism. Ophthalmology. 2014. https://doi.org/10.1016/j.ophtha.2013.10.011.

61. Wills J, Gillett R, Eastwell E, Abraham R, Coffey K, Webber A, Wood J. Effect of simulated astigmatic refractive error on reading performance in the young. Optom Vis Sci. 2012. https://doi.org/10.1097/OPX.0b013e3182429c6b.
62. Wolffsohn JS, Bhogal G, Shah S. Effect of uncorrected astigmatism on vision. J Cataract Refract Surg. 2011. https://doi.org/10.1016/j.jcrs.2010.09.022.
63. Zhou F, Jiang W, Lin Z, Li X, Li J, Lin H, et al. Comparative meta-analysis of toric intraocular lens alignment accuracy in cataract patients: Image-guided system versus manual marking. J Cataract Refract Surg. 2019. https://doi.org/10.1016/j.jcrs.2019.03.030.
64. Zhu X, He W, Zhang K, Lu Y. Factors influencing 1-year rotational stability of AcrySof Toric intraocular lenses. Br J Ophthalmol. 2016. https://doi.org/10.1136/bjophthalmol-2015-306656.

Systematic Overview of Monovision

Annika Müller-Kassner and Kleopatra Varna-Tigka

Results

Both monovision using LASIK and after lens surgery show very good visual results. Ito et al. examined the visual results and patient satisfaction of 54 patients after **pseudophakic monovision** up to five years postoperatively. The difference in the spherical equivalent of both eyes was 2.13 D on average and 98% of the patients achieved an uncorrected distance visual acuity of 0.1 logMAR (0.8 decimal visual acuity) and uncorrected near visual acuity according to Jaeger of at least J2 in 76% of the cases. Five years after surgery, 56% of patients had stereo vision within the normal range (87% of the patients when corrected by spectacles). Patient satisfaction (rated as at least acceptable to highly satisfied) increased significantly in the period between one month (78%) and three years (89%) postoperatively. After five years, 91% of the patients were satisfied with the visual outcome. 88% of the examined patients were spectacle independent postoperatively [1].

Author's recommendation

Patients with natural existing monovision via using contact lenses as well as myopic, presbyopic patients represent the most suitable patient clientele, as they are familiar with a preserved but limited near vision.

Results of **monovision after LASIK** were examined and reported by Reilly et al. Uncorrected distance visual acuity of 20/25 Snellen visual acuity (0.8 decimal visual acuity) was found in 100% of the patients. 70% of the patients achieved uncorrected near visual acuity of J1+ according to Jaeger, 25% of at least J1 and 4% of J2. For 15% of the patients a second surgery was necessary. Two of the 164 patients examined (1%) decided to have their myopic eye corrected to emmetropia;

A. Müller-Kassner (✉) · K. Varna-Tigka
Universitätsklinikum Frankfurt, Frankfurt am Main, Germany
e-mail: annikamaria.mueller-kassner@kgu.de

M. Shajari et al. (eds.), *Cataract and Lens Surgery*,
https://doi.org/10.1007/978-3-031-05394-8_75

in 6 eyes (4%) myopia and in 17 eyes (10%) emmetropia was increased [2]. In a retrospective study by Braun et al. 7% of the patients decided to abolish their monovision for binocular emmetropia postoperatively. In 28% of the cases a subsequent increase of the emmetropia of the eye adjusted to distant vision was necessary [3].

Comparing pseudophakic monovision (Akreos AO IOL (Bausch & Lomb)) with **multifocal IOLs** (Tecnis ZM900 IOL (Abbott Medical Optics)), Wilkins et al. showed a comparable uncorrected distance visual acuity (0.06 logMAR vs. 0.08 logMAR) and a significantly better near vision of multifocal IOLs (0.01 logMAR vs. −0.03 logMAR). The monovision group had a significantly better intermediate visual acuity (0.15 logMAR vs. 0.22 logMAR). After implantation of multifocal IOLs, a higher rate of complete spectacle independence was achieved (26% vs. 71%) while with pseudophakic monovision significantly fewer optical phenomena occurred (79% vs. 56%). Contrast sensitivity was higher in the monovision group while the multifocal group showed better results regarding stereo vision [4]. A Cochrane review from 2016 by de Silva et al. confirms these results. A relative risk (RR) of 0.63 for spectacle independence with multifocal IOLs was found as well as an RR of 1.41 for glare and of 3.58 for halos [5]. When looking at everyday activities, multifocal IOLs and monovision showed comparable results in a study by Labiris et al. However, the monovision group performed significantly worse with regard to demanding everyday activities at near distance [6].

Rodov et al. compared monovision with **Extended Depth of Focus** (EDOF) IOLs. The EDOF IOL provided better distance visual acuity (0.03 ± 0.08 logMAR vs. 0.08 ± 0.12 logMAR) and good intermediate visual acuity (0.08 ± 0.12 logMAR), which was not measurable in the monovision group. Monovision resulted in better near visual acuity (0.07 ± 0.12 logMAR vs. 0.23 ± 0.17 logMAR) and less optical phenomena (6% vs. 14%). The rate of spectacle-free vision was similar in both groups (70% in monovision vs. 74% in EDOF IOLs); in the group of EDOF IOLs more patients indicated that they would choose the same IOL again [7].

Complications

Postoperative patient dissatisfaction is mainly based on reduced uncorrected near visual acuity and persistent spectacle dependence. In addition, patients may report asthenopic complaints and, in cases of previous strabismus, new onset diplopia. Patients over 60 years of age are more likely to be satisfied postoperatively and to be spectacle independent [8]. Whether and for how long an adaptation to monovision takes place has not yet been sufficiently shown in studies.

Finkelman et al. examined the **contrast sensitivity** of monovision. A comparably reduced contrast sensitivity was found for both the emmetropic and myopic eye. Binocularly, better though still reduced results were obtained (1.63 ± 0.96 vs. 1.90 ± 0.11 in healthy eyes) [9]. Contrast sensitivity was reduced, especially in mesopic and scotopic conditions, and was higher in monovision than in eyes with multifocal IOLs [8]. Hayashi et al. investigated the influence of anisometropia on contrast sensitivity and found a deterioration of contrast sensitivity with higher anisometropia, although it was not statistically significant.

The same study also examined **stereo vision** in eyes with monovision. A reduction was found particularly for higher anisometropia (reduction of 29 arc seconds with 1.5 D monovision compared to isometropia and of 87 arc seconds with 2.0 D monovision) [10]. It was found that 63–86% of patients were in the normal range. Multifocal IOLs achieved better results than monovision. However, only a few studies in this area have been conducted so far [8].

Author's recommendation

Various studies argue in favor of an anisometropia of 1.0–1.5 D to maintain binocular fusion and thus ensures good stereo vision and contrast sensitivity [8]. An anisometropia of >3 D should be avoided due to excessive aniseikonia.

Conclusion

Monovision is an effective method for presbyopia correction. High patient satisfaction and good distance and intermediate visual acuity as well as less frequent optical phenomena are seen using this technique. However, it also comes with reduced near visual acuity and stereo vision as well as with a lower rate of spectacle independence compared to multifocal IOLs.

References

1. Ito M, Shimizu K, Iida Y, Amano R. Five-year clinical study of patients with pseudophakic monovision. J Cataract Refract Surg. 2012;38:1440–5.
2. Reilly CD, Lee WB, Alvarenga L, Caspar J, Garcia-Ferrer F, Mannis MJ. Surgical monovision and monovision reversal in LASIK. Cornea. 2006;25:136–8.
3. Braun EHP, Lee J, Steinert RF. Monovision in LASIK. Ophthalmology. 2008;115:1196–202.
4. Wilkins MR, Allan BD, Rubin GS, Findl O, Hollick EJ, Bunce C, Xing W. Randomized trial of multifocal intraocular lenses versus monovision after bilateral cataract surgery. Ophthalmology. 2013;120:2449-2455.e1.
5. de Silva SR, Evans JR, Kirthi V, Ziaei M, Leyland M (2016) Multifocal versus monofocal intraocular lenses after cataract extraction. Cochrane Database Syst Rev 12:CD003169
6. Labiris G, Ntonti P, Patsiamanidi M, Sideroudi H, Georgantzoglou K, Kozobolis VP. Evaluation of activities of daily living following pseudophakic presbyopic correction. Eye Vis (Lond). 2017;4:2.
7. Rodov L, Reitblat O, Levy A, Assia EI, Kleinmann G. Visual outcomes and patient satisfaction for trifocal, extended depth of focus and monofocal intraocular lenses. J Refract Surg. 2019;35:434–40.

8. Labiris G, Toli A, Perente A, Ntonti P, Kozobolis VP. A systematic review of pseudophakic monovision for presbyopia correction. Int J Ophthalmol. 2017;10:992–1000.
9. Finkelman YM, Ng JQ, Barrett GD. Patient satisfaction and visual function after pseudophakic monovision. J Cataract Refract Surg. 2009;35:998–1002.
10. Hayashi K, Yoshida M, Manabe S-I, Hayashi H. Optimal amount of anisometropia for pseudophakic monovision. J Refract Surg. 2011;27:332–8.

Systematic Overview of Multifocal Intraocular Lenses

Annika Müller-Kassner and Mehdi Shajari

Multifocal intraocular lenses (IOLs) have been available since the 1980s for presbyopia correction and are offered as part of cataract surgery or refractive lens exchange. Multifocal IOLs are characterized by the creation of **different focal points** (minimum two) and are also available with aspherical and toric designs. The selection of an IOL is mainly influenced by three factors: (1) the patient's wishes, (2) the surgeon's experience and attitude towards different techniques, and (3) the market for IOLs with the emergence of new techniques and clinical evidence.

Multifocal IOL Models

Multifocal IOLs are currently available as **bifocal** (far and near distance (40 cm), though these are rarely used), **trifocal** (additional intermediate range (about 60 to 80 cm)) and **quadrifocal** models (intermediate range divided (60 cm and 120 cm)).

Since 2016, the options for multifocal correction have been expanded by a group of lenses known as **Extended Depth of Focus (EDOF) IOLs**. These IOLs exploit various physical principles to extend the focal point, improving the depth of focus and enabling the patient to see sharply from about 50 cm into the distance. The monocular depth of focus of an EDOF lenes should be at least 0.5 D greater than that of an equivalent strength monofocal IOLs, at a visual acuity of 0.63 decimal.

Reminder
EDOF IOLs have an extended focal point and thus an improved depth of field (monocular depth of field at a visual acuity of 0.63 decimal is at least 0.5 D greater than that of monofocal IOLs). They cover the intermediate and distant vision, though patients may still need reading glasses for small text.

A. Müller-Kassner (✉) · M. Shajari
Universitätsklinikum Frankfurt, Frankfurt am Main, Germany
e-mail: annikamaria.mueller-kassner@kgu.de

M. Shajari et al. (eds.), *Cataract and Lens Surgery*,
https://doi.org/10.1007/978-3-031-05394-8_76

Different technologies exist for this purpose. The IC-8 (AcuFocus, Inc.) has a small aperture that blocks peripheral light using pin-hole technology and only allows central and paracentral light rays to reach the retina. The IC-8 is typically used in only one eye and a monofocal IOL is implanted into the contralateral, usually dominant eye. The Wichterle IOL-Continuous Focus (WIOL-CF, Medicem) has a bioanalog design that mimics the crystalline lens by decreasing refraction towards the periphery. The material adheres to the capsular bag, so no haptics are necessary. There are EDOF-IOLs lenses with step-like diffractive optics (e.g., Tecnis Symfony (Johnson & Johnson Vision Care, Inc.), AT LARA 829MP (Carl Zeiss Meditec AG)) and EDOF-IOLs with non-diffractive optics (e.g., SIFI Mini WELL (SIFI MedTech), AcrySof IQ Vivity (Alcon)).

Refractive IOLs, in particular, can be dependent on the pupil size. If the focus for the near distance is located centrally in the IOL and the focus for the distance in the periphery, a narrow pupil can cause problems in near vision, whereas a large pupil will allow all optical zones to be used, but glare and optical phenomena occur more frequently.

Some IOLs are available in aspherical form to reduce spherical and higher order aberrations or as toric multifocal IOLs in order to reduce astigmatism while also providing multifocality.

Author's recommendation

An astigmatism should be corrected to allow fully functional multifocality. This can either be at the level of the cornea or by using a toric multifocal IOL to achieve spectacle independence. When correcting astigmatism using a toric multifocal implant, it is best to use measurement devices and formulae that consider the "total corneal refractive power".

The IOLs available on the market differ in their biomaterials, optics and haptics but can also vary in their presence of UV and blue light filters. They are also available with innovative adaptations that allow the lens to be fixed onto the rhexis by an additional "haptic groove" which provides better centration and stabilization of the IOL in the capsular bag (e.g., Femtis Comfort (Oculentis GmbH)).

One further option in cases where a patient may already have a monofocal lens or where there is some doubt as to whether the patient will be satisfied with the lens, a secondary multifocal Add-On IOL (e.g., Sulcoflex (Rayner). The placement of the Add-On IOL can occur at the time of the original cataract surgery or years afterwards and provides the reassuring possibility of explantation, if needed. Multifocal implants can cause disturbing optical phenomena or over the long term, the development of retina or corneal pathology which can result in a reduction of the multifocal effect. While this can be an excellent choice in the right patients, the use of Add-On lenses can occasionally be associated with inflammation, pigment loss and raised intraocular pressure so these patients should be followed up regularly.

Table 1 gives an overview of the currently most common trifocal and EDOF IOLs.

Table 1 Overview of the most common trifocal and EDOF IOLs. (IOL = intraocular lens, EDOF = Extended depth of focus, R = refractive, D = diffractive)

Manufacturer	IOL name	Focus (optical principle)	Near addition (D)	Intermediate addition (D)	Asphericity	Blue light filter	Toric version available	Material characteristics
AcuFocus	IC-8	EDOF	–	–	+	–	–	Hydrophobic
Alcon	PanOptix	Trifocal (R)	3,25	2,17	+	+	+	Hydrophobic
Johnson & Johnson Vision Care, Inc	Tecnis Symfony	EDOF (D)	–	1,78	+	–	+	Hydrophobic
Medicem	WIOL-CF	EDOF (R)	2,5	1,5	+	–	–	Hydrophilic
Physiol	Fine Vision	Trifocal (D)	3,5	1,75	+	+	+	Hydrophilic
Oculentis	Comfort	EDOF (R)	–	1,5	+	–	+	Hydrophilic
Oculentis	Femtis Comfort	EDOF (R)	–	1,5	+	–	–	Hydrophilic
Rayner	RayOne Trifocal	Trifocal (D)	3,5	1,75	+	–	–	Hydrophilic
Rayner	Sulcoflex Trifocal	Trifocal (D)	3,5	1,75	–	–	–	Hydrophilic
Sifi Medtech	Mini Well	EDOF (R)	3	–	+	–	+	Hydrophilic
Zeiss	AT Lisa tri	Trifocal (D)	3,3	1,67	+	–	+	Hydrophilic with hydrophobic surface
Zeiss	AT Lara	EDOF (D)	1,9	0,9	+	–	+	Hydrophilic with hydrophobic surface

Results

Multifocal IOLs, in general, show very good refractive and visual outcomes which can be credited partly to the high level of technical development in modern IOLs but also to optimized preoperative diagnostics and surgical skills.

In a review of 76 studies conducted in 2016 by Alio et al., 100% of the patients with multifocal IOLs showed monocular, uncorrected distant visual acuity of at least 0.3 logMAR (0.5 decimal visual acuity) and 71% of the patients of at least 0.1 logMAR (0.8 decimal visual acuity); binocularly, 77% had uncorrected distant visual acuity of 0.1 logMAR.

Monocular uncorrected intermediate visual acuity was at least 0.3 logMAR for 95% of the patients and at least 0.1 logMAR for 23%; binocularly, 32% achieved an uncorrected intermediate visual acuity of 0.1 logMAR. Uncorrected near visual acuity was at least 0.3 logMAR monocularly in 93% of the cases and at least 0.1 logMAR in 38% of the cases; binocularly, 62% had near visual acuity of at least 0.1 logMAR. Diffractive optics showed slightly better results at all distances [1]. While monofocal aspherical IOLs showed a significantly better visual outcome than monofocal spherical IOLs, multifocal aspherical IOLs have so far only shown an equivalent to slightly better visual outcome [2].

Kohnen et al. evaluated the visual outcomes of a **trifocal IOL** and found a binocular uncorrected distance visual acuity of 0.00 ± 0.094 logMAR, an uncorrected intermediate visual acuity of 0.00 ± 0.11 logMAR and an uncorrected near visual acuity of 0.01 ± 0.09 logMAR with best visual outcomes at 0.0 and −2.0 D. The spherical equivalent in the study was -0.04 ± 0.32 D [3]. A review by Kohnen and Suryakumar described the visual outcome of **EDOF IOLs**. They showed a good distance visual acuity for all EDOF models, improved intermediate visual acuity and a functional but limited near visual acuity [4]. The IC-8 (AcuFocus, Inc.) showed a visual acuity of at least 0.63 in 90% (uncorrected distance vision), 95% (uncorrected intermediate vision) and 79% (uncorrected near vision) of the cases in a prospective study. [5]. With implantation of EDOF-IOLs, mild **monovision** is another option to improve near vision. Jackson et al. showed the best visual results were achieved when the dominant eye was set to emmetropia and the non-dominant eye to myopia (between −0.21 D and −0.63 D) [6]. The Concerto Study Group investigated a micro-monovision of −0.5 D in the non-dominant eye with implantation of the Tecnis Symfony (Johnson & Johnson Vision Care, Inc.) They showed comparable distance vision to bilateral emmetropia with significantly better intermediate and near vision ($p = 0.003$, $p = 0.11$). Spectacle independence was increased by almost 9% with monovision while 14% of the patients still needed reading glasses [7].

Author's recommendation

When implanting EDOF-IOLs, a mild monovision (−0.5 D to −0.75 D in the non-dominant eye) can achieve an improvement of near visual acuity and provides a greater degree of spectacle independence.

Cochener et al. conducted a prospective study **comparing two trifocal IOLs with the EDOF-IOL** Tecnis Symfony (Johnson & Johnson Vision Care, Inc.). Monocular and binocular distance visual acuity was equivalent in all three IOLs, while the EDOF-IOL showed better intermediate visual acuity. Near visual acuity was better in the trifocal group but the EDOF-IOL also showed satisfactory results, especially with mild monovision (<−0.25 D) (visual acuity > 0.63 in 82 and 83% vs. 53%). Contrast sensitivity was comparably reduced in all groups and no differences in patient satisfaction were found. 86–89% of the patients with trifocal IOLs and 90% of the patients with EDOF IOLs were spectacle independent postoperatively [8].

For patients with previous **myopic or hyperopic laser surgery**, preoperative calculation is difficult, but the visual results do not differ significantly from those of untreated patients. Only in cases of previously high myopic patients (>−6 D), were the postoperative outcomes less predictable [9, 10]. A review by Alio et al. showed that at least 49% of the patients had **spectacle independence**. When divided by distance, this degree of spectacle independence was found in 92% of the cases for distance vision, in 100% for intermediate vision and in 70% for near vision [1]. Rosen et al. showed a spectacle-free rate of 80% with a binocular, uncorrected distance visual acuity of 0.05 ± 0.01 logMAR (0.9 decimal visual acuity) in their meta-analysis [11]. Divided according to the IOL model, Böhm et al. found a spectacle independence in 96% (panfocal IOL), 93% (trifocal IOL), 92% (segmental refractive IOL) and 71% (EDOF-IOL) of the cases [12].

Böhm et al. also conducted a comparison of the **defocus curves** of a panfocal IOL (AcrySof PanOptix, Alcon), a trifocal diffractive IOL (AT Lisa tri 839MP, Zeiss), an EDOF IOL (TECNIS Symfony ZXR00, Johnson & Johnson Vision Care, Inc.) and a segmental refractive IOL (LENTIS Mplus X LS-313 MF30, Oculentis). A comparable distance visual acuity (2–4 m; 0.0 to −0.5 D) was obtained for all models. In the intermediate distance (0.5–1 m; −1.0 to −2.0 D) the visual results of the EDOF IOL were significantly better; in the distance of 50 cm (−2.0 D) the panfocal IOL showed the best visual acuity. In comparison, the EDOF IOL achieved worse near visual acuity than the other multifocal IOLs (40 cm, −2.5 D) [12]. Figure 1 shows the comparison of the defocus curves.

Author's recommendation

Trifocal/quadrifocal IOLs can be a promising solution for patients for whom good near vision and spectacle independence is a high priority. Patients who do a lot of computer or screen work, or those who in everyday life and who want to be spectacle independent are suitable candidates for EDOF IOLs.

The **comparison of multifocal and monofocal IOLs** showed comparable uncorrected distant visual acuity in a meta-analysis by Cao et al. Which included 21 randomised trials. Intermediate visual acuity in 63 and 80 cm was also similar in the two groups, with multifocal IOLs showing better visual results at a distance of 60 cm. Multifocal IOLs led to better near visual acuity and significantly more patients achieved complete spectacle independence (relative risk (RR) 1.85 after

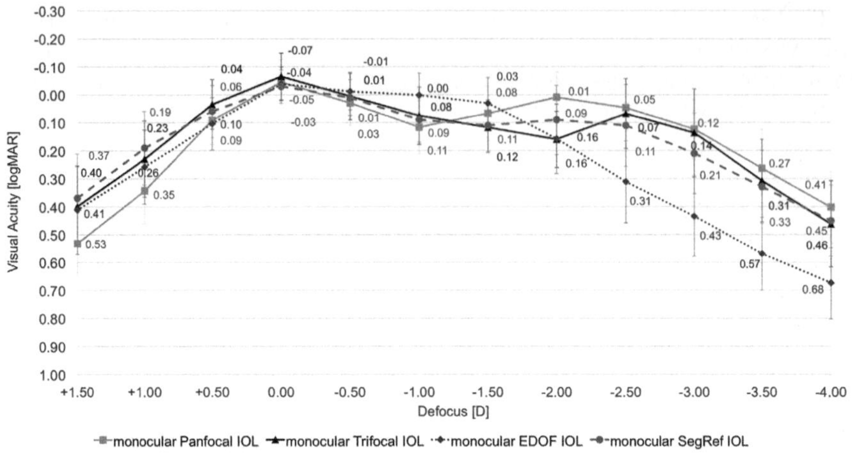

Fig. 1 Monocular, corrected defocus curves of a panfocal IOL (n = 54), a trifocal IOL (n = 54), an EDOF IOL (n = 52) and a segmental refractive IOL (n = 50) 3 months after implantation. (Böhm et al. [12]; with kind permission of © Wolters Kluwer 2020. All Rights Reserved)

3 months, 4.03 after 6 and 12 months). Optical phenomena such as glare and halos occurred more frequently with multifocal IOLs (glare: RR 1.91, halos: RR 3.08); in addition, lower contrast sensitivity was observed [13]. In patients with unilateral cataract, e.g., posttraumatic or after unilateral steroid therapy, monocular implantation of a multifocal IOL may be considered. Due to lower incidence of light on the retina in the affected eye, a neurosensory difference occurs, which requires a prolonged neuroadaptation. Although monocular suppression is discussed, monocular multifocality shows satisfactory results, more frequent spectacle independence and better stereo vision than after implantation of a monofocal IOL and can therefore be considered especially in young patients [1].

Complications and Postoperative Problems

Intra- and postoperatively, the same risks exist as with the implantation of a monofocal IOL. The patient must be informed about possible development of posterior capsular opacification, postoperative infections leading to endophthalmitis and the risk of associated blindness, as well as the risk of retinal detachment. **Postoperative dissatisfaction** after implantation of multifocal IOLs is mainly due to reduced visual acuity (95%) and disturbing optical phenomena (38–42%). De Vries et al. found the main causes to be residual refractive errors (66%), secondary cataracts (16%), wide pupils in mesopic light conditions (14.5%) and wavefront changes (12%) [14]. Woodward et al. also found the causes to be secondary cataract (54–66%), residual refractive errors (29%), dry eyes (2–15%) and IOL decentration (12%) [15].

After implantation of a multifocal IOL, the brain must become accustomed to the new optical phenomena, less light on the retina and reduced contrast sensitivity, especially in mydriasis or in situations of backlighting. In a prospective study, Rosa et al. investigated **neuroadaptation** after implantation of multifocal IOLs using functional magnetic resonance imaging. Activation of cortical areas involved in visual attention, procedural learning, cognitive control and goal-oriented behavior was shown. This level of activity normalized after six months, hence after this period of time neuroadaptation is considered complete [16].

Refractive residual errors can be reduced by accurate preoperative biometry, correct calculation and surgical precision. Treatment options for vision-limiting refractive errors include refractive laser procedures (LASIK/ PRK), IOL exchange or implantation of an Add-on/Piggyback IOL. A retrospective study examined different treatment options for refractive residual errors after implantation of a monofocal IOL and showed the best results after LASIK, whereby the correction of only minor residual errors in the study must be considered. All of the patients had a spherical equivalent within ±1 D after LASIK, while only 63% of cases after IOL exchange and 85% after implantation of a three-part Piggyback IOL achieved this outcome [17]. A study by Piñero et al. showed an improvement in uncorrected and corrected distance vision after LASIK in both monofocal and multifocal IOLs, but refraction could be adjusted more precisely in the group of monofocal IOLs. Performing hyperopic LASIK after implantation of multifocal IOLs however showed limitations in the predictability of results [18].

Another possible complication is **decentration** of the IOL or an **IOL tilt**. The average decentration after uncomplicated cataract surgery is 0.30 ± 0.16 mm and is more frequent in myopic patients with longer axial lengths. This mainly worsens the optical quality of distant and intermediate visual acuity. The effects are greater, the more complex the optics of the multifocal IOL are. Xu et al. investigated the effect of IOL decentration on the optical quality and compared a monofocal, an EDOF and a bifocal IOL. With a decentration of >0.25 mm, the bifocal IOL showed significantly more higher order aberrations; the monofocal and the EDOF IOL were more resistant to a decrease in optical quality [19]. As a treatment, argon laser iridoplasty can be considered first, to avoid IOL exchange. An IOL tilt occurs mainly in hydrophilic IOLs and IOLs with C-haptics and can be avoided by the insertion of a capsular tension ring or the implantation of an IOL with plate haptics. In a prospective study in eyes with implantation of trifocal IOLs, optical phenomena were observed when **angle kappa** exceeded 0.4 mm and a reduction of visual acuity when angle kappa exceeded 0.5 mm [20].

Based on preoperative measurements, the **pupil size** after IOL implantation is difficult to predict, as postoperative changes are often observed. A small pupil (<4.5 mm) leads to a deterioration of near visual acuity, as shown by Hayashi et al. in an interventional study [21]. Although a large pupil makes all optical zones available and provides better contrast sensitivity, it also leads to more optical phenomena. There are no values that are considered absolute contraindications for multifocal IOLs up to this date. Small pupils can be treated with cyclopentolate eye drops in mesopic and scotopic environments or a 360° argon laser iridoplasty and large pupils treated with brimonidine eye drops.

Reminder
Preoperative evaluation of pupil size with planned implantation of a multifocal IOL is important for the postoperative outcome. Postoperative changes in pupil size are frequent but difficult to predict.

After implantation of multifocal IOLs, **contrast sensitivity** can be reduced due to the fragmentation of light to the different optical zones of the multifocal IOL. In a prospective study by Mesci et al., a significantly stronger reduction of contrast sensitivity in refractive compared to diffractive multifocal IOLs could be shown in all light conditions. However, there was an increase of contrast sensitivity in the course of the months due to neuroadaptation [22].

Finally, the higher **rate of posterior capsular opacification** in multifocal IOLs should be noted (15% vs. 6% in monofocal IOLs) which occurs more frequently in hydrophilic than in hydrophobic materials. Patients are also symptomatic at an earlier stage than in the case of monofocal lenses so Nd:YAG capsulotomy is required more frequently. [1].

Explantation of the IOL should be considered the last resort for persistent reduced visual acuity and optical phenomena and is a disappointing situation for both the patient and the surgeon. The explantation rate for multifocal IOLs is 0.9–7% and is most often due to reduced contrast sensitivity (36%), optical phenomena (34%), non-objectifiable reasons such as failure of neuroadaptation (32%) or implantation of an incorrect lens power (20%). Intra- and postoperative complications such as the need for anterior vitrectomy, IOL dislocation with the need for scleral fixation, postoperative corneal decompensation or cystoid macular edema must be considered, and the expected benefit must be weighed against the surgical risk [1].

Conclusion

Multifocal IOLs represent an effective treatment option for presbyopia with a high rate of spectacle independent vision. Nowadays, trifocal and EDOF IOLs are implanted mainly, showing very good visual and refractive outcome when accurate preoperative biometry, calculation and intraoperative exact centration is achieved. The most common causes of patient dissatisfaction are residual refractive errors followed by optical phenomena and increased glare sensitivity.

References

1. Alio JL, Plaza-Puche AB, Férnandez-Buenaga R, Pikkel J, Maldonado M. Multifocal intraocular lenses: An overview. Surv Ophthalmol. 2017;62:611–34
2. de Vries NE, Nuijts RMMA. Multifocal intraocular lenses in cataract surgery: literature review of benefits and side effects. J Cataract Refract Surg. 2013;39:268–78.
3. Kohnen T, Herzog M, Hemkeppler E, Schönbrunn S, De Lorenzo N, Petermann K, Böhm M. Visual performance of a quadrifocal (trifocal) intraocular lens following removal of the crystalline lens. Am J Ophthalmol. 2017;184:52–62.
4. Kohnen T, Suryakumar R. Extended depth-of-focus technology in intraocular lenses. J Cataract Refract Surg. 2020;46:298–304.
5. Dick HB, Piovella M, Vukich J, Vilupuru S, Lin L. Prospective multicenter trial of a small-aperture intraocular lens in cataract surgery. J Cataract Refract Surg. 2017;43:956–68.
6. Jackson MA, Edmiston AM, Bedi R. Optimum refractive target in patients with bilateral implantation of extended depth of focus intraocular lenses. Clin Ophthalmol. 2020;14:455–62.
7. Cochener B. Clinical outcomes of a new extended range of vision intraocular lens: International Multicenter Concerto Study. J Cataract Refract Surg. 2016;42:1268–75.
8. Cochener B, Boutillier G, Lamard M, Auberger-Zagnoli C. A comparative evaluation of a new generation of diffractive trifocal and extended depth of focus intraocular lenses. J Refract Surg. 2018;34:507–14.
9. Vrijman V, van der Linden JW, van der Meulen IJE, Mourits MP, Lapid-Gortzak R. Multifocal intraocular lens implantation after previous corneal refractive laser surgery for myopia. J Cataract Refract Surg. 2017;43:909–14.
10. Vrijman V, van der Linden JW, van der Meulen IJE, Mourits MP, Lapid-Gortzak R. Multifocal intraocular lens implantation after previous hyperopic corneal refractive laser surgery. J Cataract Refract Surg. 2018;44:466–70.
11. Rosen E, Alió JL, Dick HB, Dell S, Slade S. Efficacy and safety of multifocal intraocular lenses following cataract and refractive lens exchange: Metaanalysis of peer-reviewed publications. J Cataract Refract Surg. 2016;42:310–28.
12. Böhm M, Petermann K, Hemkeppler E, Kohnen T. Defocus curves of 4 presbyopia-correcting IOL designs: Diffractive panfocal, diffractive trifocal, segmental refractive, and extended-depth-of-focus. J Cataract Refract Surg. 2019;45:1625–36.
13. Cao K, Friedman DS, Jin S, et al. Multifocal versus monofocal intraocular lenses for age-related cataract patients: a system review and meta-analysis based on randomized controlled trials. Surv Ophthalmol. 2019;64:647–58.
14. de Vries NE, Webers CAB, Touwslager WRH, Bauer NJC, de Brabander J, Berendschot TT, Nuijts RMMA. Dissatisfaction after implantation of multifocal intraocular lenses. J Cataract Refract Surg. 2011;37:859–65.
15. Woodward MA, Randleman JB, Stulting RD. Dissatisfaction after multifocal intraocular lens implantation. J Cataract Refract Surg. 2009;35:992–7.
16. Rosa AM, Miranda ÂC, Patrício MM, McAlinden C, Silva FL, Castelo-Branco M, Murta JN. Functional magnetic resonance imaging to assess neuroadaptation to multifocal intraocular lenses. J Cataract Refract Surg. 2017;43:1287–96.
17. Fernandez-Buenaga R, Alio JL, Perez AL, Quesada AL, Pinilla L, Barraquer RI. Resolving refractive error after cataract surgery: IOL exchange, piggyback lens, or LASIK. J Refract Surg. 2013;29:676–83.
18. Pinero DR, Ayala Espinosa MJ, Alio JL. LASIK outcomes following multifocal and monofocal intraocular lens implantation. J Refract Surg. 2010;26:569–77.
19. Xu J, Zheng T, Lu Y. Effect of decentration on the optical quality of monofocal, extended depth of focus, and bifocal intraocular lenses. J Refract Surg. 2019;35:484–92.
20. Qi Y, Lin J, Leng L, Zhao G, Wang Q, Li C, Hu L. Role of angle κ in visual quality in patients with a trifocal diffractive intraocular lens. J Cataract Refract Surg. 2018;44:949–54.

21. Hayashi K, Hayashi H, Nakao F, Hayashi F. Correlation between pupillary size and intraocular lens decentration and visual acuity of a zonal-progressive multifocal lens and a monofocal lens. Ophthalmology. 2001;108:2011–7.
22. Mesci C, Erbil H, Ozdoker L, Karakurt Y, Bilge AD. Visual acuity and contrast sensitivity function after accommodative and multifocal intraocular lens implantation. Eur J Ophthalmol. 2010;20:90–100.

Intraocular Lens Fixation in the Ciliary Sulcus: A Systematic Overview

Jakob Siedlecki

Quality of Available Data and Evidence

In contrast to the sulcus add-on IOL, the placement of a sulcus IOL in complicated cataract extraction or secondary treatment of aphakia is not a planned procedure but is usually part of a complication management plan. For this reason, no prospective randomised studies are available and long-term data on safety and complication rates are also only available from a small number of studies. Until well into the 2000s, single-piece IOLs were also implanted in the sulcus. Nowadays, many ophthalmologists strictly recommend the implantation of three-piece IOLs. Therefore, the distinction of the lens type in the sulcus is essential for the reader to assess the complication rate as the lens biomaterial and design are major determinants of the success of long-term sulcus placement.

Furthermore, the available studies do not consistently differentiate whether optic capture (i.e. placement of optic of the lens behind the rhexis) was performed during sulcus positioning. As this measure has a major influcnce on the refractive predictability of the sulcus IOL, comparison of the studies is difficult, especially as many studies report simultaneously on sulcus IOLs with and without optic capture. The comparison of the predictability of the target refraction of a sulcus IOL is complicated by the fact that the possibility of optic capture depends mainly, but not entirely, on the integrity of the anterior rhexis. Thus, it is often only apparent after implantation of a given IOL into the eye whether an optic capture is possible. Therefore, the correct choice of IOL power depending on the possibility of optic capture can be difficult.

J. Siedlecki (✉)
University of Munich, Munich, Germany
e-mail: jakob.siedlecki@med.uni-muenchen.de

M. Shajari et al. (eds.), *Cataract and Lens Surgery*,
https://doi.org/10.1007/978-3-031-05394-8_77

Choice of the IOL

A few older studies report good long-term results of single-piece acrylic or PMMA IOLs in the sulcus [1, 2]. However, the vast majority of studies (particularly the newer ones) consistently recommend that single-piece IOLs should not be placed in the sulcus [3, 4], as this type of lens causes complications in the case of acrylic design due to its greater thickness. The softer, more pliable acrylic is also less reliable in the sulcus as they are designed for the capsular bag diameter. The thinner PMMA IOLs, which are more suitable for the sulcus, are hardly represented on the market anymore as they are not foldable and require large incisions for implantation. Their rigid haptics, however, provide excellent stability in the sulcus. One of the complications of the widely used single-piece acrylic IOL is that this type of lens can lead to chafing against the iris in the sulcus [5], and thus can cause bleeding, pigment dispersion and often lead to glaucoma [6]; it can also cause cystoid macular edema [7]. In a meta-analysis by Mehta and Aref, the complication rate for single-piece acrylic IOLs in the sulcus is 83% for pigment dispersion, 80% for iris transillumination defects, 33% for an increase in intraocular pressure and 23% for hemorrhage [2, 6]. This so-called "iris chafing' can also be detected after explantation of the IOL through pigment granules on the anterior surface of the IOL; here, mainly the haptics and the area of the optic/haptic transition are affected [3]. Chronic iris contact can lead to iridocyclitis and cystoid macular edema and decentration of the IOL is also frequently observed. Currently, there are no large prospective studies on the complication rate of three-piece IOLs in the sulcus; however, it is assumed that the complication rates are lower due to the reduced thickness and added stability of the more rigid haptics.

Author's recommendation

Three-piece IOLs with thin haptics are best suited for implantation into the sulcus.

Choice of IOL Power

Due to the more anterior IOL position relative to the capsular bag, an adjustment of IOL power is necessary [8] and, in general, the IOL power must be reduced. In the studies currently available on the predictability of the target refraction, the greatest confounding factor is that some cases include optic capture while others do not. If no optic capture is performed, i.e. the entire IOL remains in the sulcus plane, Suto et al. showed myopic outcomes of mean -0.78 ± 0.47 D [9]. The capsular bag power IOL was thus 1.11 ± 0.67 D too strong, which is why a reduction of the IOL strength by 1.0 D was recommended. A similar finding was made by Bayramlar et al. [10] where, in a series of 162 eyes, a myopic shift of -1.02 ± 0.96 D was detected. Similarly, Dubey et al. were able to confirm the recommendation of reducing the power by 1.0 D in 36 eyes when "normal' IOL strengths of 18–25 D

Table 1 Rule of 9s

IOL power in the capsular bag	Adjusted IOL power in the sulcus (without optic capture)
0.0 – 9.0 D	No adjustment
9.5 – 18.0 D	Reduce by 0.50 D
18.5 – 27.0 D	Reduce by 1.00 D
> 27.5 D	Reduce by 1.50 D

were implanted; in contrast, lenses with a power > 25 D were recommended to be reduced by 1.5–2.0 D. The currently widely accepted rule of thumb is the "Rule of 9s" (Table 1) [2].

If optic capture (optics in the capsular bag, haptics in the sulcus) is possible, it can be assumed that no change in IOL power relative to positioning in the capsular bag is required [11]. In a study of 58 eyes, Millar et al. [11] compared the effect of optic capture (24 eyes; 41%) with complete placement in the sulcus (34 eyes; 59%). The difference between the two methods was reported to be 0.74 D in spherical equivalent, corresponding to about 1.0 D change in IOL power. Compared to the in-the-bag results of the same surgeon, a delta of +0.28 D was found for optic capture sulcus IOLs, so the authors recommend not to change the IOL power if optic capture is planned.

Author's recommendation

If optic capture is performed simultaneously with sulcus implantation, no adjustment of IOL power (relative to the positioning in the capsular bag) is necessary.

Results and Complication Rate

Only retrospective studies are available on the refractive results and the complication rate. It should be noted that important confounders exist with different IOL types and the inconsistent application of optic capture. As a result, most studies report "real life' results (e.g. planned optic capture that cannot be performed after implantation of the desired IOL power). Brunin et al. report in a study of 167 eyes with secondary IOL implantation that sulcus fixation (with and without optic capture) had the lowest complication rate and best visual acuity compared to anterior chamber IOLs, iris-fixated IOLs and scleral fixated IOLs. Best-corrected distance visual acuity of 20/40 and better was achieved in 98% with sulcus fixation and optic capture, 95% without optic capture, 70% with iris or scleral fixation, and 80% with anterior chamber fixation [7]. Seventy percent of eyes with sulcus fixation and no optic capture were within 0.50 D of target refraction; the percentage was 38% with optic capture. For iris, anterior chamber and scleral fixation, the percentages were 65, 63 and 37% respectively. Eighty % of sulcus fixated IOLs without optic capture were within 1.0 D, as compared to 83% with optic capture. For iris fixation, 88% were within 1.0 D, whereas anterior chamber fixation resulted in 80% and scleral fixation in 64%. The predicted residual refractive error was lowest for sulcus fixation compared to the other secondary fixation options (0.03 ± 0.75 D sulcus + optic capture; 0.02 ± 0.82 D sulcus −optic capture; −0.22 ± 0.86 D anterior chamber; −0.07 ± 0.62 D iris fixation; −0.23 ± 0.79 D transscleral fixation).

Using the SRK-T formula, Chang et al. compared the results with (9 eyes, 64%) and without optic capture (5 eyes, 36%) in 14 eyes [12]. In these cases, optic capture did not require any adjustment of IOL strength. 93% of the eyes had a visual acuity of 20/25 and better. There was no decentration in the optic capture group, while this was the case in 2 out of 5 eyes (40%) without optic capture.

Basically, the complication rate depends on the choice of the right IOL type. Common to all studies is that placement of an IOL in the sulcus can cause pigment dispersion, iris transillumination defects, ocular pressure increases, cystoid macular edema, decentration, dysphotopsia, anterior chamber/vascular hemorrhage and uveitis [3, 7]. Of all forms of secondary IOL fixation (scleral, anterior chamber, iris fixation), sulcus fixation with and without optic capture seems to be the safest if thin three-piece IOLs are used.

References

1. Taskapili M, Engin G, Kaya G, Kucuksahin H, Kocabora MS, Yilmazli C. Single-piece foldable acrylic intraocular lens implantation in the sulcus in eyes with posterior capsule tear during phacoemulsification. J Cataract Refract Surg. 2005;31(8):1593–7.
2. Mehta R, Aref AA. Intraocular Lens Implantation In The Ciliary Sulcus: Challenges And Risks. Clinical ophthalmology (Auckland, NZ). 2019;13:2317–23.
3. Chang DF, Masket S, Miller KM, Braga-Mele R, Little BC, Mamalis N, et al. Complications of sulcus placement of single-piece acrylic intraocular lenses: recommendations for backup IOL implantation following posterior capsule rupture. J Cataract Refract Surg. 2009;35 (8):1445–58.
4. Mohebbi M, Bashiri SA, Mohammadi SF, Samet B, Ghassemi F, Ashrafi E, et al. Outcome of Single-piece Intraocular Lens Sulcus Implantation following Posterior Capsular Rupture during Phacoemulsification. J Ophthalmic Vis Res. 2017;12(3):275–80.
5. Amino K, Yamakawa R. Long term results of out-of-the-bag intraocular lens implantation. J Cataract Refract Surg. 2000;26(2):266–70.
6. Uy HS, Chan PS. Pigment release and secondary glaucoma after implantation of single-piece acrylic intraocular lenses in the ciliary sulcus. At J Ophthalmol. 2006;142(2):330–2.
7. Brunin G, Sajjad A, Kim EJ, de,. Oca IM, Weikert MP, Wang L, et al Secondary intraocular lens implantation: Complication rates, visual acuity, and refractive outcomes. J Cataract Refract Surg. 2017;43(3):369–76.
8. Dubey R, Birchall W, Grigg J. Improved refractive outcome for ciliary sulcus-implanted intraocular lenses. Ophthalmology. 2012;119(2):261–5.
9. Suto C, Hori S, Fukuyama E, Akura J. Adjusting intraocular lens power for sulcus fixation. J Cataract Refract Surg. 2003;29(10):1913–7.

10. Bayramlar H, Hepsen IF, Yilmaz H. Myopic shift from the predicted refraction after sulcus fixation of PMMA posterior chamber intraocular lenses. Can J Ophthalmol. 2006;41 (1):78–82.
11. Millar ER, Allen D, Steel DH. Effect of anterior capsulorhexis optic capture of a sulcus-fixated intraocular lens on refractive outcomes. J Cataract Refract Surg. 2013;39 (6):841–4.
12. Chang JSM, Ng JCM, Chan VKC. Sulcus Fixation of a 3-Piece Diffractive Multifocal Intraocular Lens with and without Optic Capture in the Anterior Capsulorhexis. Ophthalmology. 2014;121(1):429-30.e2.

Systematic Overview on Secondary Intraocular Lenses

Daniel R. Muth and Wolfgang J. Mayer

Main Text

The number of secondary implanted intraocular lenses (IOL), often many years after the primary surgery, is currently on the rise. Since the beginnings of IOL implantation on 29th November 1949 by Sir Nicholas Harold Lloyd Ridley, the demographics of the cataract surgery patient has changed markedly. [4] While the global population has been continuously increasing, life expectancy has also increased. As a result, more people reach an age at which cataract clinically becomes clinically significant and cataract extraction with implantation of a primary IOL is performed (pseudophakic shift) [15, 31, 43, 48, 57, 69]. Moreover, as people get older and their implanted IOLs get older too (pseudophakic ageing) which increases the prevalence of IOL long-term complications [3]. The management of longer term IOL complications often includes explantation, with subsequent implantation of a secondary IOL. Many techniques and IOL models for secondary IOL implantation have been described.

Indications for secondary IOL implantation include IOL exchange due to spontaneous IOL dislocation (incidence ≈ 1,7% over 25 years) [46], IOL dislocation due to zonular weakness such as pseudoexfoliation (PEX) (prevalence ≈ 1:20) [27], Marfan's syndrome (prevalence ≈ 1:10,000) [47], Ehlers-Danlos'

D. R. Muth (✉) · W. J. Mayer
Department of Ophthalmology, University Hospital, LMU Munich, Munich, Germany
e-mail: dr-muth@t-online.de

W. J. Mayer
e-mail: wolfgang.j.mayer@med.uni-muenchen.de

D. R. Muth
Department of Ophthalmology, University Hospital Zurich (USZ), University of Zurich, Zurich, Switzerland

D. R. Muth
University of Zurich (UZH), Zurich, Switzerland

M. Shajari et al. (eds.), *Cataract and Lens Surgery*,
https://doi.org/10.1007/978-3-031-05394-8_78

syndrome (prevalence ≈ 1:10,000) [56], Weill-Marchesani's syndrome (prevalence ≈ 1:100,000) [59], homocystinuria (variable prevalence) [40, 51], high myopia [14], IOL biomaterial issues such as opacification, glistening or breaks of the haptics, induced intraocular inflammation such as uveitis glaucoma hyphema (UGH) syndrome, corneal endothelial decompensation, iris damage such as iris chafing (incidence ≈ 1% per year) [9, 11, 16] (Fig. 1). More recent indications for explantation and subsequent secondary lens implantation include dissatisfied patients because of refractive surprise, ill-fitting IOL type such as multifocal IOLs. Furthermore, a secondary IOL implantation might be necessary in aphakic patients after congenital cataract extraction, after vitrectomy, [21] after complicated previous surgery with posterior capsule rupture (PCR) (prevalence ≈ 1–3%) [8, 52] or after trauma [10, 12, 14, 24, 62].

Secondary IOL Implantation

If the patient is already pseudophakic, surgical revision with refixation of the existing IOL should be the primary goal. Depending on what anatomical structures are still intact, the existing IOL can either be put back into the capsular bag or (if the IOL model is appropriate e.g. three-piece IOLs), in the ciliary sulcus. In some cases and depending on the lens, scleral refixation of the primary IOL is sometimes possible and is usually less invasive than IOL exchange, but this should only be considered by an experienced surgeon [21]. In all other cases, when aphakia is not an option, secondary IOL implantation is the solution.

Which option to choose for secondary IOL implantation depends on the amount of residual anatomical capsular or iris support of the patient, on the material and design of the primary IOL and on the expertise of the ophthalmic surgeon.

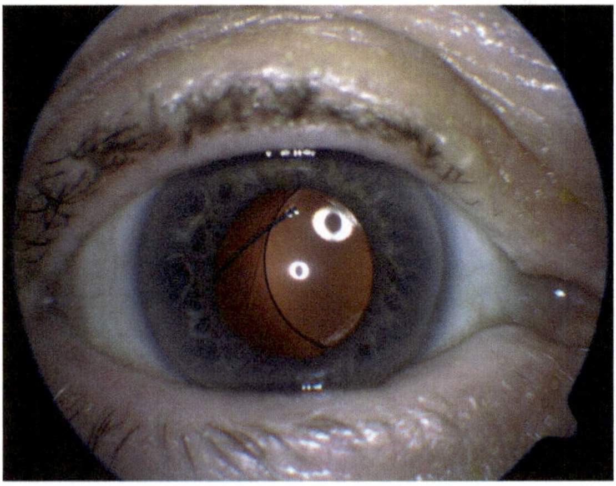

Fig. 1 Dislocated IOL

Secondary Implantation in the Capsular Bag

If the capsular bag is still intact and no posterior capsulotomy had been performed a secondary IOL implantation in the capsular bag should be possible and is considered the "golden standard" [55]. If the capsular bag turns out to be fibrotic, careful dissection of the capsular bag and gentle insertion of a capsular tension ring (CTR) may be necessary. This implantation technique has the advantage of offering the full IOL portfolio as well as the full range of proven biometric formulas without the need of estimated manual formula corrections. Centration of a secondary IOL in a highly fibrotic capsular bag, however, is not always possible. (Fig. 2)

Secondary Implantation in the Ciliary Sulcus

With an existing but compromised capsular bag (e.g. after posterior capsulotomy) secondary IOL implantation in the ciliary sulcus may be possible and should be the preferred implantation method when using the bag is not possible. Using a three-piece IOL design allows the IOL optic to be pushed through the anterior capsulorhexis into the area of capsular bag while the haptics remain within the ciliary sulcus (so called "optic capture") [19, 38, 58]. Optic capture allows to use the standard "in-the-bag" biometric calculations. If placed entirely in the ciliary sulcus the IOL optic sits approximately 0.5 mm more anteriorly then compared to an in-the-bag position leading to a myopic shift. The myopic shift has to be taken into account before IOL implantation by choosing a different IOL power. Approximation of the reduction factor are the "Rule of 9 s" or the correction table by *Warren E. Hill*. [38, 22] Advantages of the IOL implantation in the ciliary sulcus are the reliable IOL power calculation and the relative simplicity of the lens fixation. However, three-piece IOLs should be preferred as complications due to sulcus implantation are mainly described in association with using single-piece IOLs [37]. Complications include iris chafing with pigment dispersion and iris

Fig. 2 Therapeutic strategy

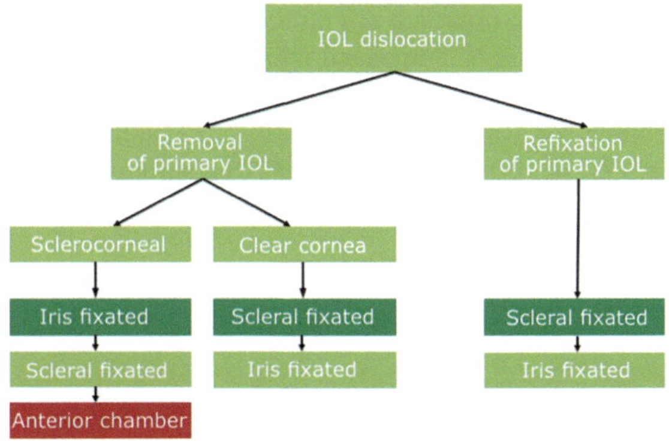

transillumination defects resulting in recurrent iridocyclitis or uveitis-glaucoma-hyphema (UGH) syndrome with rise of intraocular pressure (IOP) and cystoid macular edema (CME) [9, 38].

Iris Fixation

As IOLs made of polymethyl methacrylate (PMMA) are neither foldable nor can they be cut intraocularly they need to be explanted via a sclero-corneal tunnel. The tunnel can then be used afterwards for iris-fixated lens implantation. Two iris-fixated IOL variants exist: iris-clip IOLs based on the original designs of *Brinkhorst* and iris-claw IOLs based on the original designs of *Worst* [18]. Both can be implanted in the anteriorly on the iris(AC) or in the posterior chamber (PC), attached to the back of the iris. Complication rates with the corneal endothelium are higher with AC implantation [39].The general advantage of iris fixated IOLs is the quick and relatively easy surgical procedure. Studies to date have not shown statistically significant differences in long-term complications when compared to scleral fixation [25]. As all currently available iris fixation IOLs are made of non-foldable PMMA, a larger sclero-corneal tunnel is necessary, increasing the risk of surgically induced astigmatism (SIA) or wound healing problems.

Scleral Fixation

If a foldable primary IOL made of acrylate or silicone is extracted via a smaller incision, a scleral fixated IOL will generally be the more favorable option, as a broad range of foldable IOLs is available. Scleral fixation techniques are also useful in cases where large iris defects or an instable iris diaphragm in pseudoexfoliation (PEX) patients mean that iris fixation is not an option. Most foldable IOL types can be cut intraocularly for explantation through a clear corneal incision. Basically, any IOL type, be it single-piece or three-piece, plate haptics or loop haptics, is suitable for scleral suturing but scleral fixation via flanged haptic ends described by *Yamane* et al. can only be performed with three-piece IOLs with thin haptics [67]. Recently, scleral IOL fixation offers the possibility of implanting toric and multifocal IOLs to correct for astigmatism either by suture, sutureless with a scleral tunnel or using a specialized IOL design with “T”-shaped transscleral haptic plugs [26, 29, 42, 50, 60, 65].

Sutured IOL Scleral Fixation

First described 1981 by *Girard,* sutured sclera fixation is still a relatively young technique [20]. *Lewis* et al. described the use of polypropylene sutures in combination with scleral pockets that were later modified by Hoffman et al. [23, 34]. This so called "Hoffman technique" requires two scleral pockets on the 0°–180° axis, one at the nasal and one at the temporal side. A 10–0 or 9–0 polypropylene (e.g. Johnson and Johnson Ethicon Prolene®) suture is attached to each of the haptics via clove hitch or cow hitch and some IOL types are designed with specific eyelets to thread the suture. The ends of the sutures are armed with a straight long needle. Within the anterior chamber the straight needles are docked into a 27-gauge cannula to externalize the sutures. The suture is then knotted externally, and the knot is buried within the scleral pocket. Originally, 10–0 polypropylene sutures were used but [7] as suture-associated complications such as breaks were seen, thicker 9–0 or 8–0 polypropylene sutures are recommended [6, 64]. Alternatively, a monofilament expanded polytetrafluoroethylene (ePTFE) (GoreTex CV-8®) can be used for scleral fixation. The GoreTex CV-8® suture is about the same thickness as a 7–0 Prolene® suture and therefore should have a better long-term stability [32, 49]. Basically, the full-range IOL portfolio is suitable for the sutured scleral fixation technique. However, sutured IOL scleral fixation is a time-consuming procedure and has a steep learning curve for the ophthalmic surgeon.

Sutureless Scleral Fixation

Approaches for sutureless IOL scleral fixation have been proposed since 1997 with the goal of simplifying and speeding up scleral fixation [36, 54]. Four main types of sutureless IOL scleral fixation with slight modifications are currently used: (a) Sutureless and glueless burial of the externalized IOL haptics within a scleral tunnel [17, 63]; (b) glued IOL haptics under sclera flaps [2, 41]; (c) Transscleral externalization of haptics and flange of haptic ends using cautery ("Yamane technique"). [5, 67]; (d) specialized IOL designs with "T"-shaped transscleral haptic plugs to be externalized through a scleral pocket (e.g. Soleko Carlevale®) [60].

Long-Term Stability

Literature review on this topic reveals numerous studies having evaluated the long-term stability of secondary fixated IOLs (Table 1).

While this literature overview is not exhaustive, it does show that secondary IOL implantation provides a long-term solution for visual acuity with moderate dislocation rates. However, long-term complications such as IOL tilt, suture-associated

Table 1 Literature overview

IOL fixation technique	Study group	Eyes evaluated	Mean (minimal) follow-up time [months]	Dislocation rate (%)
Suture: Polypropylene (10–0)	Kokame et al. [33]	118	72 (24)	3.4
Suture: Polypropylene (10–0)	Vote et al. [61]	63	43.5 (12)	28.0
Suture: Polypropylene (10–0)	Sindal et al. [54]	50	12 (12)	2.0
Suture: Polypropylene (8–0)	Brandt et al. [6]	338	2 (2)	1.8
Suture: Polypropylene (10–0), Z-suture	Dimopoulos et al. [13]	66	64 (36)	16.7
Suture: Polypropylene (9–0), Z-suture	Wasiluk et al. [64]	29	60 (50)	13.8
Suture: GoreTex	Khan et al. [32]	85	11 (3)	0
Suture: GoreTex	Patel et al. [44]	49	7 (1)	0
Sutureless: scleral tunnel	Prasad [45]	6	3 (3)	16.7
Sutureless: scleral tunnel	Abbey et al. [1]	8	11.8 (3)	0
Sutureless: scleral tunnel	Shuaib et al. [53]	15	6 (6)	0
Sutureless: scleral tunnel	Kelkar et al. [28]	30	11.5 (9)	0
Sutureless: scleral tunnel	Sindal et al. [54]	59	12 (12)	0
Sutureless: scleral tunnel	Madhivanan et al. [35]	56	12 (12)	1.8
Sutureless: flanged haptics (Yamane)	Kelkar et al. [30]	60	12 (1.5)	0
Sutureless: flanged haptics (Yamane)	Yamane et al. [67]	100	20.6 (6)	0
Sutureless: flanged haptics (modified Yamane)	Kelkar et al. [28]	40	8.6 (7)	0
Sutureless: flanged haptics (modified Yamane)	Yavuzer et al. [68]	21	3 (3)	0
Sutureless: Carlevale	Veronese et al. [60]	4	6.5 (5)	0
Sutureless: Carlevale	Rossi et al. [50]	78	10.2 (*not stated*)	0

(continued)

Table 1 (continued)

IOL fixation technique	Study group	Eyes evaluated	Mean (minimal) follow-up time [months]	Dislocation rate (%)
Iris: iris clip	Kelkar et al. [30]	90	12 (1.5)	0
Iris: iris clip	Vounotrypidis et al. [62]	40	17 (3)	0
Iris: iris clip	Madhivanan et al. [35]	48	12 (12)	0

complications like suture erosion and iris-associated complications such as iris damage with pupil distortion and pigment dispersion may be underreported in current literature [25, 39, 66].

Conclusion

Currently, no concrete recommendation can be made on superiority of a single secondary IOL implantation technique. Moreover, additional factors tip the scale in the decision process such as surgical approach (clear cornea vs. sclerocorneal), IOL design (three-piece vs. single-piece), anatomical conditions (capsular bag status, iris status).

Consequently, for the ophthalmic surgeon, it is advisable to be familiar with more than one secondary IOL implantation technique. The experience of the ophthalmic surgeon with the secondary IOL technique(s) seems to be more important than the surgeon's choice of the used technique.

References

1. Abbey AM, Hussain RM, Shah AR, Faia LJ, Wolfe JD, Williams GA. Sutureless scleral fixation of intraocular lenses: outcomes of two approaches: the 2014 Yasuo Tano Memorial Lecture. Graefes Arch Clin Exp Ophthalmol. 2015;253(1):1–5. https://doi.org/10.1007/s00417-014-2834-9.
2. Agarwal A, Kumar DA, Jacob S, Baid C, Agarwal A, Srinivasan S. Fibrin glue-assisted sutureless posterior chamber intraocular lens implantation in eyes with deficient posterior capsules. J Cataract Refract Surg. 2008;34(9):1433–8. https://doi.org/10.1016/j.jcrs.2008.04.040.
3. Ascaso FJ, Huerva V, Grzybowski A. Epidemiology, etiology, and prevention of late IOL-capsular bag complex dislocation: review of the literature. J Ophthalmol. 2015;2015:805706. https://doi.org/10.1155/2015/805706.
4. Auffarth GU, Schmidbauer J, Apple DJ. The life work of Sir Nicholas Harold Lloyd Ridley. Ophthalmologe. 2001;98(11):1012–6. https://doi.org/10.1007/s003470170019.

5. Bonnell AC, Mantopoulos D, Wheatley HM, Prenner JL. Surgical technique for sutureless intrascleral fixation of a 3-piece intraocular lens using a 30-gauge needle. Retina. 2019;39 (Suppl 1):S13–5. https://doi.org/10.1097/IAE.0000000000001889.
6. Brandt L, Petersen J, Callizo J, Bemme S, Pfeiffer S, Hoerauf H, et al. Complications in sutured scleral fixation of artificial lens implantation. Ophthalmologe. 2019;116(12):1200–6. https://doi.org/10.1007/s00347-019-0896-0.
7. Buckley EG. Hanging by a thread: the long-term efficacy and safety of transscleral sutured intraocular lenses in children (an American Ophthalmological Society thesis). Trans Am Ophthalmol Soc. 2007;105:294–311. https://www.ncbi.nlm.nih.gov/pubmed/18427618.
8. Chakrabarti A, Nazm N. Posterior capsular rent: prevention and management. Indian J Ophthalmol. 2017;65(12):1359–69. https://doi.org/10.4103/ijo.IJO_1057_17.
9. Chang DF, Masket S, Miller KM, Braga-Mele R, Little BC, Mamalis N, et al. Complications of sulcus placement of single-piece acrylic intraocular lenses: recommendations for backup IOL implantation following posterior capsule rupture. J Cataract Refract Surg. 2009;35 (8):1445–58. https://doi.org/10.1016/j.jcrs.2009.04.027.
10. Clark A, Morlet N, Ng JQ, Preen DB, Semmens JB. Whole population trends in complications of cataract surgery over 22 years in Western Australia. Ophthalmology. 2011;118(6):1055–61. https://doi.org/10.1016/j.ophtha.2010.11.001.
11. Crowell EL. Uveitis-glaucoma-hyphema syndrome. eyewiki.aao.org/Uveitis-Glaucoma-Hyphema_Syndrome. Accessed 22 Dec 2019 (2019).
12. Davies EC, Pineda R 2nd. Intraocular lens exchange surgery at a tertiary referral center: indications, complications, and visual outcomes. J Cataract Refract Surg. 2016;42(9):1262–7. https://doi.org/10.1016/j.jcrs.2016.06.031.
13. Dimopoulos S, Dimopoulos V, Blumenstock G, Trevino-Rodriguez H, Bartz-Schmidt KU, Spitzer MS, et al. Long-term outcome of scleral-fixated posterior chamber intraocular lens implantation with the knotless Z-suture technique. J Cataract Refract Surg. 2018;44(2):182–5. https://doi.org/10.1016/j.jcrs.2017.11.009.
14. Fernandez-Buenaga R, Alio JL, Perez-Ardoy AL, Larrosa-Quesada A, Pinilla-Cortes L, Barraquer R, et al. Late in-the-bag intraocular lens dislocation requiring explantation: risk factors and outcomes. Eye (Lond). 2013;27(7):795–801; quiz 802. https://doi.org/10.1038/eye.2013.95.
15. Flaxman SR, Bourne RRA, Resnikoff S, Ackland P, Braithwaite T, Cicinelli MV, et al. Global causes of blindness and distance vision impairment 1990–2020: a systematic review and meta-analysis. Lancet Glob Health. 2017;5(12):e1221–34. https://doi.org/10.1016/S2214-109X(17)30393-5.
16. Foroozan R, Tabas JG, Moster ML. Recurrent microhyphema despite intracapsular fixation of a posterior chamber intraocular lens. J Cataract Refract Surg. 2003;29(8):1632–5. https://doi.org/10.1016/s0886-3350(03)00122-6.
17. Gabor SG, Pavlidis MM. Sutureless intrascleral posterior chamber intraocular lens fixation. J Cataract Refract Surg. 2007;33(11):1851–4. https://doi.org/10.1016/j.jcrs.2007.07.013.
18. Galvis V, Tello A, Rangel CM, Carreño NI, Berrospi RD, Niño CA. Letter: Iris-clip versus iris-claw intraocular lenses (Letter). J Cataract Refract Surg. 2018;44(11):1.
19. Gimbel HV, DeBroff BM. Intraocular lens optic capture. J Cataract Refract Surg. 2004;30 (1):200–6. https://doi.org/10.1016/j.jcrs.2003.11.035.
20. Girard LJ. Pars plana phacoprosthesis (aphakic intraocular implant): a preliminary report. Ophthalmic Surg. 1981;12(1):19–22. https://www.ncbi.nlm.nih.gov/pubmed/7231865.
21. Hayashi K, Hirata A, Hayashi H. Possible predisposing factors for in-the-bag and out-of-the-bag intraocular lens dislocation and outcomes of intraocular lens exchange surgery. Ophthalmology. 2007;114(5):969–75. https://doi.org/10.1016/j.ophtha.2006.09.017.
22. Hill W. Calculating bag vs. sulcus IOL power. East Valley Ophthalmology; 2020. https://doctor-hill.com/iol-power-calculations/bag-vs-sulcus/. Accessed 23 May 2020.
23. Hoffman RS, Fine IH, Packer M. Scleral fixation without conjunctival dissection. J Cataract Refract Surg. 2006;32(11):1907–12. https://doi.org/10.1016/j.jcrs.2006.05.029.

24. Jakobsson G, Zetterberg M, Lundstrom M, Stenevi U, Grenmark R, Sundelin K. Late dislocation of in-the-bag and out-of-the bag intraocular lenses: ocular and surgical characteristics and time to lens repositioning. J Cataract Refract Surg. 2010;36(10):1637–44. https://doi.org/10.1016/j.jcrs.2010.04.042.
25. Jing W, Guanlu L, Qianyin Z, Shuyi L, Fengying H, Jian L, et al. Iris-claw intraocular lens and scleral-fixated posterior chamber intraocular lens implantations in correcting aphakia: a meta-analysis. Invest Ophthalmol Vis Sci. 2017;58(9):3530–6. https://doi.org/10.1167/iovs.16-21226.
26. Jun JH, Bang SP. Transscleral fixation of a toric intraocular lens by a slipable suture technique. Can J Ophthalmol. 2018;53(1):e29–32. https://doi.org/10.1016/j.jcjo.2017.06.011.
27. Kanski JJ, Bowling B. Kanski's clinical ophthalmology. Elsevier: W.B. Saunders Ldt.; 2015.
28. Kelkar A, Kelkar J, Kothari A, Mehta H, Chitale S, Fogla R, et al. Comparison of two modified sutureless techniques of scleral fixation of intraocular lens. Ophthalmic Surg Lasers Imaging Retina. 2018;49(10):e129–34. https://doi.org/10.3928/23258160-20181002-15.
29. Kelkar A, Shah R, Kelkar J, Kelkar S, Arora E. Sutureless, glueless, scleral fixation of single-piece and toric intraocular lens: a novel technique. Case Rep Ophthalmol. 2015;6(2):239–45. https://doi.org/10.1159/000437349.
30. Kelkar AS, Kelkar JA, Kothari AA, Kelkar SB. Comparison of flanged intrascleral intraocular lens fixation versus iris claw intraocular lens fixation: a retrospective study. Indian J Ophthalmol. 2019;67(11):1838–42. https://doi.org/10.4103/ijo.IJO_300_19.
31. Khairallah M, Kahloun R, Bourne R, Limburg H, Flaxman SR, Jonas JB, et al. Number of people blind or visually impaired by cataract worldwide and in world regions, 1990 to 2010. Invest Ophthalmol Vis Sci. 2015;56(11):6762–9. https://doi.org/10.1167/iovs.15-17201.
32. Khan MA, Gupta OP, Smith RG, Ayres BD, Raber IM, Bailey RS, et al. Scleral fixation of intraocular lenses using Gore-Tex suture: clinical outcomes and safety profile. Br J Ophthalmol. 2016;100(5):638–43. https://doi.org/10.1136/bjophthalmol-2015-306839.
33. Kokame GT, Yanagihara RT, Shantha JG, Kaneko KN. Long-term outcome of pars plana vitrectomy and sutured scleral-fixated posterior chamber intraocular lens implantation or repositioning. Am J Ophthalmol. 2018;189:10–6. https://doi.org/10.1016/j.ajo.2018.01.034.
34. Lewis JS. Ab externo sulcus fixation. Ophthalmic Surg. 1991;22(11):692–5. https://www.ncbi.nlm.nih.gov/pubmed/1792035.
35. Madhivanan N, Sengupta S, Sindal M, Nivean PD, Kumar MA, Ariga M. Comparative analysis of retropupillary iris claw versus scleral-fixated intraocular lens in the management of post-cataract aphakia. Indian J Ophthalmol. 2019;67(1):59–63. https://doi.org/10.4103/ijo.IJO_326_18.
36. Maggi R, Maggi C. Sutureless scleral fixation of intraocular lenses. J Cataract Refract Surg. 1997;23(9):1289–94. https://doi.org/10.1016/s0886-3350(97)80104-6.
37. Mamalis N. Sulcus placement of single-piece acrylic intraocular lenses. J Cataract Refract Surg. 2009;35(8):1327–8. https://doi.org/10.1016/j.jcrs.2009.06.001.
38. Mehta R, Aref AA. Intraocular lens implantation in the ciliary sulcus: challenges and risks. Clin Ophthalmol. 2019;13:2317–23. https://doi.org/10.2147/OPTH.S205148.
39. Mohr A, Hengerer F, Eckardt C. [Retropupillary fixation of the iris claw lens in aphakia. 1 year outcome of a new implantation techniques]. Ophthalmologe. 2002;99(7):580–3. https://doi.org/10.1007/s00347-001-0563-z.
40. Morris AA, Kozich V, Santra S, Andria G, Ben-Omran TI, Chakrapani AB, et al. Guidelines for the diagnosis and management of cystathionine beta-synthase deficiency. J Inherit Metab Dis. 2017;40(1):49–74. https://doi.org/10.1007/s10545-016-9979-0.
41. Narang P, Agarwal A. Glued intrascleral haptic fixation of an intraocular lens. Indian J Ophthalmol. 2017;65(12):1370–80. https://doi.org/10.4103/ijo.IJO_643_17.
42. Pan Q, Yang Z, Chen X, Wei W, Ke Z, Chen D, et al. Suturing technique for scleral fixation of toric intraocular lens in the traumatic aphakic eye with corneal astigmatism. Eur J Ophthalmol. 2019;29(1):100–5. https://doi.org/10.1177/1120672118769522.
43. Pascolini D, Mariotti SP. Global estimates of visual impairment: 2010. Br J Ophthalmol. 2012;96(5):614–8. https://doi.org/10.1136/bjophthalmol-2011-300539.

44. Patel NA, Shah P, Yannuzzi NA, Ansari Z, Zaveri JS, Relhan N, et al. Clinical outcomes of 4-point scleral fixated 1-piece hydrophobic acrylic equiconvex intraocular lens using polytetrafluoroethylene suture. Clin Ophthalmol. 2018;12:2145–8. https://doi.org/10.2147/OPTH.S174211.
45. Prasad S. Transconjunctival sutureless haptic fixation of posterior chamber IOL: a minimally traumatic approach for IOL rescue or secondary implantation. Retina. 2013;33(3):657–60. https://doi.org/10.1097/IAE.0b013e31827b6499.
46. Pueringer SL, Hodge DO, Erie JC. Risk of late intraocular lens dislocation after cataract surgery, 1980–2009: a population-based study. Am J Ophthalmol. 2011;152(4):618–23. https://doi.org/10.1016/j.ajo.2011.03.009.
47. Raghunath M, Nienaber C, Kodolitsch Yv. 100 Jahre Marfan-Syndrom -eine Bestandsaufnahme. Dtsch Arztebl Int. 1997;94(13):821. https://www.aerzteblatt.de/int/article.asp?id=5694.
48. Rao GN, Khanna R, Payal A. The global burden of cataract. Curr Opin Ophthalmol. 2011;22(1):4–9. https://doi.org/10.1097/ICU.0b013e3283414fc8.
49. Roach L, Eden RA, Gupta OP, Rubenstein JB. Gore-tex: an alternative for fixation sutures. Eyenet Mag 2016:3. https://www.aao.org/eyenet/article/gore-tex-alternative-fixation-sutures.
50. Rossi T, Iannetta D, Romano V, Carlevale C, Forlini M, Telani S, et al. A novel intraocular lens designed for sutureless scleral fixation: surgical series. Graefes Arch Clin Exp Ophthalmol. 2021;259(1):257–62. https://doi.org/10.1007/s00417-020-04789-3.
51. Sacharow SJ, Picker JD, Levy HL. Homocystinuria caused by cystathionine beta-synthase deficiency. In: Adam MP, Ardinger HH, Pagon RA, Wallace SE, Bean LJH, Stephens K, et al. (eds.) GeneReviews((R)). Seattle (WA); 1993. https://www.ncbi.nlm.nih.gov/pubmed/20301697.
52. Salowi MA, Chew FLM, Adnan TH, King C, Ismail M, Goh PP. The Malaysian cataract surgery registry: risk indicators for posterior capsular rupture. Br J Ophthalmol. 2017;101(11):1466–70. https://doi.org/10.1136/bjophthalmol-2016-309902.
53. Shuaib AM, El Sayed Y, Kamal A, El Sanabary Z, Elhilali H. Transscleral sutureless intraocular lens versus retropupillary iris-claw lens fixation for paediatric aphakia without capsular support: a randomized study. Acta Ophthalmol. 2019;97(6):e850–9. https://doi.org/10.1111/aos.14090.
54. Sindal MD, Nakhwa CP, Sengupta S. Comparison of sutured versus sutureless scleral-fixated intraocular lenses. J Cataract Refract Surg. 2016;42(1):27–34. https://doi.org/10.1016/j.jcrs.2015.09.019.
55. Srinivasan VJ, Adler DC, Chen Y, Gorczynska I, Huber R, Duker JS, et al. Ultrahigh-speed optical coherence tomography for three-dimensional and en face imaging of the retina and optic nerve head. Invest Ophthalmol Vis Sci. 2008;49(11):5103–10. https://doi.org/10.1167/iovs.08-2127.
56. Steinmann B. Das Ehlers-Danlos-Syndrom: Klinik – Einteilung – Pathogenese. In: Luttkus A, editor. Das Ehlers-Danlos-Syndrom : eine interdisziplinäre Herausforderung. Berlin: Walter de Gruyter GmbH & Co. KG; 2011. p. 1–11.
57. Stevens GA, White RA, Flaxman SR, Price H, Jonas JB, Keeffe J, et al. Global prevalence of vision impairment and blindness: magnitude and temporal trends, 1990–2010. Ophthalmology. 2013;120(12):2377–84. https://doi.org/10.1016/j.ophtha.2013.05.025.
58. Tian T, Chen C, Jin H, Jiao L, Zhang Q, Zhao P. Capture of intraocular lens optic by residual capsular opening in secondary implantation: long-term follow-up. BMC Ophthalmol. 2018;18(1):84. https://doi.org/10.1186/s12886-018-0741-2.
59. Tsilou E, MacDonald IM. Weill-marchesani syndrome. In: Adam MP, Ardinger HH, Pagon RA, Wallace SE, Bean LJH, Stephens K, et al. (eds), GeneReviews((R)). Seattle (WA); 1993. https://www.ncbi.nlm.nih.gov/pubmed/20301293.
60. Veronese C, Maiolo C, Armstrong GW, Primavera L, Torrazza C, Della Mora L, et al. New surgical approach for sutureless scleral fixation. Eur J Ophthalmol. 2020;30(3):612–5. https://doi.org/10.1177/1120672120902020.

61. Vote BJ, Tranos P, Bunce C, Charteris DG, Da Cruz L. Long-term outcome of combined pars plana vitrectomy and scleral fixated sutured posterior chamber intraocular lens implantation. Am J Ophthalmol. 2006;141(2):308–12. https://doi.org/10.1016/j.ajo.2005.09.012.
62. Vounotrypidis E, Schuster I, Mackert MJ, Kook D, Priglinger S, Wolf A. Secondary intraocular lens implantation: a large retrospective analysis. Graefes Arch Clin Exp Ophthalmol. 2019;257(1):125–34. https://doi.org/10.1007/s00417-018-4178-3.
63. Walia S, Kashyap S, Bhaisare V, Rawat P, Kori N. Novel technique of sutureless glueless scleral fixated intraocular lens (SFIOL). Indian J Ophthalmol. 2019;67(1):64–8. https://doi.org/10.4103/ijo.IJO_447_18.
64. Wasiluk E, Krasnicki P, Dmuchowska DA, Proniewska-Skretek E, Mariak Z. The implantation of the scleral-fixated posterior chamber intraocular lens with 9/0 polypropylene sutures-Long-term visual outcomes and complications. Adv Med Sci. 2019;64(1):100–3. https://doi.org/10.1016/j.advms.2018.08.005.
65. Whang WJ, Kwon H, Jeon S. Application of a four-flanged intrascleral fixation technique for toric and multifocal intraocular lenses. Am J Ophthalmol Case Rep. 2020;20: 100933. https://doi.org/10.1016/j.ajoc.2020.100933.
66. Wolter-Roessler M, Kuchle M. Correction of aphakia with retroiridally fixated IOL. Klin Monbl Augenheilkd. 2008;225(12):1041–4. https://doi.org/10.1055/s-2008-1027721.
67. Yamane S, Sato S, Maruyama-Inoue M, Kadonosono K. Flanged intrascleral intraocular lens fixation with double-needle technique. Ophthalmology. 2017;124(8):1136–42. https://doi.org/10.1016/j.ophtha.2017.03.036.
68. Yavuzer K, Evcimen Y. Sutureless transconjunctival intrascleral intraocular lens fixation: the modified Yamane technique. Arq Bras Oftalmol. 2019;82(5):389–93. https://doi.org/10.5935/0004-2749.20190072.
69. Zvornicanin J, Zvornicanin E. Premium intraocular lenses: the past, present and future. J Curr Ophthalmol. 2018;30(4):287–96. https://doi.org/10.1016/j.joco.2018.04.003.

Systematic Review of Add-on Intaocular Lenses

Benedikt Schworm

Add-on intraocular lenses (IOLs) are lenses implanted into the ciliary sulcus in addition to an existing capsular bag IOL to create a state of pseudopolyphakia. The most common indications for the implantation of an add-on IOL are postoperative ametropia and treatment of pseudophakic accommodation loss (by way of adding a multifocal optic). In the literature, they are often referred to as "secondary piggy-back" IOLs. Add-on IOLs are available in all common optical variants, being monofocal, monofocal-toric, multifocal and multifocal-toric lenses. The calculation of the lens power is usually simpler than the calculation of the primary lens and is based on the patient's subjective refraction. This chapter summarizes data available in the literature on the effectiveness and safety of add-on IOLs. Only studies with a case number of $\geq$ 10 eyes were included. In addition, only studies investigating specifically designed add-on IOLs were included, as there are many publications in the older literature (before 2010) with IOLs that were not designed for the purpose of add-on implantation. The summarized studies include all lens types that are currently on the market (Sulcoflex by Rayner Intraocular Lenses, Add-On by Human Optics, Erlangen, Germany, 1stQ Add-On by 1stQ GmbH, Mannheim, Germany, Cristalens Reverso, Cristalens, Eragny, France).

B. Schworm (✉)
Department of Ophthalmology, University Hospital of Munich, LMU, München, Germany
e-mail: benedikt.schworm@med.uni-muenchen.de

M. Shajari et al. (eds.), *Cataract and Lens Surgery*,
https://doi.org/10.1007/978-3-031-05394-8_79

Data on Correction of Refractive Errors in Pseudophakic Patients by Add-on Iols

Correction of the Spherical Refractive Error

There are no systematic reviews and no prospective randomized controlled trials in the literature on these lenses. There is one prospective case series without a comparison group [9], the other studies are retrospective evaluations [4, 7, 10, 18].

Regarding refractive success, the results are consistently good and the percentage of patients reaching a target refraction in a range of ± 0.5 diopters is 89.5% on average (weighted mean, n = 163). In the two largest study collectives, uncorrected distance visual acuity improved from 0.28 ± 0.16 to 0.01 ± 0.1 (logMAR) [18] and from 0.22 ± 0.12 to 0.04 ± 0.12 (logMAR) [7]. Few postoperative complications are reported, mainly decentrations (7% and 8% in each of two studies). No lens-associated complications requiring explantation were reported in any study. The complications described in older studies than those included here – interlenticular opacification, postoperative intraocular pressure rise, optic capture in the pupil, pigment dispersion due to rubbing of edges on the posterior iris, secondary pigment dispersion glaucoma – are largely attributable to the types of lenses used at that time.

Keypoint

The add-on intraocular lenses currently on the market have been optimized with regard to their intended use (concave posterior curvature, large optics, flat profile, rounded edges, rotation-stable haptics). Therefore, the overall likelihood of lentogenic complications is considered to be low.

There is no published study comparing an add-on lens with corneal surface ablation procedures for the correction of refractive errors. The only review article on this topic dates from 2014 and concludes that in terms of refractive predictability, add-on implantation is superior to IOL exchange, but the more accurate correction is still possible with LASIK [1].

Keypoint

There is insufficient data in the existing literature to compare the effectiveness of add-on lenses versus corneal ablation procedures for postoperative refractive correction.

Correction of Astigmatism

There are four publications on the use of a toric add-on lenses to correct high postoperative residual astigmatism, all of them retrospective evaluations [5, 8, 12, 13]. In three of the four publications, the indication for an add-on implantation was high astigmatism after corneal transplantation.

The largest case series on implantation of toric add-on IOLs was published by McLintock and co-authors in 2019. The study investigates refractive correction of pseudophakic eyes with penetrating keratoplasty (n = 19) and without keratoplasty (n = 32). On average, astigmatism was reduced from 2.51 ± 2.08 to 1.32 ± 1.56 diopters in the whole group. The eyes with keratoplasty performed worse in terms of uncorrected visual acuity and achieved refraction: the percentage of patients with uncorrected visual acuity of 0.3 LogMAR (0.5 decimal) or better was 85% in the group without keratoplasty versus 56% in the group with keratoplasty, and the target refraction ± 0.5 diopters was achieved in 84% in the group without keratoplasty versus 34% in the keratoplasty group. The slightly worse refractive outcome of the eyes after keratoplasty were ultimately attributed to the irregular component of astigmatism by the authors. The high rate of IOL-rotation of 62% in the entire collective is striking, possibly indicating insufficient rotational stability of the add-on IOL used (in this case the toric variant of the Rayner Sulcoflex). In the second largest published cohort by Hassenstein and coauthors (n = 15, all after penetrating keratoplasty), astigmatism was reduced from a mean of −6.5 ± 2.85 diopters to -1.0 ± 1.34 diopters, and uncorrected visual acuity improved from 0.05 ± 0.09 (decimal) to 0.4 ± 0.23 (decimal). The toric version of 1stQ Add-on was used in this study. No IOL-rotation was reported, one lens (=6.7%) had to be exchanged due to a haptic defect.

Conclusion

Add-on intraocular lenses are an effective and safe option to correct refractive errors in pseudophakic patients. However, this statement is based on limited evidence (no randomized-controlled trials, largely retrospective case series).

Add-on Intraocular Lenses for Correction of Presbyopia

There are currently no meta-analyses in the literature on the success and safety of multifocal add-on intraocular lenses. However, there are several prospective and retrospective studies with and without comparison groups [2, 6, 11, 14–16, 19]. Here, secondary implantation in pseudophakic eyes versus primary implantation of both lenses as a “duet” in one surgical procedure have to be distinguished. The available randomized-controlled trials have both been performed for duet implantation.

The first randomized-controlled trial for duet implantation was published in 2014 by Schrecker et al. The compared groups were primary capsular bag multifocal-IOL (n = 25) vs. duet implantation (n = 29). The lenses used in each case were the capsular bag-fixed Diff-aA and the add-on model Diff-sPB combined with the monofocal Aspira-aA from the manufacturer Human Optics. Visual outcomes after one year were comparable in both groups (uncorrected visual acuity in add-on group: near 0.07 ± 0.0, intermediate 0.00 ± 0.06, distance 0.02 ± 0.04; standard multifocal group: near 0.10 ± 0.08, intermediate 0.10 ± 0.11, distance 0.02 ± 0.04; all logMAR).

Another randomized-controlled study by Liekfeld and co-authors was published in 2015. It also compared a primary duet implantation with a conventional capsular bag-fixed IOL [11], using the Human Optics Diff-sPB combined with the monofocal ASPIRA-aA as the add-on lens and the Diff-s from the same manufacturer as the primary capsular bag-fixed lens. There were no significant differences in the achieved refraction, the mean absolute error was 0.30 ± 0.31 D in the add-on group and 0.36 ± 0.39 D in the standard multifocal group (p = 0.78). Both variants showed no significant differences in visual acuity (uncorrected visual acuity in add-on group: distance 0.08 ± 0.12, intermediate 0.04 ± 0.14, near 0.13 ± 0.08; standard multifocal group: distance 0.04 ± 0.09, intermediate 0.02 ± 0.16, near 0.03 ± 0.05 all logMAR), only in near visual acuity the standard multifocal group performed better (p = 0.003). This had no effect on reading speed (tested with Radner reading charts), where there were no significant differences in both groups.

The other studies mentioned above (without randomization or case series only) also reported satisfactory visual acuity results for distance, intermediate, and near, though this will not be discussed in detail here. Regarding complications: Averaged over all available studies, surgical revisions were necessary in 4 of 277 eyes (=1.4%). The rate of cases with pigment dispersion varied between 5.9% and 8.3%.

Conclusion

Both the simultaneous implantation of a monofocal capsular bag-fixed IOL with a multifocal add-on IOL ("duet' implantation) and the additional implantation of a multifocal add-on IOL in case of pre-existing pseudophakia seem to be safe based on the available literature. Visual outcomes, defocus curves and contrast vision seem to be comparable to a primary capsular bag-fixed multifocal intraocular lens. However, long-term data on refractive stability and lens-associated complications are lacking.

Data on Dysphotopsia After Add-on Implantation

Negative optical effects due to reflections from the add-on lenses have been rarely reported. In general, contrast vision is regarded as comparable to regular pseudophakia. The only study that investigated interface reflections with and without an add-on IOL in a model concluded that no relevant increase in glare effects is to be expected due to the add-on lens compared to regular pseudophakia [17]. Another study was able to show by applying a ray tracing model that the negative dysphotopsia (shadow in periphery) of the capsular bag-fixed IOL could acutally even be improved by an additional refractive medium, because the increased distance between iris and lens leads to better illumination of the peripheral retina [3].

References

1. Alio JL, Abdelghany AA, Fernandez-Buenaga R. Management of residual refractive error after cataract surgery. Curr Opin Ophthalmol. 2014;25(4):291–7. https://doi.org/10.1097/icu.0000000000000067.
2. Cassagne M, Porterie M, Gauthier L, Chapotot E, Soler V, Malecaze F, et al. Primary sulcus implantation of a diffractive multifocal pseudophakic piggyback intraocular lens. J Cataract Refract Surg. 2018;44(3):266–73. https://doi.org/10.1016/j.jcrs.2017.11.019.
3. Erie JC, Simpson MJ, Bandhauer MH. Effect of a sulcus-fixated piggyback intraocular lens on negative dysphotopsia: Ray-tracing analysis. J Cataract Refract Surg. 2019;45(4):443–50. https://doi.org/10.1016/j.jcrs.2018.10.041.
4. Falzon K, Stewart OG. Correction of undesirable pseudophakic refractive error with the Sulcoflex intraocular lens. J Refract Surg. 2012;28(9):614–9. https://doi.org/10.3928/1081597x-20120809-01.
5. Ferreira TB, Pinheiro J. Clinical results with a supplementary toric intraocular lens for the correction of astigmatism in pseudophakic patients. Eur J Ophthalmol. 2015;25(4):302–8. https://doi.org/10.5301/ejo.5000564.
6. Gerten G, Kermani O, Schmiedt K, Farvili E, Foerster A, Oberheide U. Dual intraocular lens implantation: Monofocal lens in the bag and additional diffractive multifocal lens in the sulcus. J Cataract Refract Surg. 2009;35(12):2136–43. https://doi.org/10.1016/j.jcrs.2009.07.014.
7. Gundersen KG, Potvin R. A review of results after implantation of a secondary intraocular lens to correct residual refractive error after cataract surgery. Clin Ophthalmol. 2017;11:1791–6. https://doi.org/10.2147/opth.S144675.
8. Hassenstein A, Niemeck F, Giannakakis K, Klemm M. Toric add-on intraocular lenses for correction of high astigmatism after pseudophakic keratoplasty. Ophthalmologe. 2017;114 (6):549–55. https://doi.org/10.1007/s00347-016-0386-6.
9. Kahraman G, Amon M. New supplementary intraocular lens for refractive enhancement in pseudophakic patients. J Cataract Refract Surg. 2010;36(7):1090–4. https://doi.org/10.1016/j.jcrs.2009.12.045.
10. Levinger E, Mimouni M, Finkelman Y, Yatziv Y, Shahar J, Trivizki O. Outcomes of refractive error correction in pseudophakic patients using a sulcus piggyback intraocular lens. Eur J Ophthalmol. 2020. https://doi.org/10.1177/1120672120903560.
11. Liekfeld A, Ehmer A, Schröter U. Visual function and reading speed after bilateral implantation of 2 types of diffractive multifocal intraocular lenses: Add-on versus capsular bag design. J Cataract Refract Surg. 2015;41(10):2107–14. https://doi.org/10.1016/j.jcrs.2015.10.055.

12. McLintock CA, McKelvie J, Gatzioufas Z, Wilson JJ, Stephensen DC, Apel AJG. Outcomes of toric supplementary intraocular lenses for residual astigmatic refractive error in pseudophakic eyes. Int Ophthalmol. 2019;39(9):1965–72. https://doi.org/10.1007/s10792-018-1027-7.
13. Meyer JJ, McGhee CN. Supplementary, Sulcus-Fixated Intraocular Lens in the Treatment of Spherical and Astigmatic Refractive Errors in Pseudophakic Eyes After Keratoplasty. Cornea. 2015;34(9):1052–6. https://doi.org/10.1097/ico.0000000000000506.
14. Schrecker J, Feith A, Langenbucher A. Comparison of additional pseudophakic multifocal lenses and multifocal intraocular lens in the capsular bag. Br J Ophthalmol. 2014;98(7):915–9. https://doi.org/10.1136/bjophthalmol-2013-304591.
15. Schrecker J, Kroeber S, Eppig T, Langenbucher A. Additional multifocal sulcus-based intraocular lens: alternative to multifocal intraocular lens in the capsular bag. J Cataract Refract Surg. 2013;39(4):548–55. https://doi.org/10.1016/j.jcrs.2012.10.047.
16. Schrecker J, Langenbucher A. Visual Performance in the Long Term With Secondary Add-on Versus Primary Capsular Bag Multifocal Intraocular Lenses. J Refract Surg. 2016;32 (11):742–7. https://doi.org/10.3928/1081597x-20160630-02.
17. Schrecker J, Zoric K, Messner A, Eppig T. Effect of interface reflection in pseudophakic eyes with an additional refractive intraocular lens. J Cataract Refract Surg. 2012;38(9):1650–6. https://doi.org/10.1016/j.jcrs.2012.03.039.
18. Venter JA, Oberholster A, Schallhorn SC, Pelouskova M. Piggyback intraocular lens implantation to correct pseudophakic refractive error after segmental multifocal intraocular lens implantation. J Refract Surg. 2014;30(4):234–9. https://doi.org/10.3928/1081597x-20140321-02.
19. Wolter-Roessler M, Küchle M. Implantation of multifocal add-on IOLs simultaneously with cataract surgery: results of a prospective study. Klin Monbl Augenheilkd. 2010;227(8):653–6. https://doi.org/10.1055/s-0029-1245266.

Systemic Overview of Experimental Lens Surgery

Christian M. Wertheimer

Introduction

Cataract surgery has undergone significant development and constant evolution from its origins hundreds of years ago to the present day [28] and has become a safe and standardized procedure. But, arguably, it is still far from perfection. In an ideal scenario, even though senile cataract presumably develops slowly throughout life, the reconstruction of the physiological lens properties of a healthy emmetropic, accommodating infant would be the goal to strive for. If we pursue this idea further, the disadvantages of the current method become clear. While it may be a slight exaggeration, we injure a healthy cornea by incision and tear an intact lens capsule to reach the site of disease. We then shatter the endogenous lens protein and then squeeze a rigid intraocular lens (IOL) into the capsular bag. In order to keep the IOL fixed and axis-stable in the capsular bag, a fibrotic reaction and vision-reducing wound healing (posterior capsule opacification) is accepted. Optically, the IOL does not fit perfectly with the rest of the biological optical apparatus compared to the characteristics of the patient's own lens. Although the current procedure works well in, the self-critical surgeon can think of other disadvantages. Critical evaluation is a necessary impetus for innovation and novelty. In the following chapter, new and innovative approaches will be examined in more detail, which could perhaps accelerate the long journey that still remains to the perfect procedure. Given the large number of interesting approaches and mostly experimental research results, neither the demand for completeness nor a critical discussion can be provided in the scope of this chapter.

C. M. Wertheimer (✉)
Munich, Germany
e-mail: Christian.Wertheimer@uniklinik-ulm.de

M. Shajari et al. (eds.), *Cataract and Lens Surgery*,
https://doi.org/10.1007/978-3-031-05394-8_80

Accommodative IOL

Loss of accommodation due to presbyopia, as well as for younger patients with cataract, is a largely unsolved problem, which results in a reduction of quality of life. Current treatments are suboptimal compromise solutions that buy some depth of focus at the expense of optical aberrations. Since the earliest development of artificial lenses, there has been an intensive search for accommodative properties in IOLs to simulate the biological, functional curvature change of the patient's own lens. One example of a so-called "next-generation" IOL is the accommodative FluidVision™ IOL developed by PowerVision for in-the-bag implantation. It has achieved both CE and FDA approval and has already been evaluated in clinical trials. Fluid shifts in the soft IOL change its surface curvature and it can be injected through a 3.5 mm incision. Another example is "accommodative lens refilling", in which the empty capsular bag is filled with a high refractive index fluid. The amount of fluid determines the surface curvature [46]. The major obstacle to accommodation is fibrosis of the capsular bag in the posterior capsule opacification setting, as contraction of the capsule limits the transmission of accommodative forces from the zonular apparatus. IOL placement into the ciliary sulcus could potentially remedy this [2]. There is already an abundance of experimental models and numerous clinical studies that give hope that this problem will be solved in the foreseeable future.

Artificial Intelligence

This subfield of computer science, which deals with the automation of intelligent behavior and machine learning, is becoming increasingly important in medicine, and ophthalmology is not different. Although the main focus is currently on applications related to imaging and diseases of the posterior segment of the eye, benefits are also expected in cataract surgery [19]. Self-learning algorithms that can identify correlations from vast amounts of data (Big Data) can be used to draw conclusions about new as well as established ophthalmic treatments in the real world, among other applications [11, 32]. The computer uses these learned correlations to make accurate decisions. Clinically, this has been used to biometrically calculate dioptric power of IOLs and has also been more accurate than current formulas [27]. The use of the algorithms continues to evolve [7] and is increasingly being extended to more complex computational situations such as the post-myopic LASIK conditions [26]. The eventual goal would be an adaptable learning curve of the intelligent algorithm to individual surgeon outcomes to improve personal outcome [27]. Other applications, mostly experimental, aim at determining the exact timing for surgery [6] as well as predicting surgical complications [33].

Green Cataract Surgery and Sustainability

In the U.S., for example, the healthcare sector accounted for a significant portion of national air pollution, including acid rain (12%), greenhouse gas emissions (10%), air pollutants (9%), and carcinogenic and non-carcinogenic air toxics (1–2%) [15]. In most developed countries, the systems used in medicine, and especially their use of disposable materials, are not designed for sustainability [45]. With the increased adoption of single-use devices, cataract surgery generates large amounts of waste [37]. Cataract surgery emits 180 kg of carbon dioxide equivalents per eye, with more than half of these emissions attributable to the procurement of single-use medical devices [34]. However, when discussing the sustainability of cataract surgery, the issue of surgical safety is crucial, as there should be no compromise. An interesting study of a pilot project in the southern Indian state of Tamil Nadu shows an innovative and effective model for broad-based care of the poorer population there, focusing on time and resource efficiency. Sixty percent of the operations were performed at minimal or no cost to the patient and according to the authors—with comparable or better outcomes and comparable or lower complication rates than in the United Kingdom (one endophthalmitis and four capsular ruptures per 2942 eyes). The reduction in use of material generated only 5% of carbon dioxide equivalents per eye, compared to the UK [45]. Whether this system would also be applicable in other settings has been questioned and is not answered by the authors, but the results of the study should at least give us pause and provide an opportunity to re-think our current perceptions of single-use material.

Electrical IOL Devices

Electronic medical implants, as the retinal prosthesis or cochlear implant, are well known in the medical field. Digitalization could also influence future IOL innovations. One example active in this field are the Swiss company "SAV-IOL" which has launched the concept project "R-TASC". R-TASC is an active electronic IOL with real-time autofocus for accommodation and wireless connectivity via an antenna. It is powered by a solar cell integrated into the IOL. This electronically controlled lens is expected to be controllable with an app, provide a full visual accommodation range, and also allow computer-assisted perception or representation that adds virtual aspects to the real world—so-called "augmented reality" [44]. Other innovations with electronic extensions of the IOL include continuous intraocular pressure sensors [17], glucose sensors [31], and other accommodative lenses [23].

Lens Regeneration Following Lens Extraction

Lens regeneration refers to the recreation of a clear and functional lens after loss of the patient's own lens. The first experiments on lens regeneration in mammals after lens removal were performed as early as the beginning of the nineteenth century. It was observed that 6 months after lens removal in rabbits, there was a regrowth of a clear lens [10]. The technique was recently revisited and has been significantly developed further. Firstly, a new method of cataract extraction was developed in which the lens capsule was opened through a very small capsular opening, almost at the equator of the lens, and the lens then emulsified and aspirated through this incision. The method was first tested in primates and then in 12 infants and young children born with cataracts in both eyes. Using the technique, clear, healthy lenses developed in all 24 eyes within three months of surgery. After eight months the authors argued, these lenses were equivalent to those of children of the same age [29].

Drug Eluting IOL

Cataract surgery still brings many, albeit minor, inconveniences to the patient. One of them is the postoperative use of local anti-inflammatory eye drops. The regimens vary widely and are sometimes redefined individually and change regularly [3]. As always, patient compliance should be taken into account [22]. To counter these problems, various procedures for loading IOLs with pharmaceutical agents have been developed to use the IOL as a drug carrier with long-term delivery. Loading methods include "hypercritical fluid impregnation" [38], "dip coating" [47], and "nano matrices of poly(lactic-co-glycolic acid)" [25]. All of these methods, at least experimentally, were able to achieve a therapeutic benefit. The postoperative delivery of related substances over time and were designed to reduce postoperative inflammation, infection [37], or posterior capsule opacification formation [24]. By releasing the drug directly into the capsular bag, toxic side effects of highly concentrated eye drops are avoided on the surface and systemically. Patient compliance is not required, and surgical technique does not need to be modified. Drug-releasing intraocular lenses would also be helpful for other common ocular comorbidities such as glaucoma, diabetes, uveitis, or neovascular disease.

Pharmacological Cataract Therapy–Molecular Biology

To date, there is no consistently effective pharmacologic treatment option for cataract, making surgery the only option. Numerous groups worldwide are engaged in research into the molecular biology mechanisms of cataract development [4]. With increasing insight into the pathobiological processes of this development, there is a reasonable hope that it can be pharmacologically influenced or even reversed. There are a number of studies that have already restored clarity to cataractogenic, opacified lenses in animal models using pharmacological agents. One experimental substance, a pharmacological chaperone (substance 29), was able to clear the lens by one level on the LOCS III scoring system after 6 days in five, 118 to 263-day-old mice with age-related cataracts [30]. After artificial activation of pluripotent stem cells, clear human lenses were grown in the laboratory that could focus light [35]. Lanosterol, which occurs naturally in the lens, reduced lens opacities in dogs in vivo and in excised rabbit lenses [50]. To date, one gene therapy has been approved for subretinal injection of a viral vector in ophthalmology. In the future, genes could also be targeted that control cataract formation, and expression could be inhibited with microRNAs [8]. Furthermore, the well-known gene scissors CRISPR-Cas9 was able to cure a gene mutation leading to cataract formation in mice [49].

Political and Economic Innovation Projects

Of course, infinite resources are not available in a healthcare system. Since cataract surgery is still one of the most common procedures worldwide, economic and health policy innovations are also necessary in order to continue to make this treatment available to the general population. Not only is the performance of the surgery itself important, but socially, it is the postoperative outcomes that are essential, e.g., how many people have good or functional vision after surgery that is important, and at what cost. To measure this, macroeconomic tools available include cost-utility analyses. Here, for example, the FEMCAT study shows that while clinically there is no difference between phacoemulsification and femtosecond laser assisted cataract surgery, the femtolaser's assistance carries a great total cost to society and the patient and cannot be justified for the same outcome [42]. Other innovations include smartphone-based teleophthalmology applications that allow efficient prediction of the need for presentation to the ophthalmologist [12]. Similar to the results of a posterior segment research project at Moorfield Hospital and Google subsidiary DeepMind, Artificial Intelligence could also help with this decision, saving the hospital unnecessary visits while allowing relevant pathologies requiring treatment to be identified in a timely manner [13].

Postoperative Non-invasive Adjustment of Dioptric IOL Power

Depending on definition, refractive outcome errors still affect a certain portion of patients [32]. For refractive errors that occur due to errors in the biometric determination of IOL refractive power, the only surgical options clinically available to date, are reoperation at the lens plane or corneal refractive surgery. Several groups have attempted to use photochemical or photothermal methods to change the refractive power of the already implanted IOL in the capsular bag without reopening the eye. In the United States, the "RxSight Light Adjustable Lens" has been approved since 2017, and can be altered postoperatively using UV light irradiation [18]. Another method is the so-called "refractive index shaping" using femtosecond laser and resulted in a precise change of the dioptric refractive power without significantly affecting the quality of the IOL [36]. In addition, it was possible to torically modify a monofocal IOL and correction from multifocal to monofocal or revision the other way around was also possible [41].

Robotics

As with many surgical fields, robotics continues to make their way into ophthalmic surgery. Robotics show some advantages over human motor skills, such as accuracy, reduction or elimination of physiological hand tremor, and the possibility of manipulation on very small structures [20]. In cataract surgery, it is already used clinically in femtolaser-assisted surgery and can take over some steps of the surgery [48]. However, penetration of the bulb is not yet taken over by robot-guided instruments. In vitreoretinal surgery, however, robot-guided instruments have been somewhat more explored than in cataract surgery [39]. Experimental robots have evolved enough in the laboratory to perform microvascular procedures on retinal vessels [16]. However, there are also early developments of systems in cataract surgery such as the AXSIS with two small arms that can move in the anterior chamber [1]. The IRISS platform is another robot similar to the AXSIS platform [40]. The Da Vinci robot has four arms and is approved by the U.S. Food and Drug Administration for use in humans, and has been used clinically for capsulorhexis [5]. In some cases, robotic systems are already superior to humans in attention to detail. Superior pressure sensors can be used to precisely adjust the force used to touch sensitive structures such as the retina [21]. Other advancements, such as OCT probes in the instrument tips also allow precise measurements of the distance to an anatomical structure [9]. Overall, the systems are still in development but the potential clinical applications they offer remain exciting.

3D-Printed IOL

Today's IOLs only allow compensation of a certain range of lower order optical aberrations (astigmatism and sphere). If patients suffer from higher order aberrations (e.g. coma in keratoconus) or have particularly long or short eyes, custom-made lenses are not available or, in individual cases, only conditionally available. This is where 3D-printing of optical lenses opens up new possibilities, as it could potentially enable unlimited optical and morphological lens designs. Using widely available three-dimensional printing technology, a fully personalized IOL would be printed in the operating room and provided fitting individually for each patient's optical apparatus [14]. Recently, a 3D printable hydrogel was published for this purpose [43]. A large lens stock or ordering of special custom-made lenses could be eliminated.

Conclusion

Cataract surgery from 20 years ago is very different to how it is performed today so it is reasonable to assume that cataract surgery in 20 years from now will have evolved again. It can only be speculated which of the concepts described above, or other ideas not mentioned here, will make it into clinical use. Many are still early in experimental development and have partly obvious and also hidden accompanying problems. Ultimately, the future remains exciting in the field of cataract surgery and offers many opportunities for innovation.

References

1. Adee S. Eye, robot. Elsevier; 2016.
2. Alio JL, Simonov AN, Romero D, Angelov A, Angelov Y, van Lawick W, et al. Analysis of accommodative performance of a new accommodative intraocular lens. J Refract Surg. 2018;34(2):78–83. https://doi.org/10.3928/1081597X-20171205-01.
3. Bandello F, Coassin M, Di Zazzo A, Rizzo S, Biagini I, Pozdeyeva N, et al. One week of levofloxacin plus dexamethasone eye drops for cataract surgery: an innovative and rational therapeutic strategy. Eye (Lond). 2020. https://doi.org/10.1038/s41433-020-0869-1.
4. Berry V, Georgiou M, Fujinami K, Quinlan R, Moore A, Michaelides M. Inherited cataracts: molecular genetics, clinical features, disease mechanisms and novel therapeutic approaches. Br J Ophthalmol. 2020. https://doi.org/10.1136/bjophthalmol-2019-315282.
5. Bourla DH, Hubschman JP, Culjat M, Tsirbas A, Gupta A, Schwartz SD. Feasibility study of intraocular robotic surgery with the da Vinci surgical system. Retina. 2008;28(1):154–8. https://doi.org/10.1097/IAE.0b013e318068de46.
6. Caixinha M, Amaro J, Santos M, Perdigao F, Gomes M, Santos J. In-vivo automatic nuclear cataract detection and classification in an animal model by ultrasounds. IEEE Trans Biomed Eng. 2016;63(11):2326–35. https://doi.org/10.1109/TBME.2016.2527787.

7. Carmona Gonzalez D, Palomino Bautista C. Accuracy of a new intraocular lens power calculation method based on artificial intelligence. Eye (Lond). 2020. https://doi.org/10.1038/s41433-020-0883-3.
8. Chen X, Xiao W, Chen W, Liu X, Wu M, Bo Q, et al. MicroRNA-26a and -26b inhibit lens fibrosis and cataract by negatively regulating Jagged-1/Notch signaling pathway. Cell Death Differ. 2017;24(8):1431–42. https://doi.org/10.1038/cdd.2016.152.
9. Cheon GW, Huang Y, Cha J, Gehlbach PL, Kang JU. Accurate real-time depth control for CP-SSOCT distal sensor based handheld microsurgery tools. Biomed Opt Express. 2015;6(5):1942–53. https://doi.org/10.1364/BOE.6.001942.
10. Cocteau M, d'Etoille L. Physiology: Experiments relating to the reproduction of the crystalline lens, by MM. Cocteau and Leroy d'Etoille, Doctors of Physic. Account read at the Academy of Surgery, 10th Feb. 1825. The Lancet. 1827;8(191):117–118. https://doi.org/10.1016/S0140-6736(02)81126-6
11. Coleman AL. How big data informs us about cataract surgery: the LXXII Edward Jackson memorial lecture. Am J Ophthalmol. 2015;160(6):1091–1103 e3. https://doi.org/10.1016/j.ajo.2015.09.028.
12. Collon S, Chang D, Tabin G, Hong K, Myung D, Thapa S. Utility and feasibility of teleophthalmology using a smartphone-based ophthalmic camera in screening camps in Nepal. Asia Pac J Ophthalmol (Phila). 2020;9(1):54–8. https://doi.org/10.1097/01.APO.0000617936.16124.ba.
13. De Fauw J, Ledsam JR, Romera-Paredes B, Nikolov S, Tomasev N, Blackwell S, et al. Clinically applicable deep learning for diagnosis and referral in retinal disease. Nat Med. 2018;24(9):1342–50. https://doi.org/10.1038/s41591-018-0107-6.
14. Debellemaniere G, Flores M, Montard M, Delbosc B, Saleh M. Optical and morphological characterization of a 3D printed intraocular lens. Acta Ophthalmol. 2014;92(s253). https://doi.org/10.1111/j.1755-3768.2014.1771.x.
15. Eckelman MJ, Sherman J. Environmental impacts of the US health care system and effects on public health. PLoS ONE. 2016;11(6): e0157014.
16. Edwards TL, Xue K, Meenink HCM, Beelen MJ, Naus GJL, Simunovic MP, et al. First-in-human study of the safety and viability of intraocular robotic surgery. Nat Biomed Eng. 2018;2:649–56. https://doi.org/10.1038/s41551-018-0248-4.
17. Enders P, Cursiefen C. Device profile of the EYEMATE-IO system for intraocular pressure monitoring: overview of its safety and efficacy. Expert Rev Med Devices. 2020. https://doi.org/10.1080/17434440.2020.1761788.
18. Ford J, Werner L, Mamalis N. Adjustable intraocular lens power technology. J Cataract Refract Surg. 2014;40(7):1205–23. https://doi.org/10.1016/j.jcrs.2014.05.005.
19. Goh JHL, Lim ZW, Fang X, Anees A, Nusinovici S, Rim TH, et al. Artificial intelligence for cataract detection and management. Asia Pac J Ophthalmol (Phila). 2020;9(2):88–95. https://doi.org/10.1097/01.APO.0000656988.16221.04.
20. Gomez-Blanco M, Riviere CN, Khosla PK. Intraoperative tremor monitoring for vitreoretinal microsurgery. Stud Health Technol Inform. 2000;70:99–101.
21. Gonenc B, Handa J, Gehlbach P, Taylor RH, Iordachita I. Design of 3-DOF force sensing micro-forceps for robot assisted vitreoretinal surgery. Conf Proc IEEE Eng Med Biol Soc. 2013;2013:5686–9. https://doi.org/10.1109/EMBC.2013.6610841.
22. Hermann MM, Ustundag C, Diestelhorst M. Electronic compliance monitoring of topical treatment after ophthalmic surgery. Int Ophthalmol. 2010;30(4):385–90. https://doi.org/10.1007/s10792-010-9362-3.
23. Horiuchi T, Mihashi T, Fujikado T, Oshika T, Asaka K. Voltage-controlled accommodating IOL system using an ion polymer metal composite actuator. Opt Express. 2016;24(20):23280–8. https://doi.org/10.1364/OE.24.023280.
24. Kassumeh S, Kueres A, Hillenmayer A, von Studnitz A, Elhardt C, Ohlmann A, et al. Development of a drug-eluting intraocular lens to deliver epidermal growth factor receptor inhibitor gefitinib for posterior capsule opacification prophylaxis. Eur J Ophthalmol. 2019;1120672119891042. https://doi.org/10.1177/1120672119891042.

25. Kassumeh SA, Wertheimer CM, von Studnitz A, Hillenmayer A, Priglinger C, Wolf A, et al. Poly(lactic-co-glycolic) acid as a slow-release drug-carrying matrix for methotrexate coated onto intraocular lenses to conquer posterior capsule opacification. Curr Eye Res. 2018;43(6):702–8. https://doi.org/10.1080/02713683.2018.1437455.
26. Koprowski R, Lanza M, Irregolare C. Corneal power evaluation after myopic corneal refractive surgery using artificial neural networks. Biomed Eng Online. 2016;15(1):121. https://doi.org/10.1186/s12938-016-0243-5.
27. Ladas JG, Siddiqui AA, Devgan U, Jun AS. A 3-D "super surface" combining modern intraocular lens formulas to generate a "super formula" and maximize accuracy. JAMA Ophthalmol. 2015;133(12):1431–6. https://doi.org/10.1001/jamaophthalmol.2015.3832.
28. Leffler CT, Hadi TM, Udupa A, Schwartz SG, Schwartz D. A medieval fallacy: the crystalline lens in the center of the eye. Clin Ophthalmol. 2016;10:649–62. https://doi.org/10.2147/OPTH.S100708.
29. Lin H, Ouyang H, Zhu J, Huang S, Liu Z, Chen S, et al. Lens regeneration using endogenous stem cells with gain of visual function. Nature. 2016;531(7594):323–8. https://doi.org/10.1038/nature17181.
30. Makley LN, McMenimen KA, DeVree BT, Goldman JW, McGlasson BN, Rajagopal P, et al. Pharmacological chaperone for α-crystallin partially restores transparency in cataract models. Science. 2015;350(6261):674–7. https://doi.org/10.1126/science.aac9145.
31. March WF, Ochsner K, Horna J. Intraocular lens glucose sensor. Diabetes Technol Ther. 2000;2(1):27–30. https://doi.org/10.1089/152091500316700.
32. Melles RB, Kane JX, Olsen T, Chang WJ. Update on intraocular lens calculation formulas. Ophthalmology. 2019;126(9):1334–5. https://doi.org/10.1016/j.ophtha.2019.04.011.
33. Mohammadi S-F, Sabbaghi M, Hadi Z, Hashemi H, Alizadeh S, Majdi M, et al. Using artificial intelligence to predict the risk for posterior capsule opacification after phacoemulsification. J Cataract Refract Surg. 2012;38(3):403–8.
34. Morris DS, Wright T, Somner JE, Connor A. The carbon footprint of cataract surgery. Eye (Lond). 2013;27(4):495–501. https://doi.org/10.1038/eye.2013.9.
35. Murphy P, Kabir MH, Srivastava T, Mason ME, Dewi CU, Lim S, et al. Light-focusing human micro-lenses generated from pluripotent stem cells model lens development and drug-induced cataract in vitro. Development. 2018;145(1):dev155838. https://doi.org/10.1242/dev.155838.
36. Nguyen J, Werner L, Ludlow J, Aliancy J, Ha L, Masino B, et al. Intraocular lens power adjustment by a femtosecond laser: In vitro evaluation of power change, modulation transfer function, light transmission, and light scattering in a blue light–filtering lens. J Cataract Refract Surg. 2018;44(2):226–30.
37. Ongkasin K, Masmoudi Y, Tassaing T, Le-Bourdon G, Badens E. Supercritical loading of gatifloxacin into hydrophobic foldable intraocular lenses—process control and optimization by following in situ CO2 sorption and polymer swelling. Int J Pharm. 2020a;581: 119247. https://doi.org/10.1016/j.ijpharm.2020.119247.
38. Ongkasin K, Masmoudi Y, Wertheimer CM, Hillenmayer A, Eibl-Lindner KH, Badens E. Supercritical fluid technology for the development of innovative ophthalmic medical devices: Drug loaded intraocular lenses to mitigate posterior capsule opacification. Eur J Pharm Biopharm. 2020b;149:248–56. https://doi.org/10.1016/j.ejpb.2020.02.011.
39. Pandey SK, Sharma V. Robotics and ophthalmology: Are we there yet? Indian J Ophthalmol. 2019;67(7):988–94. https://doi.org/10.4103/ijo.IJO_1131_18.
40. Rahimy E, Wilson J, Tsao TC, Schwartz S, Hubschman JP. Robot-assisted intraocular surgery: development of the IRISS and feasibility studies in an animal model. Eye (Lond). 2013;27(8):972–8. https://doi.org/10.1038/eye.2013.105.
41. Sahler R, Bille JF. Refractive index shaping: In vivo optimization of an implanted intraocular lens (IOL). In: Bille JF (ed) High resolution imaging in microscopy and ophthalmology: new frontiers in biomedical optics. p. 319–336. Cham (CH); 2019. https://doi.org/10.1007/978-3-030-16638-0_15.

42. Schweitzer C, Brezin A, Cochener B, Monnet D, Germain C, Roseng S, et al. Femtosecond laser-assisted versus phacoemulsification cataract surgery (FEMCAT): a multicentre participant-masked randomised superiority and cost-effectiveness trial. Lancet. 2020;395 (10219):212–24. https://doi.org/10.1016/S0140-6736(19)32481-X.
43. Shiblee MNI, Ahmed K, Khosla A, Kawakami M, Furukawa H. 3D printing of shape memory hydrogels with tunable mechanical properties. Soft Matter. 2018;14(38):7809–17. https://doi.org/10.1039/c8sm01156g.
44. Swiss Advanced Vision Intraocular Lens (2020). R-Tasc. Accessed 02.05.2020 2020.
45. Thiel CL, Schehlein E, Ravilla T, Ravindran R, Robin AL, Saeedi OJ, et al. Cataract surgery and environmental sustainability: Waste and lifecycle assessment of phacoemulsification at a private healthcare facility. J Cataract Refract Surg. 2017;43(11):1391–8.
46. van Kooten TG, Koopmans SA, Terwee T, Langner S, Stachs O, Guthoff RF. Long-term prevention of capsular opacification after lens-refilling surgery in a rabbit model. Acta Ophthalmol. 2019;97(6):e860–70. https://doi.org/10.1111/aos.14096.
47. Wertheimer C, Kueres A, Siedlecki J, Braun C, Kassumeh S, Wolf A, et al. The intraocular lens as a drug delivery device for an epidermal growth factor-Receptor inhibitor for prophylaxis of posterior capsule opacification. Acta Ophthalmol. 2018a;96(7):e874–82. https://doi.org/10.1111/aos.13759.
48. Wertheimer CM, Shajari M, Kohnen T, von Studnitz A, Kassumeh S, Dimitriou S, et al. Comparison of fibrotic response in the human lens capsular bag after femtosecond laser-assisted cataract surgery and conventional phacoemulsification. J Cataract Refract Surg. 2018b;44(6):750–5. https://doi.org/10.1016/j.jcrs.2018.01.035.
49. Wu Y, Liang D, Wang Y, Bai M, Tang W, Bao S, et al. Correction of a genetic disease in mouse via use of CRISPR-Cas9. Cell Stem Cell. 2013;13(6):659–62. https://doi.org/10.1016/j.stem.2013.10.016.
50. Zhao L, Chen X-J, Zhu J, Xi Y-B, Yang X, Hu L-D, et al. Lanosterol reverses protein aggregation in cataracts. Nature. 2015;523(7562):607–11. https://doi.org/10.1038/nature14650.

Postoperative Management

Perioperative Management in Cataract Surgery

Ingo Schmack and Daniel G. Dawson

The main tasks of the therapeutic measures taken perioperatively in cataract surgery are the prophylaxis, risk reduction, and management of serious vision threatening consequences including pseudophakic cystoid macular edema (PME) and uncontrolled intraocular inflammation like endophthalmitis) in order not to jeopardize the actual goal of the cataract surgery, namely the timely and functionally best possible visual rehabilitation.

In order to achieve this goal, adequate, individually tailored preoperative preparation and perioperative management including aseptic (e.g. povidone-iodine) and drug measures are of great importance [1]. The individual therapeutic preparations can be applied locally (topical, subconjunctival, sub-tenon's, peribulbar, intracameral, intravitreal) and/or systemically (oral, intravenous) as required.

They mainly comprise the following groups of active ingredients:

- corticosteroids,
- non-steroidal anti-inflammatory drugs (NSAIDs) and.
- antibiotics.

Depending on the situation, the use of

- virustatics,
- antiglaucomatous and.
- hyperosmolar, deswelling preparations may also be required.

I. Schmack (✉) · D. G. Dawson
Department of Ophthalmology, University of Frankfurt, Frankfurt, Germany
e-mail: ingo.schmack@kgu.de

D. G. Dawson
Department of Ophthalmology, University of Florida, Florida, United States

M. Shajari et al. (eds.), *Cataract and Lens Surgery*,
https://doi.org/10.1007/978-3-031-05394-8_81

Corticosteroids

Keypoint

The most potent steroids used in cataract surgery are the classic glucocorticoids dexamethasone and (methyl)prednisolone (see Table 1). Although dexamethasone (potency approx. 30) has the strongest anti-inflammatory and analgesic properties, it is inferior to the less potent prednisolone (potency 5) in terms of its duration of action due to its galenics.

In addition to pure steroid medications, a large number of combination preparations (steroid plus broad-spectrum antibiotic) are also offered for postoperative therapy today, due to the theoretical advantage of better compliance (1 versus 2 preparations), it should always be taken into account that the antibiotic contained in the preparation, in contrast to the desired corticosteroid, is inevitably administered for a disproportionately long period of time. The prescribed eye drops are usually applied gradually over a period of 3–6 weeks (initially 4–6 times daily). In addition, corticosteroids can also be administered by intracameral, subconjunctival, parabulbar, intravitreal or systemic routes. In this application to the eye, the "off-label use" should not go unmentioned.

Non-Steroidal Anti-Inflammatory Drugs (NSAIDs)

In addition to corticosteroids, NSAIDs in the form of eye drops are routinely used in cataract surgery (see Table 1). Although there is no proven advantage between the two in terms of reducing the postoperative inflammatory response, NSAIDs have nevertheless been proven superior for the prevention of postoperative PME [2, 3]. In addition, when used pre-operatively, they have antiphlogistic and analgesic properties as well as being beneficial in maintaining intraoperative mydriasis. Depending on the active substance and concentration, recommended dosages are between 1 and 4 drops per day for a total duration of usually 4–6 weeks.

Antibiotics

Today, antibiotics are still often used as a therapeutic standard in cataract surgery as a prophylaxis for postoperative endophthalmitis (see Table 2). In contrast to topical applied eye drops, which have variable transcorneal penetrance often achieving low concentrations in the aqueous humor, the effectiveness of intracameral antibiotics has been impressively proven in the meantime, based on a large-scale prospective study by the European Society of Cataract & Refractive Surgeons (ESCRS) from 2007 and subsequent multicenter trials [4–7].

Table 1 Composition of anti-inflammatory ophthalmic drugs

Active ingredient class	Active principle / Mechanism of action	Indication(s)	Ophthalmic preparations						Side-effects	Precautions
			Generika	Brand (example)	Contration	Application form	Preservative-free	Combinations	Local	(Relative/absolut)
(Gluco)corticoids										
	Anti-inflammatory, analgesic and immunosuppressive	Prophylaxis and treatment of postoperative/ posttraumatic intraocular irritations	Dexamethasone	Dexa POS®, Dexa sine® SE	0.1%	Eye drops	Available	Gentamycin	Transient stinging and/or burning sensation in the eye	Acute herpes simplex infection (epithelial form) or other viral keratitis
		Allergic conjunctivitis/ blepharitis		Dexagel® AUG	1%	Eye gel/ ointment	Not available	Neomycin + Polymyxin B	Ocular discomfort, eye pain, headache,	Bacterial or mycotic inflammation without adequate antibacterial/mycotic coverage
		Episcleritis, scleritis, keratitis							Blurred vision	Injuries and ucerating processes of the cornea
		Uveitis (anterior, intermedia, posterior)	Prednisolon acetate	Inflanefran forte®, Predni-POS®	1%	Eye drops	Not available	Not available	Excerbation of local inflammatory conditions	Narrow and wide angle glaucoma
		Retinitis, neuritis nervi optici		Predni-Ophthal®	1%	Eye gel			Occurrence of secondary infection	Known intraocular pressure increase to glucocorticoids (steroid response)
		Blunt bulbar injuries (contusio bulbi)		Ultracortenol®	0.5%	Eye ointment			Corneal/ scleromalacia	Young, phakic patients with clear eye lens
		Ocular burns	Fluorometholone	Efflumidex®	0.1%	Eye drops	Not available	Not available	Intraocular pressure increase	Allergic disposition to the active substance
		Non-specific inflammatory eye diseases							Cataract formation	
			Loteprednoletabonat	Lotemax®	0.5%	eye drops	not available	not available		
Non-steroidal anti-inflammatory (NSAID) drops										

(continued)

Table 1 (continued)

Active ingredient class	Active principle / Mechanism of action	Indication(s)	Ophthalmic preparations						Side-effects	Precautions
			Generika	Brand (example)	Contration	Application form	Preservative-free	Combinations	Local	(Relative/absolut)
	Anti-inflammatory and analgesic via reduced prostaglandin synthesis (inhibition of cyclooxygenases)	Maintenance of intraoperative pupillary dilation (mydriasis)	Nepafanac	Nevanac®	0,1–0,3%	Eye drops	Not available	Not available	Transient stinging and/or burning sensation in the eye	Viral or bacterial eye infections
		Prophylaxis and treatment of postoperative/ posttraumatic intraocular irritations							Ocular discomfort, eye pain, headache,	Keratoconjunctivitis sicca
		Prophylaxis of postoperative changes at the ocular fundus (cystoid macular edema)							Inflammation of the ocular surface including the cornea as well as the interior of the eye (uveitis)	Corneal epithelial lesions
		Non-infectious inflammations of the anterior segment of the eye (e.g. conjunctiva, cornea, sclera)	Ketorolac	Acular®	0.50%	Eye drops	Not available	Not available	Blepharitis, dry eye (keratitis punctata superficialis)	
									Blurred vision and/or reduced vision, light sensitivity	
									Allergic reactions such as (peri-)ocular swelling, redness, itching, epiphora	
			Diclofenac	Difen® UD	0.1%	Eye drops	Available	Not available	Ocular or periocular fibrosis	
									Miosis	
									Mydriasis	
			Bromfenac	Yellox®	0.09%	Eye drops	Available	Not available		
			Flurbiprofen	Ocuflur O.K	0.1%	Eye drops	Available	Not available		

Table 2 Overview of common antibiotic ophthalmological drugs

Active ingredient class	Active principle/ Mechanism of action	Indication(s)	Active ingredients			Ophthalmic preparations					Side-effects	Precautions
			Name	Group	Profile of action	Brand (example)	Concentration	Application form	Preservative-free	Combinations	Local	(Relative/ absolut)
Fluoroquinolones /Gyrase inhibitors												
	Inhibition of supercoiling of prokaryotic DNA	Prophylaxis and treatment of infections of the anterior segment of the eye after surgical interventions and injuries of the eye	Norfloxacin	I	Gram-negative rods (e.g. E. coli)	Zoroxin	0.3%	Eye drops/ ointment	Not available	Not available	Eye discomfort (e.g. burning, itching, foreign body sensation)	Allergic reactions to individual active ingredients or excipients
	Bactericidal / bacteristatic										Allergic reactions	
											Epiphora	
											Photophobia	
			Ciprofloxacin	II	Broad spectrum of activity: gram-positive and gram-negative pathogens	Ciloxan®	0.3%	Eye drops	Not available	Not available	Hyperemia, chemosis	
					Pseudomonas aeruginosa (good efficacy)						Decrease of visual acuity, blurred vision	
					Streptococci (poor efficacy)						Corneal deposits/ precipitates	
			Ofloxacin	II	Broad spectrum of activity: gram-positive and gram-negative pathogens	Floxal®, Floxal® EDO	0.3%	Eye drops/ ointment	Available	Not available		
					Pseudomonas aeruginosa (good efficacy)	Ofloxacin-Ophtal® sine	0.3%	Eye drops				
					Streptococci (poor efficacy)	Ofloxacin-ratiopharm®	0.3%	Eye drops				

(continued)

Table 2 (continued)

Active ingredient class	Active principle/ Mechanism of action	Indication(s)	Active ingredients			Ophthalmic preparations					Side-effects	Precautions
			Name	Group	Profile of action	Brand (example)	Concentration	Application form	Preservative-free	Combinations	Local	(Relative/ absolut)
			Levofloxacin	III	Improved efficacy compared to group II	Oftaquix®	0.5%	Eye drops	Available	Not available		
					· Gram-negative cocci							
					· Atypical pathogens (e.g. chlamydia, mycoplasma)							
					Pseudomonas aeruginosa (moderate efficacy)							
			Moxifloxacin	IV	Improved efficacy compared to group III	Vigamox®	0.5%	Eye drops	Available	Not available		
					· Gram-positive cocci							
					· Atypical pathogens (e.g. chlamydia, mycoplasma)							
					· Anaerobes							
					Pseudomonas aeruginosa (no efficacy)							
Aminoglykoside												
	Inhibition of protein biosynthesis by binding to	Prevention and treatment of inflammation and to prevent possible infections of the eye after	Gentamicin		Mainly gram-negative pathogens (e.g.	Gentamycin-POS®	0.5%	Eye drops/ ointment	Available	Available	Burning, stinging,	Allergic reactions to individual

(continued)

Table 2 (continued)

Active ingredient class	Active principle/ Mechanism of action	Indication(s)	Active ingredients			Ophthalmic preparations					Side-effects	Precautions
			Name	Group	Profile of action	Brand (example)	Concentration	Application form	Preservative-free	Combinations	Local	(Relative/ absolut)
	the 30S subunit of ribosomes	cataract surgery of the lens of the eye (cataract)			enterococci, Pseudomonas aeruginosa)						foreign body sensation	active ingredients or excipients
	Bactericidal (concentration-dependent)				Gram-positive staphylococci (good efficacy)	Infectogenta®					Allergic reactions, itching	
					Anaerobic pathogens (ineffective)	Refobacin®					Epiphora	
			Kanamycin		Streptococci (ineffective)	Kan-Ophtal®	0.62%	Eye drops			Hyperemia, chemosis	
						Kanamytrex®	0.5%	Eye ointment			Wound healing disorders	
											Decrease of visual acuity, blurred vision	
											Calcification of the corneal stroma (rare)	
			Neomycin			Isopto-Max®	0.35%	Eye drops/ ointment	Not available		Secondary infections	
						Maxitrol®	0.35%	Eye drops				
			Tobramycin			Tobrex®[1]	0.3%	Eye ointment	Available	Available		
						Tobramaxin®	0.3%	Eye ointment				
Polypeptides												
	Disruption of cell membrane permeability by incorporation into the cell wall of bacteria	Prevention and treatment of inflammation and to prevent possible infections of the eye after cataract surgery of the lens of the eye (cataract)	Polymyxcin-B		Gram-negative bacteria	Polyspectran®		Eye drops	Not available	Available	Inflammation of the ocular surface	Allergic reactions to individual active ingredients or excipients

(continued)

Table 2 (continued)

Active ingredient class	Active principle/ Mechanism of action	Indication(s)	Active ingredients			Ophthalmic preparations					Side-effects	Precautions
			Name	Group	Profile of action	Brand (example)	Concentration	Application form	Preservative-free	Combinations	Local	(Relative/ absolut)
	Bactericidal (reserve antibiotic)				Bactericidal	Isopto-Max®		Eye drops			Increased intraocular pressure	
						Maxitrol®		Eye drops			Burning, stinging, foreign body sensation	
											Pruritus, epiphora	
											Blurred vision, phthophobia	
											Allergic reactions (e.g. swelling of the eyelids)	

The intraoperative administration of antibiotics is therefore often a standard part of cataract surgery and, at least the additional postoperative use of antibiotic eye drops, is increasingly becoming a matter of choice [8–10].

While in Europe cefuroxime, to which resistance to enterococci is already established, is the most widespread, in the USA, moxifloxacin is used most frequently in "off-label use". This has advantages over cefuroxime, especially in its effectiveness against gram-negative bacteria. With vancomycin, a so-called "reserve" antibiotic that can also be administered intracamerally, it should be noted that an idiopathic retinal vasculitis (e.g., hemorrhagic occlusive retinal vasculitis [HORV]) can occur in individual cases, depending on the dose [4].

Virustatics

In view of its primarily herpetic origin, acyclovir is mainly used, either as a pure substance or as a prodrug (valacyclovir). Acyclovir itself is used topically in the form of an ointment 3–5 times a day as well as systemically as a tablet (200–800 mg) or infusion (e.g. 500 mg) between 2–5 times a day, where attention should always be paid to kidney function and sufficient fluid intake.

Antiglaucoma Agents

Among the individual preparations, caution is required, especially when using prostaglandin analogues, as they have been shown to promote the occurrence of PMEs (see Table 3) [11]. It is irrelevant whether they are administered as monotherapy in combination with topical beta blockers (e.g. timolol). Patients with known diabetes mellitus, uveitis, retinal vein occlusion, pseudoexfoliation syndrome, epiretinal membrane, or vitreoretinal surgery are at increased risk and temporary cessation of prostaglandins (with alternative pressure medications) should be considered [12].

Osmotic Agents

In addition to sodium chloride (10% sodium chloride), glucose (5–10%) eye drops continue to prove effective in the supportive treatment of postoperative corneal edema due to temporary corneal endothelial decompensation. While the former, available over the counter in pharmacies, often cause a burning sensation when applied, the latter have to be specially prepared and have an unpleasant sticky effect due to their high sugar content. Depending on the corneal findings, they can be used up to every hour.

Table 3 Overview of intraocular-pressure lowering ophthalmologic preparations

Active ingredient class	Indication	Active principle/ mechanism of action	Active ingredients			IOP lowering effects	Preparations		Side-effects		Precautions	
			Generics		Application		Preservative-free	Combinations	Local	Systemic	Local	Systemic
Parasympathomimetics (cholinergics)												
Direct parasympathomimetics	Open angle glaucoma	Widening of the chamber angle	Pilocarpine	0,5–3%	AUT	20–40%	Not available	Timolol	Conjunctival hyperemia	Cardiovascular (e.g. bradycardia, increase in blood pressure, …)	Post-operative inflammation	Gastric/small intestinal ulceration
	Angle-closure glaucoma	Contraction of the trabecular meshwork	Carbachol	0,75–3%		20–40%			Visual acuity reduction, - impairment	Central nervous (e.g. headache, …)	Anterior uveitis	Higher grade bradycardia
									Disturbed accommodation	Gastrointestinal (e.g. nausea, vomiting, …)	Malignant glaucoma	Arterial hypotension
									Visual field impairment	Pulmonary (e.g. bronchial spasm, pulmonary edema, …)	Neovascularization glaucoma	Condition after myocardial infarction
									Iris cysts	Muscular (e.g. cramps, weakness, …)	Pseudoexfoliation glaucoma	Epilepsia
											Absolute glaucoma	M. Parkinson's disease
											Post retinal detachment	
											Myopia magna	
Selective alpha-2 agonists												
	All types of glaucoma	Improvement of the trabecular and uveoscleral outflow	Clonidin	0.125–0.25%	Eye drops	18–25%	Available	Timolol	Reactive vasodilatation	Cardiovascular (e.g. bradycardia, hypotension, …)	None	Heart diseases (e.g. angina pectoris, acute myocardial infarction)
		Inhibition of aqueous humor production	Brimonidine	0.2%		18–25%	Not available		Conjunctival pallor	Central nervous (e.g. fatigue, tiredness, …)		Arterial hypertension
		Reduction of episcleral venous pressure	Apraclonidine	0.5%		25–35%	Not available		Pruritus	Gastrointestinal (e.g. nausea, constipation, …)		Condition after apoplexy
		Central intraocular pressure reduction							Keratoconjunctivitis sicca	Pulmonary (e.g. dyspnea, asthma, …)		Cerebrovascular diseases

(continued)

Table 3 (continued)

Active ingredient class	Indication	Active principle/ mechanism of action	Active ingredients			IOP lowering effects	Preparations		Side-effects		Precautions	
			Generics		Application		Preservative-free	Combinations	Local	Systemic	Local	Systemic
									Epiphora	Muscular (e.g. cramps, myalgia, …)		M. Parkinson's disease
									Eyelid edema, erythema	Other (e.g. dry mouth/nose, …)		Chronic renal insufficiency
									Mydriasis			Liver dysfunction
									Miosis (clonidine)			Raynaud's syndrome
									Visual deterioration			Depression
ß-receptor antagonists												
Non-selective	All types of glaucoma	Inhibition of aqueous humor production	Timolol	0.1–0.5%	eye drops	20–25%	Available	Cholinergics	Shortening of the tear film break-up time	Cardiovascular (e.g. bradycardia, arrhythmia, …)	Keratoconjunctivitis sicca	Allergic rhinitis, bronchial asthma
		Improvement of the trabecular outflow	Metipranolol	0.1–0.6%				Selective alpha-2 agonists	Decrease in secretory tear film formation	Central venous (e.g. fatigue, headache, …)	Severe dystrophic disorders of the cornea	Chronic obstructive airway disease
			Levobunolol	0.1–0.5%				ß-blockers	Burning, itching	Pulmonary (e.g. bronchospasm, apnea, …)		Sinus bradycardia
								Carboanhydrase inhibitors	Allergic conjunctivitis	Other (e.g. urticaria, exanthema, …)		2nd and 3rd degree AV block
								Prostaglandin F2 alpha analogues	Blepharitis			Decompensated heart failure
								Prostamides	Keratitis			Cardiogenic shock
ß1-selective	All types of glaucoma	Inhibition of aqueous humor production	Betaxolol	0.10%	eye drops	± 20%	Not available		Diplopia			Cerebral perfusion disorders
		Improvement of the trabecular outflow							Ptosis			Muscular weakness
Prostaglandin F2 alpha agonists, prostamides												
Prostaglandin analogs	All types of glaucoma	Improvement of uveoscleral outflow	Latanoprost	0.005%	Eye drops	25–35%	Available	Timolol	Conjunctival hyperemia	Cardiovascular (e.g. angina pectoris, arrhythmia, …)	Pseudophakia	Bronchial asthma
		Improvement of the trabecular outflow	Tafluprost	0.0015%					Burning, itching, foreign body sensation	Central venous (e.g. fatigue, headache, …)	Aphakia	Severe cardiovascular diseases
			Travoprost	0.004%					Hyperpigmentation of the periocular skin	Gastrointestinal (e.g. peptic ulcer, constipation, …)	Posterior capsular defect	Liver dysfunction

(continued)

Table 3 (continued)

Active ingredient class	Indication	Active principle/ mechanism of action	Active ingredients			IOP lowering effects	Preparations		Side-effects		Precautions	
			Generics		Application		Preservative-free	Combinations	Local	Systemic	Local	Systemic
Prostamide	All types of glaucoma	Improvement of uveoscleral outflow	Bimatoprost	0.01–0.03%	Eye drops	25–35%	Available	Timolol	Periocular adipose tissue atrophy	Pulmonary (e.g. dyspnea, asthma, …)	Macular edema	Kidney dysfunction
		Improvement of the trabecular mashwork outflow							Hyperpigmentation of the iris	Muscular (e.g. myalgia, …)	Ocular infklammation (e.g. herpetic keratitis)	
									Eyelash extension	Other (e.g. hypertrichosis, tinnitus, …)	Secondary glaucoma (e.g. pigment dispersion or neovascularization glaucoma)	
									Cystoid macular edema	Increased PSA values	Congenital glaucoma	
									Reactivation of uveitis, herpes keratitis		All iris colors except brown	
carbonic anhydrase inhibitors												
	All types of glaucoma	Inhibition of aqueous humor production	Brinzolamide	1%	Eye drops	20–24%	Available	Brimonidine, timolol	Burning, stinging, tearing, foreign body sensation	Cardiovascular (e.g. angina pectoris, arrhythmia, …)	Low endotheial cell conut	Allergy or hypersensitivity to sulfonamides
			Dorzolamide	2%				Timolol	Ocular hyperemia	Central nervous (e.g. somnolence, amnesia, apathy, …)	Endothelial cell disorders (e.g. Fuchs' endothelial dystrophy)	Hypokalemia
									Iridocyclitis	Gastrointestinal (including taste disturbances, loss of appetite, …)		Impaired liver function
									Corneal edema	Pulmonary (e.g. cough, sinusitis, asthma, …)		Severe renal dysfunction (clearance < 30 ml/min)
									Diplopia	Muscular (e.g. functional disorders, myalgias, …)		Hyperchloremic anemia
									Transient myopia	Other (e.g. paresthesias, hearing loss, …)		
									Keratitis punctata superficialis			

(continued)

Table 3 (continued)

Active ingredient class	Indication	Active principle/ mechanism of action	Active ingredients			IOP lowering effects	Preparations		Side-effects		Precautions	
			Generics		Application		Preservative-free	Combinations	Local	Systemic	Local	Systemic
									Blurred vision			
									Madarosis			
			Acetazolamid	250 mg	Oral	30–40%	Not appropriate	Not appropriate				
Osmotics												
	All types of glaucoma	Dehydration and reduction of vitreous volume	Glycerol	1,0–1,5 g/kg BW	Oral	15–20%	Not appropriate	Not appropriate		Allergic reactions (esp. mannitol)		Diabetes mellitus (glycerol)
		Deepening of the anterior chamber								Cardiovascular (e.g. tachycardia, hypo/hypertension, …)		Persistent oliguria/anuria after trial infusion
										Central nervous (e.g. confusion, headache, …)		Cardiac decompensation
										Gastrointestinal (e.g. nausea, vomiting, …)		Dehydration states
			Mannitol	1,0–1,5 g/kg BW	Intravenously	15–30%	Not appropriate	Not appropriate		Pulmonary (e.g. rhinitis, pulmonary edema, …)		Pulmonary edema
										Muscular (e.g. cramps, convulsions, …)		Intracranial hemorrhage
										Renal (e.g. acute renal failure, …)		Blood–brain barrier disorders
										Fluid and electrolyte imbalance, electrolyte loss, acidosis		Drainage obstruction of the urinary tract

General perioperative measures and therapy recommendations for cataract patients without operative abnormalities or accompanying ocular diseases.

Table 4 summarizes basic perioperative therapeutic and diagnostic measures, treatment instructions and therapy recommendations for cataract patients without pre-operative abnormalities, ocular concomitant diseases and intraoperative complications that have been repeatedly tested in clinical studies. The authors would

Table 4 Perioperative management for uncomplicated 'standard' cataract surgery

Setting	Therapeutic measures	Frequency	Duration
Preoperative			
Surgical preparation room	Pupil dilation (e.g. tropicamide eye drops plus 2.5% neosynephrine eyed drops or mydriatic* eye drops)	2–3x	–
	Eyelid disinfection (e.g., 10% povidone-iodine or octenidine/phenoxyethanol**)		–
	Local anesthesia (e.g. proxymetacaine AUT or Conjuncain EDO* AUT)		–
	Conjunctival sac disinfection (e.g. 2% povidine-iodine or 0.04% polihexanide**)		–
Operating room	Local anesthesia (e.g., lidocaine gel "2% or proxymetacaine or conjucaine EDO* eye drops)	Once daily	–
	Eyelid skin disinfection (e.g., 10% povidone-iodine 10% or octenidine/phenoxyethanol**)	1x	3–5 min
	Conjunctival disinfection (e.g. 2% povidine-iodine or 0.04% polihexanide**)	1x	3–5 min
	Optional		
	Peri- or retrobulbar anesthesia (e.g. lidocaine 2% plus bupivacaine 0.5%)	1x	–
Intraoperative			
Operating room	Local anesthesia, intracameral (e.g. lidocaine 2%)	1x	–
	Optional		
	Pupil dilation, intracameral (e.g., epinephrine 1% or tropicamide/phenylephrine/lidocaine solution)	1x	–
	Pupil constriction, intracameral (e.g. acetylcholine 1% solution)	1x	–

(continued)

Table 4 (continued)

Setting	Therapeutic measures	Frequency	Duration
Postoperative			
Operating room	Antibiosis, intracameral (e.g. cefuroxime solution)	1-2x	–
	Corticosteroid ointment (e.g. dexamethasone)	1-2x	–
	Optional		
	Antibiotic ointment (e.g., ofloxacin or gentamycin)		
	Corticosteroids, subconjunctival (e.g., 4 mg/ml dexamethasone injection solution)	1 × 0.1–0.2 ml	
	Dressing (e.g., eye compress or perforated capsule)	1x	–
Day 1	Corticosteroidal eye drops (e.g., dexamethasone)	4 × daily	2 weeks
	Nonsteroidal antiphlogistic eye drops (e.g., diclofenac or nepafanac 0.3%)	4 × daily or 1 × daily, respectively	4–6 weeks
	Optional		
	Antibiotic eye drops (e.g., ofloxacin or gentamycin)	3–4 × daily	7–10 days
	Moisturizing eye drops (e.g. hyaluronate or dexpanthenol)	4–6 × daily	10–12 weeks
Perioperatives setting			
Outpatient or inpatient			
Follow-up schedule			
After 1 day, 1–2 weeks, 4–6 weeks, and once a year (optional)			
Diagnostic procedures			
Visual acuity measurement (with and without correction)			
Intraocular pressure measurement (non-contact or applanatory)			
Slit lamp control of the anterior and posterior segment of the eye (miosis and/or mydriasis)			
Optional			
Macular OCT (depending on clinical findings)			

like to emphasize that the individual therapy proposals are not legally binding and may serve cataract surgeons only as a guideline, without restricting their individual freedom of decision.

Specific perioperative measures and therapy recommendations for cataract operations in patients with pre-operative abnormalities, ocular concomitant diseases or intraoperative complications

Deviating from the therapy recommendations for so-called regular, complication-free "standard" cataract surgery listed in Table 4. There are a large number of specific circumstances and initial situations that require a different procedure tailored to the individual patient. For the sake of clarity, only those "additive" treatment suggestions that go beyond the so-called "general perioperative measures and therapy recommendations" are listed under the respective subitems.

(a) Cataract surgery with intraoperative complications ("complicated cataract')*

Perioperative management:

- Intraoperative
  - Acetylcholine chloride (e.g. miochol® solution) intracameral (among other things for posterior capsule rupture with and without vitreous prolapse or loss)
- Postoperative
  - Intracameral:
    - Corticosteroids (e.g. dexamethasone acetate 4 mg/ml) (alternative: subconjunctival administration)
  - Topical:
    - Antibiotic ointment bandage (e.g. ofloxacin or gentamicin) (alternative: combination with corticosteroids e.g. dexamethasone acetate) 4–6 times daily
    - If necessary, osmotically active eye drops (e.g. 10% sodium chloride every 1–2 h)
    - If necessary, pupil-constricting eye drops (e.g. 1–2% pilocarpine) 3–4 times daily
  - Systemic:
    - If necessary, corticosteroids (e.g. prednisolone acetate 30–40 mg p.o.) 1 × daily for 3–4 days (caution: systemic contraindications)

    - Acetazolamide (250 mg p.o.) 1–3 × daily for 1–3 days (caution: renal dysfunction)
  - Optional:
    - Potassium substitution, stomach protection (e.g. pantoprazole 20–40 mg p.o. per day)

Perioperative setting:

- 1–2 nights in hospital

Note: *e.g. intraoperative posterior capsule defect with and without vitreous loss b).

(b) Cataract surgery in patients with uveitis [13–17]

Timing: Generally early stage of cataract disease; inflammation-free interval of 3 to 6 months, ideally 1 year; adequate therapeutic adjustment of ocular or general underlying diseases.

Perioperative management:

- Preoperative
  - Topical:
    - Corticosteroids (e.g. prednisolone acetate 1%) 4–6 times daily and facultative NSAID eye drops (e.g. nepafenac) 1–3 times daily; caution: less protective) for 3–7 days
  - Systemic:
    - Corticosteroids (e.g. prednisolone 0.5 mg/kg bw p.o.) 1 × daily for 2–5 days (consultation with treating colleague recommended) while retaining the other immunosuppressive medication
  - Optional:
    - Acyclovir 400 mg 2 × p.o. daily or valacyclovir 0.5 g p.o. 4 × daily for 2–3 days (in patients with ocular history of herpetic keratitis/ keratouveitis; caution: ensure sufficient fluid uptake)
- Intraoperative
  - Intracameral:
    - Corticosteroids (e.g. dexamethasone acetate 4 mg/ml)
    - Alternatively: intravitreal, subconjunctival or subtenon (e.g. dexamethasone acetate 40 mg/ml)

- Systemic:
  - Corticosteroids (e.g. prednisolone 5 mg/kg bw i.v.)
- Postoperative
  - Topical:
    - Corticosteroids (e.g. prednisolone acetate 1%) 6–8 times daily and facultative NSAID eye drops (e.g. nepafenac) 1–3 times daily; caution: less protective) for 6–8 weeks
  - Systemic:
    - Corticosteroids (e.g. prednisolone acetate 0.5 mg/kg body weight p.o.) 1 time daily followed by a slow dose reduction (e.g. 5 mg/week) over several weeks (in consultation with the treating colleague)
- Optional:
  - Acyclovir 400 mg 2 × p.o. daily or valacyclovir 0.5 g p.o. 4 × daily for 2–3 days (in patients with ocular history of herpetic keratitis/ keratouveitis; caution: ensure sufficient fluid uptake)

Perioperative setting:

- 1–2 nights in hospital if necessary (depending on postop inflammatory stimulus)

General comments:

- Patients with history of uveitis should generally be treated with corticosteroids over a longer period of time than patients undergoing uncomplicated cataract surgery.
- Prophylactic administration of antiparasitic drugs (e.g. toxoplasmosis retinochorioiditis) is controversially discussed and currently not recommended.
- NSAID should be given priority over topical corticosteroids in the presence of herpetic keratouveitis.

(c) Cataract surgery in patients with diabetic retinopathy (DRP)/maculopathy (DMP) [18–20].

Timing: Patients with a well-controlled blood sugar and absence of a DRP/DMP requiring therapy.

Perioperative management:

- Preoperative*
  - Topically

    NSAID eye drops (e.g. nepafenac) 1–3 times daily and corticosteroids (e.g. prednisolone acetate 1%) 4–6 times daily for 3–5 days

- Intravitreal

  anti-VEGF preparations (e.g. Bevabizumab 1.25 mg) or corticosteroids (e.g. dexamethasone acetate 4 mg/ml)

- Intraoperative

  - Intravitreal administration of anti-VEGF preparations* (e.g. Bevabizumab 1.25 mg) or corticosteroids* (e.g. dexamethasone acetate 4 mg/ml)

- Optional:

  Intracameral, subconjunctival or subtenon's administration of dexamethasone acetate

General comments:

- *Patients with DME or high risk of developing PMEE
- The risk of PME increases as the severity of DRP increases.
- Prophylactic focal/grid laser coagulation of patients with DME is no longer routinely recommended.

(d) Cataract surgery in patients with age-related macular degeneration (AMD).

Timing: If possible, in patients without evidence of intra-/subretinal fluid or with stable macular findings; in patients with exudative AMD and current IVOM therapy between 2 injection intervals (e.g. 1 week after last injection).

Perioperative management:

- Optional:

  - Intravitreal Bevacizumab or Ranibizumab at the end of the operation

General comments:

- Patients with wet (exudative) AMD have an increased overall risk of developing PME
- Cataract surgery does not lead to significant progression of dry or wet (exudative) AMD

(e) Cataract surgery in patients with post corneal transplant condition.

Timing: At the earliest 3–6 months after keratoplasty (depending on the type of keratoplasty).

Perioperative management:

- Preoperative
  - Systemic: Acyclovir 400 mg p.o. 2 times daily or valacyclovir 0.5 g p.o. 4 × daily for 2–3 days (only in case of corresponding medical history)
- Postoperative
  - Day of surgery:
    - Prednisolone acetate 100 mg p.o. 1 × daily for 3 days
    - Pantoprazole 20–40 mg p.o. 1 × daily for 3 days
  - 1st postoperative day:
    - Topical corticosteroids (e.g. dexamethasone acetate 1%) 6 times daily for 1 week, then gradually increasing for 2–3 weeks until the preoperative dose is reached
    - Osmotically active eye drops (e.g. 10% sodium chloride) 4–6 times a day for 1–2 weeks (depending on corneal findings)
    - Artificial tears 4–6 times daily, permanent
    - optional: Acyclovir 400 mg p.o. 2 × daily or valacyclovir 0.5 g p.o. 4 times daily for 1–2 weeks (in patients with ocular history of herpetic keratitis/ keratouveitis; caution: ensure sufficient fluid uptake)

Perioperative setting:

- 1 night inpatient

General comments:

- Any existing immunomodulatory concomitant therapy should be continued.

(f) Cataract surgery in combination with corneal transplantation (pKP, DALK, DS (A)EK, DMEK) [21, 22].

Timing: see ‘Cataract surgery in patients with uveitis’

Perioperative management:

- Preoperative
  - Topical:
    - NSAID eye drops (e.g. nepafenac) 3–4 times daily for 2–3 days

- Systemic:

  Mannitol (e.g. 15% mannitol infusion solution) 1 h preoperative
  Acyclovir 400 mg p.o. 2 × daily or Valacyclovir 0.5 g p.o. 4 times daily for 2–3 days (caution: ensure sufficient fluid uptake)

- Intraoperative
  - Intracameral:
    - Acetylcholine 1% (after completion of cataract surgery)
- Postoperative
  - Day of surgery:
    - Acetazolamide 250 mg p.o. 2–3 times daily for 3–5 days
    - Potassium 600 mg p.o. every other day for 3–5 days
    - Prednisolone acetate 100 mg i.v. 1 × daily for 3 days
    - Pantoprazole 20–40 mg p.o. 1 time daily for 3–5 days
    - Optional: bandage contact lens (until epithelial closure)
  - 1st postoperative day:
    - Antibiotic eye drops (e.g. ofloxacin) 4 times daily for 7–10 days
    - Corticosteroids (e.g. dexamethasone 1%) 6 times daily for 4 weeks with subsequent monthly reduction by 1 drop/day
    - Osmotically active eye drops (e.g. 10% sodium chloride) 4–6 times daily for 1–2 weeks
    - Pilocarpine 1–2% eye drops 3–4 times daily for the duration of intracameral air/gas filling (for DALK or DMEK)
    - Artificial tears 6–8 times daily
  - Optional:
    - Acyclovir 400 mg or 800 mg p.o. 5 × daily for 2–3 months with subsequent reduction (total duration: 6–18 months) (in case of past herpetic keratouveitis (caution: ensure sufficient fluid intake)
    - Acyclovir ointment or gancyclovir ointment 5 × with monthly reduction of 1 application/day

Perioperative setting:

- 3–5 nights in hospital

General comments:

- Back support for DALK/DS(A)EK/DMEK patients for the duration of intra-cameral air/gas filling

(g) Cataract surgery in combination with filtering glaucoma surgery [23]

Perioperative management:

- Preoperative
    - Topical: Change over to preservative-free steroid-containing eye drops (e.g. dexamethasone acetate) 2–3 times daily for 1–2 weeks o
    - Systemic: Acetazolamide 250 mg p.o. (dosage depends on individual intraocular pressure) for 1–2 weeks
- Postoperative
    - Topical:
        - Corticosteroids (e.g. dexamethasone 1%) 7–8 times a day with weekly reduction by 1 eye drops
        - Antibiotic eye drops (e.g. ofloxacin) 4 times daily for 1 week
        - Artificial tears 6–8 times daily continuously

Perioperative setting:

- 2–3 nights in hospital

General comments:

- Topical ß-blockers and/or carboanhydrase inhibitors, if preservative-free can be retained.
- All other anti-glaucomatous eye drops should be discontinued if possible (in particular prostagandin analogues due to the increased risk of postoperative PME).

(h) Cataract surgery in patients with glaucoma [11, 12, 24]

General comments:

- Prostaglandin analogues (alone or in combination with beta-blockers) should be paused perioperatively for 2–3 weeks if possible due to the increased risk of postoperative PME.
- Cholinergics such as pilocarpine should be discontinued at least 3 days before surgery if possible.

(i) Cataract surgery in children [25–27]

Timing: As early and promptly as possible (caution: risk of amblyopia); in the inflammation-free interval (see "Cataract surgery in patients with uveitis").

Perioperative management:

- Postoperative
  - Corticosteroids, subconjunctival (e.g. 4 mg/ml dexamethasone acetate)
  - Alternatively: intracameral, sub-tenon or intravitreal administration of dexamethasone acetate
  - Tropicamide eye drops 2 times daily for 1–2 weeks

Perioperative setting: 1 night as an inpatient or 2 nights as an outpatient (for additional intraoperative measures such as anterior vitrectomy or synechiolysis).

General comments:

- If possible, use preservative-free preparations
- Education about the "off-label" use of drugs not yet explicitly tested on children.

(j) Cataract surgery in patients with Ocular Surface Diseases* [28].

General comments:

- *e.g. ocular cicatrising pemphigoid, Steven-Johnson syndrome, Mooren's ulcer, vernal keratoconjunctivitis, limbal stem cell insufficiency
- Cataract operations should always be performed only during the inactive period of the disease.
- Eyelid malpositions that could cause postoperative wetting disorders of the eye surface should always be corrected/surgically repaired first.
- Preoperative immunosuppressive therapy should be maintained and, if necessary, intensified in the case of active concomitant diseases after consultation with the treating specialist colleague.

Concepts of Dropless Cataract Surgery [8, 9, 29, 30].

Besides the above suggested treatment regimens there are also emerging trends, especially in the U.S., where no FDA-approved antibiotic products for intracameral injection are commercially available, focusing on reduction or complete avoidance of topical therapy after cataract surgery. The rationale behind dropless cataract surgery is based on the knowledge of poor compliance to noncompliance of the patients with health care regimes for medical (e.g. incorrect handling or insufficient eye drop application), social, and financial reasons (e.g. insurance restrictions). Currently, there are a few pre-mixed compounded solutions (e.g. TriMoxi®, TriMoxiVanc®, Dex-Moxi-Ketor®; ImprimisRx®) of antibiotics (e.g. moxifloxacin, vancomycin), steroids (e.g. triamcinolone acetonide, dexamethasone sodium phosphate), and NSAID (e.g. ketorolac tromethamine) available for intracameral and intravitreal installation in order to reduce the risk and severity of postoperative endophthalmitis inflammation, pain, and PME. They can be delivered into the anterior vitreous through a 27 or 30-gauge cannula via a transzonular or a transscleral pars plana injection just before removing of the viscoelastic.

Other surgeons prefer stromal hydration and flushing the anterior chamber with moxifloxacin 0.1 or 0.15% and subsequent subconjunctival injection of 0.4 ml triamcinolone acetate 10 mg/ml (4 mg) 5–6 mm posterior to the limbus). In addition, drug formulations combining phenylephrine, lidocaine (Phenyl-Lido Injectable; ImprimisRx®), and tropicamide (Mydrane®; Thea Pharmaceuticals Ltd.) or phenylephrine and ketorolac (Omidria®; Omeros Corporation) can be injected in the anterior chamber or added to the irrigation solution to achieve a sufficient and stable iris dilatation. Despite promising preliminary results and a lack of major side-effects (e.g. steroid-induced increase of intraocular pressure, corneal, retinal toxicity) large multicenter, prospective, randomized clinical trials are still missing confirming the safety and efficacy of dropless cataract surgery.

References

1. Speaker MG, Menikoff JA. Prophylaxis of endophthalmitis with topical povidone-iodine. Ophthalmology. 1991;98:1769–75. https://doi.org/10.1016/s0161-6420(91)32052-9.
2. Juthani VV, Clearfield E, Chuck RS. Non-steroidal anti-inflammatory drugs versus corticosteroids for controlling inflammation after uncomplicated cataract surgery. The Cochrane. 2017. https://doi.org/10.1002/14651858.CD010516.pub2.
3. Kessel L, Tendal B, Jorgensen KJ, et al. Postcataract prevention of inflammation and macular edema by steroid and nonsteroidal anti-inflammatory eye drops. Ophthalmology. 2014;121:1915–24. https://doi.org/10.1016/j.ophtha.2014.04.035.
4. Gower EW, Lindsley K, Tulenko SE et al Peri-operative antibiotics for prevention of acute endophthalmitis after cataract surgery. Cochrane Database of Systematic Reviews 2017, Issue 2. art. No.: CD006364. doi: https://doi.org/10.1002/14651858.CD006364.pub3.
5. ESCRS Endophthalmitis Study Group. Prophylaxis of postoperative endophthalmitis following cataract surgery: Results of the ESCRS multicenter study and identification of risk factors. J Cataract Refract Surgery. 2007;33:978–88. https://doi.org/10.1016/j.jcrs.2007.02.032.

6. Bowen RC, Zhou AX, Bodalapati S, et al. Comparative analysis of the safety and efficacy of intracameral cefuroxime, moxifloxacin and vancomycin at the end of cataract surgery: a meta-analysis. Br J Ophthalmol. 2018;102:1268–76. https://doi.org/10.1136/bjophthalmol-2017-311051.5.
7. Barry P. Adoption of intracameral antibiotic prophylaxis of endophthalmitis following cataract surgery update on the ESCRS Endophthalmitis Study. J Cataract Refract Surg. 2014;40:138–42. https://doi.org/10.1016/j.jcrs.2013.11.002.
8. Lindstrom RL, Galloway MS, Grzybowski A, Liegner JT. Dropless cataract surgery: an overview. Curr Pharmaceutical Design. 2017;23:558–64. https://doi.org/10.2174/1381612822666161611291.
9. Shornstein NH, Myers WG. Drop-free approaches for cataract surgery. Curr Opin Ophthalmol. 2020;31:67–73. https://doi.org/10.1097/ICU.0000000000000625.
10. Haripriya A, Chang DF. Intracameral antibiotics during cataract surgery: evidence and barriers. Curr Opin Ophthalmol. 2017;29:33–9. https://doi.org/10.1097/ICU.0000000000000445.
11. Wendel C, Zakrzewski H. Carleton B et al Association of postoperative topical prostaglandin analogue or beta-blocker use and incidence of pseudophakic cystoid macular edema. J Glaucoma. 2018;27:402–6. https://doi.org/10.1097/IJG.0000000000000929.
12. Holló G, Aung T, Cantor LB, Aihara M. Cystoid macula edema related to cataract surgery and topical prostaglandin analogues: mechanism, diagnosis, and management. Surv Ophthalmol. 2020;65:496–512. https://doi.org/10.1016/j.survophthal.2020.02.004.
13. Mehta S, Linton MM, Kempen YH. Outcomes of cataract surgery in patients with uveitis: a systematic review and meta-analysis. On J Ophthalmol. 2014;158:676–92. https://doi.org/10.1016/j.survophthal.2020.02.004.
14. Chan NS, Ti SE, Chee SP. Decision-making and management of uveitic cataract. Indian J Ophthalmol. 2017;65:1329–39. https://doi.org/10.4103/ijo.IJO_740_17.
15. Chu CJ, Dick AD, Johnston RL, Yang YC, Denniston AK UK Pseudophakic Macular Edema Study Group. Cataract surgery in uveitis: A multicentre database study. Br J Ophthalmol. 2017; 101:1132–1137. doi: https://doi.org/10.1136/bjophthalmol-2016-309047.
16. Conway MD, Star E, Enfield DB, Peyman GA. Management of cataract in uveitis patients. Curr Opin Ophthalmol. 2018;29:69–74. https://doi.org/10.1097/ICU.0000000000000438.
17. Zierhut M, Szurman P. Perioperative medical management. In: Surgical management of inflammatory eye disease. Eds. Becker, Davis; Springer-Verlag, Heidelberg 2008; 99–102.
18. Boscia F, Giancipoli E, D'Amico-Ricca G, Pinna A. Management of macular oedema in diabetic patients undergoing cataract surgery. Curr Opin Ophthalmol. 2017;28:23–8. https://doi.org/10.1097/ICU.0000000000000328
19. Sarao V, Veritti D, Maurutto E, et al. Pharmacotherapeutic management of macular edema in diabetic subjects undergoing cataract surgery. Exp Opin Pharmacother. 2018;19:1551–63. https://doi.org/10.1080/14656566.2018.1516206.
20. Peterson SR, Silva PA, Murtha TJ, Sun JK. Cataract Surgery in Patients with Diabetes: Management Strategies. Seminar Ophthalmol. 2018;33:75–82. https://doi.org/10.1080/08820538.2017.1353817.
21. Cursiefen C, Schaub F, Bachmann BO. Minimally Invasive Lamellar Keratoplasty: DMEK. DSAEK and DALK Klin Monatsbl Ophthalmology. 2016;233:1033–42. https://doi.org/10.1055/s-0041-110448.
22. Heinzelmann S, Maier P, Böhringer D et al. Cystoid macular edema following Descemet membrane endothelial. Br J Ophthalmol 2015; 99):98–102. doi: https://doi.org/10.1136/bjophthalmol-2014-305124.
23. Marchini G, Ceruti P, Vizzari G, Berzaghi D, Zampieri A. Management of Concomitant Cataract and Glaucoma. Dev Ophthalmol. 2017;59:155–64. https://doi.org/10.1159/000458494.
24. Vizzeri G, Vine RN. Cataract surgery and glaucoma. Cur Opin Ophthalmol. 2010;21:20–4. https://doi.org/10.1097/ICU.0b013e328332f562.

25. Lim ME, Buckley EG, Prakalapakorn SG. Update on congenital cataract surgery management. Curr Opin Ophthalmol. 2017;28:87–92. https://doi.org/10.1097/ICU.0000000000000324.
26. Nischal KK. State of the Art in Pediatric Cataract Surgery. Dev Ophthalmol. 2016;57:15–28. https://doi.org/10.1159/000442497.
27. Mohammadpour M, Shaabani A, Sahraian A, Momenaei B, Tayebi F, Bayat R, Mirshahi R. Updates on managements of pediatric cataract. J Curr Ophthalmol. 2018;2018(22):18–26. https://doi.org/10.1016/j.joco.2018.11.005.
28. Sangwan VS, Gupta S, The S. Cataract surgery in ocular surface diseases: clinical challenges and outcomes. Curr Opin Ophthalmol. 2018;29:81–7. https://doi.org/10.1097/ICU.0000000000000441.
29. An JA, Kasner O, Samek DA, Levesque V. Evaluation of eyedrop administration by inexperienced patients after cataract surgery. J Cataract Refract Surg. 2014;40:1857–61. https://doi.org/10.1016/j.jcrs.2014.02.037.
30. Bardoloi N, Sarkar S, Pilania A, Das H. Safety and efficacy of dropless cataract surgery. Indian J Ophthalmol. 2020;68:1081–5. https://doi.org/10.4103/ijo.IJO_1186_19.

Posterior Capsular Opacification

Pankaj Singh and Clara König

Introduction

Posterior capsule opacification (PCO) is one of the most common postoperative complications encountered after cataract surgery and occurs in 30% of adult patients. It is caused by migration and proliferation of equatorial lens epithelial cells (LECs) to cover the posterior capsule. [8] The incidence of posterior capsule opacification varies greatly. Factors that influence the incidence rate include the age of the patient (children are very prone to early and aggressive PCO), a history of intraocular inflammation or pre-operative procedures (for example, silicone oil can dramatically accelerate progression), the size of the capsulorhexis, the quality of cortical cleaning, the fixation of the implant in the capsule, the design of the lens implant (e.g. square edge optic design), and the time elapsed since surgery.

Factors influencing the formation of PCO after cataract

One of the most important factors that can significantly influence the formation of PCO formation are listed below:

- The intraocular lens material

Supplementary Information The online version contains supplementary material available at https://doi.org/10.1007/978-3-031-05394-8_82. The videos can be accessed individually by clicking the DOI link in the accompanying figure caption or by scanning this link with the SN More Media App.

P. Singh (✉) · C. König
Goethe-University Hospital Frankfurt Am Main, Frankfurt, Germany
e-mail: pankaj.singh@kgu.de

C. König
e-mail: clara.koenig@kgu.de

M. Shajari et al. (eds.), *Cataract and Lens Surgery*,
https://doi.org/10.1007/978-3-031-05394-8_82

An IOL material can be bionic or bioactive, with PMMA and silicone being considered as bionic material and acrylic as bioactive. With bioactive material such as acrylic, the rate of PCO is lower and the onset of the cloudiness after 3 years has been reported as 56% for polymethyl methacrylate, 40% for silicone and 10% for acrylic. [7]

In the case of acrylic implants, it has also been shown that bioadhesion between the capsule and the lens is created at the anterior edge of the capsule in the capsulorhexis area, which stabilizes the overall fit and reduces the formation of PCO. In addition, the edge of the lens has a decisive influence on the formation of PCO: A hard 90° ground edge of the IOL reduces the migration of cells at the posterior capsular bag and thus PCO formation [3]. A recent study also showed that the PCO rate may be higher in multifocal IOLs (15% vs. 6% in monofocal IOLs) [1].

– The position of the lens in the capsule

The position of the lens in the capsule contributes to the reduction of PCO by creating a 360° overlap between the bioactive acrylic surface and the rhexis edge to prevent cell migration. [13] The fitting of the IOL haptics in the capsular bag also promotes stability and thus reduces after cataract formation. Folds in the posterior capsule also increase the incidence of PCO as it provides a channel for cell migration. These often occur due to haptics that are too long or too stiff. A haptic that is too short and too slack can also lead to increased PCO because the capsular bag is not sufficiently stretched [11].

– Surgical technique

In addition to the position of the lens in the capsular bag, surgical factors also play an important role. Polishing the underside of the anterior capsule rim and thorough removal of cortical remnants from the posterior capsule surface leads to a lower probability of PCO. Conversely, removal of lens epithelial cells on the anterior capsule that is too aggressive may also increase the likelihood of PCO. [2] In paediatric cataract surgery, the risk of early and aggressive PCO is high. It can also be difficult to treat in this patient population so it is strongly recommended that a primary posterior continuous curvilinear capsulotomy (with or without an anterior vitrectomy) be performed during the surgery [14].

The treatment of PCO by means of Nd YAG laser capsulotomy

The Nd: YAG laser posterior capsulotomy, or YAG-CT for short, is the preferred procedure for PCO nowadays.

Treatment is typically indicated if:

- the best possible corrected visual acuity has decreased as a result of clinically significant posterior capsular opacity
- a cloudy posterior capsule which prevents a clear view to the back of the eye

- monocular diplopia or glare is caused by wrinkling of the posterior capsule or by a partially opened posterior capsule after surgery in otherwise clear refractive media
- a contraction of the anterior capsulotomy margins (capsular phimosis) occurs, which leads to a displacement of the lens and therefore requires incisions to relax the capsule.

Contraindications for YAG-CT are insufficient visualisation of the posterior capsule, as well as cases of non-cooperative patients who cannot maintain a fixation during the procedure. The use of a fixating contact lens or retrobulbar anaesthesia may improve the feasibility in such patients.

Nd:YAG laser dissection is normally painless and is performed on an outpatient basis.

The surgeon should first adjust the eyepieces of the microscope laser system so that the focal point of the helium–neon target beam is clearly focused at the level of the IOL.

The delivered energy for the capsulotomy of the posterior capsule is usually 0.8 to 2.0 mJ in either Q-switched (5–30 ns pulse length) or mode-locked (30–200 ps pulse length) systems. The surgeon should always use the lowest effective energy output to break through the posterior capsule. Higher energy levels may be required for dense fibrosis.

A clinical view of the posterior capsule through an un-dilated pupil can help the surgeon determine the position of the visual axis, as this is the desired location for opening the capsule. A capsule opening of approximately 3–4 mm is usually sufficient for a satisfactory final result. A `high-plus-power laser lens' improves the stability of the eye and increases the cone angle of the laser beam, thus reducing the depth of field. This reduces damage to structures in front of and behind the focal point by the YAG-CT at a smaller focus diameter. If light reflections from the slit lamp illumination obscure the target beam or the treated area, the position of the biomicroscope should be adjusted.

It has been shown that opening the capsule with a spiral pattern instead of a cross-shaped pattern can reduce the likelihood of damage to the lens, but does tend to cause more vitreous floaters [4, 5].

Lower energy settings reduce the risk of damage to the anterior vitreous boundary membrane. To minimise damage to the IOL, focus directly behind the capsule and then, if necessary, slowly shift the laser pulse towards the lens until the desired location on the capsule is reached. The procedure should start with non-central locations and, ideally in places where the capsule does not directly contact the lens, as YAG-CT can be performed more safely there and optic pits can be avoided. Studies show that lens damage is less likely with acrylic than with other lens materials [9].

If the opacity is exceptionally thick and dense, however, patients require invasive surgical removal using a Vit-cutter (video 1).

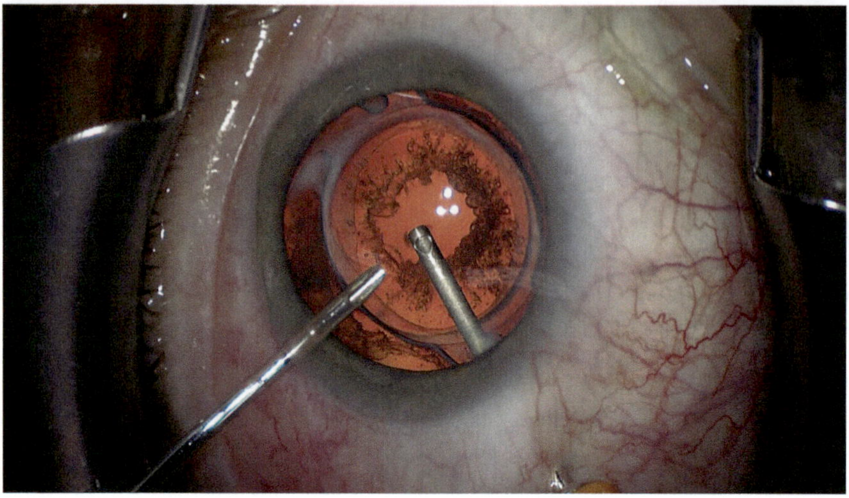

Video 1 Removal of the cataract by a Vit-cutter (MP4 37625 kb) (▶ https://doi.org/10.1007/000-8f3)

Possible complications

- A temporary increase in lOP may occur in a significant number of patients (0.2–3%). This is particularly important in patients with a background of glaucoma. [12] The pressure reaches its peak within two to three hours, probably due to blockage of the drainage channels after the laser treatment. Pressure control should therefore be carried out after the capsulotomy. Intraocular pressure increases usually respond quickly to topical pressure-reducing medication. If necessary, this can then be continued for 3–5 days after the procedure.
- Macular edema can occur after YAG capsulotomy (in 0.4 to 4.9% of cases) [12] Patients with a history of CME or in high-risk patients such as patients with diabetic retinopathy benefit from the use of topical steroids and non-steroidal anti-inflammatory drugs and are recommended.

Author's recommendation

We recommend preoperative macular OCT in high-risk patients to exclude macular edema, and in all patients the administration of Declofenac AT 3 mg/ml once daily for 2 weeks before and after capsulotomy.

- A YAG-laser capsulotomy can increase the risk of retinal detachment, usually associated with posterior detachment of the vitreous body. However, it is difficult to determine whether this is directly related to capsulotomy or cataract surgery itself.

It is recommended that particular attention should be paid to existing risk factors such as high myopia, vitreous trauma or a positive family history of retinal detachment and to inform the patient. [6]

– Another possible complication is the dislocation of the IOL into the vitreous cavity after YAG-laser capsulotomy. This complication occurs mainly with silicone implants with a plate haptic. With a longer time interval between YAG-laser capsulotomy and cataract surgery, this risk becomes smaller, because the IOL is usually already better fixed in the capsular bag. [10] Ensuring that the YAG opening is smaller than the lens optic can significantly reduce this risk.

References

1. Alio JL, Plaza-Puche AB, Férnandez-Buenaga R, Pikkel J, Maldonado M. Multifocal intraocular lenses: an overview. Surv Ophthalmol. 2017;62(5):611–34. https://doi.org/10.1016/j.survophthal.2017.03.005.
2. Bhopi J. Evidence-based approach in cataract surgery. London; New York: Taylor & Francis; 2004. http://site.ebrary.com/id/10341460. Accessed 15 June 2020.
3. Buehl W, Findl O. Effect of intraocular lens design on posterior capsule opacification. J Cataract Refract Surg. 2008;34(11):1976–85. https://doi.org/10.1016/j.jcrs.2008.07.029.
4. Min JM, Yim JH. A new technique for Nd:YAG laser posterior capsulotomy. Int J Ophthalmol. 2014; 7, 5th edn.
5. Kara N, Evcimen Y, Kirik F, Agachan A, Yigit FU. Comparison of two laser capsulotomy techniques: cruciate versus circular. Semin Ophthalmol. 2014;29(3):151–5. https://doi.org/10.3109/08820538.2013.874467.
6. Lin J-Y, Ho W-L, Ger L-P, Sheu S-J. Analysis of factors correlated with the development of pseudophakic retinal detachment - a long-term study in a single medical centre. Graefes Arch Clin Exp Ophthalmol. 2013;251(2):459–65. https://doi.org/10.1007/s00417-012-2043-3.
7. Linnola RJ. Sandwich theory: bioactivity-based explanation for posterior capsule opacification. J Cataract Refract Surg. 1997;23(10):1539–42. https://doi.org/10.1016/S0886-3350(97)80026-0.
8. Milazzo S, Grenot M, Benzerroug M. La cataracte secondaire. J Fr Ophtalmol. 2014;37 (10):825–30. https://doi.org/10.1016/j.jfo.2014.09.003.
9. Newland TJ, McDermott ML, Eliott D, Hazlett LD, Apple DJ, Lambert RJ, Barrett RP. Experimental neodymium:YAG laser damage to acrylic, poly(methyl methacrylate), and silicone intraocular lens materials. J Cataract Refract Surg. 1999; 25(1):72–76. https://doi.org/10.1016/S0886-3350(99)80014-5.
10. Petersen AM, Bluth LL, Campion M. Delayed posterior dislocation of silicone plate-haptic lenses after neodymium:YAG capsulotomy. J Cataract Refract Surg. 2000;26(12):1827–9. https://doi.org/10.1016/S0886-3350(00)00500-9.
11. Ram J, Apple DJ, Peng Q, Visessook N, Auffarth GU, Schoderbek RJ, Ready EL. Update on fixation of rigid and foldable posterior chamber intraocular lenses part II. Ophthalmology. 1999; 106(5), 891–900. https://doi.org/10.1016/S0161-6420(99)00506-0.
12. Steinert RF, Puliafito CA, Kumar SR, Dudak SD, Patel S. Cystoid macular edema, retinal detachment, and glaucoma after Nd:YAG laser posterior capsulotomy. Am J Ophthalmol. 1991;112(4):373–80. https://doi.org/10.1016/S0002-9394(14)76242-7.
13. Ursell PG, Spalton DJ, Pande MV. Anterior capsule stability in eyes with intraocular lenses made of poly(methyl methacrylate), silicone, and AcrySof: J Cataract Refract Surg. 1997;23 (10):1532–1538. https://doi.org/10.1016/S0886-3350(97)80025-9.
14. Vasavada AR, Praveen MR, Tassignon M-J, Shah SK, Vasavada VA, Vasavada VA, et al. Posterior capsule management in congenital cataract surgery. J Cataract Refract Surg. 2011;37(1):173–93. https://doi.org/10.1016/j.jcrs.2010.10.036.

Refractive Surprise After Lens Surgery—Error Prevention and Problem Management

Daniel Kook and Nino Hirnschall

Despite all of the technological advancements and innovations in cataract surgery, we still do not always achieve an uncorrected visual acuity of 20/20 due to unexpected postoperative refractive errors. We described these deviations from the planned refractive outcomes as "refractive surprises" though they are often not that surprising. According to an evaluation of the EUREQUO database, deviations from the defined target refraction by more than 2.0 dpt occur in 1.8% of all eyes after cataract surgery, and in 0.4% the error is even higher than 4.0 dpt [1]. Common causes of this problem are difficulties after corneal or intraocular surgery, ocular or systemic comorbidities, errors and problems with biometry, intra- and postoperative complications, and human or technical errors.

Cases with a History of Previous Surgery

If we consider the EUREQUO dataset, the proportion of eyes with a history of keratorefractive surgery is almost 0.2% in cataract surgery. Due to the change in the ratio of the corneal anterior to posterior surface, the corneal asphericity and the change in the refractive corneal index, errors in biometry can lead to a myopic surprise in patients with previous hyperopic laser surgery and to a hyperopic surprise after myopic laser surgery. There are numerous formulas and methods for lens

D. Kook (✉) · N. Hirnschall
Prof. Kook & Partner, Private Practice, Graefelfing, Germany
e-mail: d.kook@profkookundpartner.de

N. Hirnschall
e-mail: nino@hirnschall.at

N. Hirnschall
Department of Ophthalmology, Kepler University Clinic GmbH and Johannes Kepler University, Linz, Austria

M. Shajari et al. (eds.), *Cataract and Lens Surgery*,
https://doi.org/10.1007/978-3-031-05394-8_83

calculation in these tricky situations. A simple and pragmatic option is the lens calculation software provided on www.iolcalc.org. This site offers 2 groups of formulas. The first is the "history based" method, where the refraction after keratorefractive surgery plays a role and the second is the purely biometric based formulas. In general, and if the information is available, it is advisable to use both methods to estimate the lens power.

Biometry Errors

Numerous ocular comorbidities can lead to incorrect measurements in biometrics. For example, the presence of amblyopia or nystagmus often leads to malfixation. Media opacities such as corneal scars, an advanced cataract, especially posterior shell opacities can also significantly impair optical biometry. Tear film pathologies interfere with keratometry or tomography and cause artefacts that can mask or even engrave an existing astigmatism. This is particularly important to note as many patients experience dry eyes after refractive surgery. It is also essential to stop wearing contact lenses for an appropriate period (up to 2 weeks in the case of hard lenses) before biometry. A good recording quality is mandatory and the quality of the measurement is provided in many devices, for example by the signal to noise ratio. Another example is a "fixation check" where the foveola is also displayed, to ensure that the patient has actually fixated correctly during the measurement. In case of doubt, it is important to check against this using immersion ultrasound biometry. Immersion ultrasound is always preferable to contact ultrasound biometry, as an incorrectly low axial length is often measured when the bulb is compressed.

IOL Calculation Formulas

Modern artificial lens formulas generally lead to good refractive results, but even here, short and long eyes can result in a number of unexpected postoperative refractions. A good way to avoid this error is to compare different artificial lens formulas and always optimise the constants for the artificial lens formulas used. Another, more recent and promising biometric option is ray tracing, which is particularly beneficial for non-standard eyes.

Intraoperative and Postoperative Complications

Intraoperative complications like the upside-down implantation of an angulated IOL can induce myopic displacement, as can an accidental sulcus implantation without buttonholing. In these cases, due to the more anteriorly positioned optic of the IOL, the strength of the IOL should be weakened depending on the chosen strength to avoid a myopic surprise. For example, a thickness of 0–10 dpt should not be changed, but an IOL thickness > 25 dpt should be reduced by about 1.5 dpt.

If there is a refractive error after the operation of the first eye, a thorough diagnosis should be made to exclude possible postoperative complications or pathologies before conclusions are drawn about the choice of IOL strength for the second eye. For example, a hyperopic shift after lens surgery can be induced by postoperative complications such as corneal edema, hypotension or pseudocystoid macular edema, whereas a myopic shift can be induced by postoperative complications such as tunnel leakage with a flat anterior chamber, residual viscoelastic behind the IOL or choroidal effusion. After all these sources of error have been eliminated, it is possible to learn from the first eye in order to adapt the artificial lens calculation for the second eye. In this way, almost 40% of the error of the first eye is corrected in the second eye [2].

Sources of Error When Implanting Toric Artificial Lenses

Although the refractive results after implantation of a toric artificial lens are generally good, in some cases there is an unexpectedly high post-operative residual astigmatism. Sources of error in this context are numerous and can occur preoperatively, intraoperatively and postoperatively [3]. One of the main problems in calculating the strength of the toric artificial lens is the measurement of the cornea itself [4]. This measurement depends on many factors, including the quality of the tear film, diurnal changes in the cornea and longer-term changes in corneal radii [5]. Another possible source of error is if only the anterior corneal surface is measured, as the influence of corneal posterior surface astigmatism on total corneal astigmatism is on average about 10–15% [6]. If posterior astigmatism is not taken into account, this leads on average to an overcorrection of 0.5–0.6 dpt in the case of a rectus astigmatism and to an undercorrection of 0.2–0.3 dpt in the case of an inverse astigmatism. On the other hand, measurements that cover both the anterior and posterior corneal surface, such as Scheimpflug measurements, are not always superior to the other measurement methods [7]. The reason for this could be movement artefacts during the longer measurement period. The trend therefore, is towards methods that allow faster measurement of the anterior and posterior corneal surface. An example of this approach is swept source optical coherence tomography measurement [7].

The misalignment of toric IOLs can in general be attributed to one of three components: The pre-operative marking on the sitting patient, the intra-operative marking and the post-operative rotation of toric IOLs [3]. For each degree of misalignment, approximately three percent of astigmatism correction is lost. With regard to preoperative marking, digital marking systems seem to offer an advantage over manual marking in terms of precision [8] If a misalignment exists postoperatively, a subsequent rotation of the toric IOL can often improve the result. A good way to calculate the extent of the post-rotation is also available free of charge as a software program and is recommended: www.astigmatismfix.com. It is important that the strength of the IOL is entered here at corneal level and not at IOL level - in other words, the torus of the lens label must not simply be entered. A post-rotation should not be performed too early (risk of a 2nd post-rotation) and not too late (capsule fibrosis), so in principle is best done about 2–4 weeks postoperatively.

On average, surgically induced corneal astigmatism is often close to zero, especially with modern microincisional incision techniques. However, the variation between patients is high, so in individual cases the corneal incision can also be a relevant source of error for postoperative astigmatism [3]. It is also important in this context that the effect of surgically induced corneal astigmatism usually fades over time postoperatively and discrepancies between pre- and early postoperative corneal tomography are often not permanent. Therefore, preoperative tomography should always be included in the search for the cause of postoperative residual astigmatism. Even after implantation of a toric IOL, total astigmatism can change naturally, according to a study, on average by 0.4 dpt against the rule over a period of 10 years after cataract surgery [9]. Therefore, in the authors' view, total corneal astigmatism according to the rule should not be initially overcorrected but rather 0.25 dpt undercorrected or accepted and astigmatism against the rule should be fully corrected. At this point it should be noted that in special situations such as the presence of deep meridional amblyopia, a full astigmatism neutralization of the optical system by means of a toric IOL is not always an ideal approach.

Human and Technical Failure

Human error can never be 100% excluded. Therefore, in the case of refractive post-operative surprises, it is always important to carefully check all available measurements again and to repeat them. A very rare source of error is also the labelling of the IOL. An incorrectly labelled IOL usually leads to an even bigger surprise when an IOL is exchanged based on working from incorrect conclusions. In this context, however, even without labelling errors according to ISO 11979, the tolerance of the deviation of the IOL thickness at over 30 dpt is 1.0 dpt.

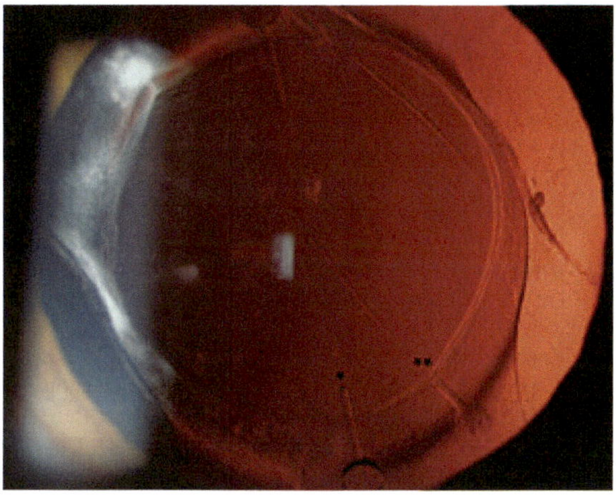

Fig. 1 Biomicroscopic image 1 day after post-rotation of a toric IOL with plate haptics 15 months after primary implantation. The asterisk marks the new axis of the lens torus, the double asterisk the old position of the lens torus as an impression in the anterior capsule leaf

Management of Refractive Surprise

Surgical options for refractive surprise can be divided into corneal and intraocular procedures. In principle, keratorefractive laser procedures are suitable for fine corrections in the indication area, i.e. mostly for myopic or anti-astigmatic post-corrections. In the case of mixed astigmatism, corneal anti-astigmatic incision procedures represent an additional option. Intraocular procedures that can be considered include IOL exchange, rotation and fixation as well as sulcus-supported add-on implants (piggy-back lenses). The correction of higher hyperopic surprises is usually reserved for intraocular procedures. In any case, it is important to check the corresponding inclusion and exclusion criteria. This includes a refractive stability, which in many cases is only performed about 3 months postoperatively. Performing a Nd:YAG-LASER for posterior capsular opacification can also cause a change in refraction by changing the IOL position, so that if a post-correction on the cornea is planned, the Nd:YAG-LASER should generally be performed before a corneal excimer laser procedure [10] If an IOL exchange or post-rotation are needed the should be performed earlier, ideally no later than 1–3 months postoperatively. However, depending on the lens material used, patient age and posterior capsular opacification formation, both IOL exchange and post-rotation are generally still possible at a later date [11] (Fig. 1).

Memo
Refractive surprises are partly avoidable, but also cannot be completely eliminated despite taking the utmost caution. In the case of non-standard eyes in particular, surprises should be anticipated and these should be carefully managed. With regard to the predictability of the target fraction, "underpromise and overdeliver" should be the goal, especially when choosing a refractive IOL.

References

1. Lundstrom M, Manning S, Barry P, Stenevi U, Henry Y, Rosen P. The European registry of quality outcomes for cataract and refractive surgery (EUREQUO): a database study of trends in volumes, surgical techniques and outcomes of refractive surgery. Eye Vis (London). 2015;2:8.
2. Olsen T, Logstrup N, Olesen H, Corydon L. Using the surgical result in the first eye to calculate intraocular lens power for the second eye. J Cataract Refract Surg. 1993;19(1):36–9.
3. Hirnshall N, Hoffmann PC, Draschl P, Maedel S, Findl O. Evaluation of factors influencing the remaining astigmatism after toric intraocular lens implantation. J Refract Surg. 2014;30 (6):394–400.
4. Roberts C. The cornea is not a piece of plastic. J Refract Surg. 2000;16(4):407–13.
5. Norrby S, Brain Sound N, Nishi Y, Findl O. Fluctuations in corneal curvature limit predictability of intraocular lens power calculations. J Cataract Refract Surg. 2013;39(2):174–9.
6. Abulafia A, Hill WE, Franchina M, Barrett GD. Comparison of methods to predict residual astigmatism after intraocular lens implantation. J Refract Surg. 2015;31(10):699–707.
7. Hoffmann PC, Abraham M, Hirnschall N, Findl O. Prediction of residual astigmatism after cataract surgery using swept source fourier domain optical coherence tomography. Current Eye Res. 2014;39(12):1178–86.
8. Mayer WJ, Kreutzer T, Dirisamer M, Kern C, Kortuem K, Vounotrypidis E, et al. Comparison of visual outcomes, alignment accuracy, and surgical time between 2 methods of corneal marking for toric intraocular lens implantation. J Cataract Refract Surg. 2017;43 (10):1281–6.
9. Hayashi K, Hirata A, Manabe S, Hayashi H. Long-term change in corneal astigmatism after sutureless cataract surgery. At J Ophthalmol. 2011;151(5):858–65.
10. Vrijman V, van der Linden JW, Nieuwendaal CP, van der Meulen IJ, Mourits MP, Lapid-Gortzak R. Effect of Nd:YAG laser capsulotomy on refraction in multifocal apodized diffractive pseudophakia. J Refract Surg. 2012;28(8):545–50.
11. Brandlhuber U, Haritoglou C, Kreutzer TC, Kook D. Reduction of a misaligned Zeiss AT TORBI 709M(R) intraocular lens 15 months after implantation. Eur J Ophthalmol. 2014;24 (5):800–2.

Management of the Unhappy Patient

Richard Packard and Wolfgang J. Mayer

Introduction

On February 8th 1950 when Harold (later Sir Harold) Ridley, a surgeon at St Thomas' Hospital in London, first implanted an intraocular lens (IOL), he was completing what he called "the cure for aphakia". The operation itself, a secondary implantation, went without any problems. The cataract had been removed from this patient on November 29th the previous year. There is no doubt that Ridley expected his operation to be a refractive success also. However due to a major miscalculation of the correct lens power, the measurement being made in air rather than water, the patient was made very myopic. Not only that, the black silk sutures, used to close the wound, induced many dioptres of astigmatism.

Today we have a wide range of instruments to assist us to achieve, what both the surgeon and the patient regard, as an excellent visual outcome. However, despite our best efforts to achieve this result patients may still be unhappy because their expectations for their surgery have not been met. This may be due to a number of reasons not the least being, as discussed later, a false impression of the outcome being generated at the informed consent. There are also patients that achieve what we as surgeons consider to be a perfect result, but still the patient is not happy. An example of this is a patient having had an aspheric IOL implanted with an excellent biometric result, seeing 6/5, 20/15, −0.1, or 1.25 unaided, but unhappy. They have great unaided distance vision but have to put glasses on to see the food on their

R. Packard
Department of Ophthalmology, University of London, London, United Kingdom
e-mail: eyequack@vossnet.co.uk

W. J. Mayer (✉)
Department of Ophthalmology, Ludwig Maximilian University, Munich, Germany
e-mail: wolfgang.j.mayer@med.uni-muenchen.de

M. Shajari et al. (eds.), *Cataract and Lens Surgery*,
https://doi.org/10.1007/978-3-031-05394-8_84

plate when they are eating. More often it is the quality or level of vision being sub-optimal which is the cause of dissatisfaction.

Let's have a look at some of the reasons why this might be. One issue which is worth exploring first, which applies to all patients, but much more particularly to those having multifocal or extended depth of focus (EDOF) IOLs is the process of neural adaptation. The ability of an individual patient to adapt to the change that has taken place in their vision.

Our visual system is essentially made up of two different components: the optical system which alters light before it reaches the retina, and the neurological system (including the retina and brain) that processes the information. This adaptation can be rapid, as when we adapt to light or darkness, but can be very slow due to altered neuronal plasticity, for example, when there is a long-term change in anatomical connections or synaptic properties due to neuronal activity or injury. Thus, axons and dendrites may grow and retract in the retina and brain and synapses may be lost or gained. We know for example that adaptation allows people to see better with their own higher-order aberrations than with corresponding optical defocus. In multifocal IOL (MFIOL) patients, neural plasticity probably explains:

- the improvement in contrast sensitivity generally observed at six months postoperatively
- better contrast sensitivity in patients with bilateral MFIOLs compared with those only unilaterally implanted
- perceptual learning from experience gained after surgery giving permanent changes in perception
- programmes aimed at deliberately improving specific functioning, such as exercises with Gabor patches or discrimination tests in orientation.

The important message is to wait at least 6 months before taking any action if there are no obvious contributory factors which might have caused problems [1, 2].

Reasons for Dissatisfaction: Monofocal IOLs

There are certain problems which can cause dissatisfaction with any type of IOL and these most often relate to biometry. Axial length measurements with optical devices are now very accurate and unlikely to be a cause of an inaccurate lens power calculation. Estimating the effective lens position is by far the most common cause followed by corneal measurements.

The commonest reasons for inaccurate corneal measurements are tear film related. It is very important to recognise an inadequate tear film when measurements are made. Using a topographer to check the corneal power will demonstrate this even when it is not obvious clinically. Missed tear film problems will also cause unhappiness post-operatively particularly with MFIOL patients.

With non-toric monofocal IOLs, if the biometry target has been hit and the tear film is good, patient complaints are uncommon. As I said above, a limited visual range with only excellent unaided distance vision, but a poor range of vision, can also be an issue.

Toric IOLs on the other hand can lead to patient complaints for other reasons which are largely related to:

- Incorrect measurement of the corneal power (including posterior corneal curvature).
- Undetected irregular astigmatism
- Wrong IOL chosen
- Surgically induced astigmatism (SIA)
- Anatomical anomalies like deep or shallow anterior chambers
- Preoperative marking
- Intraoperative misalignment
- Postoperative rotation of the IOL.

However, post-operatively the last two are the only ones that are easily dealt with by an intervention repositioning the IOL. This can be calculated using the on-line calculator astigmatismfix.com. This software programme allows the post-operative data to be entered and suggestions as to the best outcome by rotating the |IOL will be made. Of course if there are spherical inaccuracies rather than those related to astigmatism then refractive laser approaches can be used to improve the patient's vision.

Multifocal IOLs

Most of the patients that present in the post-operative period with complaints will have had MFIOLs implanted. So, let us examine the issues that cause these patients to come forward and offer solutions for them and their surgeons. Make no mistake unhappy patients will make your professional life unhappy too as these patients will come back to see you on a regular basis.

Whilst the use of multifocal and EDOF IOLs has increased very greatly in the past decade as more and varied designs come onto the market and increasing patient awareness and surgeon enthusiasm has driven demand, not every patient is happy with the result. This may, for example, be because of a suboptimal visual acuity result for either near or distance or due to the effects of the IOL design causing intolerable dysphotopsias. Very often these problems will be due to inadequate understanding by the patient of what is actually possible. Let us now will review the major causes of patient unhappiness and suggest solutions.

Avoiding Problems by Adequate Preoperative Discussions and Ocular Measurement

After having carried out a full ophthalmic examination including the following:

- Tear film
- Pupillary function
- Optical media
- Macular issues.

Make sure that there are no comorbidities like diabetic retinopathy or advanced glaucoma which will not only compromise the visual result but are contraindications for multifocal IOL use; time needs to be spent talking through what your patients are about to experience. Many of the issues which appear as a problem for these patients after their surgery would not occur with time spent in discussion prior to surgery. This includes an assessment by the surgeon and ancillary staff as to the character, patient's needs, lifestyle and expectations. It may be that unreasonable expectations for visual outcome or a particularly obsessive nature will be a contraindication for the use of these lenses. Never promise full spectacle independence but say that there is a good chance that a lot of the time glasses will not be needed. There are a number of useful questionnaires available to try to assist in this personality assessment.

From the surgeon's point of view a well-developed knowledge of the characteristics of each style of lens they plan to use is mandatory.

- Do they for example give good distance and intermediate vision at the expense of better reading vision like the current crop of new EDOF IOLs e g Eyhance (Johnson and Johnson, USA or Vivity (Alcon, USA) but with minimal effect on contrast sensitivity and dysphotopsia creation?
- Will reading require good light for the lens to work like most diffractive IOLs because the available light must be divided between the various foci?

In practice it is worth going to great lengths to emphasize such issues. All patients need to understand that whichever IOL is used a compromise will need to be made as the available light is divided and some lost. There is simultaneous vision between near and distance resulting in a second blurred image which patients need to learn to ignore. This becomes even more important when trifocal lenses like the Fine Vision (Physiol, Belgium) or the Lisa Tri (Zeiss, Germany) are being considered. In the past, most multifocal IOLs were actually bifocal and the relatively poorer intermediate vision available needed to be emphasized. There are now a number of newer trifocals including those from Rayner in the UK, Care Group in India and VSY in Turkey. All diffractive IOLs will lead to haloes at night and patients need to know this in advance and preferably get some idea of what this means by a simulation. Many patients with cataracts will have been aware of these anyway. Patients should be informed that this phenomenon is a function of the design of the lens and that the vast majority of people get used to them very quickly. Also emphasize that when driving at night it is important to look at the near side kerb where the dipped headlight beam falls.

Patients should have a clear idea of the process and time frame of adaptation to their new lenses. Although most patients will be comfortable with their near and distance vision within a week, but some may take much longer, up to several months. Say to all my patients that they will be happy quicker if they do not try to deconstruct every aspect of their vision because this will lead to a much slower neural adaptation and potential dissatisfaction. The same can be said of constantly comparing one eye with the other if the patient has not been bilaterally implanted [3–5]. All of the multifocal lenses like trifocals available have a fixed reading distance which has a limited range on either side of the sweet spot. Patients need to realise that finding the focal length at an early stage post operatively will lead to a quicker adaptation to their new visual status. Emphasise that from day one they should try to find this distance and try to place whatever they are reading in the same position until it becomes second nature. The same is true of intermediate distance with trifocal and EDOF IOLs. But both of these will blend as time goes on as part of the neural adaptation. One reason one of the authors (RP) likes to carry out same day surgery is that there is no opportunity to compare eyes and also because of the enhancement to vision of binocular implantation from day one. Certainly, there are advantages of doing the surgery to both eyes in close temporal proximity even if not on the same day.

Optimisation of A constants and careful biometry with a modern optical device like the latest IOL Master (Zeiss, Germany) or LenStar (Haag Streit, Germany) will help to avoid refractive surprises. The Zeiss Lisa Tri has been optimised for the Haegis formula, but whichever formula is used the surgeon must optimise from their refractive outcomes. Using the calculator on Dr Warren Hill's website makes this a simple exercise. The Hill-RBF 3.0 calculator, the new Kane formula and the Barrett suite are now generally recommended for the most accurate calculations. If it is not possible to use an optical device for biometry it is preferable to use immersion A scan as this is more accurate than using the direct contact method.

It is critical that the corneal characteristics are also assessed. Using topography and aberrometry will not only pick up corneal abnormalities like forme fruste keratoconus and coma which will be contraindications for multifocal IOL implantation but using a Scheimpflug device like the Pentacam (Oculus, Germany) enables the surgeon to determine the posterior corneal power. The Barrett True-K formula has proven very useful. This last has been shown to be important in determining the amount of cylindrical error requiring correction by a toric IOL of any sort. With a multifocal IOL astigmatism of 0.5 dioptres or more should be corrected. With very small amounts of cylinder limbal relaxing incisions may be a better option than a toric lens especially if done with the precision of the femtosecond laser.

Having made the patient aware of what they should expect from their new lens and given them a fully informed consent form to sign it is now time to arrange their surgery. Be aware that despite the best efforts of you and your staff to prepare your patients for their surgery and recovery they will forget most of what has been told them. It is thus very important that you give patients written information about their lenses. Most companies will have some patient literature available but you may wish to create your own.

When the time comes for surgery, apart from the obvious need to make a central capsulorhexis overlapping the IOL, making every effort to place a toric lens accurately is even more important when using a multifocal. Even small inaccuracies of placement will result in degradation of the image for the patient.

Why are Patients Unhappy?

Let us assume in the first instance that the surgery has gone well, the lenses are implanted as expected and the patient has come for their first postoperative visit. Despite all that you and your staff have told them they are not happy. At this point it is important to try and assess what is disturbing them. What are the potential problems?

- Distance vision less than expected
- Distance vision “waxy”
- Reading vision less than expected
- Inability to read in poor light
- Poor intermediate vision
- Dark shadow in the temporal field
- Glare and haloes at night
- Poor night vision
- Foreign body sensation.

Let us consider these in turn.

Distance Vision Less Than Expected or “Waxy”

If seen at one week postoperatively the effects of the surgery on ocular tissues are normally mostly gone. By this stage the patient should be getting a fair idea of their distance vision. Complaints of poor distance vision at this point generally fall into three categories:

- Failure to adapt to the presence of combinations of near, intermediate and distance vision at the same time. Patients report that they can see a long way down the chart but somehow it seems blurred. This is generally more of a problem in diffractive multifocals like the PanOptix (Alcon,USA) or FineVision (Physiol, Belgium) than zonal refractive lenses like the MPlus or EDOF IOLs like Eyhance or Vivity. If the spherical correction is accurate i.e. less than 0.5 dioptres from desired outcome patients will generally adjust pretty quickly and

learn to ignore any blur and concentrate on the clear image. Although some may always complain that their vision seems "waxy".
- Inability to see clearly down the chart beyond 20/40 or 6/12. This is due to two issues, either the biometry has been inaccurate or a toric lens has not been correctly placed or has shifted position. These patients will generally require some remediation, and this will be discussed below.
- The patient has a comorbidity in the eye which was not picked up preoperatively. For example in cataract patients a preretinal membrane may not have been visible through the lens opacity. An OCT before surgery is recommended for all patients for MFIOLs. In the presence of an epiretinal membrane referral to a vitreoretinal surgeon is required. A poor tear film is often missed and can have a profound effect on the vision with multifocal IOLs. Checking tear osmolarity and break up time preoperatively even when patients are asymptomatic is a useful, exercise which can avoid later disappointment. As already stated Placido disc topography is also a good way to assess the integrity of the tear film. Dosing with lubricants and repeating the measurements will normally improve things considerably.

Reading Vision Less Than Expected and Poor in Low Light

One of the main reasons that patients opt for a multifocal IOL is to be able to read without glasses. Thus, when they cannot even in good light, they are not happy. This may occur for several reasons.

- At one week postop however one of the commonest reasons for less than expected reading vision is that the reading material is not being held in the optimal position. A little time spent demonstrating that reading is actually good when the right position is used generally solves the problem particularly when the patient has shown you that they have good unaided distance vision. This is where a device like Vivior (Vivior, Switzerland) which enables the focal distances used by a patient to be analysed by a device worn on a pair of glasses. Thus, real reading distance before surgery will be known for example and the optimal reading addition in the IOL can be utilised.
- It may be that the reading addition is not sufficient for the patient to resolve small print. Often this is because the lens has been chosen for distance and intermediate vision according to the patient's claimed needs. The spherical correction is not correct. This will mean that if myopic the reading distance may be too close or too far if the patient has ended up hyperopic. As for distance vision a toric lens may be malpositioned. Solutions for this will be discussed below.
- As above ocular comorbidity may be present and will need to be dealt with as before.

Reading in poor light is generally not very good with most multifocal lenses. When patients complain of this they need to be reminded that they were told this before surgery. It is worth suggesting the use of the flashlight on a mobile phone if they need to read for short periods. For extended reading using a good halogen or LED light works very well.

Early and seemingly minimal posterior capsular changes can with MFIOLs lead to loss of reading vision and such patients will need a capsulotomy much sooner than in a monofocal implantee. A wide capsular opening is essential here to enable the IOL to function properly again.

Poor Intermediate Vision

As already stated most multifocal IOLs were in the past in fact bifocals but whilst some with lower adds have good intermediate vision for most it is much poorer than near or distance. Happily the availability of trifocal MFIOLs and the new EDOF lenses has really eliminated this as an issue.

Dark Shadows or Flickering Lights in the Temporal Field

The shadow is a common complaint in the early postoperative period due a negative dysphotpsia but there may also be a positive change in the temporal visual field as in shards of light, positive dysphotpsias. There are many theories as to why these occur but no clear answers. The good news is that these usually disappear with time. As far as negative dysphotopsia is concerned some say that it is when the anterior capsule covering the edge of the IOL opacifies others that the patient adapts. Others still say that it is the anterior capsule itself which causes the problem. It may be due to a space between the edge of the lens and the iris allowing stray light to create an internal reflection from the sharp edge of the IOL. Another theory says that when the pupil is small a penumbra is created in the nasal field of vision which is seen as dark arc [6–9]. In some patients it can persist because either they are unable to adapt to it or it just has not get better. In any event they complain bitterly leading to frequent office visits. The prevalence is up to 19% with decrease to 3% after one year. Solutions will be discussed below.

Glare and Haloes

Inherent in the design of all MFIOLs whether they are diffractive or refractive is the likelihood of some unwanted optical effects like glare and haloes. However, some designs have been shown to have more problems in this regard than others.

Diffractive designs, due to the concentric rings on their surface that enable near, intermediate and distance vision to be achieved, will inevitably create haloes at night. The use of apodisation and an aspheric base lens does lessen the effect considerably but despite this patients will complain. The good news is that in the vast majority of cases time will allow them to adapt. However, if they feel they cannot manage then lens exchange has to be considered. Make sure that no one has tried to improve the situation by carrying out a YAG capsulotomy as this will make any lens exchange much more hazardous. As above, a trial for the patient of loss of reading vision can help them to decide if it is a worthwhile price for getting less visual problems at night. It is important to distinguish between glare which may occur with any IOL for some patients and issues relating to their MFIOL. Unfortunately, even after lens exchange patients may still be troubled by unwanted glare. If lens exchange is contemplated it is important to have warned the patient that there may be surgical complications which could worsen their vision and that they may still have some symptoms. Most patients will adapt in time but be aware in younger patients where the entry pupil at night is large, haloes may be a problem. Here the use of a mild miotic at night like brimonidine can be helpful. Finally, in IOLs made of a hydrophilic acrylic, opacification of the optic (Fig. 1) can induce haloes. This has been found most often in MFIOLs from Oculentis (now Teleon, Germany) due to packaging and manufacturing issues. It is said these have now been resolved but it is something to bear in mind as this takes years to develop.

Other issues to bear in mind concern such things as higher order aberrations. Thus, a corneal Root Mean Square (RMS HOA) of 0.3 microns should not be exceeded for the central 4 mm zone. Coma (blurred vision, double vision), spherical aberration (glare and haloes), and trefoil (starburst and comet tail) are particularly notable as common aberrations that negatively affect corneal multifocal intraocular optics in particular and are perceived as positive dysphotopsias [10–14].

In hyperopic eyes angle kappa is important in relation to IOL centration. Less than 0.5 mm here is the critical "offset" for multifocal optics implantation [15].

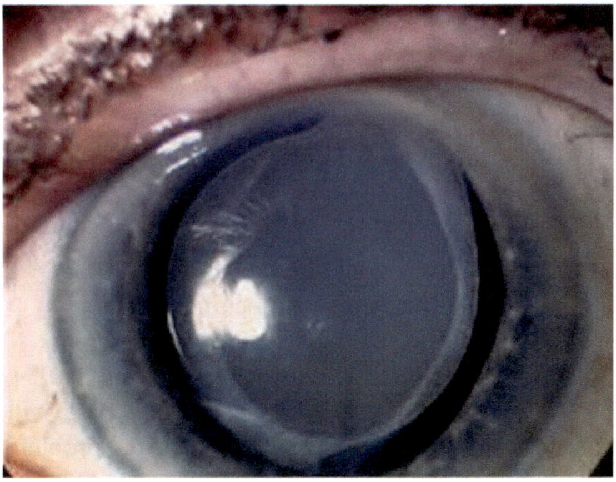

Fig. 1 Opacification of a hydrophilic IOL

A Structured Approach to Provide Solutions for the Unhappy Patient

When the unhappy patient returns to see you, it is best to have clear and logical approach to help both you and them. For the patient, their problem seems to them very real and they want a solution. Often as we have seen above this will be very obvious and straightforward. However, spending time listening to the complaints is very important in maintaining the patient's trust in you to deal with their issues as well as your understanding of how to make things better. Members of your staff need to know that this patient is not happy and thus be supportive.

- Less than hoped for far vision
- Less than hoped for near vision
- Less than hoped for intermediate vision
- Dysphotopsias whether negative or positive
- Glare and haloes.

Many of these issues have already been referred to but it is useful at this stage to review solutions.

Distance Vision Issues

With modern optical devices for biometry refractive surprises are not a common problem but with MFIOLs small errors of refraction can diminish the effectiveness of the lens. Normally being within 0.5D of intended refraction should ensure a good result. Many patients will tolerate up to 1D of spherical error but at this level especially with diffractive IOLs haloes at night are likely to be more troublesome and awareness of a second blurred image. Distance vision may also be affected by failure to correct astigmatism fully. Increasingly there are devices to help the surgeon place the lens more accurately in the correct meridian, but the corneal measurements are still not completely accurate. If the residual astigmatism is less than 0.5D patients will normally be happy.

What solutions can be offered to patients to enhance their distance vision? The need to do this depends partly on the degree of refractive error but also on the patient's expectation as far as spectacle independence is concerned. Thus, whilst some will accept a situation which means that for many tasks they do not need glasses, others will deem this unacceptable. Often this latter group have had unrealistic expectations from the outset despite preoperative discussions. It is important that this has been documented.

A number of patients implanted with diffractive MFIOLs initially have difficulty, even with a good refractive result, complaining that their vision seems not clear or "waxy". Almost all of these patients, given time, will adapt. As already states do not consider any action for at least 6 months. A problem here may be that only one eye has been implanted and the patient is hesitant to have a similar lens in the second eye. One of the reasons one of the authors (RP) likes to do same day surgery for both eyes is that with both eyes open this visual effect is much diminished. However, another solution is to use a lens in the second eye which has less effect on distance vision like an MPlus or an enhanced monofocal which acts like an EDOF lens like Eyhance or Vivity.

Finally, a good tear film is essential for MF but also important for EDOF IOLS to work properly. This is much more critical than with purely monofocal IOLs. This ideally should be picked up at preoperative examination and the patient advised accordingly. Checking tear film break up time and performing preoperatively a Schirmer test and tear osmolarity are very useful. If a patient with less-than-ideal tear film still wishes for an MFIOL; lubricants will be required.

Here is an algorithm for correction of postop refractive errors:

- Counselling to assess the patient's attitude with assurances, and if required, of solutions.
- Offer glasses for occasional use such as in driving or watching movies. For many people being able to do most things around the house without glasses is a good result.
- Offer contact lenses because with full distance correction reading glasses usually are not needed. This may work for people who previously wore contact lenses.
- Surgical solutions to include excimer laser, SMILE, piggyback sulcus lenses, toric lens adjustment.
- The advantage of excimer laser, SMILE or piggybacking is that you are correcting a known error. Lens exchange unless the reason for the refractive error is a recognised lens error is not advised.

Near Vision Problems

The commonest difficulty that patients experience with their near vision is their failure to understand the limited range of focus that MFIOLs like trifocals generally provide. Patients need to learn to find their ideal reading distance which may be different from that which they had preoperatively. We emphasize this preoperatively and especially in the immediate postoperative period. Once that has been dealt with the importance of good lighting with most MFIOLs must be highlighted. Making patients aware in advance of surgery of the capabilities of the proposed lens they are receiving helps greatly in avoiding disappointment. Some lenses like the Symfony (Johnson and Johnson, USA) and the Lentis Comfort (Teleon, Germany) lens will give good distance and intermediate vision but only poor reading unless some sort of monovision has been used. Despite all of this some patients are not satisfied and this is generally due to residual refractive error either spherical or cylindrical. A myopic error may mean the reading distance is too close and the opposite if the patient is left hyperopic. As above tear film is also very important. If the poor reading is due to the actual lens design the simplest solution really is reading glasses about which the patient has probably been warned anyway. It is possible that a patient would ask for different IOL with a stronger reading addition but great care needs to be taken in this situation. The patient may swap their better reading vision for less clear distance vision. If the refractive error is either due to incorrect spherical power or failure to correct astigmatism the solutions mentioned above for distance vision can be utilised.

Poor Intermediate Vision

One of the drawbacks until recently with MFIOLs is that they were actually bifocal with two distinct peaks on the defocus curve. As stated above there are now trifocal IOLs available that offer better intermediate vision, but the available light now needs to be divided three ways. Finding out in advance if intermediate rather than near vision is more important preoperatively is helpful. This the opens up a range extended depth of focus (EDOF) IOLs like the Symfony (J and J. USA) or Lara (Zeiss, Germany) and the enhanced monofocals.

Negative and Positive Dysphotopsias

As already mentioned, dysphotopsias are a common complaint in the early post-operative period. Fortunately for most patients the reassurance that these will pass or seem to disappear will be sufficient. However, some patients will be extremely disturbed by these phenomena. The cause is not by any means fully understood nor is it possible to predict which patients will have problems. Both negative and positive dysphotopsias may have the same root cause. There is a general feeling that the sharp edge of a hydrophobic acrylic IOL is more likely to produce a problem but there are many theories as to why [16, 17]. Miotics may help with positive dysphotopsias but do not with negative ones. In patients that insist on some remedial action after allowing time for adaptation or resolution there are two courses of action. The IOL can be removed and replaced with one of a different design and material. Often this may mean that they lose their multifocal lens in favour of a monofocal with a round edge. A trial for the patient by placing a −3 lens in front of them when they try to read will remind the patient what it is like not to have unaided reading vision. A better alternative is to implant sulcus lens [18] like the Rayner Sulcoflex. This has a 6.5 mm optic and a round edge it fills the space behind the iris and redirects the light away from the sharp edge of the multifocal lens. The Sulcoflex IOL can also be used to correct any residual refractive error if present. It has also been suggested that in fact prolapsing the IOL optic out of the capsular bag can help [7].

Glare and Haloes

MFIOLs by virtue of their complex designs are highly likely to produce some unwanted visual phenomena as we have seen already. These include glare and haloes (Fig. 2). It is not unusual for any patient having lens implant surgery whether mono or multifocal to experience some photophobia in the immediate postoperative period. There is greater light scatter with MFIOLs which may make this more prominent but it generally passes. Haloes are normally associated with MFIOLs because of their design whether diffractive or refractive. Patients should be made aware in advance of surgery that they will see this. Again, almost all patients adapt to this and do not find that there is a permanent problem. Some patients feel relief of these symptoms when driving at night while the cabin light is on, causing a reduction in pupil size and hence a relief of glare and haloes. The later designs of lens have made haloes less obvious. However, some patients find these intolerable and for them lens exchange is probably the only option. Fortunately the newer enhanced monofocals have no more photic phenomena than a normal monofocal so for patients concerned by the idea of any glare or haloes who still would like some degree of independence this type of lens is a safer solution.

It is important that no one carries out a YAG laser capsulotomy which makes lens exchange surgery much more difficult and potentially hazardous. Remember to have a trial with each potential lens exchange patient of what losing their unaided reading vision will mean.

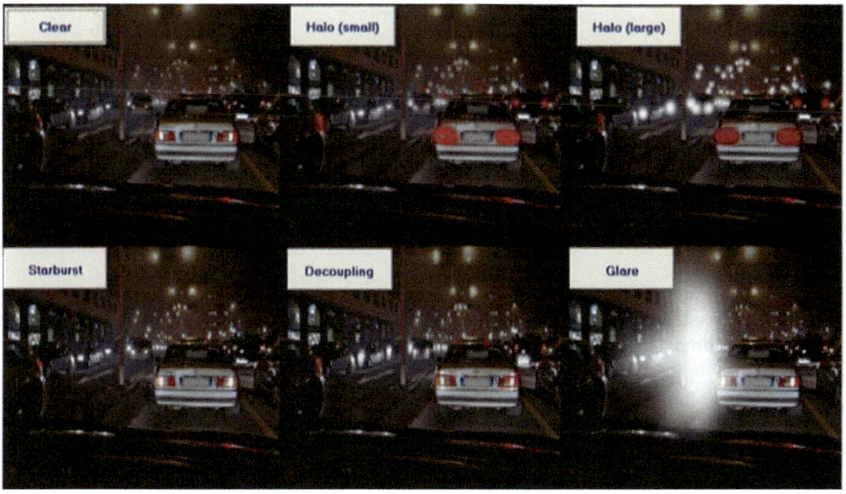

Fig. 2 Various types of positive dysphotopsia

In Summary

Thankfully, most patients implanted with standard monofocal lenses, providing the biometry has been correct, will complain little.

Multifocal IOLs of whatever design are a compromise with which most patients manage admirably provided that they have been suitably counselled in advance of their surgery and are motivated to do so for spectacle independence. However, when the biometry has not yielded the desired result or the toric lens has not adequately corrected astigmatism the visual result may be suboptimal and patients are unhappy. Visual phenomena due to lens design and individual patient perception may also lead to patient dissatisfaction. By taking a measured and rational approach and making the patient understand that there are, in most cases, solutions which may be simply time or adjunctive surgery long term unhappiness may be averted.

References

1. Yang E, Blake R, McDonald JE 2nd. A new interocular suppression technique for measuring sensory eye dominance. Invest Ophthalmol Vis Sci. 2010;51(1):588–93. https://doi.org/10.1167/iovs.08-3076.
2. Kaymak H, Fahle M, Ott G, Mester U. Intraindividual comparison of the effect of training on visual performance with ReSTOR and Tecnis diffractive multifocal IOLs. J Refract Surg. 2008;24(3):287–93. https://doi.org/10.3928/1081597X-20080301-11.
3. Alió JL, Pikkel J. Multifocal intraocular lenses-the art and the practice. Switzerland: Springer; 2020.
4. Simpson MJ. Simulated images of intraocular lens negative dysphotopsia and visual phenomena. J Opt Soc Am A Opt Image Sci Vis. 2019;36(4):B44–51. https://doi.org/10.1364/JOSAA.36.000B44.
5. Shajari M, Mayer WJ, Priglinger S. Lens Surgery: implantation of Multifocal Intraocular Lenses. Klin Monbl Augenheilkd. 2019;236(12):1461–71. https://doi.org/10.1055/a-1023-9795.
6. Holladay JT, Simpson MJ. Negative dysphotopsia: Causes and rationale for prevention and treatment. J Cataract Refract Surg. 2017;43(2):263–75. https://doi.org/10.1016/j.jcrs.2016.11.049.
7. Masket S, Fram NR. Sulcus-fixated IOLs for negative dysphotopsia. J Cataract Refract Surg. 2015;41(2):478. https://doi.org/10.1016/j.jcrs.2014.12.040.
8. Masket S, Fram NR, Cho A, Park I, Pham D. Surgical management of negative dysphotopsia. J Cataract Refract Surg. 2018;44(1):6–16. https://doi.org/10.1016/j.jcrs.2017.10.038.
9. Osher RH. Differentiating transient and permanent negative dysphotopsia. J Cataract Refract Surg. 2010;36(9):1619; author reply 161–9. https://doi.org/10.1016/j.jcrs.2010.06.018.
10. Lee S, Choi M, Xu Z, Zhao Z, Alexander E, Liu Y. Optical bench performance of a novel trifocal intraocular lens compared with a multifocal intraocular lens. Clin Ophthalmol. 2016;10:1031–8. https://doi.org/10.2147/OPTH.S106646.
11. Ferreira TB, Marques EF, Rodrigues A, Montes-Mico R. Visual and optical outcomes of a diffractive multifocal toric intraocular lens. J Cataract Refract Surg. 2013;39(7):1029–35. https://doi.org/10.1016/j.jcrs.2013.02.037.

12. Alio JL, Pinero DP, Plaza-Puche AB, Amparo F, Jimenez R, Rodriguez-Prats JL, et al. Visual and optical performance with two different diffractive multifocal intraocular lenses compared to a monofocal lens. J Refract Surg. 2011;27(8):570–81. https://doi.org/10.3928/1081597X-20101223-01.
13. Alio JL, Pinero DP, Plaza-Puche AB, Chan MJ. Visual outcomes and optical performance of a monofocal intraocular lens and a new-generation multifocal intraocular lens. J Cataract Refract Surg. 2011;37(2):241–50. https://doi.org/10.1016/j.jcrs.2010.08.043.
14. Alio JL, Plaza-Puche AB, Pinero DP, Amparo F, Jimenez R, Rodriguez-Prats JL, et al. Optical analysis, reading performance, and quality-of-life evaluation after implantation of a diffractive multifocal intraocular lens. J Cataract Refract Surg. 2011;37(1):27–37. https://doi.org/10.1016/j.jcrs.2010.07.035.
15. Fu Y, Kou J, Chen D, Wang D, Zhao Y, Hu M, et al. Influence of angle kappa and angle alpha on visual quality after implantation of multifocal intraocular lenses. J Cataract Refract Surg. 2019;45(9):1258–64. https://doi.org/10.1016/j.jcrs.2019.04.003.
16. Henderson BA, Geneva II. Negative dysphotopsia: A perfect storm. J Cataract Refract Surg. 2015;41(10):2291–312. https://doi.org/10.1016/j.jcrs.2015.09.002.
17. Hong X, Liu Y, Karakelle M, Masket S, Fram NR. Ray-tracing optical modeling of negative dysphotopsia. J Biomed Opt. 2011;16(12): 125001. https://doi.org/10.1117/1.3656745.
18. Ernest P. Severe photic phenomena. J Cataract Refract Surg. 2006;32(4):685–686.

Management After Opacification of Intraocular Lenses

Ramin Khoramnia

Introduction

Implantation of intraocular lenses is one of the most commonly performed surgical procedures worldwide. Advances in surgical techniques and the resulting improvements in postoperative outcomes have led to surgeries being performed at earlier stages of cataract development, even to the point of refractive lens exchange in presbyopia. In addition, due to increased life expectancy, the expected length of time that an intraocular lens (IOL) remains in the eye is also increasing. IOL implantation is routinely performed in patients undergoing refractive lens exchange and is also common in the treatment of cataract in children so it is reasonable to expect an IOL to remain in situ for several decades. The material of the IOL should remain inert and transparent over all of these years so it should be as resistant to material changes as possible. When an implant is no longer fit for its purpose, the only therapeutic option would be an explantation of the impant. The surgical indications for the explantation of artificial lenses have changed when looking at the literature on the subject. In the 1980s and 1990s, IOL dislocation, inflammatory reactions and incorrect IOL powers were major reasons for explantation. Proportionally, these reasons are now increasingly fading into the background as IOL designs have improved but opacifications have increased worldwide. In a recently published paper on 200 explanted intraocular lenses, IOL opacification was the cause of explantation in 76.5% of cases while dislocation only accounted for 13.5% [9].

R. Khoramnia (✉)
München, Germany
e-mail: ramin.khoramnia@med.uni-heidelberg.de

M. Shajari et al. (eds.), *Cataract and Lens Surgery*,
https://doi.org/10.1007/978-3-031-05394-8_85

Keypoint

While with hydrophilic IOLs, it is mainly calcification of the material that causes lens opacification, with IOLs made of hydrophobic material the problem of glistenings predominates.

Calcification in Hydrophilic IOLs

With hydrophilic acrylic intraocular lenses, there is a risk that they will calcify under certain circumstances. In this form of lens opacity, a distinction is made between primary and secondary IOL calcification and pseudocalcification.

Primary IOL Calcification

The primary form of IOL calcification refers to those cases where the cause of the opacity lies in the lens manufacture itself. For example, faulty polymer fabrication or the packaging of the IOL can lead to opacification [4, 11, 15]. Thus, this type of calcification tends to occur relatively early postoperatively in eyes where there are usually no associated diseases. The problem of primary calcification often affects entire batches of IOLs, which then (almost) all show opacification. Macroscopically, the optics and the haptics may even become opacified, if they are made of the same material as the optics. Light and scanning electron microscopy can often reveal numerous fine granular deposits of calcium phosphate arranged in a parallel line a few μm below the surface on both the anterior and posterior surfaces. When these opacifications occur, serial numbers and lot numbers of the lenses should be collected and the opacifications should be reported to the company and national or international competent authority.

Secondary IOL Calcification

Secondary IOL calcification is the term used for cases in which calcium deposits are most likely to occur as a result of specific ocular or systemic diseases or as a result of other operations.

Secondary IOL calcification can generally occur in any hydrophilic IOL, regardless of its manufacturer.

It is assumed that a change in the composition of the aqueous humour is primarily responsible for the development.

Concomitant diseases or surgical procedures performed after lens surgery (e.g. posterior lamellar keratoplasty, vitrectomy, intravitreal injections, rtPA injection into the anterior chamber) are often responsible for secondary calcification [1, 7, 10, 14].

Macroscopically, the opacities of the IOL in this form of calcification are usually concentrated only in the central area of the optic, i.e. the area left out by the capsulorhexis. It is possible that the lens surface is altered by contact with the altered aqueous humour and/or the triggering noxious agent (e.g. gas) in the area in such a way that the formation of crystallisation nuclei is favoured [8]. Light and scanning electron microscopy can also detect numerous fine, granular, crystal-like deposits of calcium phosphate below the surface of secondary calcified IOLs, which are arranged in a line parallel to the surface [3]. Typically, however, in contrast to primary IOL calcification, only one of the surfaces, usually the anterior surface of the IOL, is affected. By means of energy dispersive X-ray spectroscopy, it can be shown that the embedded material is calcium phosphate.

Pseudocalcification

The term pseudocalcification refers to those cases in which other pathologies (e.g. a liquefied after-cataract) are mistaken for calcification [2]. False positive results in histological staining are also referred to as pseudocalcification.

Keypoint

Calcification of IOLs leads to a significant decrease in light transmission, which significantly deteriorates the optical quality of the IOL and causes a marked increase in stray light and a loss of contrast [6, 15]. In most cases, IOL replacement is the only way to improve vision.

Explantation techniques are discussed in Chap. 57. Unfortunately, the occurrence of complications (e.g. zonular dehiscence, rupture of the posterior lens capsule, corneal decompensation) cannot always be avoided. In particular, a pronounced adhesion of the haptics and optics to the lens capsule can complicate the surgery. An IOL exchange should therefore only be carried out in the case of clear symptoms and after particularly careful explanation to the patient with regard to the high risk.

Author's recommendation

Patients with opacified artificial lenses often undergo Nd:YAG laser capsulotomy because the opacity is misinterpreted as secondary cataract. However, this should be avoided, as an opened posterior capsule unnecessarily increases the risk of complications during an IOL exchange. Attempts to remove the opacities with a "laser polish' are also not promising in the case of lens calcification, as the opacities lie below the intraocular lens surface.

After removal of the opacified IOL (reference to Chap. 57), depending on the condition of the capsular apparatus, a new IOL can be implanted in the capsular bag or the ciliary sulcus (ideally by performing an optic capture, i.e. "tying" the optic into the rhexis). Otherwise, the IOL can also be fixated to the iris or to the sclera.

Glistenings

Glistenings are small fluid-filled microvacuoles that can develop in the IOL optic when it is placed in an aqueous environment and exposed to temperature fluctuations. They occur most frequently and severely in hydrophobic acrylic IOLs (Fig. 1). It is known that the low water content of hydrophobic materials can favour the formation of glistenings. Studies have shown that IOLs differ in their resistance

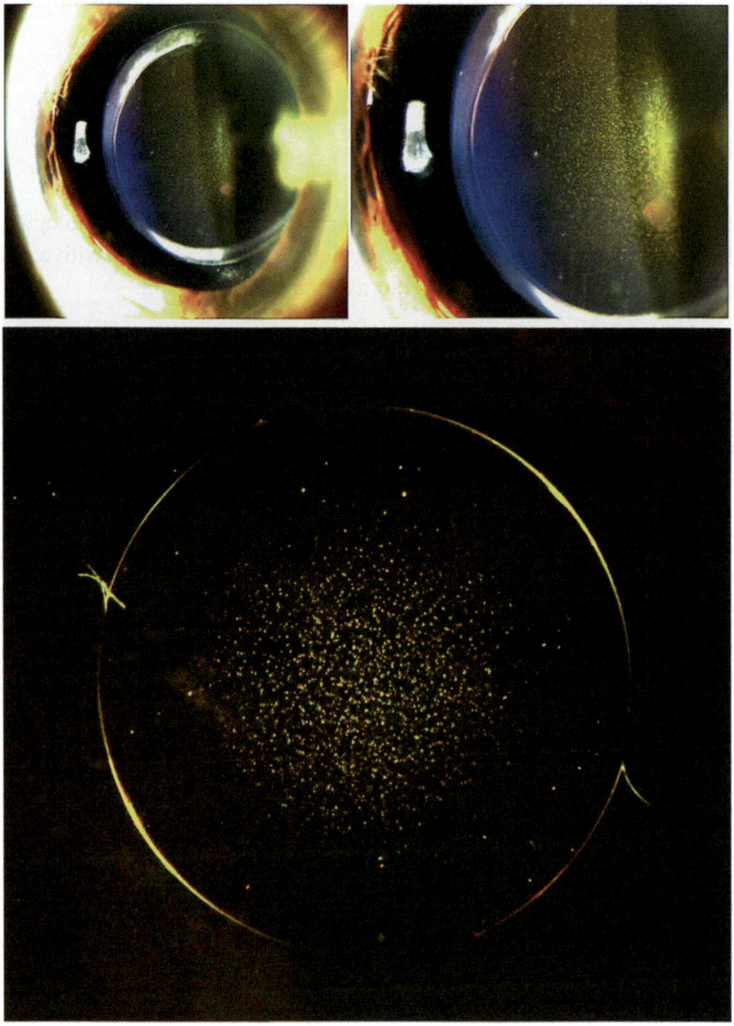

Fig. 1 Legend: Top: Anterior segment of the eye in a patient with a hydrophobic acrylic IOL showing significant glistenings. Bottom: Glistenings produced in vitro with a hydrophobic acrylic IOL

to glistenings and as a result, the arrangement and number of glistenings is different in different IOL materials. Continuous improvement in the manufacturing process has significantly reduced the density of glistenings in newer IOLs [12]; some IOL models have even been described as "glistening-free".

The impact of glistenings on visual function is still not fully understood, but the need for IOL explantation is rarely reported.

Ophthalmologists may tend to underestimate the importance of glistenings during slit lamp examination of the anterior segment of the eye; this may be because the forward scatter of light perceived by the patient is more than 300 times greater than the observed backward scatter.

Clinical studies show that glistenings have little effect on visual acuity, but can cause glare symptoms, especially when driving at night with backlighting or on a sunny day. The influence of glistenings on visual quality has also been investigated using in vitro models. For example, studies on the optical bench showed that a fairly high number of glistenings is required to reduce optical quality (modulation transfer function and Strehl ratio) [13].

Keypoint

Glistenings, however, seem to cause light scattering and could thus certainly impair the quality of vision. In this case, the scattered light increases proportionally to the number of microvacuoles within the IOL optics [5].

References

1. Fung SS, Sykakis E, Islam NM, Zambarakji HJ, Khoramnia R, Auffarth GU, et al. Intraocular lens opacification following intracameral injection of recombinant tissue plasminogen activator to treat inflammatory membranes after cataract surgery. J Ophthalmol. 2015;2015: 975075. https://doi.org/10.1155/2015/975075.
2. Giers BC, Khoramnia R, Tandogan T, Auffarth GU. Liquefied aftercataract mimicking IOL-opacification. Klin Monbl Augenheilkd. 2017a;234(8):988–90. https://doi.org/10.1055/s-0042-121808.
3. Giers BC, Tandogan T, Auffarth GU, Choi CY, Auerbach FN, Sel S, et al. Hydrophilic intraocular lens opacification after posterior lamellar keratoplasty. BMC Ophthalmol. 2017b;17(1):150. https://doi.org/10.1186/s12886-017-0546-8.
4. Khoramnia R, Salgado JP, Auffarth GU, Schmidt S, Wegner A, Kobuch KA et al. Opacification of a hydrophilic intraocular lens 4 years after cataract surgery: a biomaterial analysis. Ophthalmologe. 2012;109(5), 483–6. https://doi.org/10.1007/s00347-011-2487-6.
5. Labuz G, Knebel D, Auffarth GU, Fang H, van den Berg TJ, Yildirim TM, et al. Glistening formation and light scattering in six hydrophobic-acrylic intraocular lenses. Am J Ophthalmol. 2018a;196:112–20. https://doi.org/10.1016/j.ajo.2018.08.032.
6. Labuz G, Yildirim TM, van den Berg T, Khoramnia R, Auffarth GU. Assessment of straylight and the modulation transfer function of intraocular lenses with centrally localized opacification associated with the intraocular injection of gas. J Cataract Refract Surg. 2018b;44(5):615–22. https://doi.org/10.1016/j.jcrs.2018.01.033.
7. Marcovich AL, Tandogan T, Bareket M, Eting E, Kaplan-Ashiri I, Bukelman A, et al. Opacification of hydrophilic intraocular lenses associated with vitrectomy and injection of

intraocular gas. BMJ Open Ophthalmol. 2018;3(1): e000157. https://doi.org/10.1136/bmjophth-2018-000157.
8. Milojcic C, Latz C, Tandogan T, Auffarth GU, Holz FG, Choi CY, et al. Opacification of a hydrophilic acrylic intraocular lens after DMEK : A material analysis. Ophthalmologe. 2017;114(9):832–7. https://doi.org/10.1007/s00347-016-0394-6.
9. Neuhann T, Yildirim TM, Son HS, Merz PR, Khoramnia R, Auffarth GU. Reasons for explantation, demographics, and material analysis of 200 intraocular lens explants. J Cataract Refract Surg. 2020;46(1):20–6. https://doi.org/10.1016/j.jcrs.2019.08.045.
10. Roland S, Khoramnia R, Auffarth GU, Son HS, Yildirim TM, Schoenherr U. Opacification of hydrophilic intraocular lens after multiple injections of bevacizumab. Ophthalmologe. 2019;116(9):882–6. https://doi.org/10.1007/s00347-018-0829-3.
11. Tandogan T, Khoramnia R, Choi CY, Scheuerle A, Wenzel M, Hugger P, et al. Optical and material analysis of opacified hydrophilic intraocular lenses after explantation: a laboratory study. BMC Ophthalmol. 2015;15:170. https://doi.org/10.1186/s12886-015-0149-1.
12. Wang Q, Yildirim TM, Schickhardt SK, Łabuz G, Khoramnia R, Merz PR, Son HS, Munro DJ, Friedmann E, Auffarth GU (2021) Quantification of the in vitro predisposition to glistening formation in one manufacturer's acrylic intraocular lenses made in different decades. Ophthalmol Ther 10(1):165–174. https://doi.org/10.1007/s40123-020-00329-8. Epub 2021 Feb 5. PMID: 33544374; PMCID: PMC7886932
13. Weindler JN, Labuz G, Yildirim TM, Tandogan T, Khoramnia R, Auffarth GU. The impact of glistenings on the optical quality of a hydrophobic acrylic intraocular lens. J Cataract Refract Surg. 2019;45(7):1020–5. https://doi.org/10.1016/j.jcrs.2019.01.025.
14. Yildirim TM, Auffarth GU, Labuz G, Bopp S, Son HS, Khoramnia R. Material analysis and optical quality assessment of opacified hydrophilic acrylic intraocular lenses after pars plana vitrectomy. Am J Ophthalmol. 2018;193:10–9. https://doi.org/10.1016/j.ajo.2018.06.002.
15. Yildirim TM, Labuz G, Khoramnia R, Son HS, Schickhardt SK, Lieberwirth I, et al. Impact of primary calcification in segmented refractive bifocal intraocular lenses on optical performance including straylight. J Refract Surg. 2020;36(1):20–7. https://doi.org/10.3928/1081597X-20191119-01.

Management After Dislocation of an Intraocular Lens

Ramin Khoramnia

Introduction

Subluxation or luxation of posterior chamber IOLs is rare but represents one of the most serious complications after cataract surgery. A distinction should always be made between early and late cases of dislocation (Table 1).

Early IOL Dislocation

This early complication (Fig. 1) often occurs due to inadequate fixation of the IOL in the capsular bag.

keypoint

Although a zonular defect may be present preoperatively (e.g. in traumatic cataracts), dislocation is usually iatrogenic and caused by intraoperative posterior capsular rupture or zonulolysis [1].

Supplementary Information The online version contains supplementary material available at https://doi.org/10.1007/978-3-031-05394-8_86. The videos can be accessed individually by clicking the DOI link in the accompanying figure caption or by scanning this link with the SN More Media App.

R. Khoramnia (✉)
Heidelberg, Germany
e-mail: ramin.khoramnia@med.uni-heidelberg.de

M. Shajari et al. (eds.), *Cataract and Lens Surgery*,
https://doi.org/10.1007/978-3-031-05394-8_86

Table 1 According to Ascaso et al. [1]

	Early cases	Late cases
Time after the surgical procedure	<3 months	≥3 months (also in cases after uncomplicated cataract surgery)
Pathogenesis	Insufficient IOL fixation in the capsular bag	Increasing insufficiency of the zonular apparatus and contraction of the capsular bag
Predisposing factors	Posterior capsule rupture, zonulolysis	Increasing age, PEX, high myopia, trauma, uveitis, pigmentous retinopathy, diabetes mellitus, atopic dermatitis, connective tissue diseases, e.g. Marfan syndrome, post vitreoretinal surgery, post angle closure glaucoma

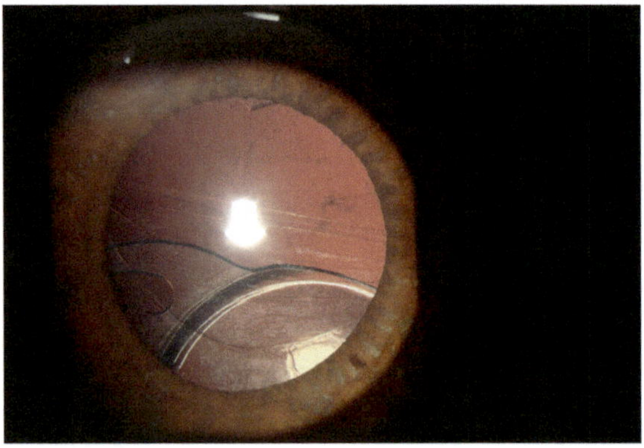

Fig. 1 Early inferior dislocation of an IOL

Late Spontaneous IOL Dislocation

Late spontaneous IOL dislocation occurs three months or later after cataract surgery.

keypoint

In contrast to early lens dislocation, late spontaneous IOL dislocation usually occurs many years after even uncomplicated cataract surgery as a result of progressive zonular weakness and contraction of the capsular bag.

It is not typically due to inadequate fixation of the IOL intraoperatively (e.g. in the case of a defective capsular bag) but rather due to postoperative factors. Factors such as zonular weakness and/or stress on the zonular apparatus (intraoperatively iatrogenic or postoperatively due to the development of anterior capsular fibrosis/ shrinkage up to capsular phimosis, e.g. in pseudoexfoliation or myotonic dystrophy) seem to be causative. [1, 2]

keypoint

Late spontaneous IOL dislocation usually results in dislocation of the entire IOL/capsular bag complex.

A large retrospective cohort study identified a cumulative risk of IOL dislocation after cataract surgery of 0.1% at 5 years, 0.1% at 10 years, 0.2% at 15 years, 0.7% at 20 years and 1.7% at 25 years [3]. Pseudoexfoliation and zonular insufficiency at surgery were significantly associated with late IOL dislocation. However, the long-term cumulative risk of late IOL dislocation after cataract extraction was low and did not change significantly over the almost 30-year study period [3]. However, the proportion of people with pseudophakia is increasing rapidly due to improvements in the quality and safety of surgical procedures, expanded indications, new IOL options and increased life expectancy. Therefore, the incidence of late IOL dislocation may increase in the future [1].

Prevention

In the case of existing risk factors, certain measures can be considered to prevent dislocation of the IOL capsular bag complex.

Author's recommendation

A particularly small capsulorhexis should be avoided as this increases the risk of capsular fibrosis and shrinkage.

However, it is still recommended to choose the diameter of the rhexis smaller than that of the IOL optic so that overlapping of the optic by the rhexis over 360° is still ensured. During phacoemulsification, care should always be taken to maintain the integrity of the zonular fibres. It has been postulated that chopping techniques, for example, are less traumatic in this regard. Some authors recommend that the cortex should not be removed perpendicularly, but tangentially to the alignment of the zonule fibres to minimise stress on them. In addition, care should be taken to remove the cortex carefully and completely. However, this is not always technically easy in eyes with pseudoexfoliation (e.g. due to poor dilatation of the pupil and/or instability of the zonula). Surgeons should take special care when implanting a posterior chamber IOL into the capsular bag in eyes with a weak zonular apparatus. Some authors go so far as to plan primary implantation of the IOL into the ciliary sulcus with "tying" of the optic into the capsulorhexis (so-called "optic capture") in eyes with risk factors [1].

Author's recommendation

It is essential to emphasise at this point that three-piece models should be used without exception when placing an IOL in the sulcus. The use of one-piece IOLs, that are designed for the capsular bag, in the sulcus leads to serious problems due to the presence of sharp edges, such as pigment dispersion (due to "rubbing" against the iris), intraocular pressure increase and chronic inflammatory conditions (often accompanied by macular edema).

Although there is no evidence that capsular tension rings prevent IOL dislocation, their use seems to be a useful preventive measure according to some authors. It may reduce the extent of damage to the zonules during surgery. Although capsular tension rings probably reduce the extent of postoperative capsular shrinkage, they do not prevent it completely. However, an implanted capsular tension ring may facilitate secondary suturing of a dislocated IOL [1].

Author's recommendation

If fibrosis and shrinkage of the capsulorhexis is detected, radial relaxing incisions can be made with the Nd:YAG laser [1]. This should minimise further stress on the zonular fibres by reducing the tensile forces.

Procedure for Dislocated IOL

In the case of a dislocated IOL, there is the option of refixation using sutures (Video 1).

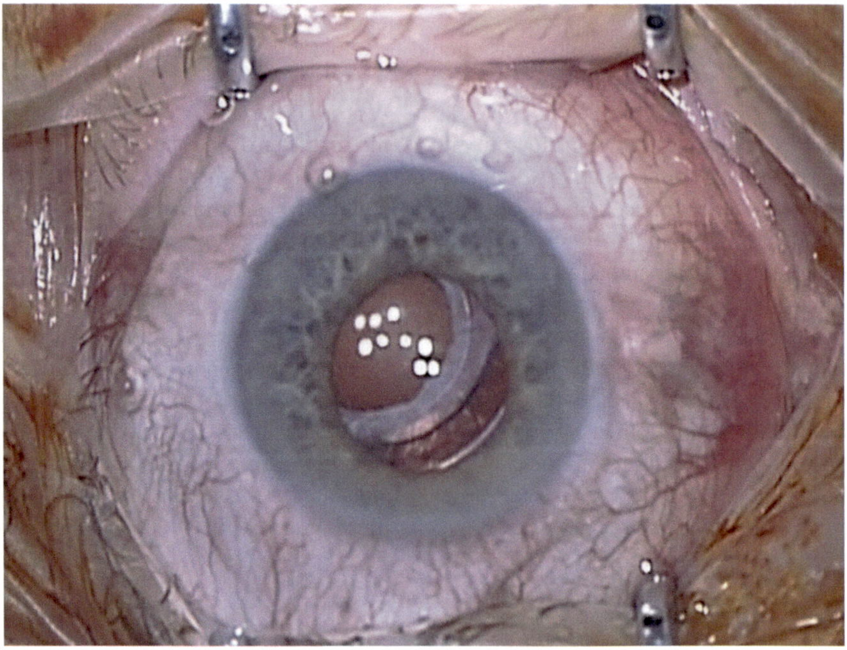

Video 1 A dislocated IOL is centred using a scleral suture (M4V 14777 kb) (▶ https://doi.org/10.1007/000-8f4)

However, depending on the type of IOL (e.g. IOLs with plate haptics), this is not always easily possible. In such cases, explantation of the affected IOL remains the only reasonable option, which should usually be done via a corneoscleral tunnel. The new IOL can then be fixed to the iris or to the sclera.

References

1. Ascaso FJ, Huerva V, Grzybowski A. Epidemiology, etiology, and prevention of late IOL-capsular bag complex dislocation: review of the literature. J Ophthalmol. 2015;2015: 805706. https://doi.org/10.1155/2015/805706.
2. Mayer C, Cordeiro SA, Khoramnia R. Cataract in a young patient. Ophthalmologe. 2011;108 (10):976–9. https://doi.org/10.1007/s00347-011-2374-1.
3. Pueringer SL, Hodge DO, Erie JC. Risk of late intraocular lens dislocation after cataract surgery, 1980–2009: a population-based study. Am J Ophthalmol. 2011;152(4):618–23. https://doi.org/10.1016/j.ajo.2011.03.009.

Treatment of Postoperative Intraocular Pressure Increase

Christoph Hirneiß

Classical cataract surgery with phacoemulsification using viscoelastic agents with implantation of a foldable intraocular lens may be accompanied by an increase in intraocular pressure in the early postoperative phase [1].

Keypoint

A postoperative pressure increase is common: one quarter of the operated eyes experience pressure increases of more than 30 mmHg within the first 24 h [2].

However, there is no clear evidence regarding the significance of these pressure spikes and there is no clear consensus for the active management of postoperative pressure increases for otherwise healthy eyes when a typical cataract surgery has been performed without complications [3]. In general, the question arises whether prophylactic treatment should be used to compensate for potential pressure peaks. Many surgeons routinely use systemic antiglaucomatous drugs such as acetazolamide or local antiglaucomatous drugs such as beta-blockers, alpha-2 agonists or local carboanhydrase inhibitors as part of their routine postoperative medications [4]. A single dose directly after surgery can be sufficient. A review of this topic showed that timolol (as monotherapy or in combination with dorzolamide, brinzolamide or brimonidine) has a good prophylactic pressure-lowering effect in the early postoperative period after cataract surgery [5].

Special care must be exercised during and after cataract surgery in eyes with a history of glaucoma. Cataract surgery alone is often a useful augmentation for long-term reduction of intraocular pressure in glaucoma, especially in eyes with narrow chamber angle conditions [6]. These eyes may be subject to more severe early postoperative pressure problems and this can also occur even after completely uncomplicated surgeries. The frequency of pressure spikes is up to 35%, and eyes with pseudoexfoliation glaucoma are at particular risk [7]. In 17% of eyes, this

C. Hirneiß (✉)
München, Germany
e-mail: christoph.hirneiss@med.uni-muenchen.de

M. Shajari et al. (eds.), *Cataract and Lens Surgery*,
https://doi.org/10.1007/978-3-031-05394-8_87

pressure increase can be more than 50% of the initial pressure. The most common cause is residual viscoelastic substances in the anterior chamber or a steroid response [8].

Author's recommendation

In glaucoma patients, in addition to complete removal of the viscoelastic agent and close monitoring, a prophylactic pressure medication should be given. Systemic carbonic anhydrase inhibitors are generally preferred for reasons of practicality [9].

If there are no contraindications to systemic carbonic anhydrase inhibitors, there is, in the author's view, no reason why a prophylactic administration of 250 mg of acetazolamide should not be given postoperatively, particularly if the intraocular lens was implanted under viscoelastic protection or if there is coexisting glaucoma. If there is no glaucoma, prophylaxis may not be necessary, especially if the intraocular lens is implanted under pure irrigation without the use of viscoelastics.

Pressure increases above 25–30 mmHg one day after surgery should be treated with medication, ideally with a local beta-blocker such as timolol (possibly in combination with a topical carbonic anhydrase inhibitor); if the pressure increases are more severe, acetazolamide should also be administered systemically.

In non-glaucomatous eyes, both the protection of the optic nerve and avoiding the risk of retinal vessel occlusion is pivotal. Further control of the pressure must be decided individually, as must the duration of the medical therapy. In glaucoma patients especially, this observation time should be of longer duration until it is certain that a stable postoperative pressure level has been reached.

Glaucoma patients often experience changes in their medications immediately after cataract surgery. Some may think that their normal medications are on hold and many have their eyes patched until the following day. In addition, glaucoma patients using topical prostaglandin may have had their therapy stopped (typically one week or more prior to the surgery) to avoid the possible increased risk of cystoid macular oedema. In these patients, the local therapy can be bridged well with systemic carboanhydrase inhibitors. As these patients also have to administer anti-inflammatory therapy, very clear information should be provided about the exact application of the drops. Ideally, an individual eye drop plan is given to these patients.

In case of a very high increase in pressure, (which is usually due to retained viscoelastic material in the anterior chamber), an acute decompression of viscoelastic may be required. This can be performed at the slit lamp as follows. A drop topical anaesthesia and a drop of 5% isobetadine is instill into the eye to prepare the ocular surface and an eyelid speculum can be placed, if needed. A sterile cannula or similar instrument is then gently pressed on the posterior lip of the paracentesis. This should allow some OVD to exit without having to enter the wound with the instrument. When effective, the patient usually experiences immediate relief. Decompression using the main incision should be avoided as this has a higher risk of iris prolapse and this cannot be safely managed at the slit-lamp. If a large amount of remaining viscoelastic material is still in the anterior chamber and cannot be gently decompressed, however, removal should be carried out by irrigation/aspiration under sterile conditions.

References

1. Thirumalai B, Baranyovits PR. Intraocular pressure changes and the implications on patient review after phacoemulsification. J Cataract Refract Surg. 2003;29(3):504–7.
2. Balsak S, Kaydu A, Erdem S, Fuat Alakus M, Ozkurt ZG. Brimonidine-timolol versus brinzolamide-timololol for treatment of elevated intraocular pressure after phacoemulsification surgery. Int Ophthalmol. 2018;38(4):1583–9.
3. kettle L, Andresen J, Erngaard D, Flesner P, Tendal B, Hjortdal J. Safety of deferring review after uneventful cataract surgery until 2 weeks postoperatively. J Cataract Refract Surg. 2015;41(12):2755–64.
4. Crawley L, Zamir SM, Cordeiro MF, Guo L. Clinical options for the reduction of elevated intraocular pressure. Ophthalmol Eye Dis. 2012;4:43–64.
5. 5th Holm JL, Bach Holm D, Holm LM, Vestergaard AH. Prophylactic treatment of intraocular pressure elevation after uncomplicated cataract surgery in nonglaucomatous eyes - a systematic review. Acta Ophthalmol. 2019;97(6):545–57.
6. 6th Young CEC, Seibold LK, Kahook MY. Cataract surgery and intraocular pressure in glaucoma. Curr Opin Ophthalmol. 2020;31(1):15–22.
7. Chen PP, Lin SC, Junk AK, Radhakrishnan S, Singh K, Chen TC. The Effect of Phacoemulsification on Intraocular Pressure in Glaucoma Patients: A Report by the American Academy of Ophthalmology. Ophthalmology. 2015;122(7):1294–307.
8. Slabaugh MA, Bojikian KD, Moore DB, Chen PP. Risk factors for acute postoperative intraocular pressure elevation after phacoemulsification in glaucoma patients. J Cataract Refract Surg. 2014;40(4):538–44.
9. Hayashi K, Yoshida M, Manabe SI, Yoshimura K. Prophylactic Effect of Oral Acetazolamide against Intraocular Pressure Elevation after Cataract Surgery in Eyes with Glaucoma Ophthalmology. 2017;124(5):701–8.

Treatment of Postoperative Cystoid Macular Edema

Nikolaus Luft

Etiology

Cystoid macular edema (CME) after lens surgery is also known as Irvine-Gass Syndrome after the first description of this entity in the 1950's and -60's [1, 2]. The entity was originally described as macular edema associated with intracapsular cataract extraction and was far more frequently seen with that technique. Although the exact pathophysiology at the cellular level is not yet fully understood, intraocular inflammatory mediators, which increase the permeability of the blood-retina barrier and thus the vascular permeability, are believed to be mainly responsible for postoperative edema formation.

Diagnostics

Initially diagnosed purely funduscopically (loss of the foveal light reflex) or by means of fluorescence angiography ("petaloid" hyperfluorescence pattern in the late phase), optical coherence tomography (OCT; see also "OCT-Based Corneal Measurements": OCT of the posterior segment of the eye) represents the current gold standard imaging modality for the diagnosis of postoperative macular edema. There are no exact OCT morphological diagnostic criteria for postoperative CME. Often, foveal and peri-foveal intraretinal cystic hyporeflective vacuoles are found, which are preferentially located in the outer nuclear and outer plexiform layers, but this is by no means always the case. Inner retinal layers (e.g. inner nuclear layer) and the subretinal space can also be affected by fluid accumulation (see Fig. 1a).

N. Luft (✉)
Munich, Germany
e-mail: nikolaus.luft@med.uni-muenchen.de

M. Shajari et al. (eds.), *Cataract and Lens Surgery*,
https://doi.org/10.1007/978-3-031-05394-8_88

Course

Postoperative macular edema is a quite common cause of postoperative loss of visual acuity after lens surgery with an incidence of approximately 0.1–3.8% [3, 4]. The incidence of postoperative CME peaks about five weeks after cataract surgery, is extremely variable in duration and commonly shows spontaneous remission. In contrast, chronic recurrent cases may also occur.

Keypoint

The incidence of postoperative CME peaks approximately five weeks after cataract surgery. Routine OCT monitoring between 4 and 6 weeks postoperatively is therefore recommended for patients at risk.

Remarkably, despite successful treatment (see below) and "dry" OCT morphology of the macula, more than a quarter of patients do not recover to 20/20 visual acuity after postoperative CME [5]. This phenomenon is presumably due to degenerative remodeling processes in the area of the outer retinal layers, especially in the case of prolonged CME. It is essential therefore to identify high-risk patients before cataract surgery and to initiate more intensive measures regarding patient education, CME prophylaxis and postoperative follow-up.

Even after complete remission of CME, more than a quarter of patients do not recover to 20/20 visual acuity.

Risk Factors

The association with intraocular inflammation mentioned above suggests that pro-inflammatory ophthalmic comorbidities (e.g. diabetic retinal disease) may be a contributive factor to postoperative CME. In fact, multiple clinical studies in cataract patients with diabetes mellitus have shown a fourfold increased risk of postoperative CME development, which increases to more than sixfold and ninefold in the presence of non-proliferative diabetic retinopathy and proliferative diabetic retinopathy, respectively. Patients that already suffered from diabetic macular edema (DME) before cataract surgery are at particular risk. A similar increase in risk is known for patients with uveitis (approx. threefold), which is particularly evident in cases of recent inflammatory episodes (over sixfold). Another well-known risk factor is a history of retinal vein occlusion (approx. fourfold increased risk) as well as the presence of an epiretinal membrane or previous vitreoretinal surgery (e.g. retinal detachment surgery). Posterior capsule rupture also increases CME risk approx. threefold. Topical prostaglandin derivatives to lower intraocular pressure are also suspected to increase the risk of CME.

Therapy

To date, there are no commonly accepted guidelines for the treatment of postoperative CME. The body of evidence from randomized controlled trials is rather sparse considering the relatively high incidence of the disease. Following the assumed strong association with intraocular inflammatory mediators, non-steroidal anti-inflammatory substances (NSAIDs) are traditionally used as first line treatment of postoperative CME (see Table 87.1: Level 1). The highest level of evidence exists for this class of drugs. Useful topical preparations include, for example, ketorolac 0.5% as well as nepafenac 0.1 and 0.3% eye drops. Another class of anti-inflammatory agents often used in combination with NSAIDs are topical corticosteroids (e.g. prednisolone 1%, dexamethasone 0.1%). Due to the heterogeneity of the available studies and the frequently combined use, it is currently not possible to assess which of the two drug classes has a better benefit/risk profile when used topically. Oral acetazolamide is anecdotally administered by some authorities (e.g. 250 mg three times a day), but the degree of evidence for this approach is relatively low.

If topical treatment fails to elicit an improvement over a period of 4 weeks or, in cases of very pronounced CME, a parabulbar triamcinolone injection (40 mg) can be administered (stage 2). Although the degree of evidence for this intervention is also considered low, this method is very popular in clinical practice and is considered very effective in the author's experience.

If this measure does not lead to a sufficient clinical and OCT-morphological response of the CME, the next step can be an intravitreal injection of a corticosteroid preparation. In the case of a first-time, therapy-refractory CME, the authors recommend an intravitreal injection of 4 mg triamcinolone (Step 3). In case of recurrence thereafter, an intravitreal corticosteroid depot administered by means of a dexamethasone implant (Ozurdex®) can be administered [6], which offers both a high efficiency as well as a three-month duration of action (stage 4).

Prophylaxis

Similar to the treatment of CME, the prophylaxis of CME is mainly based on anti-inflammatory agents—above all NSAID-containing and corticosteroid-containing topical preparations. The recent, multi-center "PREvention of Macular EDema after cataract surgery" (PREMED) study showed an additive effect of both

Table 87.1 Treatment of postoperative CME: escalation scheme

Step 1: NSAID eyedrops ± corticosteroid eyedrops AT ± acetazolamide p.o. (for 4 weeks)
Step 2: Triamcinolone 40 mg parabulbar
Step 3: Triamcinolone 4 mg intravitreal
Step 4: Dexamethasone implant intravitreal

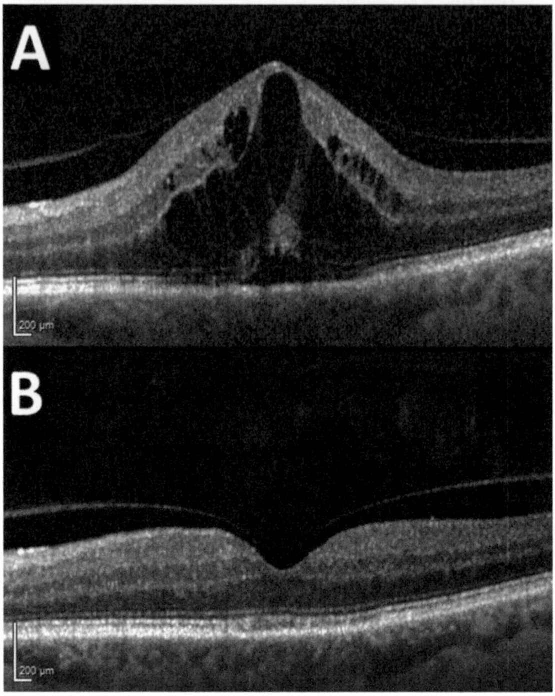

Fig. 87.1 Here: **a** Pronounced recurrent macular edema 8 weeks after cataract surgery with intra- and subretinal fluid accumulation. **b** The same eye 4 weeks after parabulbar injection of 40 mg triamcinolone.

drug classes in the prophylaxis of the CME in 914 eyes of non-diabetic cataract patients. In the group that received a combination therapy (bromfenac + dexamethasone eye drops), the incidence of postoperative CME (1.5%) was significantly lower than after bromfenac (3.6%) or dexamethasone monotherapy (5.1%) [7]. One arm of the PREMED study also investigated various prophylactic measures regarding CME development in 213 eyes of diabetic cataract patients. There was a significant reduction in central retinal thickness 6 and 12 weeks postoperatively and not a single case of clinically significant CME was encountered in patients that received a perioperative subconjunctival triamcinolone injection (40 mg) in addition to the aforementioned topical combination therapy [8]. The downside of this means of preventing CME was that 6% of patients experienced intraocular pressure (IOP) rises of $\geq$25 mmHg after 12 weeks. In the presence of other risk factors than diabetes mellitus (see above), extending the administration of topical NSAID-containing preparations over a longer period of time (e.g. 3 months) may be prudent [9]. Furthermore, evidence exists that initiating topical NSAID prophylaxis 1–3 days before cataract surgery can be effect-enhancing [10].

Author's recommendation

For CME prophylaxis in patients without particular risk factors, corticosteroid-containing eye drops should be used for one week in combination with NSAID-containing eye drops for 4 weeks after cataract surgery. In patients with diabetes mellitus, a perioperative subconjunctival injection of triamcinolone is an extremely efficient prophylaxis but requires increased vigilance with regard to postoperative IOP rises.

References

1. Gass JD, Norton EW. Fluorescein studies of patients with macular edema and papilledema following cataract extraction. Trans Am Ophthalmol Soc. 1966;64:232–49.
2. Irvine SR. A newly defined vitreous syndrome following cataract surgery. Am J Ophthalmol. 1953;36(5):599–619.
3. Packer M, Lowe J, Fine H. Incidence of acute postoperative cystoid macular edema in clinical practice. J Cataract Refract Surg. 2012;38(12):2108–11.
4. Riley AF, Malik TY, Grupcheva CN, Fisk MJ, Craig JP, McGhee CN. The Auckland cataract study: co-morbidity, surgical techniques, and clinical outcomes in a public hospital service. Br J Ophthalmol. 2002;86(2):185–90.
5. Hunter AA, Modjtahedi SP, Long K, Zawadzki R, Chin EK, Caspar JJ, et al. Improving visual outcomes by preserving outer retina morphology in eyes with resolved pseudophakic cystoid macular edema. J Cataract Refract Surg. 2014;40(4):626–31.
6. Mayer WJ, Kurz S, Wolf A, Kook D, Kreutzer T, Kampik A, et al. Dexamethasone implant as an effective treatment option for macular edema due to Irvine-Gass syndrome. J Cataract Refract Surg. 2015;41(9):1954–61.
7. Wielders LHP, Schouten J, Winkens B, van den, Biggelaar F, Veldhuizen CA, Findl O, et al European multicenter trial of the prevention of cystoid macular edema after cataract surgery in nondiabetics: ESCRS PREMED study report 1. J Cataract Refract Surg. 2018;44(4):429–39.
8. Wielders LHP, Schouten J, Winkens B, van den,. Biggelaar F, Veldhuizen CA, Murta JCN, et al Randomized controlled European multicenter trial on the prevention of cystoid macular edema after cataract surgery in diabetics: ESCRS PREMED Study Report 2. J Cataract Refract Surg. 2018;44(7):836–47.
9. Henderson BA, Kim JY, Ament CS, Ferrufino-Ponce ZK, Grabowska A, Cremers SL Clinical pseudophakic cystoid macular edema. Risk factors for development and duration after treatment. J Cataract Refract Surg. 2007;33(9):1550–8
10. Donnenfeld ED, Perry HD, Wittpenn JR, Solomon R, Nattis A, Chou T Preoperative ketorolac tromethamine 0.4% in phacoemulsification outcomes: pharmacokinetic-response curve. J Cataract Refract Surg. 2006;32(9):1474–82

Postoperative Inflammation

Thomas C. Kreutzer

Postoperative endophthalmitis is of the most serious and potentially devastating complication seen after lens surgery. Fortunately, it is rare, with an estimated incidence of 0.03–0.2% [1] It should be distinguished from non-infectious post-operative inflammatory reaction after complex lens surgery and the very rare occasion of "toxic anterior chamber syndrome" (TASS). Post-operative endophthalmitis after lens surgery usually clinically manifests between the third and seventh post-operative day. The main causative pathogens are gram positive bacteria of the conjunctival flora such as Staphylococcus epidermidis, Staphylococcus aureus, Streptococcus sp. and rarely Enterococcus sp. and Propioni bacteria sp. Less common, are gram negative pathogens such as Proteus sp., Haemophilus influenzae and Serratia sp [2].

Consistent pretreatment of the conjunctiva with 1–5% povidone-iodine solution and disinfection of the periorbital structures with 10% povidone-iodine has been shown to reduce the risk of postoperative infection. Irrigation of the conjunctiva is preferable to dripping alone with povidone-iodine [3]. Another measure to reduce postoperative infection is sterile draping of the eyelids with a particular emphasis on keeping the eyelashes away from the surgical field. A prospective, randomized study by the ESCRS (European Society of Cataract and Refractive Surgery) on the effectiveness of povidone-only disinfection versus additional local post-operative treatment with levofloxacin eye drops and/or intracameral administration of cefuroxime at the end of surgery showed the greatest effectiveness in reducing the

Supplementary Information The online version contains supplementary material available at https://doi.org/10.1007/978-3-031-05394-8_89. The videos can be accessed individually by clicking the DOI link in the accompanying figure caption or by scanning this link with the SN More Media App.

T. C. Kreutzer (✉)
Munich, Germany
e-mail: thomas.kreutzer@med.uni-muenchen.de

M. Shajari et al. (eds.), *Cataract and Lens Surgery*,
https://doi.org/10.1007/978-3-031-05394-8_89

risk of endophthalmitis in the groups with intracameral antibiotic administration [4]. Consequently, intracameral use of Cefuroxime at the end of cataract surgery is now recommended by many professional societies. It is especially recommended in situations where a known increased risk of infection exists, as in patients with immunosuppression, after intraoperative complications such as posterior capsule rupture and in cases of particularly long cataract surgery. Clinical signs of acute postoperative endophthalmitis are increased inflammation 3–7 days postoperatively. It presents itself usually with symptoms like a painful eye, significantly reduced visual acuity, mixed conjunctival and episcleral injection, fibrin reaction in the anterior chamber (AC) with the finding of inflammatory cells in the AC and anterior vitreous cavity and a hypopyon (Video 1).

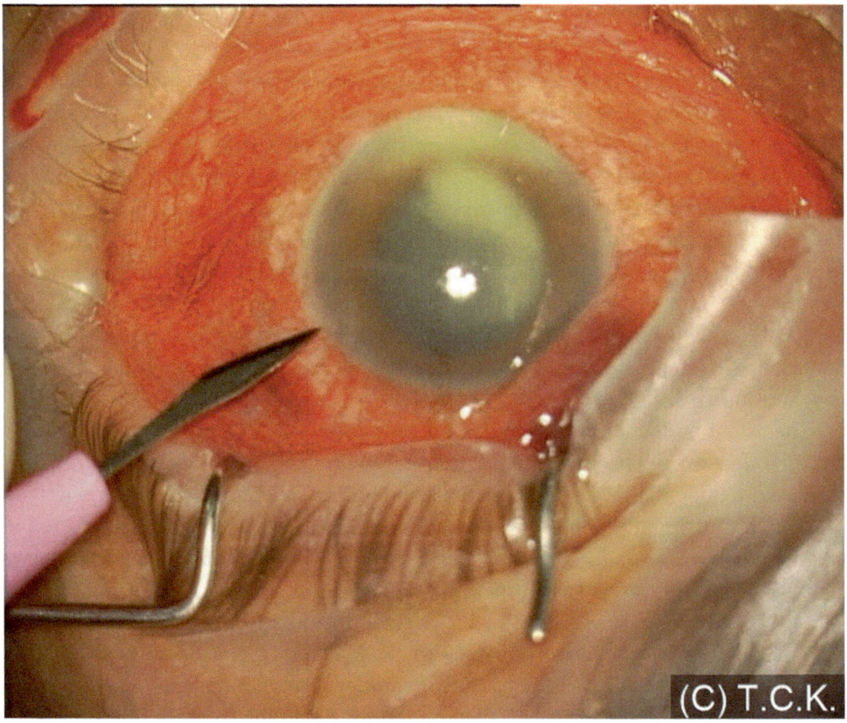

Video 1 White-colored vitreous cavity in fulminant endophthalmitis after lens surgery (▶ https://doi.org/10.1007/000-8f6)

Fibrin threads often extend from the paracentheses or the clear cornea incision into the anterior chamber. Lack of a clear fundus view indicates a more severe or advanced course.

The results of the "Endophthalmitis Vitrectomy Study" [5], which determined the therapeutic necessity of vitrectomy only in severe cases with missing fundus red reflex and a visual acuity of light perception (LP) and worse as opposed to a sole intravitreal antibiotic administration, are to be viewed critically today due to the progress in vitreoretinal surgery [6, 7] Vitrectomy should, ideally, be performed as soon as possible as it allows the most extensive removal of infectious agents in the vitreous cavity and is considered as the gold standard of endophthalmitis management. Rapid referral of a patient with postoperative endophthalmitis to a retinal surgery center is recommended. Endophthalmitis can demonstrably neither be prevented nor treated by the sole topical application of antibiotics. A sole systemic antibiotic administration is also not sufficient for treatment.

The postoperative irritation following complicated lens surgery usually manifests with corneal edema and distinct folds in Descemet's membrane, increased intraocular pressure, sometimes associated with fibrin reaction and cells in the anterior chamber, but without hypopyon. An intensified steroid administration usually leads to an improvement within days. TASS, a now rare complication, is seen as a massive inflammation of the anterior chamber after lens surgery. It typically occurs within one day, sooner than endophthalmitis. Clinical signs are a complete corneal edema, increased intraocular pressure, anterior chamber cells, fibrin, rather little pain and only very rarely a hypopyon [8]. The therapy consists of an intensified topical steroid eye drop therapy (1% prednisolone), and parabulbar steroid injections (32 mg prednisolone) can be given for severe inflammatory

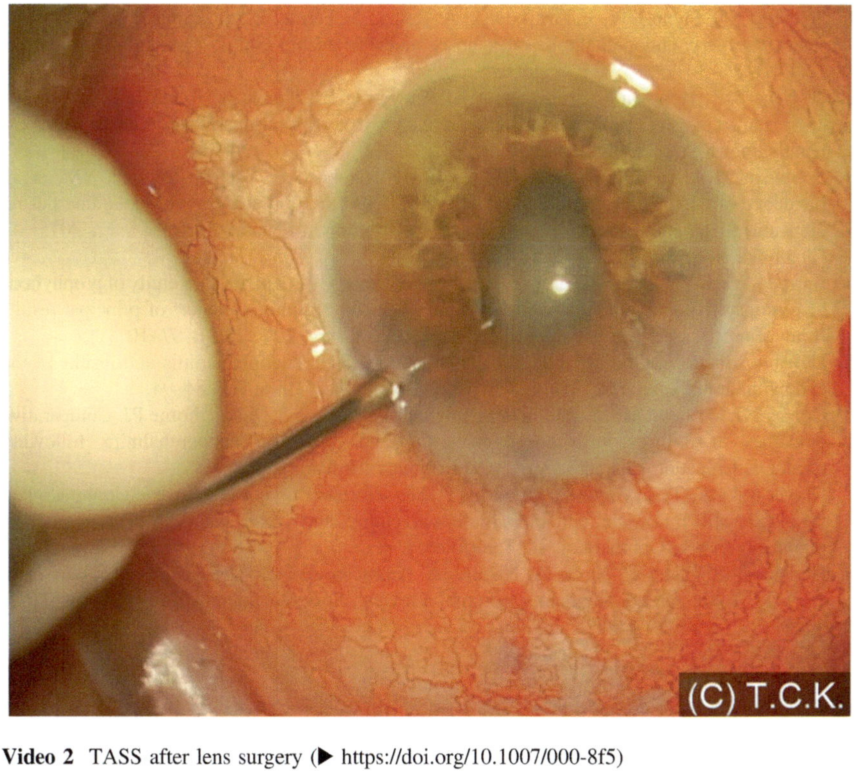

Video 2 TASS after lens surgery (▶ https://doi.org/10.1007/000-8f5)

conditions. In the past, the use of enzymatic cleaning solutions and ultrasound cleaning of instruments played a role, but this rarely occurs today in the preparation of instruments to be used intraocularly. Chemical impurities on intraocular lenses, in viscoelastics and rinsing solutions as well as preservatives in intraocularly administered drugs can still trigger TASS today however (Video 2). In case of doubt, TASS should always be treated as endophthalmitis.

Keypoint

In case of doubt, an increased intraocular inflammation after three days of lens surgery is to be managed as endophthalmitis and should be referred to a vitreoretinal surgeon.

Author's recommendation

Consistent antisepsis with povidone-iodine is the key factor for the prophylaxis of endophthalmitis. It is essential that the povidone-iodine's action time of at least 30 s—or better 40 s—be maintained. An irrigation of the conjunctiva including the fornices with 1–5% povidone-iodine is preferable to application of povidone iodine drops.

References

1. Schwartz SG, Flynn HW, Jr, Grzybowski A, Relhan N, Ferris FL. Intracameral antibiotics and cataract surgery: endophthalmitis rates, costs, and stewardship, 3rd ed. Ophthalmology. 2016; 123(7):1411–3.
2. de Geus SJR, Hopman J, Bruggemann RJ, Klevering BJ, Crama N. Acute Endophthalmitis after cataract surgery: clinical characteristics and the role of intracameral antibiotic prophylaxis. Ophthalmol Retin. 2020.
3. Nentwich MM, Ta CN, Kreutzer TC, Li B, Schwarzbach F, Yactayo-Miranda YM, et al. Incidence of postoperative endophthalmitis from 1990 to 2009 using povidone-iodine but no intracameral antibiotics at a single academic institution. J Cataract Refract Surg. 2015; 41 (1):58–66.
4. Barry P, Seal DV, Gettinby G, Lees F, Peterson M, Revie CW, et al. ESCRS study of prophylaxis of postoperative endophthalmitis after cataract surgery: preliminary report of principal results from a European multicenter study. J Cataract Refract Surg. 2006;32(3):407–10.
5. Doft bra, Barza M. Optimal management of postoperative endophthalmitis and results of the endophthalmitis vitrectomy study. Curr Opin Ophthalmol. 1996; 7(3):84–94.
6. Crosby NJ, Westcott M, Michael E, Cunningham WJ, Welch S, Polkinghorne PJ. Comparative outcomes of primary vitrectomy versus tap and inject for endophthalmitis following phacoemulsification cataract surgery. Ocul Immunol Inflamm. 2020: 1–7.
7. Grzybowski A, Turczynowska M, Kuhn F. The treatment of postoperative endophthalmitis: should we still follow the endophthalmitis vitrectomy study more than two decades after its publication? Acta Ophthalmol. 2018;96(5):e651–4.
8. Hernandez-Bogantes E, Navas A, Naranjo A, Amescua G, Gray-Hernandez EO, Flynn HW, Jr., et al. Toxic anterior segment syndrome: a review. Surv Ophthalmol. 2019; 64(4):463–76.

Dry Eye Management in Patients Undergoing Cataract Surgery

Elisabeth M. Messmer

Epidemiology

Dry Eye Disease (DED) following cataract surgery may be the reason for a patient being dissatisfied with the postoperative result (Fig. 1). Multiple studies have shown that subjective symptoms and clinical signs of DED increase following cataract surgery. In most cases, the ocular surface improves slowly within 3 months post-operatively, but ocular surface disease may persist chronically for longer than 3 months [1–4]. DED after cataract surgery is typically associated with significantly lower levels in quality of life and the patients should be counselled preoperatively [4].

Keypoint

Dry eye is frequently present preoperatively but goes often unrecognized or is inadequately treated.

In a cohort of 136 patients before cataract surgery, Trattler et al. demonstrated relatively few subjective symptoms (foreign body sensation > 50% of the time in 13% of the patients), but reduced tear film stability in 63%, corneal staining in 77% and a Schirmer test below 5 mm in 5 min in 21% of their patients preoperatively [5]. In addition, Gupta et al. observed an increased tear film osmolarity in 57% of their preoperative cataract clients, and a positive MMP-9 test as sign of ocular surface inflammation in 63% of their patients [6]. Meibomian gland dysfunction (MGD) is also a common finding in patients before cataract surgery. Cochener et al. found clinically evident MGD with partly pronounced changes in meibography in 52% of their patients preoperatively [7]. It is important to note that the patients themselves may be unaware of the baseline dryness associate an exacerbation of

E. M. Messmer (✉)
Department of Ophthalmology, University of Munich, Munich, Germany
e-mail: emessmer@med.uni-muenchen.de

M. Shajari et al. (eds.), *Cataract and Lens Surgery*,
https://doi.org/10.1007/978-3-031-05394-8_90

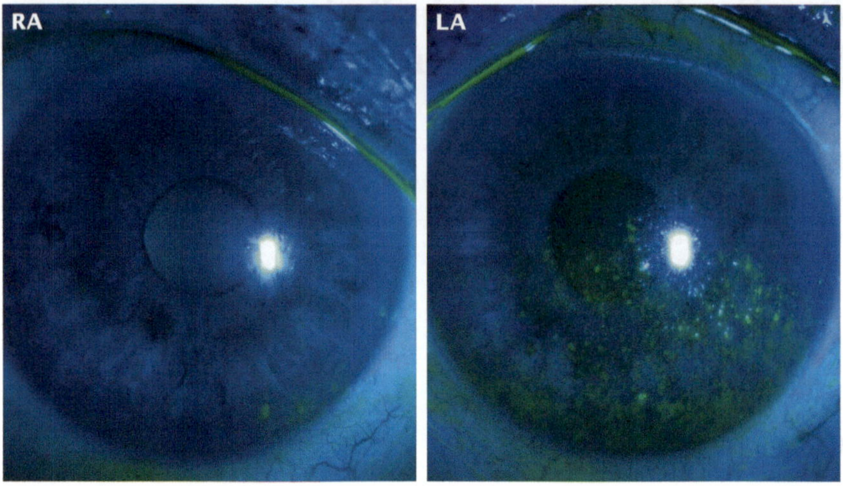

Fig. 1 Left eye (LA): s/p cataract surgery 2 years ago with sustained discomfort and pronounced corneal staining postoperatively. Unoperated right eye (RA) with cataract and mild DED with minimal ocular surface staining

underlying dry eye disease solely with the cataract surgery. Thorough preoperative examination, counselling and documentation is strongly recommended to help avoid dissatisfied patients.

An increase in subjective dry eye symptoms such as dryness, foreign body sensation, burning, itching, epiphora etc. is also known to occur as a result of the lens surgery itself. Objectively, there is a reduction in tear production, reduced tear film stability and an increase in MGD [1, 3]. Denervation caused by the corneal incisions, a reduced blinking reflex, an increase in inflammation, a loss of goblet cells, the eyelid speculum, intraoperative light damage, and intraoperative irrigation procedures as well as postoperative use of toxic, mostly preserved topical medications have all been described as pathogenetic factors. [1, 8–12].Femtosecond laser-assisted cataract surgery is associated with an increased postoperative ocular surface damage compared to conventional cataract surgery. The additional trauma caused by the suction ring appears to elicit damage to the goblet cells is thought to be responsible [12–14].

Diagnosis of Dry Eye

The diagnosis of DED is discussed in Chap. 18. In principle, two forms of DED have been described, though there is often considerable overlap of the pathological mechanisms particular in more severe dry eye. The two forms are: [1] aqueous tear deficiency with reduced tear meniscus, reduced Schirmer test and frequent ocular surface staining and [2] hyperevaporative DED, usually caused by meibomian gland dysfunction with changes in eyelid margins, blocked meibomian gland ducts and a reduced tear film break up time. New diagnostic options, including the analysis of tear film osmolarity and the evaluation of matrix metalloproteinase 9 (MMP9) in the tear film, are becoming increasingly important [15, 16]. The evaluation of tear film osmolarity and MMP9 in the tear film are recommended by the ASCRS (American Society of Cataract and Refractive Surgery) as screening tests prior to corneal refractive and cataract surgery [17].

Treatment of DED in Patients Undergoing Cataract Surgery

General Treatment Principles

Keypoint

The Dry Eye Workshop II (DEWS II) published novel guidelines for the treatment of DED in its 2017 report.

Many national and international ophthalmological associations use the DEWSII report as a guideline for the management of DED including the German Professional Association of Ophthalmologists (BVA) and the German Ophthalmological Society (DOG) [18] (Table 1). A large chapter in the DEWSII report is devoted to "iatrogenic dry eye", which of course includes dry eye following cataract surgery [19].

Basic treatment of DED includes reducing exposure to triggering (environmental) factors (smoke, dust, dry heating air, topical and systemic medication, etc.) and treatment with tear substitutes. Preferably, unpreserved artificial tears should be used. In cases of MGD, eyelid hygiene (hot compresses, lid massage) should be advised and must be carried out twice daily. This can be supported by lipid-containing tear substitutes. If this basic step 1 treatment is insufficient, anti-inflammatory drugs are initiated. A 2- to 4-week tapering course with unpreserved so called "soft" corticosteroids (e.g., hydrocortisone) can be used for a short period of time to counteract inflammation. In chronic disease with clear-cut ocular surface damage, 0.1% cyclosporine eye drops are available in Europe. These should be administered once a day, preferably at bedtime. The patient must be notified of the delayed onset of action (approx. 6–8 weeks) and that a typical burning sensation during application is normal (though this typically decreases with time). In the US, Lifitegrast, an integrin antagonist, is topically available on the market for the treatment of DED. In cases of a pronounced aqueous tear deficiency, partial closure of the tear ducts with silicone plugs can be very beneficial. In MGD, systemic doxycycline preparations (e.g. doxycycline 40–100 mg/d for at least 3 months) can also be used. The DEWS report, stage 2, recommends adding professional lid hygiene by microblepharoexfoliation as well as professional lid warming and meibomian gland expression by the ophthalmologist, intensive pulsed light therapy (IPL), thermodynamic therapy and meibomian gland probing where needed. If these measures are not sufficient, the DEWSII treatment algorithm stage 3 suggests the use of autologous serum eye drops and the application of bandage contact lenses or scleral lenses. More extensive treatment options such as surgical closure of the lacrimal puncti, amniotic membrane transplantation, and tarsorrhapy for persistent epithelial defects as well as salivary gland transplants are reserved for the most severe cases [18].

Preoperative Management

It is of utmost importance not to overlook DED preoperatively and to treat it accordingly.

Severe DED with pronounced ocular surface damage or severe DED associated with an uncontrolled underlying systemic disease (e.g., Sjögren's syndrome, s/p bone marrow transplantation etc.) should only be operated on after initiation of an effective treatment resulting in an improved ocular surface. Severe blepharitis/meibomitis/meibomian gland dysfunction should also be treated before cataract surgery and it may even be necessary to delay elective surgery until later on. Special attention must be paid to patients with diabetes mellitus with frequent neurotrophic keratopathy and epithelial healing disorders as well as patients with systemic autoimmune disease [10, 20]. Patients with increased tear film osmolarity or a positive MMP-9 test in the tear film seem to develop DED more often postoperatively [15, 16, 21]. The patient must also be advised of the possibility of developing and/or worsening of DED after surgery. Patients for premium intraocular lenses must be carefully selected and intensively advised; DED can significantly hamper preoperative intraocular lens calculation and thus the success of cataract surgery in these cases [22].

Intraoperative Management

Intraoperatively, topical anesthesia should be limited to the minimum necessary. The operation must be performed minimally invasive and quick. The ocular surface should be well moistened throughout the operation. Careful use of the speculum must be ensured.

Author's recommendation

Intraoperatively, care must be taken to ensure adequate moistening of the ocular surface throughout the procedure.

Postoperative Management

The recognition of postoperative DED as a reason for postoperative visual function disturbances and subjective symptoms is of utmost importance. Take the patient's complaints seriously. A routine application of unpreserved tear substitutes together with the postoperative antibiotic-anti-inflammatory therapy is often very useful. Several studies have demonstrated that the additional administration of artificial tears significantly reduced both the subjective complaints and the objective signs of DED, including tear film break-up time, corneal staining, and ocular surface inflammation compared to a postoperative control group without additional tear substitutes to the postoperative standard treatment [23, 24]. Patients with multifocal intraocular lenses in particular seem to benefit from intensive postoperative surface care including topical cyclosporine A [25].

Author's recommendation

The standard postoperative treatment after cataract surgery should include tear substitutes.

The use of topical non-steroidal anti-inflammatory drugs should be restricted to situations when needed. Moreover, the topical administration of antibiotics often toxic to the ocular surface should be minimized. Even in patients with severe DED, e.g. in the context of a chronic graft-versus-host disease after bone marrow transplantation or with associated autoimmune disease, cataract surgery can be successfully performed following careful preoperative preparation and intensive postoperative treatment of the ocular surface [10, 26, 27].

References

1. Han KE, Yoon SC, Ahn JM, Nam SM, Stulting RD, Kim EK, et al. Evaluation of dry eye and meibomian gland dysfunction after cataract surgery. Am J Ophthalmol. 2014;157(6):1144-50.e1.
2. Kasetsuwan N, Satitpitakul V, Changul T, Jariyakosol S. Incidence and pattern of dry eye after cataract surgery. PLoS ONE. 2013;8(11): e78657.
3. Li XM, Hu L, Hu J, Wang W. Investigation of dry eye disease and analysis of the pathogenic factors in patients after cataract surgery. Cornea. 2007;26(9 Suppl 1):S16–20.
4. Xue W, Zhu MM, Zhu BJ, Huang JN, Sun Q, Miao YY, et al. Long-term impact of dry eye symptoms on vision-related quality of life after phacoemulsification surgery. Int Ophthalmol. 2019;39(2):419–29.
5. Trattler WB, Majmudar PA, Donnenfeld ED, McDonald MB, Stonecipher KG, Goldberg DF. The Prospective Health Assessment of Cataract Patients' Ocular Surface (PHACO) study: the effect of dry eye. Clinical ophthalmology (Auckland, NZ). 2017;11:1423–30.
6. Gupta PK, Drinkwater OJ, VanDusen KW, Brissette AR, Starr CE. Prevalence of ocular surface dysfunction in patients presenting for cataract surgery evaluation. J Cataract Refract Surg. 2018;44(9):1090–6.
7. Cochener B, Cassan A, Omiel L. Prevalence of meibomian gland dysfunction at the time of cataract surgery. J Cataract Refract Surg. 2018;44(2):144–8.

8. Kwon JW, Chung YW, Choi JA, La TY, Jee DH, Cho YK. Comparison of postoperative corneal changes between dry eye and non-dry eye in a murine cataract surgery model. Int J Ophthalmol. 2016;9(2):218–24.
9. Oh T, Jung Y, Chang D, Kim J, Kim H. Changes in the tear film and ocular surface after cataract surgery. Jpn J Ophthalmol. 2012;56(2):113–8.
10. Ram J, Gupta A, Brar G, Kaushik S, Gupta A. Outcomes of phacoemulsification in patients with dry eye. J Cataract Refract Surg. 2002;28(8):1386–9.
11. Sitompul R, Sancoyo GS, Hutauruk JA, Gondhowiardjo TD. Sensitivity change in cornea and tear layer due to incision difference on cataract surgery with either manual small-incision cataract surgery or phacoemulsification. Cornea. 2008;27(Suppl 1):S13–8.
12. Yu Y, Hua H, Wu M, Yu Y, Yu W, Lai K, et al. Evaluation of dry eye after femtosecond laser-assisted cataract surgery. J Cataract Refract Surg. 2015;41(12):2614–23.
13. Ju RH, Chen Y, Chen HS, Zhou WJ, Yang W, Lin ZD, et al. Changes in ocular surface status and dry eye symptoms following femtosecond laser-assisted cataract surgery. Int J Ophthalmol. 2019;12(7):1122–6.
14. Shao D, Zhu X, Sun W, Cheng P, Chen W, Wang H. Effects of femtosecond laser-assisted cataract surgery on dry eye. Exp Ther Med. 2018;16(6):5073–8.
15. Gonzalez-Mesa A, Moreno-Arrones JP, Ferrari D, Teus MA. Role of Tear Osmolarity in Dry Eye Symptoms After Cataract Surgery. Am J Ophthalmol. 2016;170:128–32.
16. Messmer EM, by Lindenfels V, Garbe A, Kampik A. Matrix Metalloproteinase 9 Testing in Dry Eye Disease Using a Commercially Available Point-of-Care Immunoassay. Ophthalmology. 2016;123(11):2300–8.
17. Starr CE, Gupta PK, Farid M, Beckman KA, Chan CC, Yeu E, et al. An algorithm for the preoperative diagnosis and treatment of ocular surface disorders. J Cataract Refract Surg. 2019;45(5):669–84.
18. Jones L, Downie LE, Korb D, Benitez-Del-Castillo JM, Dana R, Deng SX, et al. TFOS DEWS II Management and Therapy Report. Ocul Surf. 2017;15(3):575–628.
19. Gomes JAP, Azar DT, Baudouin C, Efron N, Hirayama M, Horwath-Winter J, et al. TFOS DEWS II iatrogenic report. Ocul Surf. 2017;15(3):511–38.
20. Messmer EM, Schmid-Tannwald C, Zapp D, Kampik A. In vivo confocal microscopy of corneal small fiber damage in diabetes mellitus. Graefe's archive for clinical and experimental ophthalmology = Albrecht von Graefe's archive for clinical and experimental ophthalmology 2010;248(9):1307–12.
21. Lanza NL, Valenzuela F, Perez VL, Galor A. The Matrix Metalloproteinase 9 Point-of-Care Test in Dry Eye. Ocul Surf. 2016;14(2):189–95.
22. Woodward MA, Randleman JB, Stulting RD. Dissatisfaction after multifocal intraocular lens implantation. J Cataract Refract Surg. 2009;35(6):992–7.
23. Mencucci R, Boccalini C, Caputo R, Favuzza E. Effect of a hyaluronic acid and carboxymethylcellulose ophthalmic solution on ocular comfort and tear-film instability after cataract surgery. J Cataract Refract Surg. 2015;41(8):1699–704.
24. Sanchez MA, Arriola-Villalobos P, Torralbo-Jimenez P, Giron N, de la Heras B, Herrero Vanrell R, et al. The effect of preservative-free HP-Guar on dry eye after phacoemulsification: a flow cytometric study. Eye (Lond). 2010;24(8):1331–7.
25. Donnenfeld ED, Solomon R, Roberts CW, Wittpenn JR, McDonald MB, Perry HD. Cyclosporins 0.05% to improve visual outcomes after multifocal intraocular lens implantation. Journal of cataract and refractive surgery. 2010;36(7):1095–100.
26. Balaram M, Dana MR. Phacoemulsification in patients after allogeneic bone marrow transplantation. Ophthalmology. 2001;108(9):1682–7.
27. de Melo FR, Kron-Gray MM, De la Parra-Colin P, He Y, Musch DC, Mian SI, et al. Outcomes of cataract surgery in graft-versus-host disease. Cornea. 2015;34(5):506–11.

Femtoseconds Laser-Assisted Lens Surgery

Basic Principles of the Femtosecond Laser-Based Tissue Surgery

Georg Schuele and Daniel Palanker

Introduction

The development of the laser in 1960 [17] revolutionized precision and control of the light delivery due to several key distinctions from the previous non-coherent sources: (1) photons are emitted at the same phase (coherence), (2) the wavelength range is very narrow (monochromatic light); (3) the beam is very directional (well collimated), and hence can be tightly focused; and (4) pulse duration can be precisely controlled in a wide range. With the further development of laser technology, four different laser-tissue interaction mechanisms have been identified, as illustrated in Fig. 1.

With sufficiently short wavelengths (in ultraviolet (UV) range, below 400 nm), photon energy is high enough (>3 eV) to induce direct photochemical reactions in proteins. To avoid any significant temperature rise, photochemical treatments are administered at a low light intensity, and to deliver a sufficient dose of irradiation, such procedures typically require long (tens of seconds) exposures. These interactions can be enhanced using photosensitizer, such as riboflavin for example, which converts photon energy into singlet oxygen, leading to efficient corneal crosslinking. In the milliseconds (ms) to seconds range of pulse durations, the dominant mechanism of tissue damage is the thermal denaturation of proteins. At pulse durations below tens of microseconds, heating is so rapid that the dominant mechanism of tissue damage becomes explosive vaporization, leading to mechanical rupture and ejection of tissue, such as corneal ablation with ns pulses of excimer laser. At pulse durations in the sub-ns range (down to femtoseconds), light

G. Schuele (✉) · D. Palanker
Portola Consulting, Portola Valley, USA
e-mail: gwschuele@gmail.com

D. Palanker
Stanford University, Stanford, USA
e-mail: palanker@stanford.edu

M. Shajari et al. (eds.), *Cataract and Lens Surgery*,
https://doi.org/10.1007/978-3-031-05394-8_91

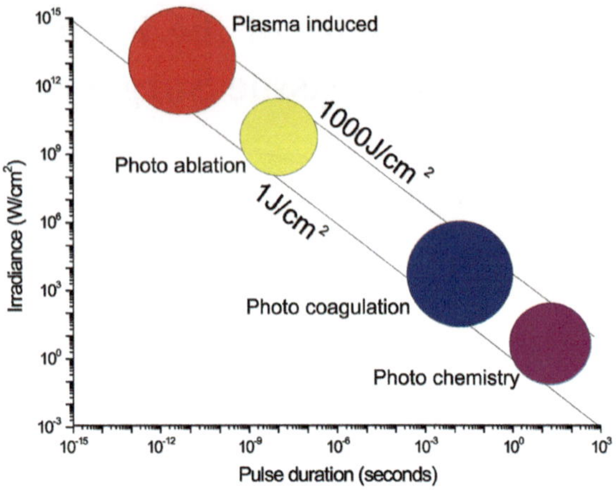

Fig. 1 Distribution of the four basic laser-tissue interaction mechanisms as a function of pulse duration and required irradiance. Plasma-mediated interactions are only achieved with very short (<ns) laser pulses and high irradiance levels

intensity in the tightly focused laser beam can be sufficiently high for photo-ionization to occur. This technique is of special interest for cataract surgery as it enables energy deposition into the optically transparent tissues like the cornea and crystalline lens, with their subsequent disruption. The first clinical use of photoionization was the removal of the posterior capsular opacification, which remains the standard of care for the treatment of secondary cataracts until today.

Laser Beam Propagation

A light beam generated by lasers comes typically with a high beam quality factor, which allows focusing of the light in a diffraction-limited spot. The diameter of the focal spot d increases linearly with the wavelength λ, and depends reciprocally on the focusing angle, which is often characterized by numerical aperture $NA = \sin(D/2f)$, where D is the beam diameter and f—is the focal length of the lens. Hence $d \cong (2 * \lambda)/(\pi * NA)$. The second important parameter to consider is the focal depth, or the length F of the laser focus waist along the propagation axes, also called the Rayleigh range. It is described as $F \cong (2 * \lambda)/(\pi * NA^2)$. Figure 2 illustrates these relationships.

For low NAs, the laser focus is very elongated along the beam axis. The aspect ratio of the Rayleigh length to focal diameter is shown in Fig. 3 for different NAs. This plot also includes a visual representation of the beam shapes in the laser focus.

Clinical cataract laser systems have NAs in the range of 0.1–0.35, which corresponds to spot sizes of 3–7 μm and Rayleigh ranges of 7–20 μm. The higher the focusing angle of the optics (NA) the smaller the laser spot and the shorter the Rayleigh range. This translates to the higher precision of the tissue cutting but also slower processing speed since more spots are needed to process the same area in the sample.

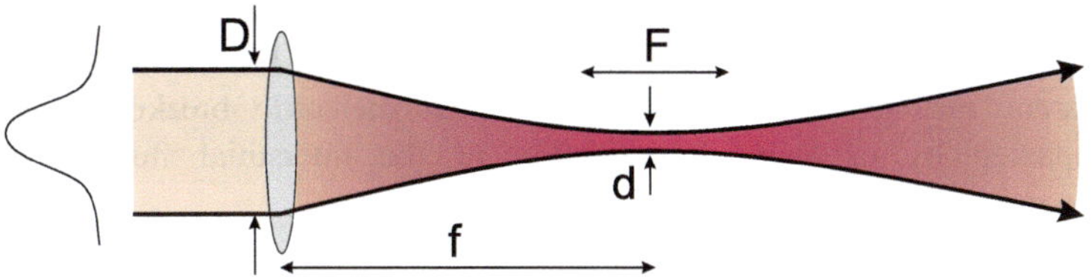

Numerical aperture NA = sin (D/2f)

For a Gaussian laser beam:

Diameter of the focal spot:

$$d = \frac{4 \cdot f}{\pi \cdot D}\lambda \cong \frac{2 \cdot \lambda}{\pi \cdot NA}$$

Focal depth:

$$F = \frac{8 \cdot f^2}{\pi \cdot D^2}\lambda \cong \frac{2 \cdot \lambda}{\pi \cdot NA^2}$$

Fig. 2 Graphical representation of a focused laser beam and the formulas describing the focal spot diameter and focal depth

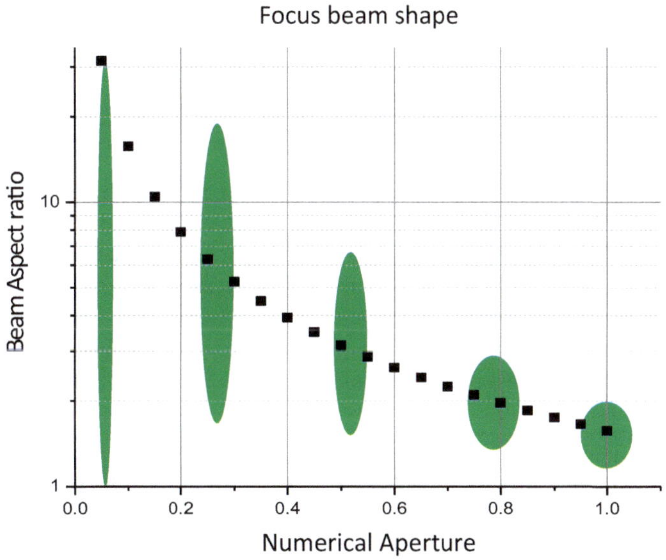

Fig. 3 Beam shape (aspect ratio of length to width of the focal zone) as a function of the numerical aperture (NA) of the focusing optics

Dielectric Breakdown

At extremely high irradiances (10^8–10^{11} W/cm^2), which can be achieved in a short-pulsed (ns-fs) tightly focused laser beam, the electric field is so intense that electrons can be stripped from atoms, creating an ionized state of matter, called plasma. If the cloud of plasma is dense enough, it in turn can absorb the laser light, which allows energy deposition at the focal point of the laser beam even inside a transparent material. This mechanism, called dielectric breakdown, is often accompanied by explosive vaporization of the interstitial fluid, leading to mechanical rupture of the tissue in the focal zone.

The energy threshold of dielectric breakdown depends on the pulse duration and spot size of the laser beam. The threshold decreases with decreasing pulse duration and reaches a plateau around 100 femtoseconds [16]. Changing the pulse duration from a few nanoseconds (like a laser used for posterior capsule opacification) to a 350 fs laser (typically used for LASIK flaps and cataract surgery) reduces the breakdown threshold energy by a factor of 1000: from about 1 mJ to 1 μJ [20, 36].

Shock Waves and Cavitation Bubble

Following the absorption of the laser pulse, a plasma is formed typically within the focal volume of the laser beam. Upon explosive vaporization, part of the absorbed energy is transferred to mechanical energy of the tissue expansion and formation of a shock wave and a cavitation bubble [35]. Figure 4 shows the sequence of events in plasma-mediated energy deposition in tissues.

The size of a cavitation bubble increases with the absorbed laser energy [34]. While the plasma itself disrupts a small volume of tissue, most of the tissue splitting

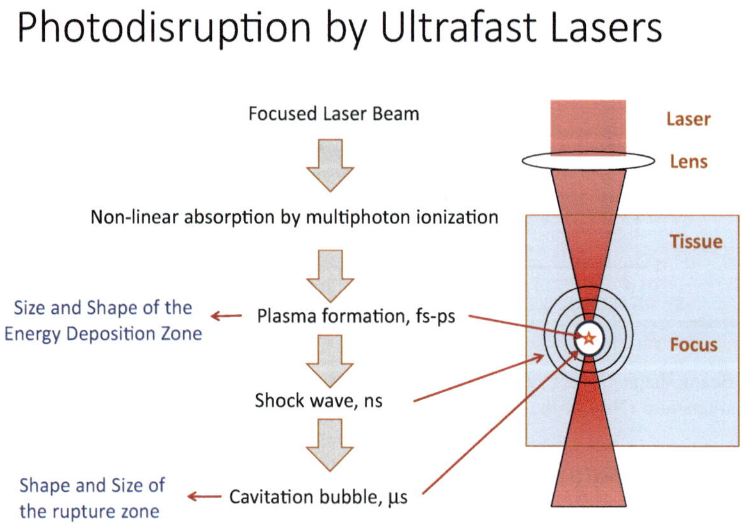

Fig. 4 The sequence of effects following dielectric breakdown-mediated energy absorption into transparent tissue. The size and shape of plasma define the energy deposition zone while the size of the cavitation bubble defines the size and shape of the mechanical rupture zone in tissue

occurs due to the cavitation bubble. To minimize the tissue disruption zone, the threshold energy of the dielectric breakdown should be reduced to a minimum, which can be accomplished by either tighter focusing or by decreasing the pulse duration. Therefore, the most delicate surgical procedures are performed with lasers having a pulse duration in the range of a few hundred femtoseconds and extremely tight laser focus.

This optimization allows reducing the tissue disruption zone from a millimeter scale (like with a ns-YAG laser for posterior capsulotomy) down to a micrometer scale (like in a lenticule cutting laser system). Scanning of the laser focus allows merging the single craters into two-dimensional tissue cuts, tailored for various applications.

System Optimization

For specific clinical applications, one needs to balance the tradeoffs between the demand for high precision, duration of the procedure, and geometrical accessibility of the target tissue. For corneal applications, high axial precision is required to ensure accurate placement of the cuts in depth, smooth separation of the tissue planes, and minimum damage zone along the edges of the cuts. A high focusing angle (NA) on the cornea enables very tight focusing of the laser beam, thereby reducing the threshold energy and improving surgical precision. Optical access to the lens, however, is more limited. Low focusing angle results in a wider and deeper focal zone, which can be suitable for lens fragmentation if the pulse duration is sufficiently short. On the other hand, the elongated focal zone of the low-NA beam enables rapid treatment of large tissue volume. These considerations are illustrated in Fig. 5.

Femtosecond Laser Cataract Laser Systems

Currently, 5 different laser technology platforms are approved by the FDA/CE for femtosecond cataract surgery: Catalys Precision Laser System (JnJ), LenSx Laser (Alcon), LENSAR (LENSAR), Femto LDV Z8 (Ziemer), and Victus (BnL). Characteristics of these systems are summarized in Table 1.

Patient Interface and Docking

All systems provide a patient interface for stable docking of the patient's eye to the system. This minimizes the eye movement during the procedure and enables precise placement of the intended cuts. The surgeon needs to ensure that the patient is

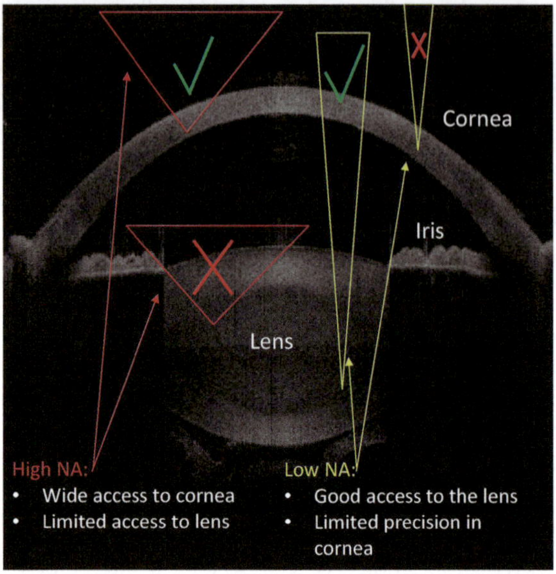

Fig. 5 Geometrical limitations on focusing of the laser beam in the eye. High NAs (high angles) are good for corneal applications with tight depth localization, while low NAs are good for lens applications, providing a long focus and effective volumetric treatment of the lens

placed comfortably in the treatment bed and the head oriented such that the eyebrow does not interfere with the interface. This is achieved by slightly tilting the patient's head, so the operated eye is in a higher plane and the chin faces slightly upwards. The surgeon should also ensure a well-centered placement of the optical interface onto the patient's eye and minimize potential forces onto the eye during docking of the system. Some systems do this automatically by monitoring the force vectors.

Even though patient interfaces differ in specifics, as outlined in Table 1, they all are designed to minimize the forces on the cornea and formation of posterior corneal folds, which distort the laser beam and result in incomplete capsulotomies [21, 31]. Most systems utilize water immersion of the cornea for optical coupling to reduce the corneal tissue deformation, as suction is only applied to a scleral ring.

The IOP rise under dock ranges from about 16–59 mmHg in different systems [9, 14, 26, 38]. High IOP rise is contraindicated for glaucoma patients. High suction can also result in subconjunctival hemorrhage under the scleral suction ring [31]. While the water immersion interfaces fit all patients, the LenSx patient interface comes in three sizes and needs to be selected depending on the patients' individual corneal curvature (steep, normal, flat) to minimize the chance of posterior corneal folds. Figure 6 shows the patient interfaces of the different systems.

After a successful dock, the optical path must be clear and free of bubbles and no haze or condensation should be visible at any timepoint. The patient should remain still while the tissue images are gathered, the treatment plan is generated, approved, and executed.

Table 1 Summary table of commercially available femtosecond laser cataract systems. Core features and functionality of these systems are summarized as reported by March 2020

Laser System	JnJ-Catalys	Alcon-LenSx	LensAR	Ziemer-LDV Z8	BnL-Victus
	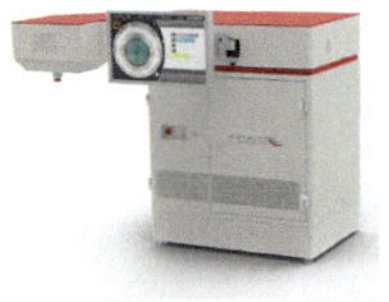	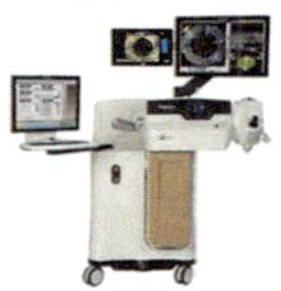	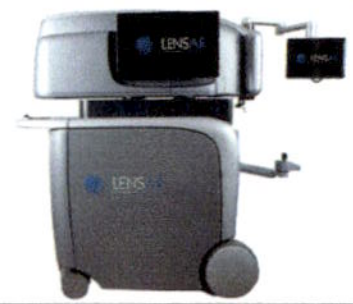	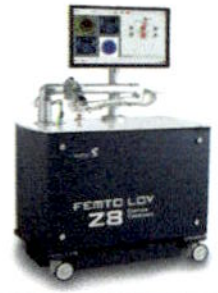	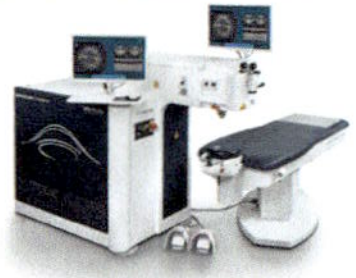
Indications	**Lens**: Capsulotomy and fragmentation; **Cornea**:Incisions and arcuates	**Lens**: Capsulotomy and fragmentation; **Cornea** : Incisions, arcuates and flap	**Lens**: Capsulotomy and fragmentation; **Cornea**: Incisions, arcuates, pocket and flap	**Lens**: Capsulotomy and fragmentation; **Cornea**: Incisions, arcuates and flap	**Lens**: Capsulotomy and fragmentation; **Cornea**: Incisions, arcuates, flap and others
Laser repetition rate	120 kHz, variable	50 kHz for cataract, 150 kHz for conreal treatments	80 kHz	1 MHz for capsulotomy, 2 MHz for lens segmentation	160 kHz, variable
Guidance	SD-OCT and Video Microscope	SD-OCT and Video Microscope	Scheimpflug and Video Microscope	SD-OCT and Video Microscope	SS-OCT and Video Microscope
Interface	Non-applanating 2-piece, vacuum docking	Curved interface 1-piece, vaccum docking	Non-applanating 2-piece, vacuum docking	Central curved-applanating 2-piece for lens based procedures, flat applanation for cornea, vacuum docking	Non-applanating for lens based procedures, curved applanating for cornea, 2-piece, vacuum docking
Docking	Water bath, No corneal applanation, no glaucoma contraindication	Curvature matching soft hydogel contact lens, minimal corneal deformation, no glaucoma contraindication	Water bath, No corneal applanation	Water bath, No corneal applanation	Water bath, No corneal applanation, no glaucoma contraindication

(continued)

Table 1 (continued)

Laser System	JnJ-Catalys	Alcon-LenSx	LensAR	Ziemer-LDV Z8	BnL-Victus
IOP rise under dock	15.6 mmHg	28 mmHg		59.3 mmHg	28 mmHg
Integrated bed	Yes	No	No	No	Yes
Lens pattern	Segmentation and grid fragmentation combinations	Segmentation; ring, grid and plane fragmentation	Segmentation, ring and grid fragmentation	Segmentation	Segmentation; ring, grid and plane fragmentation
Capsulotomy duration	~1 s, full lens tilt compensation	~3–5 s depending on lens tilt	~2–3 s, full tilt compensation	10–15 s depending on lens tilt	~2s, tilt compensation
Cut sequence	Capsulotomy, fragmentation, corneal incisions	Capsulotomy, fragmentation, corneal incisions	Capsulotomy, fragmentation, corneal incisions	Fragmentation, capsulotomy, corneal incision	Capsulotomy, fragmentation, corneal incisions
Laser visualization	Full video during laser	Full video during laser	Reduced video rate during laser	No video during laser	Full video during laser
Install/mobile	Fixed install	Install with wheels	Install with wheels	Mobile	Fixed install

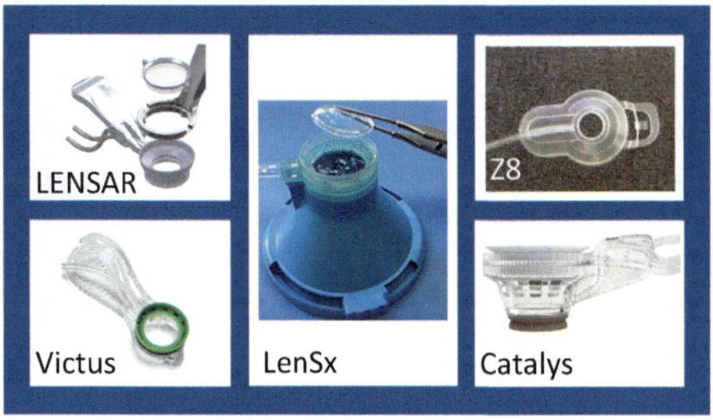

Fig. 6 Patient interfaces for the laser systems listed in Table 1. The LenSx interface uses soft and flexible hydrogel inserts, which need to be assembled and matched to the patient's corneal curvatures. All others utilize water immersion with a scleral suction ring

Imaging

All systems provide image-guided planning of the surgical procedures, with en-face video for all planning in the XY plane. All, except for the Ziemer Z8 system, also use the video system to visualize and monitor the treatment progress while the laser is active. Cross-sectional images of the tissue are provided by OCT or Scheimpflug imaging, as illustrated in Fig. 7.

Information about each patient's anterior chamber allows customized planning of capsulotomy, lens fragmentation, and corneal incisions. Following the evaluation of the image quality, the surgeon confirms the identified structures or corrects the treatment plan accordingly. Safety zones around the posterior and anterior lens capsule, iris, and cornea require special attention. It is also important to validate that the liquid interface is still correctly filled and there are no bubbles in view since proper co-registration of the OCT and the laser is based on assumptions of the refractive index of the medium in the scan path. Once all the adjustments are made and confirmed, the surgeon can proceed to the treatment, which typically begins with capsulotomy, followed by the lens fragmentation and corneal incisions.

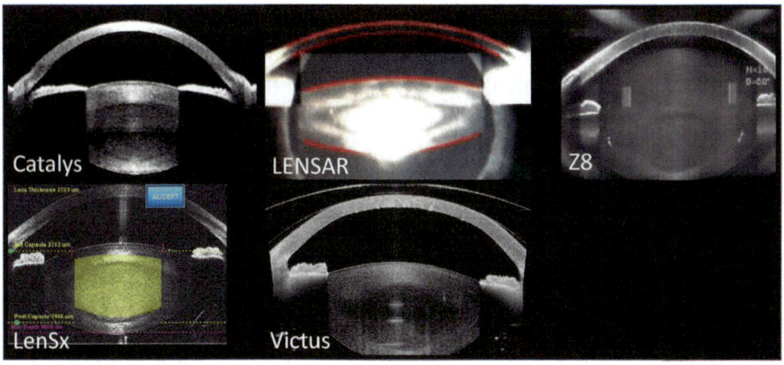

Fig. 7 Typical image quality provided by the laser systems listed in Table 1. The LENSAR system utilizes Scheimpflug imaging while all other systems use either spectral-domain (Catalys, LenSx, Z8) or swept-source (Victus) OCT

All the OCT-based systems perform treatment planning on overlays of the 3-D image, with a true visual interpretation of the distances and tissue structures [22]. The LENSAR system uses Scheimpflug principle-based imaging technology with structured scanning illumination. Using ray-tracing techniques, the software collates the multiple acquired Scheimpflug images to generate a 3D model of the anterior segment with integrated treatment patterns. Visual confirmation of the treatment plan is displayed on a 2D ocular profile of this model. The LENSAR system also utilizes the Scheimpflug image data for automatic cataract LOCS grading, which affects the lens fragmentation patterns [19, 33].

Real-time OCT imaging of the treatment progress is currently enabled only in the Victus system. The Catalys system offers a low frame rate OCT streaming only for confirmation of the corneal incision right before the treatment, but not during the treatment.

Capsulotomy

A capsulotomy is the opening of the capsular bag using a femtosecond laser. The cut is achieved by adjacent placement of the laser spots within the capsular tissue. While manual capsulorhexis creates a perfectly smooth edge (Fig. 8), SEM evaluation of the laser capsulotomy reveals a sawtooth-like structure with the distance between craters matching the laser spot spacing (see Fig. 8, middle picture) [4, 5, 27, 29, 37]. Lowering the pulse energy and providing a tighter spot overlap helps to smooth the sawtooth pattern. Such a pattern can be completely eliminated by the use of UV fs laser, which enables the photochemical decomposition of the capsular tissue instead of tissue rupture by NIR laser [37]. Figure 8 shows SEM images of the manual capsulorhexis, as well as plasma- and photochemical-mediated cuts in the porcine lens capsule.

The effect of the sawtooth edge and generation of the aberrant (out of line) spots due to tissue movements led to the controversy regarding the capsular strength after capsulotomy. Opinions on both sides of the argument have been published, i.e. claims that laser capsulotomy is stronger or weaker than the manual capsulorhexis. [1, 3, 10, 18, 25, 32]. Clinical studies are also divided regarding the rates of capsular tears [2, 23, 24, 30]. In this regard, the initial learning curve in managing laser surgery with reduced red reflex seems to be an important factor [12, 23].

The natural lens capsule is under slight tension, and therefore, upon tissue cutting, slippage of up to 200 μm has been observed clinically [27, 29]. This may result in the erroneous placement of the laser craters on capsular tissue, leading to incomplete cutting (capsular tags) or the formation of double cuts [27–29]. Since a complete capsulotomy is critically important, to minimize the tissue slippage, capsulotomy is performed before lens fragmentation because gas bubbles forming during the latter step greatly increase the tissue tension. At first glance, it would be more logical to perform all the cutting from the bottom upwards to avoid interference of the beam with the created bubbles, i.e. lens fragmentation would be the

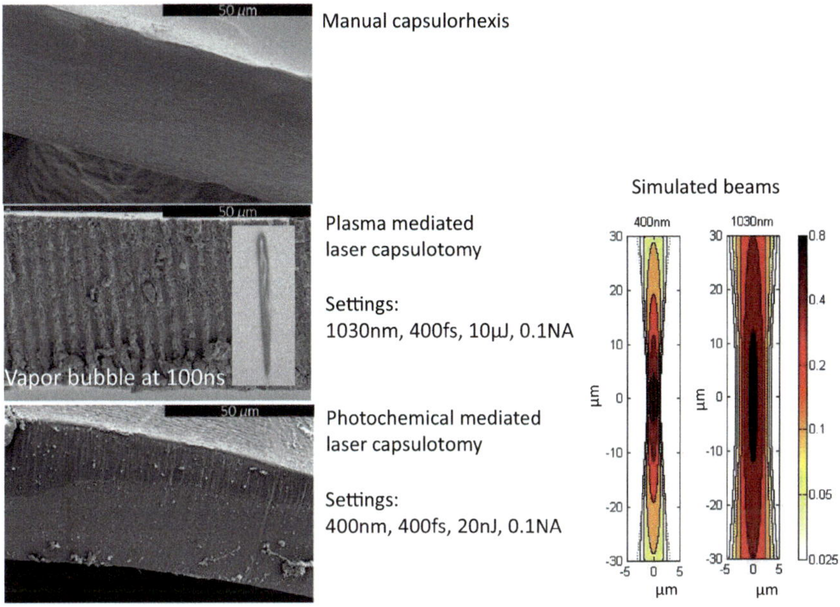

Fig. 8 Edge of the porcine lens capsules processed by manual capsulorhexis (top); plasma-mediated capsulotomy performed by IR femtosecond laser (middle), and by a photochemical process using a fs UV laser. The right panel depicts the simulated beam profiles for these two laser systems

first step, followed by capsulotomy. But the very significant volume of gas bubbles created during the lens fragmentation leads to tissue expansion and stretching of the lens capsule. This tension can lead to massive tissue slippage upon cutting, resulting in incomplete capsulotomies. To minimize these effects, capsulotomy is performed first, even though its bubbles may slightly degrade the lens fragmentation pattern.

To minimize the lens capsule slippage, it is also important to minimize the capsulotomy duration. This is especially challenging if the eye is docked under a slight tilt, so there is a large variation in depth between the capsulotomy high and low points. The systems use different technical solutions to provide a fast transition of the laser focus through the capsular tissue. The Catalys, Victus, and LENSAR systems dynamically adjust the axial position of each laser spot, so the scanning pattern follows the capsule surface even if it is tilted. The LenSx system with its slow focus adjustment gates the laser emission such that it only allows cutting when the laser beam is focused on the capsule. Therefore, the more tilted is a lens, the longer the cutting will take. Capsulotomy takes a long time with Ziemer Z8 since its small axial scan field is mitigated by cutting only small sections of the capsule at a time.

All femtosecond laser systems have demonstrated superiority in sizing, uniformity, and centration of the capsulotomy, compared to manual capsulorhexis [11, 13, 15]. Figure 9 shows examples of stained capsular discs that were removed by either manual capsulorhexis or femtosecond capsulotomy.

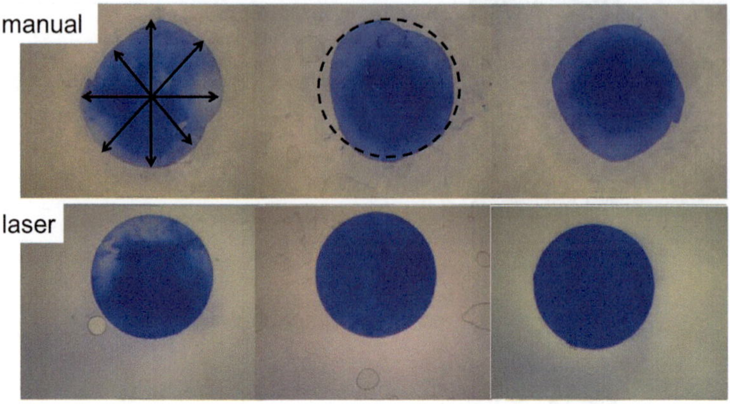

Fig. 9 Capsular discs removed during cataract surgery. The samples were stained with trypan blue to enhance image contrast. The top row is the outcome of manual capsulorhexis, while the bottom row was excised utilizing a femtosecond laser

Lens Fragmentation

The femtosecond laser is also used to pre-cut the cataract lens and thereby minimize the need for active phacoemulsification. Laser platforms allow pattern selection for lens segmentation and fragmentation based on the LOCS grade, surgeon preference, and the individual patient needs.

Segmentation: dissection of the lens into 4, 6, or 8 sections with or without the use of lens softening. These radial cuts facilitate easier splitting of the lens into smaller sections and full-depth penetration of the crack to the posterior side of the lens (see Fig. 10).

Fragmentation: softening of the lens by patterned laser treatment throughout its volume. The patterns in the different systems include cylindrical rings or

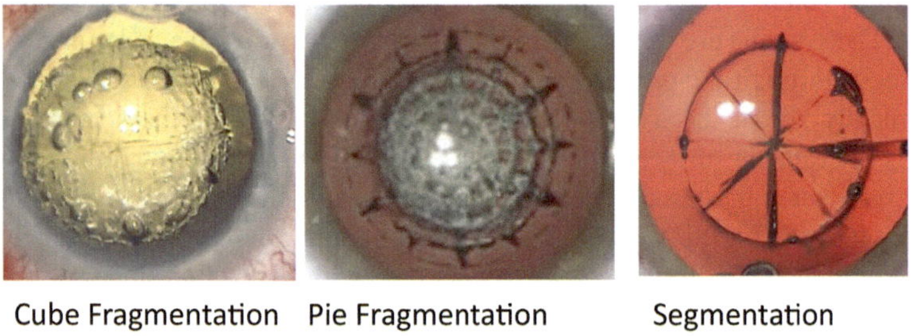

Fig. 10 Different lens segmentation and fragmentation patterns available on various laser platforms

rectangular grids, and currently, no data is available demonstrating the advantages of one over the other. The systems first define the posterior and anterior safety zones, and laser patterns are then applied in-between these boundaries. Figure 10 shows the different segmentation and fragmentation patterns available in different systems.

In addition to the easier manipulation of the lens tissue, the reduction of the phaco energy during the removal of the pre-fragmented lens is the biggest benefit of the laser in cataract surgery [7]. This also leads to better preservation of the corneal endothelium during cataract surgery [6] and faster visual recovery after cataract surgery [8].

Corneal Incisions

All systems also support the creation of corneal incisions. These include the multiplanar main incisions and paracenteses, as well as relaxing incisions for correction of astigmatism. This aspect of the treatment planning is also based on the available imaging data.

Relaxing incisions need to be placed on the correct axial orientation to correct low astigmatism. Planning of the refractive aspect of the treatment can be done separately using the surgeon-preferred nomogram, before the cataract surgery. The LENSAR and Catalys systems are currently the only available system with a system-integrated nomogram calculation. In the LENSAR, Catalys, and LenSx system, axial orientation of the relaxing incision can be based on preoperative diagnostic devices and is typically applied using an automatic iris registration. Other systems require pre-surgical manual marking of the eye to indicate the orientation as a part of the treatment planning. One unique feature of the femtosecond laser is the creation of intrastromal cuts without dissection of the anterior corneal surface, which prevents the ingrowth of corneal epithelial cells.

Main incisions and paracentesis: All systems offer multiplane main corneal incisions for a self-sealing corneal wound. With all systems, the incision needs to be placed in a transparent section of the corneal-limbal interface. Light scattering in the cornea too close to the limbus degrades the beam quality and limits the dissectability of the tissue. Some systems provide surgeons with some guidance regarding this optical transition zone, based on the OCT data.

Newer Technologies

The current systems were all first-generation introductions to the marketplace, and relatively minor iterations of the devices occurred after the approval. There is still plenty of opportunities to further optimize the systems and develop new concepts that would overcome the limitations of the existing laser platforms. For example, there have been multiple attempts to develop microscope-mounted laser systems with full integration into the surgical OR workflow, but they have not been commercialized. Other concrete concepts are:

Multispot femto laser: Keranova is currently developing a multisport femtosecond laser for cataract surgery. It utilizes a phase modulator to create an array of laser foci which are scanned in 3 dimensions, allowing faster tissue processing. The system is currently in development and does not have FDA or CE approval.

Capsulaser: This is a laser-based device for thermal capsulotomy, which uses staining of the lens capsule with trypan blue to enable absorption of visible laser light, leading to thermal cutting. A circular opening is created by scanning the laser beam. Currently, the Capsulaser only has a CE mark approval.

Zepto: Is an electrosurgical device, in which an electrically heated nitinol ring is used to thermally cut the capsule. It comes with a suction skirt which attaches to the lens to ensure good apposition of the nitinol ring to the capsule. The Zepto system is FDA and CE-approved.

In conclusion, femtosecond lasers enabled surgeons to perform more precise and reproducible cataract surgery as well as astigmatic corrections on the cornea. This technology has proven especially useful in difficult surgical cases, such as patients with weak zonules, and opalescent cataracts. More than 10 years since its introduction into the clinical practice, utilization of femtosecond laser-assisted cataract surgery is still growing in market share, and clinicians continue to discern its utility and clinical benefits. This technology has the potential to enable new generations of intraocular lenses, either injectable via a small incision, or mounted onto a perfectly micromachined lens capsule matching the IOL body features.

References

1. Abell RG, Darian-Smith E, Kan JB, Allen PL, Ewe SYP, Vote BJ. Femtosecond laser-assisted cataract surgery versus standard phacoemulsification cataract surgery: Outcomes and safety in more than 4000 cases at a single center. J Cataract Refract Surg. 2015;41(1):47–52. https://doi.org/10.1016/j.jcrs.2014.06.025.
2. Abell RG, Davies PEJ, Phelan D, Goemann K, McPherson ZE, Vote BJ. Anterior capsulotomy integrity after femtosecond laser-assisted cataract surgery. Ophthalmology. 2014;121(1):17–24. https://doi.org/10.1016/j.ophtha.2013.08.013.
3. Auffarth GU, Reddy KP, Ritter R, Holzer MP, Rabsilber TM. Comparison of the maximum applicable stretch force after femtosecond laser-assisted and manual anterior capsulotomy. J Cataract Refract Surg. 2013;39(1):105–9. https://doi.org/10.1016/j.jcrs.2012.08.065.
4. Bala C, Xia Y, Meades K. Electron microscopy of laser capsulotomy edge: interplatform comparison. J Cataract Refract Surg. 2014;40(8):1382–9. https://doi.org/10.1016/j.jcrs.2013.11.045.
5. Chan T, Pattamatta U, Butlin M, Meades K, Bala C. Intereye comparison of femtosecond laser–assisted cataract surgery capsulotomy and manual capsulorhexis edge strength. J Cataract Refract Surg. 2017;43(4):480–5. https://doi.org/10.1016/j.jcrs.2016.12.033.
6. Conrad-Hengerer I, al Juburi M, Schultz T, Hengerer FH, Dick HB Corneal endothelial cell loss and corneal thickness in conventional compared with femtosecond laser-assisted cataract

surgery: Three-month follow-up. J Cataract Refract Surg. 2013;39(9):1307–13. https://doi.org/10.1016/j.jcrs.2013.05.033.
7. Conrad-Hengerer I, Hengerer FH, Schultz T, Dick HB. Effect of femtosecond laser fragmentation of the nucleus with different softening grid sizes on effective phaco time in cataract surgery. J Cataract Refract Surg. 2012;38(11):1888–94. https://doi.org/10.1016/j.jcrs.2012.07.023.
8. Dick HB, Schultz T. A review of laser-assisted versus traditional phacoemulsification cataract surgery. In Ophthalmology and Therapy. 2017 (Vol. 6, Issue 1, pp. 7–18). Springer Healthcare. https://doi.org/10.1007/s40123-017-0080-z.
9. Donaldson KE, Braga-Mele R, Cabot F, Davidson R, Dhaliwal DK, Hamilton R, Jackson M, Patterson L, Stonecipher K, Yoo SH. Femtosecond laser-assisted cataract surgery. J Cataract Refractive Surg. 2013;39(11):1753–1763. https://doi.org/10.1016/j.jcrs.2013.09.002.
10. Friedman NJ, Palanker DV, Schuele G, Andersen D, Marcellino G, Seibel BS, Batlle J, Feliz R, Talamo JH, Blumenkranz MS, Culbertson WW (n.d.) Femtosecond laser capsulotomy ARTICLE. https://doi.org/10.1016/j.jcrs.2011.04.022.
11. Friedman NJ, Palanker DV, Schuele G, Andersen D, Marcellino G, Seibel BS, Batlle J, Feliz R, Talamo JH, Blumenkranz MS Culbertson WW Femtosecond laser capsulotomy. J Cataract Refract Surg. 2011;37(7):1189–98. https://doi.org/10.1016/j.jcrs.2011.04.022.
12. Grewal DS, Dalal RR, Jun S, Chou J, Basti S. Impact of the learning curve on intraoperative surgical time in femtosecond laser-assisted cataract surgery. J Refract Surg. 2016;32(5):311–7. https://doi.org/10.3928/1081597X-20160217-02.
13. He L, Sheehy K, Culbertson W. Femtosecond laser-assisted cataract surgery. Curr Opin Ophthalmol. 2011;1040(8738):1–10. https://doi.org/10.1097/ICU.0b013e3283414f76.
14. Kerr NM, Abell RG, Vote BJ, Toh T. Intraocular pressure during femtosecond laser pretreatment of cataract. J Cataract Refract Surg. 2013;39(3):339–42. https://doi.org/10.1016/j.jcrs.2012.12.008.
15. Kránitz K, Takacs A, Miháltz K, Kovács I, Knorz MC, Nagy ZZ (n.d.) Femtosecond laser capsulotomy and manual continuous curvilinear Capsulorrhexis parameters and their effects on intraocular lens centration. https://doi.org/10.3928/1081597X-20110623-03.
16. Lenzner M, Krüger J, Sartania S, Cheng Z, Spielmann C, Mourou G, Kautek F. Femtosecond optical breakdown in dielectrics. Phys Rev Lett. 1998;80(18):4076–9. https://doi.org/10.1103/PhysRevLett.80.4076.
17. Maiman TH. Stimulated optical radiation in Ruby. Nature. 1960;187(4736):493–4. https://doi.org/10.1038/187493a0.
18. Mastropasqua L, Toto L, Calienno R, Mattei PA, Mastropasqua A, Vecchiarino L, di Iorio D. Scanning electron microscopy evaluation of capsulorhexis in femtosecond laser-assisted cataract surgery. J Cataract Refract Surg. 2013;39(10):1581–6. https://doi.org/10.1016/j.jcrs.2013.06.016.
19. Morley D, Pillai A, Olmstead R. Development and Evaluation of an Objective Cataract Grading Metric. Invest Ophthalmol Visual Sci. 2013. https://iovs.arvojournals.org/article.aspx?articleid=2151629.
20. Noack J, Vogel A. Laser-induced plasma formation in water at nanosecond to femtosecond time scales: calculation of thresholds, absorption coefficients, and energy density. In IEEE Journal Of Quantum Electronics; 1999, Vol. 35, Issue 8.
21. Ostovic M, Klaproth OK, Hengerer FH, Mayer WJ, Kohnen T. Light microscopy and scanning electron microscopy analysis of rigid curved interface femtosecond laser-assisted and manual anterior capsulotomy. J Cataract Refract Surg. 2013;39(10):1587–92. https://doi.org/10.1016/j.jcrs.2013.07.024.
22. Palanker DV, Blumenkranz MS, Andersen D, Wiltberger M, Marcellino G, Gooding P, Angeley D, Schuele G, Woodley B, Simoneau M, Friedman NJ, Seibel B, Batlle J, Feliz R, Talamo J, Culbertson W. Femtosecond laser-assisted cataract surgery with integrated optical coherence tomography. Sci Transl Med. 2010;2(58):58ra85–58ra85. https://doi.org/10.1126/scitranslmed.3001305.

23. Roberts Tv, Lawless M, Bali SJ, Hodge C, Sutton G. Surgical outcomes and safety of femtosecond laser cataract surgery: A prospective study of 1500 consecutive cases. Ophthalmology. 2013;120(2):227–33. https://doi.org/10.1016/j.ophtha.2012.10.026.
24. Roberts Tv, Lawless M, Sutton G, Hodge C. Anterior capsule integrity after femtosecond laser–assisted cataract surgery. J Cataract Refract Surg. 2015;41(5):1109–10. https://doi.org/10.1016/j.jcrs.2014.11.044.
25. Schuele G, Palanker D, Friedman N (2011) Capsular strength and ultrastructural appearance of Femtosecond Laser Capsulotomy and Manual Capsulorhexis | IOVS | ARVO Journals. Investigative Ophthalmology & Visual Science. https://iovs.arvojournals.org/article.aspx?articleid=2361761.
26. Schultz T, Conrad-Hengerer I, … F. H.-J. of C. &, & 2013, undefined. (n.d.). Intraocular pressure variation during femtosecond laser–assisted cataract surgery using a fluid-filled interface. *Elsevier*. Retrieved March 30, 2020, from https://www.sciencedirect.com/science/article/pii/S0886335012015362.
27. Schultz T, Joachim SC, Noristani R, Scott W, Dick HB. Greater vertical spot spacing to improve femtosecond laser capsulotomy quality. J Cataract Refract Surg. 2017;43(3):353–7. https://doi.org/10.1016/j.jcrs.2016.12.028.
28. Schultz T, Joachim SC, Tischoff I, Dick HB. Histologic evaluation of in vivo femtosecond laser-generated capsulotomies reveals a potential cause for radial capsular tears. Eur J Ophthalmol. 2014;25(2):112–8. https://doi.org/10.5301/ejo.5000484.
29. Schultz T, Joachim SC, Tischoff I, Dick HB. Histologic evaluation of in vivo femtosecond laser-generated capsulotomies reveals a potential cause for radial capsular tears. Eur J Ophthalmol. 2015;25(2):112–8. https://doi.org/10.5301/ejo.5000484.
30. Scott WJ. Re: Abell et al. Anterior capsulotomy integrity after femtosecond laser-assisted cataract surgery (Ophthalmology 2014;121:17–24). In *Ophthalmology.* 2014 (Vol. 121, Issue 7). Elsevier Inc. https://doi.org/10.1016/j.ophtha.2014.02.014.
31. Talamo JH, Gooding P, Angeley D, Culbertson WW, Schuele G, Andersen D, Marcellino G, Essock E, Batlle J, Feliz R, Friedman NJ, Palanker D. Optical patient interface in femtosecond laser-assisted cataract surgery: contact corneal applanation versus liquid immersion. J Cataract Refract Surg. 2013;39(4):501–10. https://doi.org/10.1016/j.jcrs.2013.01.021.
32. Thompson V, Chang DF. Comparison of manual, femtosecond laser, and precision pulse capsulotomy edge tear strength in paired human cadaver eyes. Ophthalmology. 2016;265–274. https://doi.org/10.1016/j.ophtha.2015.10.019.
33. Uy H (2013) Grading system holds promise for improved efficiency, safety. Ophthalmology Times.
34. Vogel A, Busch S, Parlitz U. Shock wave emission and cavitation bubble generation by picosecond and nanosecond optical breakdown in water. J Acoust Soc Am. 1996;100(1):148–65. https://doi.org/10.1121/1.415878.
35. Vogel A, Noack J, Hüttman G, Paltauf G. Mechanisms of femtosecond laser nanosurgery of cells and tissues. In Applied Physics B: Lasers and Optics. 2005 (Vol. 81, Issue 8, pp. 1015–1047). https://doi.org/10.1007/s00340-005-2036-6.
36. Vogel A, Venugopalan V. Pulsed laser ablation of soft biological tissues. In Optical-Thermal Response of Laser-Irradiated Tissue. 2011 (pp. 551–615). Springer Netherlands. https://doi.org/10.1007/978-90-481-8831-4_14.
37. Wang J, Schuele G, Palanker D. Finesse of transparent tissue cutting by ultrafast lasers at various wavelengths. J Biomed Opt. 2015;20(12): 125004. https://doi.org/10.1117/1.jbo.20.12.125004.
38. Williams GP, Ang HP, George BL, Liu YC, Peh G, Izquierdo L, Tan DT, Mehta JS. Comparison of intra-ocular pressure changes with liquid or flat applanation interfaces in a femtosecond laser platform. Sci Rep. 2015;5. https://doi.org/10.1038/srep14742.

Corneal Incisions with the Femtosecond Laser

Karl Boden

The main incision and paracenteses using the femtosecond laser

Corneal incisions made as part of cataract surgery can have an impact on postoperative outcome and image quality, although the type of surgical technique used with the different incision positions and sizes plays an important role [1]. Due to the high precision and reproducibility of the laser, one might assume that the predictability of the surgically induced astigmatism produced would be more accurate compared to manual incisions. However, reports in the literature are inconsistent and comparisons are difficult due to the data collection on different laser platforms and different laser settings. The influence and quality of limbal detection of the different devices in particular was not considered in all publications.

Due to the high precision and the digital incision planning, it is also not possible to inadvertently make a too short clear cornea incision, which also results in fewer intraoperative difficulties (e.g. unstable anterior chamber or iris prolapse) or a lower rate of postoperative problems (hypotension or endophthalmitis), and thus could potentially lead to a greater safety for the patient (though this has not been verified).

Another advantage of femtosecond laser-assisted corneal incisions was found by Grewal and colleagues using anterior segment OCT [2]. They were able to demonstrate smoother inner wound edges than manual incisions, which leads to less lift-off or defects of the Descemet at the inner wound edges. The explanation for these results is that the femto-cavitation spots cause disruption of the tissue and as

Supplementary Information The online version contains supplementary material available at https://doi.org/10.1007/978-3-031-05394-8_92. The videos can be accessed individually by clicking the DOI link in the accompanying figure caption or by scanning this link with the SN More Media App.

K. Boden (✉)
Sulzbach, Germany
e-mail: drkarlboden@googlemail.com

M. Shajari et al. (eds.), *Cataract and Lens Surgery*,
https://doi.org/10.1007/978-3-031-05394-8_92

the manual blade is advanced through the tissue, it pushes the Descemet membrane slightly away from the stroma, forming a small gap before it penetrates it.

Author's recommendation

An Arcus lipoides has a much smaller influence on the patency of the incisions than vascularization does. An increase in the incision energy in the preoperative setting should be taken earlier with vascularization in the incision area than is the case with an arcus lipoides.

An advanced vessel edge loop on the limbus can produce inadequate cut qualities even at lower levels. This is most likely due to the vessels filled with haemoglobin which shows a higher absorption of the laser, compared to the arcus lipoides. Due to the media turbidity of the arcus lipoid, there is only a slight scattering of the laser light, which has less influence on the effect of the laser than absorption of the laser beam.

The lower prevalence of an arcus lipoid and prominent vessels in the temporal quadrant and the lower surgically induced astigmatism to be expected suggest that the main incision should also be made in the temporal quadrant. This is also consistent with the general findings from other FLACS studies and manual cataract surgery.

Keypoint

As with manual cataract surgery, the main incision should be created with the smallest possible cut width with a temporal access is the preferred technique for femtosecond cataract surgery.

Anti-astigmatic keratotomies as part of cataract surgery.

In the treatment of cataract, we cannot only take a curative approach, but should also consider the refractive needs of patients. In the vast majority of patients, however, we can detect an astigmatism below 1.5 dpt preoperatively, which, if left untreated, can lead to insufficient uncorrected visual acuity. In these cases, arcuate shaped keratotomies or limbal relaxing incisions are an effective treatment option in cataract surgery (Fig. 1).

Keypoint

The anti-astigmatic keratotomies are an effective treatment option for astigmatism up to 1.5 dpt. For higher values of astigmatism (>1.5 dpt) toric intraocular lenses are clearly superior to keratotomies.

Anti-astigmatic keratotomies have the advantage that the preoperative operation logistics do not have to be changed. After a detailed diagnosis, in theory, an immediate operation can be performed without having to order a special intraocular lens. The treatment is also possible with all forms of anaesthesia, however, before general anaesthesia when using laser platforms without automatic alignment, the axial position should be marked preoperatively in a sitting position. In these cases it is important to make sure that the markings lie outside the treatment zone, as some coloured marks can block the application of the laser, resulting in incomplete cuts.

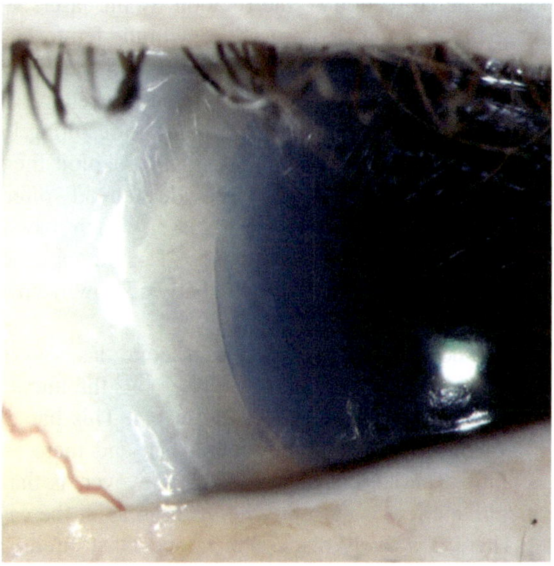

Fig. 1 Postoperative aspect of an arcuate corneal incision 4 weeks postoperative

Author's recommendation

If manual marking of the axis is required, it should be ensured that the marking is placed outside of the treatment zone, otherwise the laser may be blocked by the colour pigments.

The anti-astigmatic keratotomies are positioned in the steep meridian of corneal astigmatism. Ideally, a regular astigmatism is treated. In special cases—in case of irregular astigmatism with e.g. an asymmetrical bowtie or a symmetrical bowtie with axial tilt—a treatment with a toric IOL will not achieve a satisfactory result. Planning the femtosecond laser with different cut positioning and cut lengths offers a good option to perform an individual and customizable treatment.

It is recommended that the surgeon be flexible with regard to the main access, as the anti-astigmatic keratotomies should not overlap with the corneal incisions. Overlapping of these incisions must be avoided, as otherwise the incision architecture and the self-closing effect of the main access cannot be guaranteed.

Keypoint

Overlapping of the anti-astigmatic keratotomies with the corneal incisions should be avoided at the planning stage. The surgeon should therefore be flexible with regard to the main access in order to be able to treat these forms of astigmatism safely.

It should also be noted that a very large source of error can lie in the cyclorotation of the eye, which is not insignificant between the upright and supine positions of the patient. According to studies, this can be up to 17°. On average, however, a cyclorotation of 4–5° can be assumed. Even docking with the patient interface can increase a rotation error. Some providers recommend manual colour marking and automatic correction of the rotation by the laser. When we consider the demands made on an automated procedure with the femtosecond laser, a reliance on manual marking is ultimately not satisfactory and therefore does not meet the qualitative requirements of an automated surgical procedure. The connection of preoperative diagnostics to the laser platform and the resulting loss-free transfer of information into the operative setting is essential to exploit the full potential and speed of the femtosecond laser. Individual providers already offer the integration of preoperative diagnostics with the femtosecond laser, which may also lead to better postoperative results. The combination of diagnostics and application ultimately allows the same level of automation and quality that we know from corneal refractive surgery to be applied in cataract surgery.

Another benefit of the femtosecond laser system is that it enables purely intrastromal incisions. Here, the laser cuts the intrastromal collagen fasciae without the involvement of the epithelial layers. This has the advantage that no epithelial ingrowth can occur in the wound gap and there is also a lower risk of bacterial keratitis. The current disadvantage, however, is that the predictability of the post-operative effect is currently not as high as in the case of penetrating keratotomies.

There is a lively discussion in specialist circles as to whether a manual, blunt opening of the keratotomies on the following day postoperatively can have a further effect if the result is insufficient. The author cannot recommend this, as it must be assumed that there is a high risk of epithelial invasion into the wound gap. Furthermore, the effect and the deviation from the calculations of the nomograms cannot be calculated (Video 1).

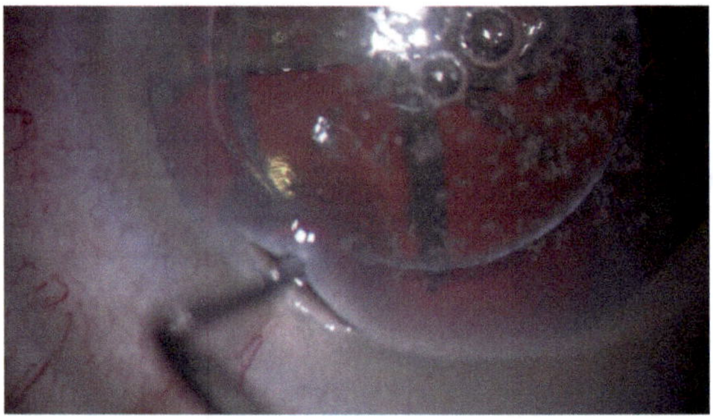

Video 1 The video shows how correct and complete the incision of the arcuate incisions is. A routine check of the incisions is not necessary or not recommended
(▶ https://doi.org/10.1007/000-8f7)

A further component in future treatments will also be the consideration of individual tissue specifications. In this case, the individual data are entered pre-operatively into a web-based application and various corneal incisions are calculated using a complex algorithm, and thus the individually optimal incision is recommended based on the calculation [3].

Nomograms

On the basis of a nomogram, values are read off which give the desired postoperative effect. The variables that influence the treatment are comparable to those of manual astigmatic keratotomy. Influenceable and non-influenceable variables include the incision length and depth, distance of the incisions from the centre of the cornea and the age of the patient. The experience and rule regarding the effect of these incisions say that the longer, deeper and the more central the incisions are, the higher the effect. Older patients respond better to anti-astigmatic keratotomies than younger patients. For incision lengths between 30° and 90°, a coupling ratio of 1 can be assumed. In case of a coupling effect, the incisions have no influence on the spherical equivalent. Larger incisions however can have an influence on the spherical equivalent.

Most nomograms recommend an incision depth between 80 and 90% of the corneal thickness and an incision position that varies with an optical zone of between 8 and 9 mm. Depending on the laser platform, the incisions are checked by means of OCT or Scheimpflug technique. The incisions themselves are usually performed perpendicularly. Some nomograms distinguish the position of the preoperative astigmatism. In general, an astigmatism “with the rule” is treated with shorter incisions than an astigmatism “against the rule”. Oblique astigmatism is treated with a mean of the two values with a tendency towards the values of the “with the rule” astigmatism. The most commonly used nomogram in the literature is the modified Lindstrom nomogram in cataract surgery. However, the author uses the “Castrop” nomogram developed by Hoffmann for anti-astigmatic keratotomies in femtosecond laser-assisted cataract surgery.

Keypoint record

Astigmatism “with the rule” is treated with shorter cuts than “against the rule”.

Conclusion

In summary, femtosecond laser is an ideal instrument to perform both corneal incisions and anti-astigmatic keratotomies in cataract surgery with high precision and reproducibility. Anti-astigmatic keratotomies are an effective and safe treatment option, especially for astigmatisms up to 1.5 dpt in cataract surgery, but can also be considered for higher astigmatisms after penetrating keratoplasty.

The sources of error in the treatment with anti-astigmatic keratotomies should be known and avoided. Intrastromal anti-astigmatic keratotomies may be less effective than penetrating but they show a lower complication rate. An appropriate adapted nomogram should be selected for intrastromal or penetrating keratotomies.

References

1. Denoyer A, Denoyer L, Marotte D, Georget M, Pisella PJ. Intraindividual comparative study of corneal and ocular wavefront aberrations after biaxial microincision versus coaxial small incision cataract surgery. Br J Ophthalmol. 2008. https://doi.org/10.1136/bjo.2007.137067.
2. Grewal DS, Basti S. Comparison of morphologic features of clear corneal incisions created with a femtosecond laser or a keratome. J Cataract Refract Surg. 2014. https://doi.org/10.1016/j.jcrs.2013.11.028.
3. Studer HP, Riedwyl H, Amstutz CA, Hanson JVM, Büchler P. Patient-specific finite-element simulation of the human cornea: A clinical validation study on cataract surgery. J Biomech. 2013. https://doi.org/10.1016/j.jbiomech.2012.11.018.

Capsulotomy Using the Femtosecond Laser

Wolfgang J. Mayer and Imad Hakim

The advantages of the femtosecond laser in performing capsulotomy include the high reproducibility, the excellent circularity and the possibility of adjusting or customizing different diameters based on needs of both patients and IOLs alike [1] Electron microscopic analyses have shown that the cut configuration of the capsulotomy edge can vary depending on the pulse energy and frequency used and this is one of the main differences between femtosecond laser and the manual alternative. The type of applanation via the patient interface also seems to play a role [2, 3].

When performing laser anterior capsulotomy it is advised that one take advantage of the adjustment possibilities of the imaging unit on the femtosecond laser (e.g. OCT) to achieve the best possible results. The overlapping of the optics also appears to have a protective effect on the development of posterior capsular opacification (PCO) [4]. Optimal centration of intraocular lenses is also thought to be more consistent due to the precise technology which appears to offer some added-value for premium lenses [5].

Performing a femtolaser-assisted anterior capsule opening requires optimal planning and the use of the integrated imaging and is typically performed with the inclusion of margin of safety. This margin of safety should be as large as necessary but as small as possible in order to allow a precise cutting configuration, depending on the selected pulse energy. It is also important that the interface is optimally aligned with the patient's eye to prevent the eye from tilting during the application of the aspiration. Care should also be taken to ensure sufficient mydriasis, as a small pupil can obscure the capsule and render it inappropriate for laser. Once the laser procedure is complete, it is essential to check that the anterior rhexis blade has been completely cut and does not contain any residual points of attachment to the rest of

W. J. Mayer (✉)
Munich, Germany
e-mail: wolfgang.j.mayer@med.uni-muenchen.de

I. Hakim
Dubai, UAE

M. Shajari et al. (eds.), *Cataract and Lens Surgery*,
https://doi.org/10.1007/978-3-031-05394-8_93

the lens capsule. This check only takes a moment but is important as it and can minimize the risk of radial tearing of the capsule.

Tip

Dimple-down technique

In rare cases, when using the femtosecond laser, so-called "skip areas" may occur where the laser perforation is not complete. Such fluctuations in the laser energy can be caused by Descemet wrinkles, for example and sometimes the smallest attachments may not be immediately visible under the surgical microscope. To be absolutely certain, in the dimple-down maneuver the surgeon makes a corneal incision and the using the OVD cannula, adjusts the anterior chamber evenly with viscoelastic and then gently presses down on the centre of the capsule with the tip of the cannula. If there are residual minimal attachments ("tags"), these can be separated by the manoeuvre—even if there is no red-reflex. This ensure that the central capsule in the area of the opening is entirely "free floating".

Special Techniques

Mature Lenses

Mature or intumescent cataracts are a particular challenge for the femto-second cataract surgeon. In these cases, the capsules are usually under a higher intralenticular pressure due to an often largely liquefied cortex often surrounding a hard or brownish core. Manual capsulorhexis in these cases can lead to tearing, and the dreaded Argentinian flag sign and as a result, the proportion of successful capsule openings in white cataracts is significantly lower than that of normal cases. Incomplete capsulorhexis is reported in 28% of cases of intumescent cataracts, while under normal circumstances this happens in 0.8–4% of normal cataracts with manual capsulorhexis.

A 2 mm minicapsulotomy at the beginning of the laser application has proven to be a safe method to remove these white lenses and to avoid the Argentinian flag sign. The material that exudes through this opening can then be removed, and after docking with the laser system again a 2nd, a 4.5–5.0 mm regular capsulotomy can then be created [6].

Posterior Capsulotomy

If required, a primary posterior capsulotomy can be performed before or after IOL implantation. If the capsulotomy is to be performed following IOL implantation, a small amount of dispersive viscoelasticity is injected between the implanted lens and the posterior capsule. The final step of the surgery is the posterior capsulotomy with the laser. The method makes use of a little-known anatomical structure, the space of Berger, between the posterior capsule and the anterior vitreous boundary membrane. This invisible structure can be easily visualized in the OCT of the femtosecond laser and prevents contact of the opened posterior capsule with the vitreous. After decompression of the crystalline lens and implantation of the IOL, the Berger space is usually clearly visible and larger than preoperatively. This is due to the supine position of the patient (and thus the effect of gravity) as well as the thinner artificial lens. In contrast to Nd:YAG capsulotomy, the anterior vitreous boundary membrane remains completely intact according to previous experience. Posterior capsulotomy can be performed successfully on all IOL types [7].

References

1. Abell RG, Davies PEJ, Phelan D, Goemann K, McPherson ZE, Vote BJ. Anterior capsulotomy integrity after femtosecond laser-assisted cataract surgery. Ophthalmology. 2014;121(1):17–24.
2. Kohnen T, Klaproth OK, Ostovic M, Hengerer FH, Mayer WJ. Morphological changes in the edge structures following femtosecond laser capsulotomy with varied patient interfaces and different energy settings. Graefes Arch Clin Exp Ophthalmol. 2014;252(2):293–8.
3. Ostovic M, Klaproth OK, Hengerer FH, Mayer WJ, Kohnen T. Light microscopy and scanning electron microscopy analysis of rigid curved interface femtosecond laser-assisted and manual anterior capsulotomy. J Cataract Refract Surg. 2013;39(10):1587–92.
4. Wertheimer C, Kreutzer TC, Dirisamer M, Eibl-Lindner K, Kook D, Priglinger S, et al. Effect of femtosecond laser-assisted lens surgery on posterior capsule opacification in the human capsular bag in vitro Acta. Ophthalmol. 2017;95(2):e85–8.
5. Kolb CM, Shajari M, Mathys L, Herrmann E, Petermann K, Mayer WJ, et al Comparison of femtosecond laser-assisted cataract surgery and conventional cataract surgery: meta-analysis and systematic review. J Cataract Refract Surg. 2020.
6. Schultz T, Dick HB. Laser-assisted mini-capsulotomy: a new technique for intumescent white cataracts. J Refract Surg. 2014;30(11):742–5.
7. Dick HB, Schultz T. Primary posterior laser-assisted capsulotomy. J Refract Surg. 2014;30 (2):128–33.

Fragmentation with the Femtolaser

Ke Yao and Mehdi Shajari

Fragmentation of the crystalline cataract lens is necessary for efficient and safe removal of an advanced cataract. To achieve this, the surgeon has various techniques at their disposal, such as the divide and conquer technique. The ultrasound energy that is delivered to the eye when forming the initial grooves in particular can lead to corneal endothelial damage and the degree of damage correlates strongly with the amount of ultrasound energy delivered. Surgeons therefore strive to keep the ultrasound energy delivered as low as possible in order to protect the ocular tissue. The femtosecond laser can be used to pre-fragment the natural lens which can save a significant amount of ultrasound energy, depending on the fragmentation pattern. The most frequently used fragmentation patterns include the pie pattern and the cube pattern.

In the pie pattern, the lens is usually divided into four or six equally sized "pie pieces" (Video 1), whereas in the cube pattern, the lens is pre-fragmented into several small cubes (Video 2). In this section, the fragmentation patterns are discussed, and a comparison is made with conventional cataract surgery.

The effective phacoemulsification time (EPT) is the product of the average "phaco-power" multiplied by the "phaco-time". It is an approximation of the ultrasound energy delivered and varies between different surgeons regardless of phacoemulsification settings. Mayer et al. found that EPT was significantly lower in femtosecond laser-assisted cataract surgery than in conventional cataract surgery

Supplementary Information The online version contains supplementary material available at https://doi.org/10.1007/978-3-031-05394-8_94. The videos can be accessed individually by clicking the DOI link in the accompanying figure caption or by scanning this link with the SN More Media App.

K. Yao (✉)
Hangzhou, China
e-mail: xlren@zju.edu.cn

M. Shajari
Frankfurt, Deutschland

M. Shajari et al. (eds.), *Cataract and Lens Surgery*,
https://doi.org/10.1007/978-3-031-05394-8_94

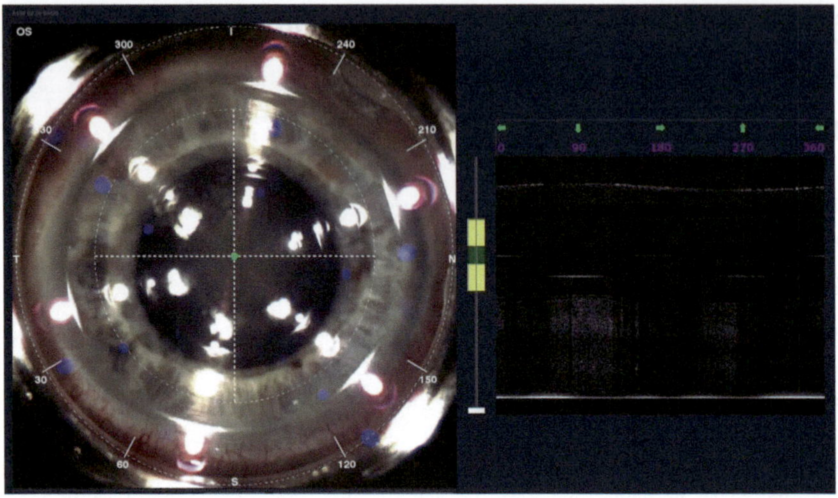

Video 1 Use of the femtolaser and fragmentation by pie pattern (▶ https://doi.org/10.1007/000-8f9)

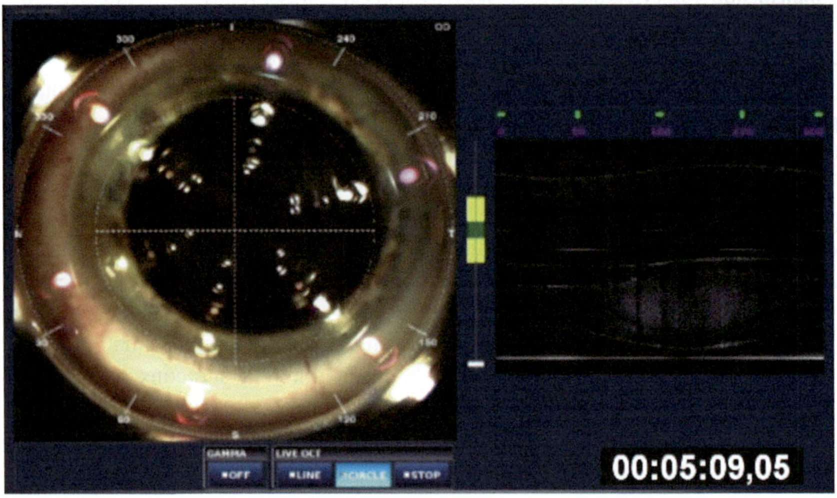

Video 2 Use of the femtolaser and fragmentation using a cube pattern (▶ https://doi.org/10.1007/000-8f8)

(1.58 s ±1.02 vs 4.17 s ±2.06, $P < 0.001$) [1]. Lens density was measured preoperatively with a Scheimpflug camera (Pentacam, Oculus) and it was found that the required ultrasound energy was higher in the conventional group for all lens densities. Hatch et al. and Ang et al. investigated the influence of the laser in mature lenses [2, 3]. They found reduced EPT, corneal oedema, anterior chamber irritation

Study or Subgroup	FLACS Mean	FLACS SD	FLACS Total	CCS Mean	CCS SD	CCS Total	Weight	Mean Difference IV, Random, 95% CI
Catalys								
Abell 2013a	0.94	3.47	100	6.5	4.3	76	3.6%	-5.56 [-6.74, -4.38]
Abell 2013c	2.33	2.28	150	14.24	10.9	51	1.0%	-11.91 [-14.92, -8.90]
Abell 2014a	1.99	5.24	405	8.69	7.47	215	3.8%	-6.70 [-7.82, -5.58]
Conrad-Hengerer 2012	0.16	1.21	57	4.07	3.14	52	4.4%	-3.91 [-4.82, -3.00]
Conrad-Hengerer 2013	0	0.1	73	1.4	0.1	73	6.6%	-1.40 [-1.43, -1.37]
Conrad-Hengerer 2014a	0.21	0.87	400	2.8	2.44	400	6.3%	-2.59 [-2.84, -2.34]
Conrad-Hengerer 2014b	0.035	0.11	104	1.39	0.13	104	6.6%	-1.35 [-1.39, -1.32]
Conrad-Hengerer 2015	0	0.1	100	1.3	1.1	100	6.4%	-1.30 [-1.52, -1.08]
Dick 2014	0.03	0.01	53	1.25	1.06	53	6.3%	-1.22 [-1.51, -0.93]
Subtotal (95% CI)			**1442**			**1124**	**44.8%**	**-2.06 [-2.30, -1.83]**
Heterogeneity: Tau² = 0.08; Chi² = 302.86, df = 8 (P < 0.00001); I² = 97%								
Test for overall effect: Z = 16.97 (P < 0.00001)								
LenSx								
Asena 2017	1.98	1.01	25	4.23	1.96	27	4.6%	-2.25 [-3.09, -1.41]
Chen 2017	12.19	6.1	47	19.08	7.13	48	1.3%	-6.89 [-9.56, -4.22]
Mastropasqua 2014a	9.1	4.8	30	11.2	5.7	30	1.3%	-2.10 [-4.77, 0.57]
Mayer 2014	1.58	1.02	88	4.17	2.06	62	5.5%	-2.59 [-3.15, -2.03]
Ranjini 2017	49.61	38.38	55	96.43	65.36	55	0.0%	-46.82 [-66.85, -26.79]
Takács 2012	0.1	0.12	38	0.12	0.13	38	6.6%	-0.02 [-0.08, 0.04]
Wang 2018	17	9	58	32	13	34	0.4%	-15.00 [-19.95, -10.05]
Yu 2016	5.632	4.904	70	7.317	5.583	54	2.1%	-1.69 [-3.57, 0.20]
Subtotal (95% CI)			**411**			**348**	**21.8%**	**-3.69 [-5.46, -1.91]**
Heterogeneity: Tau² = 4.68; Chi² = 194.18, df = 7 (P < 0.00001); I² = 96%								
Test for overall effect: Z = 4.06 (P < 0.0001)								
Victus								
Daya 2014	0.57	0.51	108	0.87	0.85	108	6.4%	-0.30 [-0.49, -0.11]
Mursch-Edlmayr 2017	2.51	1.7	50	2.82	1.6	50	5.3%	-0.31 [-0.96, 0.34]
Reddy 2013	5.2	5.7	56	7.7	6	63	1.8%	-2.50 [-4.60, -0.40]
Subtotal (95% CI)			**214**			**221**	**13.5%**	**-0.44 [-0.98, 0.11]**
Heterogeneity: Tau² = 0.12; Chi² = 4.17, df = 2 (P = 0.12); I² = 52%								
Test for overall effect: Z = 1.58 (P = 0.11)								
LDV Z8								
Cavallini 2018	3.8	2.2	70	4.5	1.8	70	5.2%	-0.70 [-1.37, -0.03]
Liu 2018	3.3	1.4	35	4.9	2.3	35	4.5%	-1.60 [-2.49, -0.71]
Pajic 2017	1.48	1.8	68	1.81	1.93	62	5.3%	-0.33 [-0.97, 0.31]
Vasquez-Peres 2018	1	0.6	45	0.1	2.4	45	5.0%	0.90 [0.18, 1.62]
Subtotal (95% CI)			**218**			**212**	**19.9%**	**-0.41 [-1.35, 0.52]**
Heterogeneity: Tau² = 0.77; Chi² = 20.09, df = 3 (P = 0.0002); I² = 85%								
Test for overall effect: Z = 0.86 (P = 0.39)								
Total (95% CI)			**2285**			**1905**	**100.0%**	**-1.88 [-2.21, -1.55]**
Heterogeneity: Tau² = 0.44; Chi² = 2502.80, df = 23 (P < 0.00001); I² = 99%								
Test for overall effect: Z = 11.12 (P < 0.00001)								

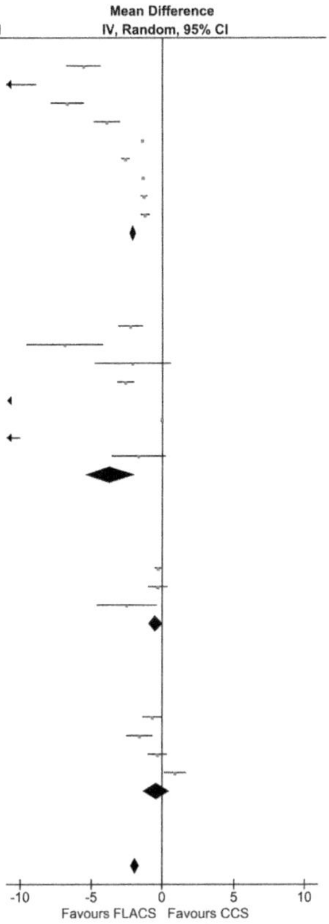

Fig. 1 Results of a meta-analysis examining effective phacoemulsification time. Compared to conventional cataract surgery, pre-fragmentation significantly reduced the effective phacoemulsification time

and endothelial cell loss when the laser was used. These results were confirmed in a meta-analysis conducted by our group. A total of 24 studies (2285 eyes pre-fragmented with laser vs 1905 conventional cataract surgery) were included, however, there were differences between the laser systems (Fig. 1) [4].

To investigate whether the fragmentation pattern had an influence on EPT, two groups (75 eyes each) were formed in which the lens was prefragmented with the pie or cube pattern. The groups were matched on the basis of lens density (10.5% ±1.52) as measured with a Scheimpflug camera (Oculus, Pentacam) [5]. In soft lenses, EPT was significantly lower in the cube fragmentation group. Also, the number of eyes in which no ultrasound energy was required during cataract surgery ("zero phacos") was significantly higher (37 eyes in the cube pattern vs 1 eye in the pie pattern). However, at high lens densities (12% and higher), the pie pattern was superior in regards to the EPT and this result was confirmed in a randomized controlled trial by Lyu et al. [6]. A total of 894 eyes were included (267 pie pattern four-split, 330 pie pattern six-split, 297 cube pattern). For low lens density, cube fragmentation resulted in significantly lower EPT and for high lens densities, the pie pattern was superior. Interestingly, dividing the nucleus into four parts led to a lower EPT than pre-fragmentation into six parts, though no significant discrepancy in operative difficulty was indicated according to their clinical practice. Furthermore, the influence of the fragmentation pattern on intraocular pressure after one day and endothelial cell loss after one week was measured. It was found that the cube pattern led to a significantly higher incidence of raised postoperative intraocular pressure in particularly hard lenses.

Author's recommendation

Since the cube pattern in hard lenses leads to increased postoperative intraocular pressure and is inferior to the pie pattern in terms of EPT, the author recommends not using the cube pattern in hard lenses.

Endothelial cell loss was dependent on lens hardness for all fragmentation patterns and varied on average from 4.85% ±7.46 for very soft lenses to 19.35% ±17.8 for very hard lenses. The fragmentation pattern had no effect on endothelial cell loss despite differences in EPT.

References

1. Mayer WJ, Klaproth OK, Hengerer FH, Kohnen T. Impact of crystalline lens opacification on effective phacoemulsification time in femtosecond laser-assisted cataract surgery. Am J Ophthalmol. 2014;157(2):426-32.e1.
2. Ang RET, Quinto MMS, Cruz EM, Rivera MCR, Martinez GHA. Comparison of clinical outcomes between femtosecond laser-assisted versus conventional phacoemulsification. Eye Vis (Lond). 2018;5:8.
3. Hatch KM, Schultz T, Talamo JH, Dick HB. Femtosecond laser-assisted compared with standard cataract surgery for removal of advanced cataracts. J Cataract Refract Surg. 2015;41 (9):1833–8.
4. Kolb CM, Shajari M, Mathys L, Herrmann E, Petermann K, Mayer WJ, et al. Comparison of femtosecond laser-assisted cataract surgery and conventional cataract surgery: a meta-analysis and systematic review. J Cataract Refract Surg. 2020;46(8):1075–85.
5. Shajari M, Khalil S, Mayer WJ, Al-Khateeb G, Bohm M, Petermann K, et al. Comparison of 2 laser fragmentation patterns used in femtosecond laser-assisted cataract surgery. J Cataract Refract Surg. 2017;43(12):1571–4.
6. Lyu D, Shen Z, Zhang L, Qin Z, Ni S, Wang W, et al. Comparison of perioperative parameters in femtosecond laser-assisted cataract surgery using three nuclear fragmentation patterns. Am J Ophthalmol. 2019.

Special Features of Cataract Surgery Using the Femtosecond Laser

Karl Boden

The surgical procedure of planning and performing femtosecond laser assisted cataract surgery differs, in some ways considerably, from manual cataract surgery with phacoemulsification. The assumption that femtolaser-assisted cataract surgery (FCS) can be performed easily by untrained surgeons is not correct, as a high level of experience and a close attention to key points are essential for a successful surgical outcome. The different types of tissue encountered during cataract surgery may behave differently when treated with femtosecond laser than with manual cataract surgery (MCS). The differences, as well as the characteristics by which an impending complication can be recognized and avoided, are described in the following sections.

Docking the Patient

The safe application of the femtosecond laser requires a fixation of the eye, which is done by means of a patient interface. It is necessary, therefore, that the patient interface docks to the eye by means of vacuum. In some cases, the high vacuum can cause subconjunctival haemorrhage, which can vary from a slight petechial haemorrhage to a pronounced extensive bleed. Immediate intervention should be carried out, especially in the case of active, heavy bleeding. An incision of the conjunctiva followed by the expression of the clot by two cigarrette swabs is usually sufficient. Subconjunctival irrigation is not typically effective here.

Supplementary Information The online version contains supplementary material available at https://doi.org/10.1007/978-3-031-05394-8_95. The videos can be accessed individually by clicking the DOI link in the accompanying figure caption or by scanning this link with the SN More Media App.

K. Boden (✉)
Sulzbach, Germany
e-mail: drkarlboden@googlemail.com

M. Shajari et al. (eds.), *Cataract and Lens Surgery*,
https://doi.org/10.1007/978-3-031-05394-8_95

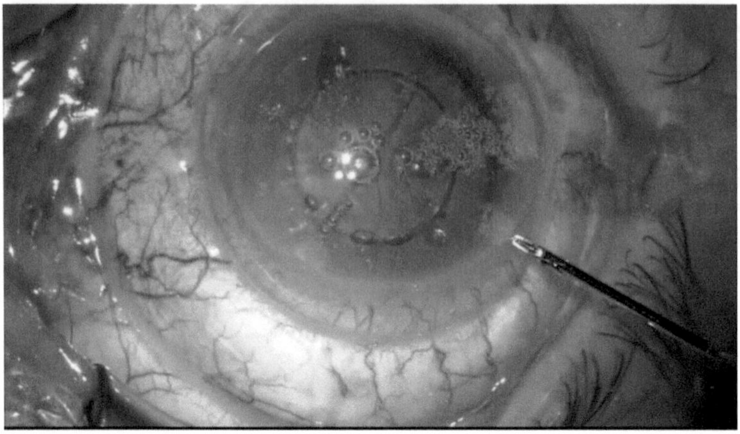

Video 1 Opening of femtolaser-assisted corneal incisions with a specially designed cannula (▶ https://doi.org/10.1007/000-8fb)

Opening of the corneal incision (Video 1)

The corneal incisions, including the main incision and the one or two paracenteses, are lasered but not yet completely opened. There are various possibilities to achieve complete patency. The incisions can be opened bluntly with an iris spatula or a similarly fine instrument. As seen in the video clip (A 82.1), the opening of femtolaser-assisted corneal incisions can also be performed using a specially developed cannula. The "FLACS' cannula is characterized by a prolonged flattening at the tip, which can be nicely inserted into the primary narrow gap of the incision. Even light adhesions caused by vessels or an arcus lipoides can be opened well and in the given incision plane.

The location of the incisions is sometimes difficult to detect. In some cases, an opaque bubble layer (OBL) forms through the incisions. OBL is caused by an accumulation of cavitation gas bubbles within the stroma and is recognizable as a white-greyish, often bubble-like cloudiness. This turbidity can be used to locate the incisions.

Opening of the anti-astigmatic keratotomies

In the case of penetrating keratotomies, it should be considered whether these should be extended with a blunt instrument. The main argument for opening the incisions is that small tissue bridges can be safely bluntly separated so that the full anti-astigmatic effect can be achieved. A danger here, however, is the chance of possible iatrogenic epithelial ingrowth into the wound gap. A further danger can be unintentional perforation if the procedure is not carried out carefully. No general conclusions can be made at this time as to how clinically relevant these tissue bridges are, but it likely depends on the laser platform. In the case of intrastromal keratotomies, this issue of persistent tissue bridges also arises. It is not uncommon for some surgeons to cut these at a later stage to enhance the antiastigmatic effect. However, even in this case there is a risk of epithelial cell invasion and an anti-astigmatic effect which is difficult to calculate.

Places of the anterior chamber

Depending on the surgical procedure, the anterior chamber can be formed with irrigation or with a viscoelastic. A dispersive viscoelastic offers the advantage of less abrupt intraocular pressure fluctuations. This allows a controlled chamber to inspect the capsulotomy margin and to treat imminent tears better. Although viscoelastic do add a significant cost factor, the procedure has been extensively validated in terms of safety.

Author's recommendation

In order to be able to carry out a precise inspection of the femtolaser-assisted capsulotomy, we recommend that the anterior chamber be stabilized, preferably with a dispersive viscoelastic.

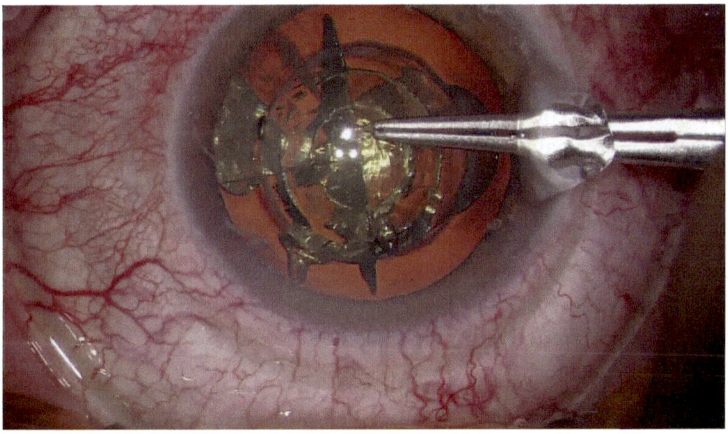

Video 2 Procedure of an FCS operation after undocking the patient interface (▶ https://doi.org/10.1007/000-8fa)

Removing the capsule (Video 2)

Removal of the central capsule leaf is probably one of the most important steps in femtosecond laser assisted cataract surgery (FCS). If this procedure is performed too fast or too carelessly, a previously simple procedure can change rapidly into a complicated operation. In contrast to manual capsulorhexis, which is controlled by one's own movements, laser treatment involves placing the patient in front of a completed cutting pattern. In the majority of cases, a free-floating capsule disc in the centre is loose and ready to be removed. However, before the capsule can be safely removed, a thorough visual inspection of the cut edges of the capsulotomy must be carried out. In this phase, it is advisable to increase the magnification on the microscope significantly to allow for an accurate assessment. In the unmanipulated state, tension wrinkles of the capsule leaf can indicate adhesions. These adhesions can occur regardless of the laser platform and regardless of whether the capsulotomy was performed before or after the core fragmentation.

Author's recommendation

If there are tension wrinkles, the capsule should be carefully pulled centrally at that point using rhexis forceps to avoid tearing the anterior capsulotomy, or if necessary, to complete it manually. The so-called "dimple down' technique is widely used in this case. The capsule is pressed in the centre towards the lens equator to create an even distribution of force to the centre which prevents radial tears in the capsulotomy [1].

After the central capsulotomy disc has been removed, small tissue threads can become visible at the capsulotomy margin, especially after the lens has been removed. These capsule remnants, so-called "tags', are remnants of the central capsule disc that are still attached to the peripheral capsulotomy. Any further manipulation of these tags should be avoided, as this may result in a higher risk of tearing the anterior capsule.

Hydrodissection

The separation of the cortex from the capsule (hydrodissection) is recommended in most cases, as in manual cataract surgery. If the capsulotomy is torn, however, this can be omitted to prevent further extension of the capsular tear across the equator.

Author's recommendation

Hydrodissection should always be performed at low pressure, as gas from fragmentation may have collected behind the lens, which can exert an additional pressure component on the posterior capsule.

In general, during hydrodissection, the gas can also rise into the anterior chamber and create a confusing view of the operating field for a short time. The hydrodilation depends on the laser platform or the fragmentation pattern chosen. With a very small "grid' pattern, as seen with the Catalys or the Victus, for example, it is even possible to do without it completely. In the case of a fragmentation pattern with slices, it may be useful to apply hydrodilation within the slices.

Author's recommendation

With FCS, hydrodissection should be carried out as a rule in the same way as with MCS.

Lens removal (Video 2)

Lens material removal is highly dependent on nucleus density and fragmentation pattern. Eyes with particularly hard lens cores are known to benefit most from FCS as it reduces phaco energy. However, the declared aim of FCS is to remove the lens without any phacoemulsification [2].

The pure aspiration handpieces specially developed for the FCS are not recommended, because in cases where aspiration alone is not sufficient, changing the handpiece unnecessarily prolongs the duration of the operation. The surgeon is much more flexible from the outset if the conventional phako handpiece is used in a pure I/A mode.

The reduction in phaco energy when changing from an MCS to the FCS is highly dependent on the surgical technique previously favoured by the surgeon. A very good phaco/chop technique will allow a lower percentage reduction in phaco energy than switching from a Divide&Conquer technique to the FCS. When changing from manual phacoemulsification to the use of femtosecond lasers, it also makes sense to change the surgical technique to a chop technique. Chopping makes it easier to remove the individual fragments from the core and aspirate them with the handpiece. Crushing the larger fragments at the tip of the phaco handpiece can help to avoid phacoemulsification completely in borderline hard lens pieces.

Polishing of the capsule

Overpressure polishing of the posterior capsule with BSS on a Sauter cannula is also useful for cataract surgery with the femtosecond laser. This cleans the posterior capsule and possibly reduce the rate of posterior capsular opacification.

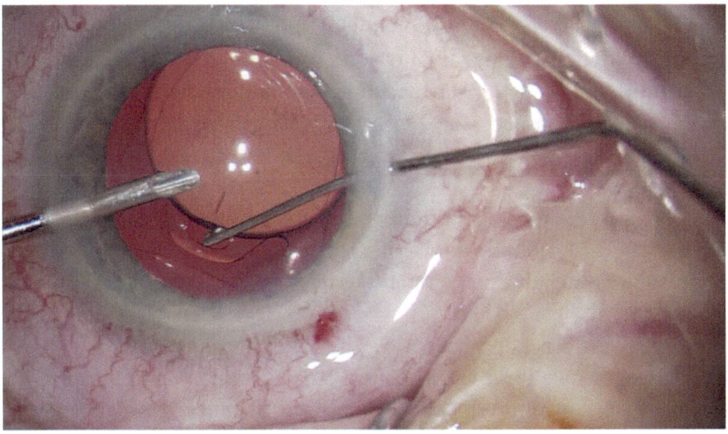

Video 3 Enclavation of a special femtolaser adapted IOL into the anterior capsulotomy (▶ https://doi.org/10.1007/000-8fc)

IOL implantation (Videos 2 and 3)

The option of exact centring of the lens should be emphasised. Thanks to the femtosecond laser technology, with the exact positioning on the apex of the lens or, in the future, other desired parameters, we are able to produce a precision in lens positioning that no surgeon in the world is able to produce. This precise positioning of the capsulotomy in combination with a capsulotomy-fixed intraocular lens can create added value for the patient. This is because lenses with additional functions (multifocal lenses/toric/aspherical IOL) in particular can benefit from less tilt or permanent centring despite capsular bag shrinkage [3].

In addition to the potentially better centration, it can be assumed that negative dysphotopsies occur less frequently postoperatively than is the case with the capsular bag supported IOL. If the surgeon decides in favour of a capsulotomy-fixed intraocular lens, the larger anterior haptics can first be uncovered with irrigation and a push–pull hook. Once this has been done, enclaving the smaller lateral haptics into the capsulotomy is much easier.

Subsequently, acetylcholine should be applied intracameral to reliably rule out postoperative iris capture (A 82.3).

Keypoint

Only the femtosecond laser technique precision in the exact positioning of the capsulotomy to a desired parameter, which no surgeon can manually reproduce permanently.

Hydration of the paracenteses

In manual cataract surgery, it is generally recommended to hydrate the incisions in order to achieve watertight closure. This is identical for femtolaser-assisted incisions, but it is noticeable that this is somewhat more difficult for the very smooth incisions, which means that more stromal hydration may be necessary from case to case. Stromal hydration of the main incision is not recommended for both MCS and FCS. With the femtosecond laser, an unintentionally short main incision, which makes stromal hydration necessary, is not expected.

Which operation logistics are reasonable?

There are considerable technical differences between the laser platforms. From the outside, the devices differ in terms of space requirements and mobility, which generally results in two different operation scenarios for femtosecond laser-assisted cataract surgery.

In the so-called "one-step scenario', the patient can be pre-treated with the femtosecond laser as well as the subsequent lens aspiration and implantation of the artificial lens in an operating theatre in the usual manner. The advantage of this operation logistic structure is that the laser is used like an instrument and no repositioning of the patient is necessary. The disadvantages include the high space requirement and the ventilation noise during the operation, which should not be underestimated. Particularly with static models, it can be problematic if the OR is heavily frequented and should also be used for operations without the use of a laser. For mobile and space-saving models, this operation logistics is preferred, as it saves time and patient repositioning.

The "two-step scenario' should be considered especially for static models that require permanent cooling. In this case, the pre-treatment of the patient is carried out in a separate room. The patient is then transferred to the operating theatre, where lens aspiration and IOL implantation is performed in the usual manner. The pre-treatment can be carried out by another surgeon and at the same time the actual operating theatre can be used for other purposes. The disadvantage here is that the patient has to be repositioned again. We do not consider the uncertainty about the interim opening of the eye during this procedure to be justified. Both the clinical aspect and iOCT images of the FS incisions show that they are stable enough that a "two-step scenario' is possible without issue. (Masket, Sarayba, Ignacio, & Fram, 2010).

Author's recommendation

For small mobile laser platforms, a one-step surgery scenario is preferable. For large static laser platforms that require air conditioning, we recommend a separate laser surgery or a two-step surgery scenario. When repositioning the patient, an opening of the eye is not expected if the parameters are correctly selected.

Conclusion

The use of the femtosecond laser in cataract surgery is a safe and gentle procedure. The precision and reproducibility of the incisions in combination with preoperative diagnostics makes it possible to transfer the same standards that we have known for years in refractive corneal surgery to cataract surgery. At first glance, femtosecond laser-assisted cataract surgery does not appear to require great manual skills. This is not correct, as this procedure also has its individual pitfalls. Every surgeon who starts with this technique should be well informed about the tissue-specific signs of impending complications in order to be able to carry out the most successful surgery on every patient.

References

1. Arbisser LB, Schultz T, Dick HB. Central dimple-down maneuver for consistent continuous femtosecond laser capsulotomy. J Cataract Refract Surg. 2013. https://doi.org/10.1016/j.jcrs.2013.09.009.
2. Conrad-Hengerer I, Hengerer FH, Joachim SC, Schultz T, Dick HB. Femtosecond laser-assisted cataract surgery in intumescent white cataracts. J Cataract Refract Surg. 2014. https://doi.org/10.1016/j.jcrs.2013.08.044.
3. Shajari M, Sonntag R, Niermann T, Holland D, Kohnen T, Priglinger S, Mayer WJ. Determining and comparing the effective lens position and refractive outcome of a novel rhexis-fixated lens to established lens designs. Am J Ophthalmol. 2020. https://doi.org/10.1016/j.ajo.2020.01.009.

Comparison of Conventional Lens Surgery to Femtosecond Laser-Assisted Lens Surgery

Mehdi Shajari and Béatrice Cochener

Studies comparing conventional lens surgery ("Manual Cataract Surgery"—MCS) with femtosecond laser-assisted lens surgery ("Laser Cataract Surgery"—LCS) were considered for the meta-analysis in this chapter [1]. Accordingly, for the sake of completeness, studies from the early days of LCS, when the laser parameters were not yet optimized, are also included. A total of 73 studies, 25 of which were randomized controlled, were included. In summary, in these studies a total of 12,274 eyes which underwent MCS and 12,769 eyes which underwent LCS were included.

Visual outcome and refraction

Both uncorrected and corrected distance visual acuity showed no significant difference at one week (P = 0.28/0.07) or at six months (P = 0.3/0.12). The postoperative spherical equivalent and the refractive prediction error also showed no significant difference after six months (P = 0.08 and P = 0.96, respectively). Chen et al. compared the two methods in very hard lenses and found no significant difference in postoperative uncorrected and corrected distance visual acuity [2]. The induced astigmatism also showed no difference between the two procedures (P = 0.43).

Keypoint

Both procedures achieve similar good results in visual outcome and refraction.

M. Shajari (✉)
Goethe Universität Frankfurt, Frankfurt, Deutschland
e-mail: gms400@gmail.com

B. Cochener
University Hospital of Brest—Hospital Morvan, Brest, France
e-mail: beatrice.cochener@ophthalmologie-chu29.fr

M. Shajari et al. (eds.), *Cataract and Lens Surgery*,
https://doi.org/10.1007/978-3-031-05394-8_96

Ultrasound energy and circularity

The effective phacoemulsification time (EPT) is the product of the average "phaco power" multiplied by the "phaco time". It allows the ultrasound energy delivered by different device settings to be comparted with each other. The higher the value, the more ultrasound energy is delivered to the eye during the operation. The "Cumulative dissipated energy" (CDE) is a similar measure for this purpose.

In femtosecond laser surgery, a reduction in EPT and CDE is achieved by pre-fragmenting the lens nucleus. The meta-analysis showed a significant reduction in EPT and CDE ($P < 0.01$ for both). Pre-fragmentation by laser leads to a reduction of EPT especially in cases of a dense lens nucleus [3].

Author's recommendation

The fragmentation pattern should be adapted to the lens density. A soft lens nucleus should be pre-fragmented in the "cube pattern" and a dense lens nucleus in the "pie pattern". It was shown that this can further reduce the CDE. An optical lens density of 12%, measured with a Scheimpflug device, (Pentacam, Oculus—limits are not yet set for OCT images) has been reported in the literature as a threshold value to help make this decision [4].

The circularity of the rhexis is also know to play a role in IOL positioning. Here it could be shown that compared to manually guided rhexiseven for experienced surgeons—the circularity with the laser is significantly better ($P < 0.01$). In addition, there are intraocular lenses whose optics are fixed with "wings" in the rhexis. When using these lenses, it is not only the circularity that plays a role, but also the exact diameter of the rhexis. Therefore, the use of a femtolaser is recommended in these cases. Femto-rhexis has also been shown to reduce the occurrence of IOL tilt or decentration—this is essential for a good visual result, especially in aspheric IOLs and those with multifocal optics [5].

Complication of capsular rupture

One of the most important complications during cataract surgery is capsular rupture. In our meta-analysis, anterior capsular rupture occurred in 78 of 8,022 eyes treated with LCS (Fig. 1). This was significantly more frequent than in MCS (16 of 7,951 eyes, $P < 0.01$). However, it is important to mention that this rate decreased with refinements of energy delivery to the anterior capsule. No significant difference was found in the incidence of posterior capsular rupture between the two procedures (0.42% in LCS and 0.27% in MCS, $P = 0.13$).

Author's recommendation

When performing hydrodissection in particular, the rhexis margin should be checked under high magnification. Sometimes a tiny tear can be seen, which can quickly widen due to the pressure during hydrodissection. Manual evacuation of gas that puts the bag in tension should be performed carefully. It should also be mentioned that in many cases, due to the pre-fragmentation in LCS, hydrodissection is no longer necessary as the lens is already detached from the capsule.

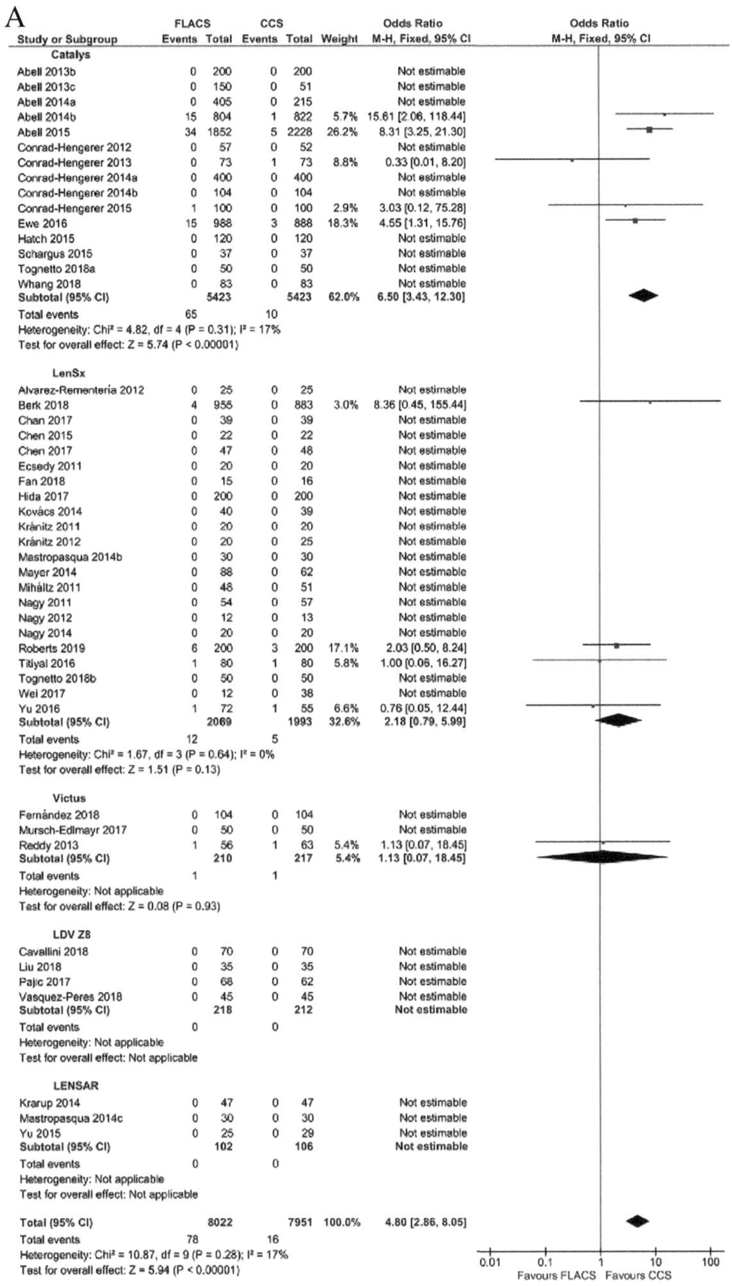

Fig. 1 Meta-analysis of anterior capsular rupture divided by laser system used. With the Catalys laser, 5,423 LCS procedures were performed and 65 anterior capsular ruptures occurred (vs. 10 with MCS). With the LenSx laser, 2,069 eyes were treated and 12 ruptures occurred (vs. 5 with MCS). If we only look at the most recent studies with a case number of more than 100 eyes (Roberts 2019, Berk 2018), we notice that the anterior capsule rupture rate is still significantly higher than in MCS. The other laser systems (Victus, LDV Z8, Lensar) were used too rarely to be evaluated separately. Nevertheless, it is important to mention that complication rate depends on the platform generation for each laser model and of the evolution of imaging systems guiding the surgery

B

Study or Subgroup	FLACS Events	FLACS Total	CCS Events	CCS Total	Weight	Odds Ratio M-H, Fixed, 95% CI
Catalys						
Abell 2013b	1	200	1	200	4.8%	1.00 [0.06, 16.10]
Abell 2013c	0	150	0	51		Not estimable
Abell 2014a	0	405	0	215		Not estimable
Abell 2015	8	1852	4	2228	17.4%	2.41 [0.73, 8.02]
Conrad-Hengerer 2012	0	67	0	52		Not estimable
Conrad-Hengerer 2013	0	73	0	73		Not estimable
Conrad-Hengerer 2014a	0	400	0	400		Not estimable
Conrad-Hengerer 2014b	0	104	0	104		Not estimable
Conrad-Hengerer 2015	0	100	0	100		Not estimable
Ewe 2016	11	988	2	888	10.1%	4.99 [1.10, 22.56]
Hatch 2015	0	120	0	120		Not estimable
Schargus 2015	0	37	1	37	7.1%	0.32 [0.01, 8.23]
Tognetto 2018a	0	50	0	50		Not estimable
Whang 2018	0	83	0	83		Not estimable
Subtotal (95% CI)		**4619**		**4601**	**39.4%**	**2.52 [1.12, 5.64]**
Total events	20		8			
Heterogeneity: Chi² = 2.76, df = 3 (P = 0.43); I² = 0%						
Test for overall effect: Z = 2.24 (P = 0.02)						
LenSx						
Alvarez-Rementería 2012	0	25	0	25		Not estimable
Berk 2018	9	965	4	883	19.9%	2.09 [0.64, 6.81]
Chan 2017	0	39	0	39		Not estimable
Chen 2015	0	22	0	22		Not estimable
Chen 2017	0	47	0	48		Not estimable
Ecsedy 2011	0	20	0	20		Not estimable
Fan 2018	0	15	0	16		Not estimable
Hida 2017	0	200	0	200		Not estimable
Kovács 2014	0	40	0	39		Not estimable
Kránitz 2011	1	20	0	20	2.2%	3.15 [0.12, 82.16]
Kránitz 2012	0	20	0	25		Not estimable
Mayer 2014	0	88	0	62		Not estimable
Miháltz 2011	0	48	0	51		Not estimable
Nagy 2011	0	54	0	57		Not estimable
Nagy 2012	0	12	0	13		Not estimable
Nagy 2014	0	20	0	20		Not estimable
Roberts 2019	0	200	6	200	31.3%	0.07 [0.00, 1.33]
Titiyal 2016	0	80	0	80		Not estimable
Tognetto 2018b	0	50	0	50		Not estimable
Wei 2017	0	12	0	38		Not estimable
Yu 2016	0	72	0	55		Not estimable
Subtotal (95% CI)		**2039**		**1963**	**53.4%**	**0.95 [0.41, 2.22]**
Total events	10		10			
Heterogeneity: Chi² = 5.21, df = 2 (P = 0.07); I² = 62%						
Test for overall effect: Z = 0.11 (P = 0.91)						
Victus						
Fernández 2018	0	104	0	104		Not estimable
Mursch-Edlmayr 2017	0	50	0	50		Not estimable
Panthier 2017	0	33	0	33		Not estimable
Reddy 2013	0	56	0	63		Not estimable
Subtotal (95% CI)		**243**		**250**		**Not estimable**
Total events	0		0			
Heterogeneity: Not applicable						
Test for overall effect: Not applicable						
LDV Z8						
Cavallini 2018	0	70	0	70		Not estimable
Liu 2018	0	35	0	35		Not estimable
Pajic 2017	0	68	0	62		Not estimable
Vasquez-Peres 2018	0	45	0	45		Not estimable
Subtotal (95% CI)		**218**		**212**		**Not estimable**
Total events	0		0			
Heterogeneity: Not applicable						
Test for overall effect: Not applicable						
LENSAR						
Krarup 2014	0	47	1	47	7.2%	0.33 [0.01, 8.22]
Yu 2015	0	25	0	29		Not estimable
Subtotal (95% CI)		**72**		**76**	**7.2%**	**0.33 [0.01, 8.22]**
Total events	0		1			
Heterogeneity: Not applicable						
Test for overall effect: Z = 0.68 (P = 0.50)						
Total (95% CI)		**7191**		**7102**	**100.0%**	**1.53 [0.88, 2.66]**
Total events	30		19			
Heterogeneity: Chi² = 9.44, df = 7 (P = 0.22); I² = 26%						
Test for overall effect: Z = 1.50 (P = 0.13)						

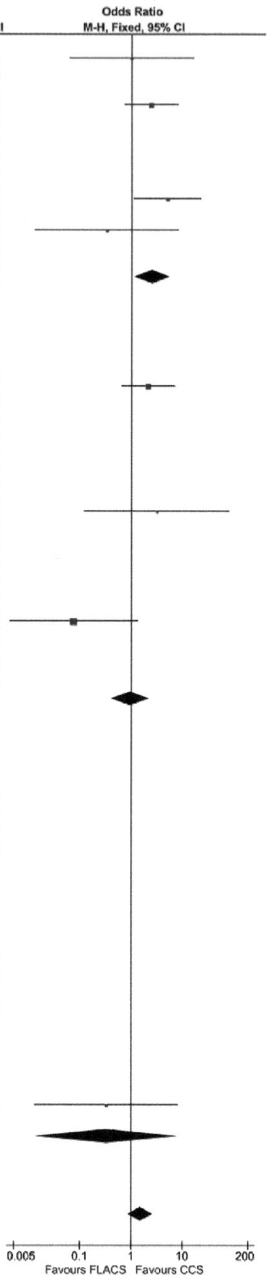

Fig. 1 (continued)

Furthermore, it is required to mention that all of these intraoperative complications are depending on the learning curve, as shown in the FEMCAT study [6].

Postoperative complications

No significant difference was found in the number of eyes with intraocular pressure above 30 mmHg one day after surgery (P = 0.79). There was also no significant difference in the incidence of cystoid macular oedema between the two cohorts (P = 0.4). Similarly, no difference was found in the incidence of significant corneal oedema during follow-up (P = 0.24 at six months). However, Abell et al. found that corneal volume one day after surgery was significantly smaller in LCS than in MCS [7]. This is consistent with a significantly greater increase in central corneal thickness one day postoperatively in MCS (P < 0.01).

Endothelial cell loss was greater one day, one week, one month and three months postoperatively in the MCS cohort than in the LCS cohort. Analysis of the randomized controlled trials alone confirmed this difference (P = 0.03; P = 0.02; P = 0.04). For example, Yong et al. found an endothelial cell loss in the MCS cohort of 347 $\pm$ 321 and 112 $\pm$ 435 cells/mm^2 in the LCS cohort [8]. This suggests that the endothelium is less affected in LCS due to the pre-fragmentation.

The posterior capsular opacification rate and the incidence of lens tilt (measured by Scheimpflug imaging) after 18 months were investigated by Kovacs et al. The incidence of both complications was found to be lower with LCS. The difference was significant but marginal and it is important to mention that using Scheimpflug images for this purpose might not be sufficiently accurate [9]. Many of the results of this meta-analysis were also confirmed in the randomized controlled FEMCAT trial published in the Lancet. However, while the LCS and MCS performed comparably well, the authors pointed out that the cost-effectiveness ratio was in favor of the MCS [6].

Currently, there are no significant benefits provided by LCS that would justify the additional costs in the case of standard cataract surgery. However, when implanting toric or multifocal IOLs LCS should be considered as it seems to lead to a better IOL positioning. In addition, some types of modern IOLs are fixated directly into the capsular opening providing a higher stability and better predictability of the refractive outcome [10]. For these kinds of IOLs a precise opening of the capsular bag with a femtosecond laser is mandatory. Furthermore, it is worth mentioning that LCS is becoming more and more popular in challenging situations like mature cataract, bag in the lens implantation, floppy iris syndrome etc. [11]. Consequently, it can be said, that LCS seems to be rather a valuable option in specific circumstances rather than a superior option in general to MCS when considering the costs.

It is also worth mentioning that the systems available today still require a second system for irrigation/aspiration at least and in many cases for phacoemulsification. So femtocataract-surgery can rather be regarded as “enhanced phacoemulsification” rather than a true standalone alternative.

Conclusion

The visual and refractive outcome after LCS are similar to MCS. When implanting special lenses, the use of the laser can be useful, as less tilt and better centration can have a positive effect on the final result, particularly with complex multifocal optics.

The postoperative complication profile is very similar for both procedures and differences are usually of no clinical relevance. The main difference is that LCS requires less ultrasound energy and there is less endothelial cell loss due to surgery. On the other hand, however, the anterior capsular rupture rate is increased with LCS and, accordingly, the advantages and disadvantages of both procedures must be discussed in detail with each patient before the procedure.

For all these reasons, including the economic considerations, the current tendency for the femto-cataract users is to dedicate this procedure to refractive and special cases, mainly.

References

1. Kolb CM, Shajari M, Mathys L, Herrmann E, Petermann K, Mayer WJ, et al. Comparison of femtosecond laser-assisted cataract surgery and conventional cataract surgery: a meta-analysis and systematic review. J Cataract Refract Surg. 2020;46(8):1075–85.
2. Chen X, Yu Y, Song X, Zhu Y, Wang W, Yao K. Clinical outcomes of femtosecond laser-assisted cataract surgery versus conventional phacoemulsification surgery for hard nuclear cataracts. J Cataract Refract Surg. 2017;43(4):486–91.
3. Mayer WJ, Klaproth OK, Hengerer FH, Kohnen T. Impact of crystalline lens opacification on effective phacoemulsification time in femtosecond laser-assisted cataract surgery. Am J Ophthalmol. 2014;157(2):426-32.e1.
4. Shajari M, Khalil S, Mayer WJ, Al-Khateeb G, Bohm M, Petermann K, et al. Comparison of 2 laser fragmentation patterns used in femtosecond laser-assisted cataract surgery. J Cataract Refract Surg. 2017;43(12):1571–4.
5. Lee JA, Song WK, Kim JY, Kim MJ, Tchah H. Femtosecond laser-assisted cataract surgery versus conventional phacoemulsification: refractive and aberrometric outcomes with a diffractive multifocal intraocular lens. J Cataract Refract Surg. 2019;45(1):21–7.
6. Schweitzer C, Brezin A, Cochener B, Monnet D, Germain C, Roseng S, et al. Femtosecond laser-assisted versus phacoemulsification cataract surgery (FEMCAT): a multicentre participant-masked randomised superiority and cost-effectiveness trial. Lancet. 2020;395(10219):212–24.
7. Abell RG, Kerr NM, Howie AR, Mustaffa Kamal MAA, Allen PL, Vote BJ. Effect of femtosecond laser-assisted cataract surgery on the corneal endothelium. J Cataract Refract Surg. 2014;40(11):1777–83.
8. Yong WWD, Chai H-CC, Shen L, Manotosh R, Anna Tan WT. Comparing outcomes of phacoemulsification with femtosecond laser-assisted cataract surgery in patients with fuchs endothelial dystrophy. Am J Ophthalmol. 2018; 196:173–80.
9. Kovács I, Kránitz K, Sándor GL, Knorz MC, Donnenfeld ED, Nuijts RM, et al. The effect of femtosecond laser capsulotomy on the development of posterior capsule opacification. J Refract Surg (Thorofare, NJ: 1995). 2014; 30(3):154–8.
10. Shajari M, Sonntag R, Niermann T, Holland D, Kohnen T, Priglinger S, et al. Determining and comparing the effective lens position and refractive outcome of a novel rhexis-fixated lens to established lens designs. Am J Ophthalmol. 2020;213:62–8.
11. Roberts TV, Lawless M, Sutton G, Hodge C. Update and clinical utility of the LenSx femtosecond laser in cataract surgery. Clin Ophthalmol. 2016;10:2021–9.

Phakic Intraocular Lenses

Overview and Indications of Phakic IOL

Martin Bechmann

Overview of Phakic IOL

The concept of the correction of ametropia using phakic lenses (pIOL) dates back to Strampelli, who implanted the first chamber angle supported pIOL (Strampelli 1954). This lens design let to serious complications so a different implantation principle was required. The iris claw lens, developed by Binkhorst in the 1950s, was used in 1986 by Fechner and Worst in a phakic version [3] (Fig. 1a) but as the technology evolved there was clearly a trend to moving more towards the posterior chamber. In 1986, the first prototype of this sort was presented by [4]. His design relocated the IOL to behind the iris and a number of problems of the implantation in the anterior chamber were improved. The risk of long-term endothelial damage decreases with increasing distance to the endothelium and the IOL is significantly closer to the main nodal point of the eye, which has a positive effect on the imaging quality and on the effective optical zone, which is significantly larger due to the more posterior position of the implant.

The Implantable Collamer Lens (ICL, Staar Surgical), is the result of continuous improvement of this type of lens. The material used, called collamer, consists of cross-linked collagen in combination with a hydrophilic acrylate and has an excellent biocompatibility. The foreign body reactions seen from previous generations of anterior chamber lenses did not occur here and the dreaded pigment dispersion hardly ever occurred. The main complication was premature cataract formation.

Some modifications of the ICL, such as increasing the distance (or vaulting" from the ICL to the crystalline lens (version V4), but the main improvement appears to be the introduction of an opening centrally located in the optic in 2012 (Aquaport). Since in introduction of the Aquaport, the occurrence of ICL induced

M. Bechmann (✉)
Munich, Germany
e-mail: martin.bechmann@smileeyes.de

M. Shajari et al. (eds.), *Cataract and Lens Surgery*,
https://doi.org/10.1007/978-3-031-05394-8_97

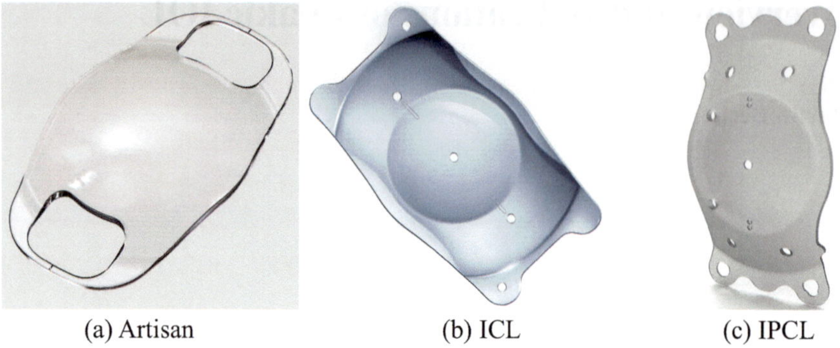

Fig. 1 **a** Phakic claw lens "Artisan" (Figure approved by Ophtec). **b** Sulcus-supported phake IOL "ICL" (Figure approved by Staar Surgical). **c** Sulcus supported phake IOL "IPCL" (Figure approved by Domilens)

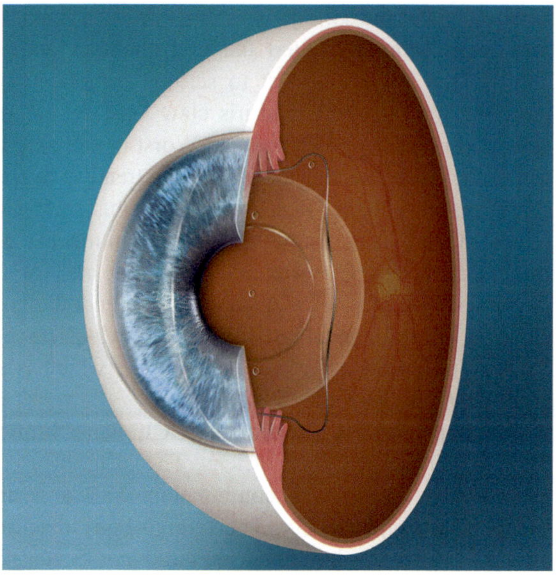

Fig. 2 Here: Position of the ICL in the ciliary sulcus. The ratio between the diameter of the sulcus and the length of the ICL results in the protrusion of the ICL and thus the distance to the lens and cornea (Fig. approved by Staar Surgical)

cataract has been significantly reduced [1, 8]. The central opening in the ICL now allows the physiological flow of aqueous humour around the crystalline lens through the centre of the ICL and from there through the pupil. The previous unphysiological diversion of the aqueous humour through an iridectomy/iridotomy is thus no longer necessary. This no longer seems to affect the nutrition of the crystalline lens via the aqueous humour to the same extent as it was without Aquaport. However, the Aquaport and magnified optics are only present in myopia-correcting lenses (Fig. 1b). Another model of a phakic posterior chamber lens, under the name of IPCL (implantable phakic contact lens) has recently been

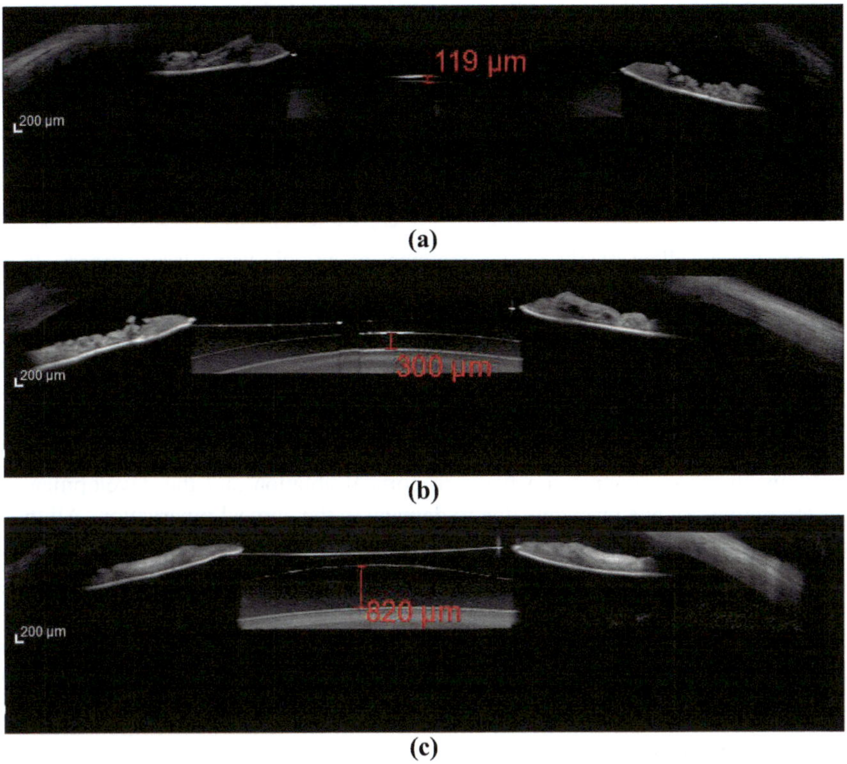

Fig. 3 **a** Small distance between ICL and the crystalline lens. **b** Normal distance between ICL and the crystalline lens. **c** Large distance between ICL and the crystalline lens

launched on the market. Some of the features known from ICL, such as Aquaport and haptic/optical design, seem to be very similar, but the material used is a classic hydrophilic acrylic without the addition of collagen [12] (Fig. 1c).

Posterior chamber pIOL

Phakic IOL Versus LVC

In principle, there are two different approaches in refractive surgery: Changing the corneal refractive power by removing corneal tissue using laser surgery and implanting a phakic IOL. As there are natural limits to the removal of corneal tissue, phakic IOLs are classically used for the treatment of higher ametropia. In recent years, however, there has been a tendency towards the implantation of phakic IOLs in cases of lower refractive errors (particularly in myopia). The reason for this change is the improvement of the ICL and significant reduction in complication rates. The current recommendations of the Commission for Refractive Surgery in Germany (KRC) define the scope of application for LASIK/SMILE in myopia to −8 dpt, the borderline area to −10 dpt. For pIOL, the range of application starts from −3 dpt, the limited range from −1 to −3 dpt. The ICL is available in a range from +10 dpt to −18 dpt, each of which can also be combined with a torus of up to 6 dpt.

ICL versus Corneal Refractive Laser for high myopia

Despite the excellent results in the treatment of myopia using laser surgery, there are certain limitations. As tissue is removed, the biomechanics of the cornea are weakened, with a corresponding increase in the risk of corneal ectasia, especially if more tissue has to be removed in higher corrections. The optical problems also increase with higher laser ablation. Thus, the quality of vision decreases significantly with treatments beyond approximately −8 dpt. The reasons for this are the excessive flattening of the cornea and reduction of the effective optical zone. In addition, there is a connection between corneal ablation and the development of postoperative dry eye problems due to damage to the corneal innervation. All these problems do not exist with the implantation of a phakic IOL, so this procedure can be considered the method of choice for high myopia. This can also be seen in a direct comparison of the two procedures, where ICL in the higher dioptric range were the preferred method both in terms of subjective quality of vision and objective parameters such as refractive accuracy, uncorrected visual acuity and higher order aberrations [11].

ICL versus Corneal Refractive Laser in low myopia

According to the recommendations of the German Commission for Refractive Surgery (KRC), the range of application of corneal laser surgery for myopia is up to -8 dpt. Below this limit, however, the implantation of a pIOL may still be the preferred procedure. In principle, the results in the lower dioptric range are excellent both with laser procedures and with the implantation of an ICL. In a direct comparison between ICL, topography-guided LASIK and SMILE in the FDA approval studies, the three techniques were found to be equivalent in terms of refractive outcome [7]. In a direct comparison between LASIK and ICL, significantly better low luminance contrast sensitivity and night vision was found in the ICL group [9]. However, the implantation of a phakic IOL is recommended in particular for corneal changes that show an increased risk of ectasia. The development of corneal ectasia is a very serious complication after corneal refractive laser. The classification scheme proposed by Randleman allows a classification of the individual risk of ectasia [10]. The main influencing factors are a preoperatively suspicious cornea in the sense of a forme fruste keratoconus, the amount of tissue ablation, preoperative corneal thickness, reduced stromal residual bed and the age of the patient. In general, modern corneal examination methods such as corneal tomography and measurement of corneal biomechanics allow a much more sensitive detection of an increased risk of ectasia. In these cases, corneal laser surgery should not be performed. In order to avoid these problems, tissue-saving PRK was often used, but it is associated with problems of a prolonged healing process and postoperative pain. Thus, the group of patients who were classically treated with PRK because of an existing corneal problem now represents the largest proportion of ICL implantations in low myopia.

Author's recommendation

In low myopia, the results of ICL and Femto LASIK/SMILE are basically comparable. However, as soon as corneal abnormalities resulting in a higher risk of ectasia become apparent, ICL implantation is the procedure of choice. The threshold, at which a phakic IOL should generally be preferred is considered to be very individual. The author recommends not to use laser refractive correction beyond -7 dpt and to give preference to ICLs in these cases.

ICL in hyperopia

The treatment of hyperopia with phakic lenses is different from the treatment of myopia, and represents a unique category of treatment. In general, phakic IOLs require a certain amount of space and space is naturally more limited in the short, hyperopic eyes than in long, myopic eyes. Nevertheless, even stricter requirements for the depth of the anterior chamber apply here compared to myopia correction. The hyperopic ICL requires an internal anterior chamber depth (distance from the endothelium to the lens anterior surface) of 3.0 mm, compared to 2.8 mm in myopia. Due to the greater material thickness of the hyperopic pIOL in the centre of the optic (the lenses are biconvex instead of biconcave and therefore have their thickest part in the center), the space requirement is greater. Because space is naturally limited in hyperopic eyes, many patients are therefore excluded from the treatment on these grounds alone. In addition, the hyperopic ICL has no Aquaport so far, so that the application of an iridotomy/iridectomy to avoid a pupillary block is absolutely necessary. This brings the well-known cataract problem with it, because without an Aquaport the physiological flow of the aqueous humour in the eye must be diverted through the iridectomy. Overall, the implantation of a hyperopic ICL seems to be more prone to complications than that in myopic cases [2]. In the end, a very careful consideration must be made here against corneal laser treatment. The results of both ICL and refractive cornea laser are also significantly worse in hyperopia, so refractive lens exchange is often the only remaining alternative. Depending on the anatomy, however, wearing glasses or contact lenses may still be the most reasonable option.

Presbyopia, Reversibility and Effects on Biometry

Regardless of the implantation of an ICL, the natural ageing process in the eye continues. With the onset of presbyopia, a slight myopic undercorrection of one eye may be recommended to improve the depth of field (monovision). For the correction of presbyopia, the IPCL is already available in a multifocal (diffractive) version, whereas the VIVA ICL uses an hyperaspheric lens profile to achieve better near vision in the presbyopic eye. An undisputed advantage of a phakic IOL is that the cornea remains unaffected for the biometric examinations for later IOL calculation if cataract surgery should become necessary. The larger postoperative refraction error known to occur in cataract surgery with a history of refractive laser correction is completely avoided. Furthermore, no additional aberrations are induced, which would complicate the later use of multifocal IOLs. Finally, phakic lenses can be removed from the eye and are therefore reversible—an advantage over laser procedures, which irreversibly changes the refractive power of the cornea, a fact that should not be underestimated in the long term.

Choosing the Right Implant—Sizing and Vaulting

After careful consideration of the indication for surgery, the choice of the right implant is of crucial importance. The ICL is implanted in the ciliary sulcus and comes to rest on the ciliary body (Fig. 2). Depending on the anatomical diameter of the ciliary sulcus, the ICL is thus subjected to a compressive force that directs the center of the ICL more or less forward, away from the crystalline lens and towards the endothelium. The final position of the ICL is thus determined by the ratio of the diameter of the ciliary sulcus and the diameter of the ICL. If the ICL is too large in relation to the diameter of the sulcus, it will be bent forward strongly. The distance between the ICL and crystalline lens, the so-called vault, becomes relatively large. Conversely, if the ICL is too small, the ICL bulges only slightly, the vault is reduced and the ICL lies close to the lens. The ICL is therefore available in different diameters in gradations of 0.5 mm.

Ideally, the ICL and the ciliary sulcus would be approximately the same size, but unfortunately there is currently no practical method for measuring the diameter of the sulcus available. Due to its anatomical position behind the iris, all measurements based on optical methods are useless. Occasionally, measurement by OCT seems possible, but only in very weakly pigmented eyes and therefore it is not routinely applicable to all patients in clinical practice. Only ultrasound can provide a direct measurement of the space, however, this is very uncomfortable for the patient because of the need for a water bath around the eye and is therefore not very common. A much more frequently used method is the indirect estimation of the sulcus diameter from the horizontal corneal diameter (white to white). Although there is no direct correlation between corneal diameter and the sulcus diameter, the use of the horizontal WTW is by far the most practical method for determining the size of ICL. The lens length is then calculated using the current white-to-white value of the cornea and the internal anterior chamber depth.

Author's recommendation

In order to obtain the most valid value possible for determining the horizontal corneal diameter, it is important to collect values with 2 different devices. The author uses the IOL Master (Zeiss) and the Pentacam (Oculus). However, the values of the IOL Master must be reduced by 0.3 mm, before comparing them with the Pentacam. The Pentacam values for the white to white distance are then compared with the modified values from the IOL Master. For deviations of up to 0.2 mm, the Pentacam value is assumed to be the most plausible. For deviations greater than 0.2 mm, the measurements must be repeated.

WZW IOL Master −0.3 mm = WZW Pentacam ± 0.2 mm.

The modified value can then be used to calculate the correct ICL size. With this step-by-step procedure, the number of necessary reoperations with exchange of the implant can be minimized.

Hypervault

The target corridor for the distance between ICL and crystalline lens is between 250 and 750 µm and a value above 1000 µm is called a Hypervault. If the vault of the lens pushes the ICL anteriorly, the chamber angle is successively narrowed and in extreme cases can be completely occluded. This possibility of an angle closure glaucoma is therefore still possible despite presence of the Aquaport and must be prevented at all costs. In this case, the anatomical conditions after removal of the viscoelastic must be taken into account during implantation. The decisive parameter here is the chamber angle and not the vault itself. In addition to OCT, Pentacam imaging of the chamber angle is also suitable for chamber angle measurement. A hypervault also has the problem of an increased glare effect since an excessive anterior curvature of the ICL stretches the iris forward and can no longer cover the edge of the optic.

Author's recommendation

A slit lamp check of the operated eye is generally recommended after approximately 2 h postop. However, this check is mandatory if there is any intraoperative suspicion that the implant could be too large by showing a pronounced bulge and a consequent flattening of the anterior chamber.

Hypovault

If the Vault measurement is below 100 µm, it is called a Hypovault. In extreme cases, the gap between the ICL and the lens can even be completely eliminated. The concern, that the proximity between implant and crystalline lens inevitably results in an increased cataract rate, seems to have become less important with the introduction of the Aquaport however. Even at very close distances, there seems to be sufficient circulation around the crystalline lens, so that nutrition and therefore the clarity of the lens remains intact.

Author's recommendation

A very small or non-existent gap between ICL and lens is no longer a compelling indication for ICL exchange in models with the Aquaport. It is recommended to wait and check regularly.

Special Features of Toric ICL

Since 2002, the ICL is has also been available in a toric version. The results with additional astigmatic correction are just as good here as with a pure spherical correction [5]. Despite the positioning in the ciliary sulcus, the ICL is usually rotationally stable over time, at least when the proportions fit. However, if the ICL is too small, it can practically float in the sulcus and then rotate out of the desired axis. Occasionally, however, a residual refraction may be present even if the ICL is stable. In this case, similar to toric IOLs used in cataract surgery, a change in the astigmatic effect can be achieved by rotating the ICL. In this case, the method described by Lege and Neuhann is recommended, which allows a simple calculation of the post-rotation to be performed [6]. The spherical equivalent of refraction remains naturally unaffected.

Conclusion

Today, ICL implantation is the procedure of choice in the treatment of high myopia and an equivalent alternative in the treatment of lower myopia. The reasons for this are both the reversibility and maintaining accommodation (as opposed to refractive lens exchange) and the avoidance of the corneal problems associated with refractive corneal laser (corneal ectasia, dry eye, induction of corneal aberrations and later problems with biometry).

References

1. Alfonso JF, Fernández-Vega-Cueto L Alfonso-Bartolozzi B et al. Five-year follow-up of correction of Myopia: posterior ChamberPhakic intraocular lens with a central port design. J Refract Surg. 2019;35(3):169–176. https://doi.org/10.3928/1081597X-20190118-01.
2. Alshamrani AA, Alharbi SS. Phakic intraocular lens implantation for the correction of hyperopia. J Cataract Refract Surg. 2019;45(10):1503–11. https://doi.org/10.1016/j.jcrs.2019.05.051.

3. Fechner PU, Worst JGF. A new concave intraocular lens for the correction of myopia. Eur J Implant Refract Surg. 1989;1:41–3.
4. Fyodorov SN, Zuyev UK, Aznabayev BM. Intraocular correction of high myopia with negative posterior chamber lens]. Oftalmokhirurgiia. 1991;3:57–8.
5. Ganesh S, Brar S, Pawar A. Matched population comparison of visual outcomes and patient satisfaction between 3 modalities for the correction of low to moderate myopic astigmatism. Clin Ophthalmol. 2017;11(1253–1263):2017. https://doi.org/10.2147/OPTH.S127101. eCollection.
6. Lege BAM, Neuhann TF. Easy method for correcting misalignment of a toric phakic intraocular lens using vector analysis. J Cataract Refract Surg. 2017;43(11):1476–7.
7. Majid Moshirfar MD, FACS; Anisha N. Somani, BS; Mahsaw N. Motlagh, BA; Uma Vaidyanathan, BS; Jorgen S. Sumsion, BS; James R. Barnes, BS; Yasmyne C. Ronquillo, MD, MSc,. Comparison of FDA-reported visual and refractive outcomes of the Toric ICL Lens, SMILE, and Topography-Guided LASIK for the correction of Myopia and Myopic Astigmatism. J Refract Surg. 2019;35(11):699–706. https://doi.org/10.3928/1081597X-20190930-01.
8. Packer M. The implantable collamer lens with a central port: review of the literature. Clin Ophthalmol. 2018;27(12):2427–38.
9. Parkhurst GD. A prospective comparison of phakic collamer lenses and wavefront-optimized laser-assisted in situ keratomileusis for correction of myopia. Clin Ophthalmol. 2016. 29;10, 1209–15. https://doi.org/10.2147/OPTH.S106120. eCollection 2016.
10. Randleman RW, et al. Risk factors and prognosis for corneal ectasia after LASIK. Ophthalmology. 2003;110:267–75.
11. Siedlecki J, Schmelter V, Mayer WJ et al (2020). SMILE versus implantable collamer lens implantation for HighMyopia: a matched comparative study. J Refract Surg. 1;36(3), 150–159. https://doi.org/10.3928/1081597X-20200210-02.
12. Stodulka P, Slovak M, Sramka M, Polisensky J, Liska K. Posterior chamber phakic intraocular lens for the correction of presbyopia in highly myopic patients. J Cataract Refract Surg. 2020;46(1):40–4. https://doi.org/10.1097/j.jcrs.0000000000000033.

Surgical Techniques for the Use of Phakic Intraocular Lenses

Suphi Taneri

A. **Introduction**

Keypoint

Requirements for an ideal phakic intraocular lens:

An ideal phakic intraocular lens (pIOL) would not only provide excellent optical image quality and a wide range of correction, but would also fulfil the following criteria directly or indirectly related to the surgical technique:

- Uniform size for all eyes (no sizing problems)
- Easy implantation
- No induction of astigmatism
- Self-centering
- Spatial stability
- Rotational stability
- Gentle for the endothelium
- Biocompatibility
- No induction of glaucoma (also no postoperative pressure peaks)
- No cataract induction

Supplementary Information The online version contains supplementary material available at https://doi.org/10.1007/978-3-031-05394-8_98. The videos can be accessed individually by clicking the DOI link in the accompanying figure caption or by scanning this link with the SN More Media App.

S. Taneri (✉)
Center for Refractive Surgery, Münster, Germany
e-mail: taneri@refraktives-zentrum.de

M. Shajari et al. (eds.), *Cataract and Lens Surgery*,
https://doi.org/10.1007/978-3-031-05394-8_98

- No induction of uveitis
- No risk of endophthalmitis [11]
- Simple to explant.

Currently, no pIOL meets all of these requirements. However, many modern pIOLs come very close to these ideals.

The first pIOL implanted in the posterior chamber was presented in 1986 by Svyatoslav Fyodorov, who was known primarily for his corneal incisions (radial keratotomies) for myopia correction [6]. The original design resembled a collar button, with the haptic behind the iris and an optic protruding through the pupil into the anterior chamber. The most popular pIOL currently, the Visian Implantable Collamer Lens (ICL, Staar Surgical), will be discussed in detail in this chapter, but was also based on this design [5]. Another posterior chamber lens, the Phakic Refractive Lens (PRL, CIBA Vision), was a one-piece pIOL made of hydrophobic silicone. It was supposed to "float" above the surface of the crystalline lens and was only supported by the zonula fibers [7]. Unfortunately, this often led to dehiscence of the zonula fibers and to a subluxation of the pIOL into the vitreous space [2]. As a result, this lens is no longer on the market.

Currently, the Staar Collamer ICL is the only phakic posterior chamber lens approved by the FDA in the USA. The first 3 versions of the ICL required a peripheral iridotomy or iridectomy to prevent a pupillary block. However, the ICLs for the correction of hyperopia still require these iridotomies. These could be applied with a YAG laser a few weeks before implantation or with micro scissors or with a vitrectome during implantation. In its current form (EVO Visian V4c) the ICL has a hole with a diameter of 360 μm exactly in the center of the optic (KS-AquaPORT), through which aqueous humour can flow into the anterior chamber (Fig. 1).

This central hole eliminates the need for a bypass through the iris, at least for the meniscus shaped ICLs used to correct myopia. Although visual acuity and contrast sensitivity are rated as very good by the patient despite the opening in the optic zone [9, 10], dysphotopsia has been reported [3, 4]. The role of the exact centration of the central opening in relation to the pupil center and in relation to the angle kappa has been described by Martinez-Plaza et al. [8]. The convex shaped ICL models for hyperopia correction have no central openings and therefore still require iridotomy or iridectomy. Choi et al. recently reported the 10-year results of the ICL and found stable visual acuity and high safety in highly myopic eyes [1]. The authors could show that the vault of ICL decreases over time, however, and as a result, the risk of cataract increases [1].

For a few years now, a posterior chamber lens very similar to the ICL called Implantable Phakic Contact Lens (IPCL, Care Group, India) has been commercially available outside the U.S. [14]. The IPCL is made of acrylic and is available in a toric version as well as with various near-additions for presbyopia correction (Fig. 2).

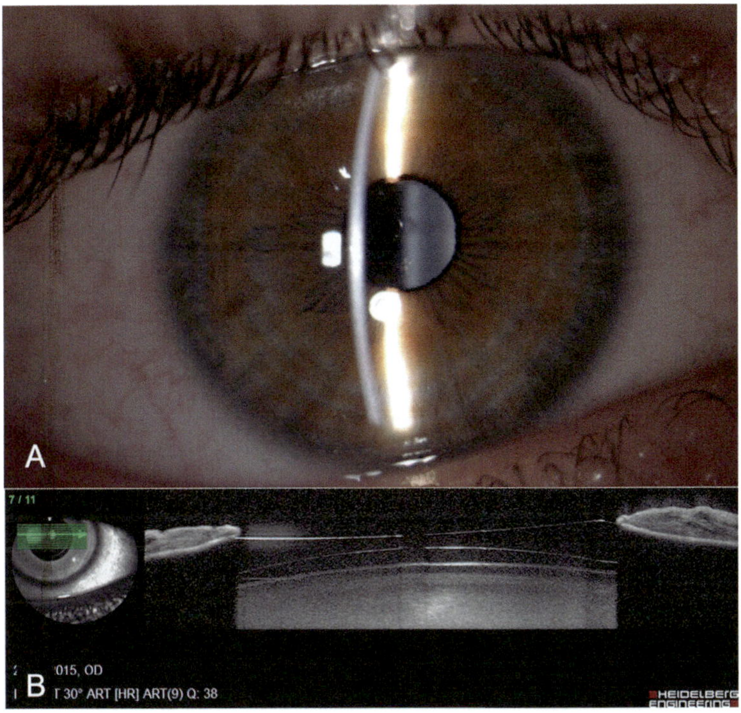

Fig. 1 **a** Regular vaulting of an ICL (Staar Surgical). **b** Regular vaulting of an ICL in optical coherence tomography (with central opening for aqueous humour circulation = Aquaport®)

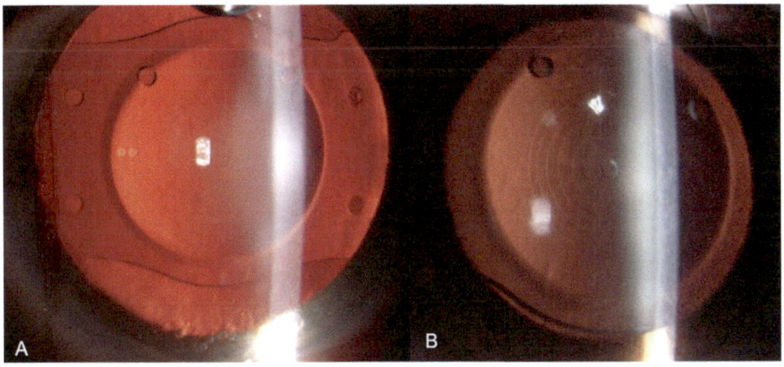

Fig. 2 **a** Regular position of an IPCL-toric (IPCL, Care Group, India) with horizontal alignment (note torus markings on the edge of the optic) 1 h after implantation. **b** Regular position of an IPCL-presbyopic 1 h after implantation. The diffractive optics provide multifocality

B. Surgical technique of chamber angle supported pIOLs

Although no chamber angle pIOL is commercially available at present, the implantation technique is briefly described for didactic reasons due to its elegant simplicity (Video 1).

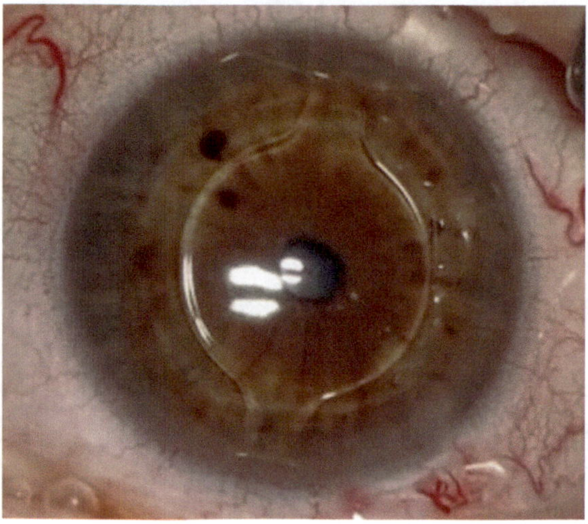

Video 1 Implantation of an ACRYSOF CACHET pIOL (Note—this lens was taken off of the market due to endothelial cell loss) (▶ https://doi.org/10.1007/000-8fg)

1. **Preoperative miosis**

Pilocarpine eye drops are applied several times before surgery.

2. **Paracenteses**

Paracenteses are not necessary.

3. **Tunnel incision**

A "clear-cornea" or limbal tunnel with a width of approx. 2.8 mm is created preferably at the steepest meridian and can reduce astigmatism.

4. **Viscoelastic device**

A viscoelastic device is injected through the tunnel to safely form the anterior chamber.

5. **Insertion of the IOL into the anterior chamber**

The IOL is injected into the anterior chamber using a shooter and the trailing haptics are positioned at the chamber angle using a push–pull instrument.

6. **Centration**

The IOL centers itself.

7. **Iridotomy/iridectomy**

Due to the anteriorly angled haptics (AcrySof cachet, Alcon), the optic has no contact with the pupil and the circulation of aqueous humour was not impaired. An iridotomy or iridectomy was therefore not necessary. For other chamber angle supported pIOLs (e.g. I-Care, Pharmacia) a surgical iridectomy was recommended. (Note: These lenses are currently not available for phakic correction. These surgeries are for illustration purposes only)

8. **Removal of the viscoelastic device**

The viscoelastic device should be removed as completely as possible to avoid obstructing the chamber angle and thus a consequent postoperative pressure spike. Manual irrigation with a Sauter cannula may be better suited to this than the use of an irrigation-aspiration handpiece.

9. **Wound closure**

A watertight closure is usually achieved without sutures.

Postoperative management

In this minimally traumatic procedure, a five-day application of dexamethasone and antibiotic eye drops, 4 times a day each, is sufficient.

Patients should be instructed to avoid rubbing their eyes and to return for follow-ups (especially of the endothelium) at least every six months. If cell density decreases over a short period, the lens should be explanted.

C. Surgical technique of iris-fixated pIOL (Artisan/Artiflex)

1. **Preoperative miosis**

During implantation, a drug-induced miosis acts as a protective shield for the crystalline lens and avoids potentially cataractogenic contact with it. For this purpose, pilocarpine eye drops should be applied several times before surgery. Alternatively, acetylcholine (e.g. Miochol-E) can be injected intracamerally at the beginning of the implantation.

2. **Paracenteses**

The paracenteses should be created in addition to a superior tunnel at 10 and 2 o'clock and be about 1 mm wide. The enclavation needles can be inserted through these later to capture or enclavate the iris in the claw-shaped haptics.

3. **Viscoelastic device**

It is recommended to use a highly viscous sodium hyaluronate solution to achieve a stable anterior chamber formation. Low-viscosity or dispersive substances can escape through the fairly wide tunnel and lead to an undesirable flattening of the anterior chamber with potential damage to the endothelium. A small bolus of the viscoelastic on top of the optic is recommended after insertion of the IOL and before enclavation of the haptics, to protect the endothelium.

4. **Tunnel incision**

Different incisions are possible: either "clear-corneal" or sclerocorneal tunnels. The incision width should be at least 5.2 mm for rigid PMMA IOLs with 5 mm optics and 6.2 mm for those with 6 mm optics to avoid difficulties during insertion. The position of these tunnels should be as superior as possible so that the upper eyelid covers the wide incision. A "frown-incision" is recommended because it causes the least amount of astigmatism. For the foldable IOLs (Artiflex/Veriflex), the incision width should not be less than 3.2 mm. In these situations the tunnel can also be created temporarily (Video 2).

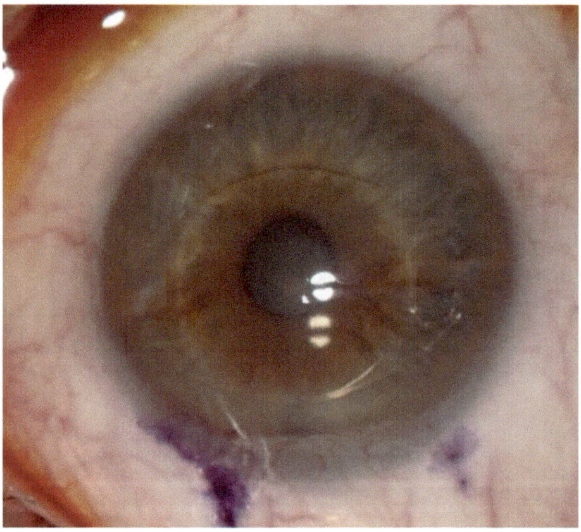

Video 2 Explantation of an Artisan lens followed by cataract surgery (▶ https://doi.org/10.1007/000-8fe)

5. **Insertion of the IOL into the anterior chamber**

The IOL is typically inserted into the anterior chamber through the superior incision with a special forceps, and rotated 90° into a horizontal position after replenishing viscoelastic device. Since the chamber angle is wider horizontally, a horizontal position of the iris fixated IOL provides the greatest distance to the endothelium.

6. **Centration**

Correct centration of the IOL is one of the most critical steps of this method because it can have a significant impact on the postoperative visual outcome. The center of the pupil serves as a reference.

Author's recommendation

The correct axial alignment of the surgical microscope can help to avoid postoperative parallax error.

7. **Enclavation**

While the IOL is held centered over the pupil with special forceps, a fold in the iris tissue is made with the help of special blunt needles inserted successively through the paracenteses. The iris fold is guided through the two claws of the nasal or temporal haptics, respectively, by an upward movement of the needle. The hands are then changed, and the procedure is repeated through the other paracentesis on the opposite side. If too little iris tissue has been fixated in the haptic during the first pass, the process can be repeated. It is important to grasp sufficient iris tissue, otherwise the iris fibers can quickly elongate and the IOL can disenclavate, even after a minor trauma [13] (Video 3).

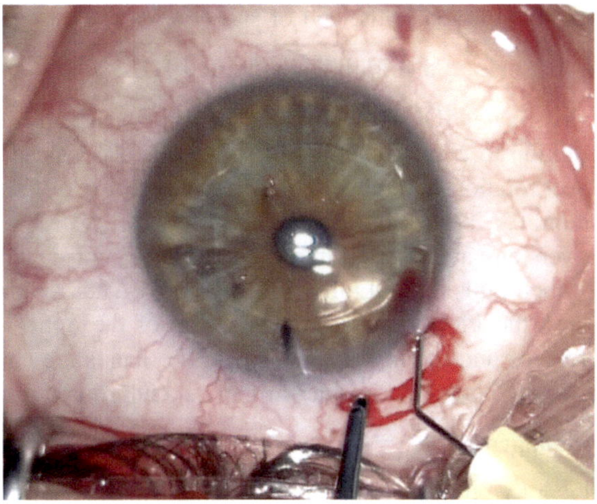

Video 3 Re-enclavation of an Artisan lens (▶ https://doi.org/10.1007/000-8ff)

8. **Iridotomy/iridectomy**

Due to the anteriorly angled haptics, the optic has no contact with the pupil and the aqueous humour circulation should not be impaired. Therefore, an iridotomy or iridectomy is not necessary, though some surgeons prefer it.

9. **Removal of the viscoelastic device**

Immediately before the tunnel is closed, the viscoelastic material should be removed as thoroughly as possible in order to prevent obstruction of the chamber angle and thus a postoperative pressure spike.

10. **Wound closure**

A watertight wound closure is of course necessary to prevent flattening of the anterior chamber leading to contact of the anterior chamber lens with the endothelium. A good closure is also required to avoid contamination with pathogens of the ocular surface in the early postoperative period. In wide tunnels in particularly, suturing with 10–0 nylon (continuous or as single tying sutures) can provide additional security against leakage.

Author's recommendation

For tunnel widths over 5 mm, considerable surgically induced astigmatism is occasionally to be expected. However, it may take up to 2–3 months before the final result is achieved. Therefore, an excessively early intervention should be avoided.

11. **Intracameral anticiotics**

In accordance with current recommendations for cataract surgery, we inject 1 mg of cefuroxime in 0.1 ml solution at the end of surgery.

Special features of toric and foldable iris-fixated IOLs

In cases of toric iris-fixated IOLs, attention must also be paid to the exact horizontal alignment (in addition to correct centration), as the torus is placed individually in the optic. To detect rotation of the eye, preoperative marking of the horizontal axis in a sitting position, e.g. at the slit lamp, is helpful.

The foldable versions are inserted into the anterior chamber with the help of a special spatula, which pulls the IOL almost like a hook. After rotating the IOL to a horizontal position, the PMMA haptic on one side of the optic is grasped with dedicated bent forceps and the iris is enclavated. The hands are changed, and this step is repeated on the contralateral side. In general, suture is not necessary.

Postoperative management

For PMMA IOLs, a five-day course of topical dexamethasone administration (four times a day) and a six-week course of non-steroidal anti-inflammatory eye drops is recommended. For foldable IOLs with a silicone compound optic, we recommend fluorometholone eye drops for 12 weeks given as a tapering dose to prevent deposition of giant cells [12]. Antibiotic eye drops for at least 5 days are standard. Patients should be instructed not to rub their eyes and to have at least annual check-ups.

D. Surgical technique of posterior chamber PIOL (ICL, IPCL)

The videos show the implantation of two posterior chamber pIOLs; ICL and IPCL (Videos 4 and 5).

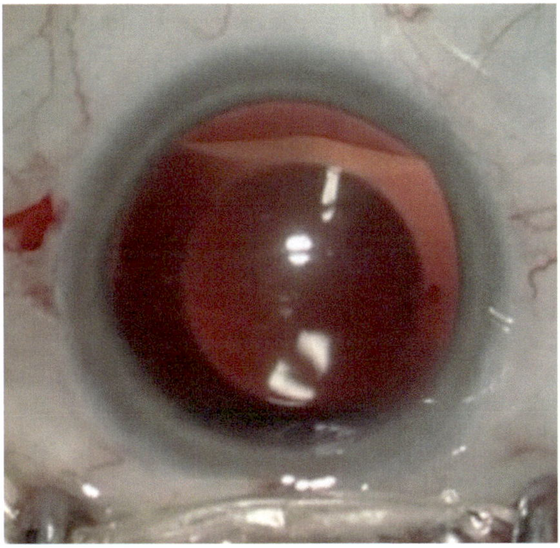

Video 4 Implantation of an ICL (▶ https://doi.org/10.1007/000-8fd)

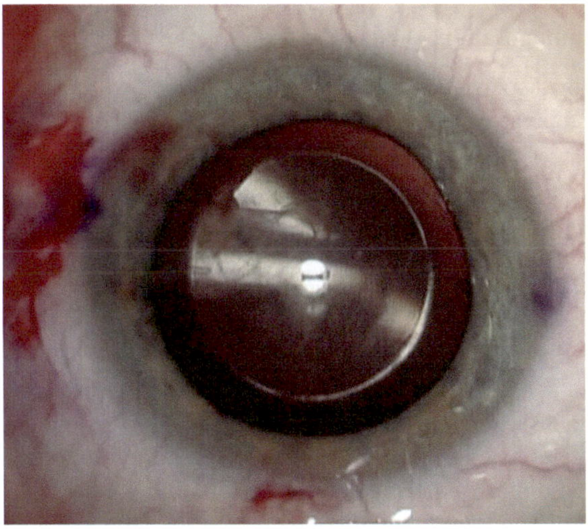

Video 5 Implantation of an IPCL (▶ https://doi.org/10.1007/000-8fh)

1. **Preoperative mydriasis**

Maximum mydriasis facilitates subsequent positioning of the haptics behind the iris. Mydriatic drops (phenylephrine, tropicamide) should be administered several times as preparations before surgery. Alternatively, a mydriatic agent (e.g., adrenaline or a CE-approved compound, Mydrane, Thea Pharma) can be injected intracamerally.

2. **Paracenteses**

The manufacturer recommends two paracenteses but we prefer to use only one at 12 o'clock. A spatula can be inserted through this paracentesis later to position the anterior haptic.

3. **Tunnel incision**

Different incisions are possible: "clear-corneal" or sclerocorneal tunnel. The incision width should be at least 3.2 mm for ICL, and 2.8 mm for IPCL. The position of the tunnel should be temporal, because from there the IOL can be inserted at a flat angle, avoiding contact to the crystalline lens.

4. **Viscoelastic device**

We inject a highly viscous viscoelastic device after the tunnel has been created in order to achieve a very stable anterior chamber. This is to protect both the endothelium and the crystalline lens from contact with the pIOL. Care should be taken not to overfill the anterior chamber as this could provoke an iris prolapse and complicate the surgery.

Author's recommendation

Low viscosity or dispersive substances can be difficult to remove completely and can lead to postoperative pressure peaks.

5. **Insertion of the pIOL into the anterior chamber**

The pIOL is carefully injected into the anterior chamber using the IOL injector. Inserting the ICL into its special cartridge can sometimes be time-consuming but should always be done under a microscope to ensure that the rear haptics are not entrapped in the cartridge. The IPCL is easier to insert, in the same way as a capsular bag IOL in cataract surgery (see also the beginning of Video 6).

It is important to ensure that the orientation of the pIOL is correct at the beginning of the insertion (the optic is bent upwards). If it is not correctly oriented, the pIOL can be retracted back into the cartridge before it unfolds completely. We also apply a small bolus of the viscoelastic on top of the optic, after insertion of the IOL, before positioning the haptics in order to protect the endothelium.

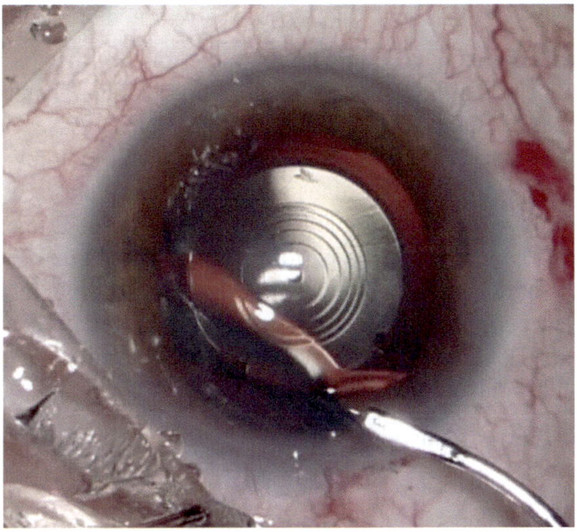

Video 6 Implantation of an IPCL presbyopic (▶ https://doi.org/10.1007/000-8fj)

6. **Positioning of the haptics**

We position the nasal haptic by inserting a spatula through the paracentesis and then the temporal haptics through the tunnel.

Author's recommendation

A dedicated spatula designed by Vukich is particularly useful for this purpose. It has a spoon-like protrusion at the end and has a roughened texture at the bottom. This allows the haptics to be guided in a very controlled way.

7. **Centration and alignment**

The ICL and IPCL are self-centering in the ciliary sulcus, while the center of the pupil is usually located slightly nasally below it. This has to be taken into account preoperatively, especially when using the presbyopic IPCL with its diffractive optics (Video 6). As a rule, these lenses are implanted horizontally, as the sulcus diameter is usually largest here.

Special features of toric IOLs

With toric sulcus supported IOLs, it is important to ensure exact horizontal alignment, as the torus is individually placed in the optic. To detect rotation of the eye during surgery, preoperative marking of the horizontal axis in a sitting position, e.g. at the slit lamp, is helpful.

8. **Iridotomy/iridectomy**

Due to the anteriorly angulated haptics, the optic touches the iris margin and the aqueous humour circulation can occasionally be impaired. Therefore, the current posterior chamber lens models for myopia correction have several holes which reliably allow the passage of the aqueous humour and an iridotomy or iridectomy is no longer necessary. However, this does not apply to the plus lenses used to correct hyperopia. With these there is no hole in the center of the IOL, therefore two laser iridotomies at 80° intervals must be performed a few weeks before implantation or alternatively, a surgical iridotomy can be performed during implantation. This should not be too peripheral, so that it cannot be displaced by haptics even in the event of rotation. IPCLs up to + 3 diopter are recently available with central holes, however, the author has no personal experience with their use.

9. **Removal of the viscoelastic device**

The viscoelastic device should be removed as thoroughly as possible in order to prevent obstructing the chamber angle and a postoperative pressure spike. However, this rinsing is much more difficult than with anterior chamber lenses, as viscoelastic may be trapped behind the iris or behind the pIOL. Extremely careful manipulation of the pIOL with a rinsing cannula can help to mobilize these hidden remnants.

10. **Pupil constriction after implantation**

To prevent the optic from being pushed forward through the pupil, a miotic agent can be injected at the end of the operation, if needed. The author usually refrains from doing this in order to avoid interaction with intracameral antibiotics.

11. **Wound closure**

A watertight wound closure is mandatory to avoid contamination by pathogens of the ocular surface in the early postoperative period. This is usually achieved by hydration of the incision and sutures are not typically required.

Author's recommendation

With tunnel widths around 3 mm, clinically relevant surgically induced astigmatism is to be expected. In the author's case this is 0.25 D and is taken into account in the preoperative lens calculation.

12. **Intracameral anticiotics**

In accordance with current recommendations for cataract surgery, we inject 1 mg of cefuroxime in 0.1 ml solution at the end of surgery.

Postoperative management

A first check at the slit lamp 1–2 h after implantation is essential to verify the correct position of the pIOL and to detect potential pressure fluctuations. A five-day course of dexamethasone four times a day and a six-week course of non-steroidal antiphlogistic eye drops is sufficient. Antibiotic eye drops for at least 5 days are also recommended as standard. Patients should be instructed not to rub their eyes and to have postoperative follow-up visits at least once a year.

Conclusion

Both modern phakic posterior chamber IOLs and iris-fixated anterior chamber IOLs allow a safe and effective correction of especially high ametropia. This is particularly helpful when laser refractive surgery is contraindicated, e.g. in case of keratoconus. Both implantation and explantation can be surgically demanding and postoperative check-ups at least once a year to follow up the clear lens and endothelial cell density are recommended.

References

1. Choi JH, Lim DH, Nam SW, Yang CM, Chung ES, Chung T-Y. Ten-year clinical outcomes after implantation of a posterior chamber phakic intraocular lens for myopia. J Cataract Refract Surg. 2019;45(11):1555–61. https://doi.org/10.1016/j.jcrs.2019.06.015.
2. Donoso R, Castillo P. Correction of high myopia with the PRL phakic intraocular lens. J Cataract Refract Surg. 2006;32(8):1296–300. https://doi.org/10.1016/j.jcrs.2006.03.035.
3. Eom Y, Kim DW, Ryu D, Kim J-H, Yang SK, Song JS, Kim S-W, Kim HM. Ring-shaped dysphotopsia associated with posterior chamber phakic implantable collamer lenses with a central hole. Acta Ophthalmol. 2017;95(3):e170–8. https://doi.org/10.1111/aos.13248.
4. Eppig T, Spira C, Tsintarakis T, El-Husseiny M, Cayless A, Müller M, Seitz B, Langenbucher A. Ghost-image analysis in phakic intraocular lenses with central hole as a potential cause of dysphotopsia. J Cataract Refract Surg. 2015;41(11):2552–9. https://doi.org/10.1016/j.jcrs.2015.05.034.
5. Huang D, Schallhorn SC, Sugar A, Farjo AA, Majmudar PA, Trattler WB, Tanzer DJ. Phakic intraocular lens implantation for the correction of myopia: a report by the American Academy of Ophthalmology. Ophthalmology. 2009;116(11):2244–58. https://doi.org/10.1016/j.ophtha.2009.08.018.
6. Jiménez-Alfaro I, del Castillo JMB, García-Feijoó J, de Bernabé JGG, de la Iglesia JMS. Safety of posterior chamber phakic intraocular lenses for the correction of high myopia: anterior segment changes after posterior chamber phakic intraocular lens implantation. Ophthalmology. 2001;108(1):90–9. https://doi.org/10.1016/S0161-6420(00)00403-6.
7. Koivula A, Taube M, Zetterström C. Phakic refractive lens: two-year results. J Refract Surg. 2008;24(5):507–15. https://doi.org/10.3928/1081597X-20080501-09.
8. Martínez-Plaza E, López-Miguel A, Fernández I, Blázquez-Arauzo F, Maldonado MJ. Effect of central hole location in phakic intraocular lenses on visual function under progressive headlight glare sources. J Cataract Refract Surg. 2019;45(11):1591–6. https://doi.org/10.1016/j.jcrs.2019.06.022.
9. Shimizu K, Kamiya K, Igarashi A, Kobashi H. Long-Term Comparison of posterior chamber phakic intraocular lens with and without a central hole (hole ICL and conventional ICL) implantation for moderate to high myopia and myopic astigmatism. Medicine. 2016;95(14):e3270. https://doi.org/10.1097/MD.0000000000003270.

10. Shimizu K, Kamiya K, Igarashi A, Shiratani T. Intraindividual comparison of visual performance after posterior chamber phakic intraocular lens with and without a central hole implantation for moderate to high myopia. Am J Ophthalmol. 2012;154(3):486-494.e1. https://doi.org/10.1016/j.ajo.2012.04.001.
11. Taneri S, Kießler S, Rost A, Schultz T, Elling M, Dick HB (Online video). Atypical endophthalmitis after intraocular collamer lens implantation. 2018. https://doi.org/10.1016/j.jcrs.2018.08.010.
12. Taneri S, Oehler S, Heinz C. Inflammatory response in the anterior chamber after implantation of an angle-supported lens in phakic myopic eyes. J Ophthalmol. 2014;2014:923691. https://doi.org/10.1155/2014/923691.
13. Taneri S, Oehler S, Koch JM, Heiligenhaus A. Hypermotility of an iris-fixated anterior chamber phakic intraocular lens due to nontraumatic iris laxity. Eur J Ophthalmol. 2012;22(3):481–4. https://doi.org/10.5301/ejo.5000059.
14. Vasavada V, Srivastava S, Vasavada SA, Sudhalkar A, Vasavada AR, Vasavada VA. Safety and efficacy of a new phakic posterior chamber IOL for correction of myopia: 3 years of follow-up. Journal of Refractive Surgery (Thorofare, N.J.: 1995). 2018;34(12):817–23. https://doi.org/10.3928/1081597X-20181105-01.

Management of Surgical Complications When Implanting Phakic IOLs

Karel Van Keer, Caroline Dauwe, and Erik Mertens

Wound construction

As with cataract surgery, well constructed incisions are of key importance in phakic IOL surgery. Depending on the size and properties of the implanted lens, the surgeon may opt for a clear corneal, limbal or scleral incision. The ideal incision provides optimal access to the anterior chamber whilst preserving the eyes' structural integrity. Poor wound construction may result in excessive astigmatism, iris prolapse and post-operative wound leakage. To avoid these complications, the surgeon should master the technique of creating reproducible incisions of adequate positioning, tunnel length and depth [1].

Tight incisions can be enlarged manually to the desired width using the keratome. In the case of inadequately sealing incisions, care should be taken to prevent iris prolapse through the main incision. Should this complication occur, one should try to reduce and redirect the pressure gradient pushing the iris through the incision. This can be achieved by reducing the IOP and/or sweeping the iris out of the main incision through the side port [2]. At the end of the surgery, all incisions should be watertight. Non-sealing wounds should be sutured using one or more sutures as needed.

Supplementary Information The online version contains supplementary material available at https://doi.org/10.1007/978-3-031-05394-8_99. The videos can be accessed individually by clicking the DOI link in the accompanying figure caption or by scanning this link with the SN More Media App.

K. Van Keer (✉)
Emmetropia, Leuven, Belgium
e-mail: karel@vankeer.org

C. Dauwe · E. Mertens
Medipolis Eye Centre, Wilrijk, Belgium
e-mail: e.mertens@medipolis.be

M. Shajari et al. (eds.), *Cataract and Lens Surgery*,
https://doi.org/10.1007/978-3-031-05394-8_99

Intraocular manipulation

The delicacy of the ocular tissues demands for skillful manipulation. Touching the anterior lens capsule and corneal endothelium should be avoided and manipulation of the cornea and iris should be minimized.

The incisions should therefore be placed such that they provide optimal access to the anterior chamber and instruments should be inserted along the axis of the incisions. Failure to respect the incision plane can result in corneal trauma, such as Descemet membrane detachment. In most cases, a conservative approach is appropriate for Descemet membrane detachments. More extensive detachments can be treated with air/gas tamponade, repositioning with viscoelastic material or corneal stab incision to drain the pre Descemet aqueous [3].

Manipulation of the iris should be minimized. In the absence of an aqueous drainage hole in the lens, a peripheral iridotomy should be performed either pre- or peroperatively. Peroperative surgical iridotomies, created using scissors or a vitrector, can result in intracameral bleeding. When this occurs, temporarily increasing the IOP will result in adequate tamponade of the bleeding [4].

To reduce the risk of cataract induction, the crystalline lens should remain untouched during surgery. For anterior chamber pIOLs, pharmacological miosis can help to protect the crystalline lens. Unlike in cataract surgery, it's not recommended to remove the OVD from behind the implanted pIOL unless irrigation can be directed through the Aquaport to push the viscoelastic from behind the pIOL into the anterior chamber [5].

Implant lens-related problems

The importance of correct positioning of the lens is imperative. It is necessary to take time to load the lens correctly. First remove the ICL from the sealed glass container and load it inside the cartridge under the surgical microscope. The inner side of the cartridge is then lubricated with methylcellulose and balanced salt solution. The ICL has 2 tiny holes on the footplates (distal right and proximal left) that allow correct anterior–posterior orientation. The ICL is loaded making sure that both longitudinal edges of the haptic are symmetrically tucked under the edge of the cartridge with the lens vaulted anteriorly. Coaxial forceps are used to pull the lens through the cartridge tunnel. Inspection of the lens inside the tunnel is necessary to

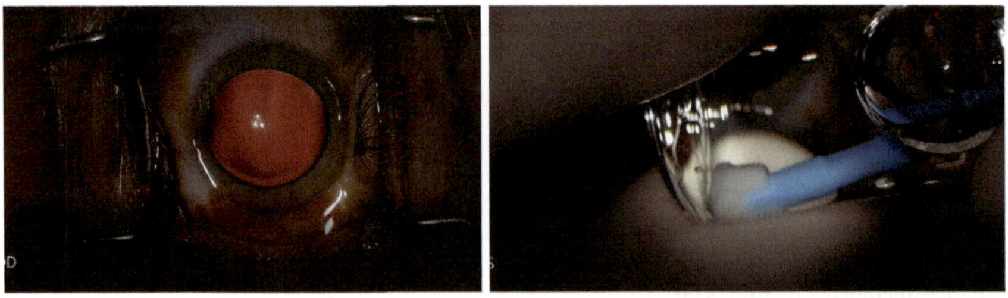

Video 1 Properly loading ICL (▶ https://doi.org/10.1007/000-8fm)

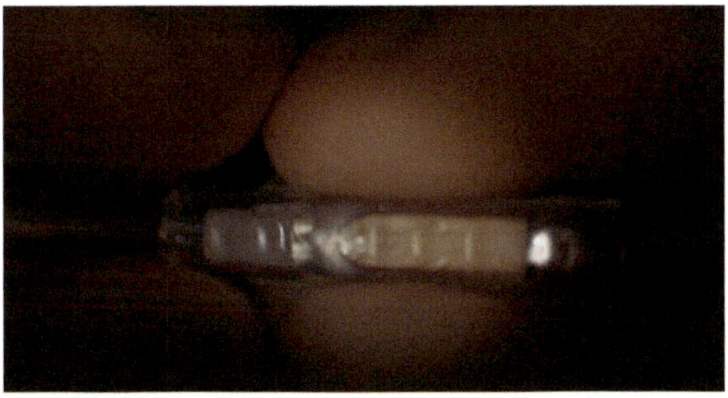

Video 2 Reloading ICL (▶ https://doi.org/10.1007/000-8fk)

exclude twisting of the lens which helps making the injection inside the anterior chamber symmetrical, smooth, and reproducible. A piece of soft material, the micro-Staar foam tip, is positioned to protect the ICL from contact with the plunger of the shooter.

When placing the lens, it is important to fixate and stabilise the eye, then placing the tip of the cartridge at the edge of the incision, after which the lens can be injected slowly. The surgeon must pay attention to the distal footplate to unfold in the anterior chamber before the trailing footplate is injected out of the cartridge. This prevents the lens from unfolding upside down in the anterior chamber. Once the lens is unfolded in the anterior chamber the marks on the distal and proximal footplates are checked for proper orientation. Using the side-port and with a manipulator, the distal haptics are tucked under the iris. Care should be taken to keep all manipulations as peripheral as possible with no instruments touching the optic or crossing the pupillary zone. The proximal footplates are then tucked under the iris through the main incision. Inspect the orientation under the operating microscope. The clear funnel of the cartridge enables identification of the center marks on each side of the optic. These marks should be visible at the 12 o'clock position and be in straight alignment down the shaft. If the ICL is not aligned or properly oriented, the ICL may be twisted in the cartridge leading to a possible upside-down injection and position in the anterior chamber which requires immediate explantation and re-injection of a correct positioned ICL [6].

The importance of correct sizing of the lens is critical [7]. Sizing represents the methodology by which the appropriate overall lens diameter is selected for implantation in order to achieve a safe level of vault, which is the axial distance between the ICL and the crystalline lens. Perfectly fitting the ICL in the posterior chamber depends on the lens design and lens sizing. The phakic lens should neither touch the natural lens, nor obstruct the normal circulation of the aqueous humor. Optimal ICL sizing is important as excessive vault is associated with problems such as angle closure glaucoma, pupil dilatation and anisocoria and too low a vault with increased risk of cataract formation. The larger ICL size can lead to angle closure and subsequent intraocular pressure elevation. The vaulting must not cause excessive contact with the posterior surface of the iris, which could lead to pigment dispersion, and subsequent glaucoma, especially in highly myopic eyes. Insufficient vaulting can lead to toric ICL rotation and cataract formation [8, 9]. To avoid these complications, improperly sized ICLs should be exchanged for an alternative size. In the case of non-toric ICLs, ICL rotation to the vertical meridian can provide an easy surgical solution for reducing the vault [10].

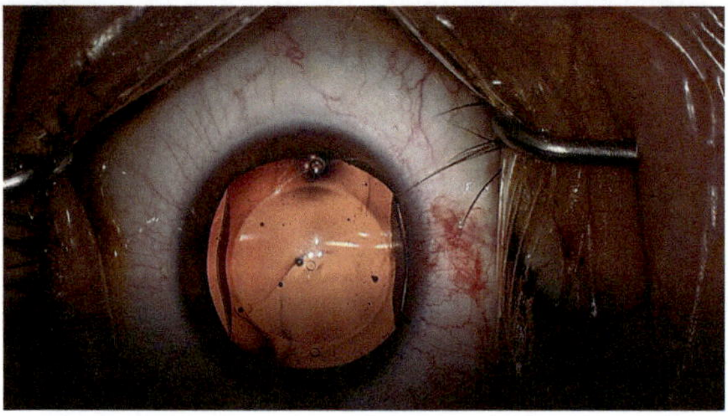

Video 3 Vertical ICL rotation (▶ https://doi.org/10.1007/000-8fn)

OVD-related problems

After making a 1.0-mm side-port at 10 o'clock in the left eye and at 5 o'clock in the right eye, followed by injection of intracameral preservative-free lidocaine 1%, the anterior chamber is filled with viscoelastic preferably methylcellulose. This is done with caution to not overfill the anterior chamber to avoid excessively high intraoperative intraocular pressure. It is important to remove most of the methylcellulose at the end of surgery, as retained viscoelastic can result in IOP spikes in the immediate postoperative period. The rheological properties of the OVD determine the ease by which the OVD can be removed from the anterior chamber and should therefore be carefully considered. To further prevent postoperative pressure spikes, topical carbonic anhydrase inhibitors and/or beta-blockers and a tablet of acetazolamide 250 mg can be administered post-operatively. It is recommended to measure the IOP before discharging the patient. Certain OVDs containing chondroitin sulphate can lead to anterior subcapsular opacities of the crystalline lens and should be avoided [6, 11].

Post-operative endophthalmitis

To prevent endophthalmitis a good standard protocol is imperative. On the day of surgery, one drop of 0.5% tropicamide and 5% phenylephrine HCl are serially instilled for pupil dilation. We apply 15 min before surgery a drop of preservative-free oxybuprocaine HCl 0.4% to the eye followed by povidone iodine 10% to the eyelid and two drops of povidone iodine 5% in the eye. Afterwards the patient is draped and a lid speculum inserted. Three drops of preservative-free oxybuprocaine HCl 0.4% is used to further anaesthetize each eye. Three minutes before the start of surgery povidone iodine 5% is again applied to the ocular surface. At the completion of the procedure intracameral preservative-free antibiotics (0.1 cc of cefuroxime 1 mg/mL) are injected and topical antibiotics (for example Ofloxacin 3 mg/mL 4 times daily) are started for the course of one week [6, 12].

In the rare but unfortunate event of postoperative infectious endophthalmitis, appropriate measures should be taken to identify and treat the causal infection [13, 14].

References

1. Kohnen T. Corneal shape changes and astigmatic aspects of scleral and corneal tunnel incisions. J Cataract Refract Surg. 1997;23(3):301–2.
2. Allan BDS. Mechanism of iris prolapse: a qualitative analysis and implications for surgical technique. J Cataract Refract Surg. 1995;21(2):182–6.
3. Sharma N, et al. Incision-site descemet membrane detachment during and after phacoemulsification: risk factors and management. Eye Contact Lens. 2015;41(5):273–6.
4. Wu Y, et al. Comparison of peripheral iridectomy methods for posterior chamber phakic intraocular lens implantation in patients with brown irides. BMC Ophthalmol. 2016;16 (1):1–7.
5. Smith RJ, et al. Lens opacities after posterior chamber phakic intraocular lens implantation. Ophthalmology. 2003;110(4):781–5.
6. Mertens EL. Toric phakic implantable collamer lens for correction of astigmatism: 1-year outcomes. Clin Ophthalmol (Auckland, NZ). 2011;5:369.
7. Igarashi A, et al. Predictability of the vault after posterior chamber phakic intraocular lens implantation using anterior segment optical coherence tomography. J Cataract Refract Surg. 2019;45(8):1099–104.
8. Packer M. The implantable collamer lens with a central port: review of the literature. Clin Ophthalmol (Auckland, NZ). 2018;12:2427.
9. Jiménez-Alfaro I, et al. Safety of posterior chamber phakic intraocular lenses for the correction of high myopia: anterior segment changes after posterior chamber phakic intraocular lens implantation. Ophthalmology. 2001;108(1):90–9.
10. Matarazzo F, et al. Vertical implantable collamer lens (ICL) rotation for the management of high vault due to lens oversizing. Int Ophthalmol. 2018;38(6):2689–92.
11. Hayashi K, et al. Prophylactic effect of oral acetazolamide against intraocular pressure elevation after cataract surgery in eyes with glaucoma. Ophthalmology. 2017;124(5):701–8.
12. Barry P, et al. ESCRS study of prophylaxis of postoperative endophthalmitis after cataract surgery: preliminary report of principal results from a European multicenter study. J Cataract Refract Surg. 2006;32(3):407–10.
13. Allan BD, Argeles-Sabate I, Mamalis N. Endophthalmitis rates after implantation of the intraocular collamer lens: survey of users between 1998 and 2006. J Cataract Refract Surg. 2009;35(4):766–9.
14. Lemley CA, Han DP. Endophthalmitis: a review of current evaluation and management. Retina. 2007;27(6):662–80.

Systematic Overview of Phakic Intraocular Lenses

Christoph Lwowski and Daniel Kook

Overview Phakic Intraocular Lenses

When considering the results after implantation of phakic intraocular lenses (pIOL) and with regard to intra- or postoperative complications, a distinction must be made between anterior and posterior chamber lenses and how each lens type is fixated in the eye.

Anterior chamber angle-supported phakic lenses (AC-pIOL)
Since the last chamber angle-supported VK-pIOL was discontinued due to progressive endothelial cell loss in 2014 (AcrySof© Cachet, Alcon, Texas, USA), no AC-pIOL is currently commercially available. Nevertheless, knowledge regarding potential long-term complications is relevant, as a large proportion of implanted AC-pIOLs are still in the eyes of patients and may be encountered during clinical practice.

Iris-fixed phakic intraocular lens (IF-pIOL)
IF-pIOLs are pIOLs that are fixed into the iris tissue by means of iris claws. The currently available models are the Artisan/Verisyse and Artiflex/Veriflex (Ophtec BV, NL and Abott Medical Optics, Inc., CA, USA, respectively). Both models are also suitable as intraocular lenses for aphakia correction.

Phakic posterior chamber lens (pIOL)
Phakic posterior chamber lenses are implanted between the natural lens and iris. The models currently available on the market are the Implantable Collamer® Lens (ICL, Staar Surgical, CA, USA), the Phakic Refractive Lens (PRL, Carl Zeiss

C. Lwowski (✉) · D. Kook
Frankfurt, Germany
e-mail: christoph.lwowski@kgu.de

D. Kook
e-mail: daniel.kook@med.uni-muenchen.de

M. Shajari et al. (eds.), *Cataract and Lens Surgery*,
https://doi.org/10.1007/978-3-031-05394-8_100

Meditec, Jena, Germany) and the Implantable Phakic Contact Lens (IPCL, Polytech Domilens, Roßdorf, Germany), with the latter pending CE certification or FDA approval.

Results After Implantation of Phakic Intraocular Lenses

In the following section, we provide with an overview of the current state of studies on outcomes after successful implantation of pIOLs.

Safety/Effectiveness

Safety and efficacy are essential for the evaluation of refractive surgery. Since the goal for the patient is to achieve freedom from spectacles, the effectiveness is defined by the ratio of the preoperative corrected visual acuity to the postoperative uncorrected visual acuity (Efficiency Index, EI). To evaluate safety, the pre- and postoperative corrected visual acuity is compared accordingly (Safety Index, SI).

A systematic review and meta-analysis of Artisan IF-pIOL (published in the Journal of Cataract and Refractive Surgery in 2020) evaluated more than 30 studies with a follow-up of at least 2 years. It showed good to very good efficacy with a mean EI of 0.8 to 0.96 and excellent safety with an SI of 1.02 to 1.39 [63]. Similar good results were also demonstrated for Artiflex IF-pIOL [14].

In a 2018 review of ICL with a total of 67 original papers, the authors reported equally excellent results and a mean EI of 1.04 with a mean follow-up of more than 12 months and a mean SI of 1.15 [56]. More recent publications also show comparable results for both ICL and PRL and IPCL [19, 37, 77, 78], suggesting equivalence of phakic anterior and posterior chamber lenses in terms of safety and efficacy [8]. Even in children with high myopia, the ICL and Artisan pIOLs provide good outcomes with a low risk profile [25].

Predictability/Stability

The predictability of the postoperative outcome is defined by deviation of the calculated residual refraction (target refraction, ZR) from the achieved refraction after implantation of the pIOL, or the number of eyes within ±0.5dpt or ±1.0dpt. Stability of the postoperative outcome is defined by statistically significant changes in spherical equivalent (SE) over time. Both the Artisan and Artiflex pIOL show comparable Menezoresults with the ICL and PRL in this regard [6, 8, 37, 50, 53, 54, 70, 77, 78]. With an average of 90.8% and 98.7% of eyes within ± 0.5 and

1.0dpt, respectively, ICL appears to be superior to Artisan (68.1% and 89.1%) in the literature [56, 63]. However, it should be mentioned that the duration of follow-up, the type of statistical analysis, and also the timing of surgery could cause bias here. Thus, it may be that postoperative outcomes are influenced by modern calculation formulas and advancement in ocular measurement.

Regarding the stability of the SE, posterior and anterior chamber lenses also seem to be equivalent. Changes in refraction during postoperative follow-up are rarely significant [28, 37, 43, 54, 63, 78]. However, in the long-term, progression of axial length or myopic nuclear sclerosis may occur in high myopes.

Patient Satisfaction and Optical Phenomena

Thanks to developments in tools and questionnaires on optical quality and subjective patient satisfaction, the focus of refractive surgery has shifted somewhat from the "hard numbers" such as high contrast visual acuity and refraction, to softer criteria. This is particularly relevant because patients may be dissatisfied with visual acuity especially optical phenomena—despite having full visual acuity and being spectacle-free. Patient-completed, validated questionnaires are the gold standard of PROMs (Patient Reported Outcome Measures) here. Eom et al reported a cohort of 29 eyes after ICL implantation, of which 18 noticed glare, 16 halos, 10 starburst and 15 negative dysphotopsia though these regressed after a mean of three months, according to the authors [23]. This could be evidence that—similar to multifocal IOLsneuroadaptation takes place, compensating for optical phenomena. Other studies confirm this assumption. For example, Liu et al reported halos in 58% of patients, but these regressed after three months [45]. This is also reflected in the manufacturer's own registry with PROMs, where 92.1% of patients reported being very satisfied and 7.3% satisfied [a]. Similar results can be found for patients after implantation of an IF-pIOL. Moshirfar et al, for example, reported that only 2.7% reported halo or glare postoperatively, compared with 6% one month postoperatively. The trend that optical phenomena disappear with time seems to apply accordingly to IF-pIOL as well [53]. A scotopic pupil diameter larger than the lens optic may have a negative effect which underlines the relevance of preoperative pupillometry.

Keypoint

Halos and optical phenomena are usually self-limiting or regress by neuroadaptation.

Postoperative and Long-term Complications of Phakic Intraocular Lenses

In addition to the above-mentioned risks of the surgery, the potential long-term consequences after implantation of a pIOL—should be consistently monitored by the treating ophthalmologist. In particular, the possible loss of endothelial (more often seen with the older designs), cataract, or pressure increases or pupillary block must be diagnosed and treated accordingly.

Surgically Induced Astigmatism (SIA)

Since phakic lens implantation is a refractive procedure, the SIA is of paramount importance for both surgeon and patient. In view of this, the refractive surgeon may need to adjust the size and location or axis of the incision, as well as the selection of the pIOL, to the given corneal conditions. Alternatively, postoperative visually relevant astigmatism can be corrected with a second procedure (e.g., corneal) or a toric pIOL. In general, it can be summarized that a large optic or a large lens—which may not be foldable—causes a larger SIA and an induced astigmatism of up to 2.0dpt [6] has been observed with Artisan/Verisyse lenses. Of course, this amount varies depending on the incision axis and the preoperative values and may even reduce the preoperative astigmatism if necessary [46, 53, 70]. With the foldable Artiflex/Veriflex IOL the SIA seems to be lower—corresponding to the smaller incision width (Coullet et al., SIA: 0.3 vs. 0.7dpt [17]). In foldable pIOL, the SIA is not a clinically relevant problem due to the incision width of only 3mm.

Corneal Endothelial Cell Loss

Corneal endothelial cells are one of the primary targets of postoperative checkups after implantation of a pIOL [41]. This also explains why pIOLs are not suitable for patients with a flat anterior chamber or endothelial damage. For example, Alio et al showed that patients had 8.4% endothelial cell loss after seven years following implantation of a AC-IOL [5]. Similar results were published by Kohnen et al in a long-term study with 11% after seven years [43] and Alleman et al with a loss of 12% [7].

The problem also applies to IF-pIOLs, where cell loss of up to 21.5% after ten years has been reported [61] or 29% after 12 years as currently published [71]. Overall, however, cell loss here appears to be less pronounced than that of AC-IOLs ([13, 18, 28], "Initial results of endothelial cell counts after Artisan lens for phakic eyes: an evaluation of the United States Food and Drug Administration Opht...—PubMed—NCBI" n.d.; [49]) and dependent on the depth of the anterior chamber or the distance between pIOL and endothelium [61]. In addition, the initial surgical trauma at implantation of a pIOL should not be neglected, and may account for a large part of the cell loss [5]. For pIOLs, progressive endothelial cell loss above the physiological (0.6% per annum [12]) has also been demonstrated. Endothelial cell losses of 3.7% after 4 [39], 8.4% after 4 years [21], 6.4% after 7 years have been reported [73]. Moya et al. in 2015 reported an endothelial cell loss of 19.8% after 12 years in myopic patients [54]. Regarding endothelial cell loss in the current version of ICL with aquaport, a 2018 literature review by Packer reported a loss of 2.6%- after a mean of 14.7 months (1476 eyes from 21 studies [56]). Thus, an annual check of the endothelial cell count is mandatory. This is also underlined by Jonker et al with a paper from 2019 with over 1000 eyes evaluating explantation reasons of pIOL. Here, the reason for 32% of explanted lenses was progressive endothelial cell loss [35].

Keypoint

Depending on the findings, the endothelial cell count should be checked at least once a year.

Pigment Dispersion and Lens Coatings

Pigment dispersion with consecutive lens fogging and a potential IOP increase, is primarily caused by contact of the pIOL with the iris. Menezo et al found a consecutive pressure increase of 1.5mmHg up to 3 years postoperatively [50], but other studies found no IOP increase after implantation of a pIOL [39, 57]. Due to the pre-curved optics, contact of IF-pIOL and the iris seems to be rather rare. Thus, pigmentary fogging seems to be mostly due to the surgical trauma. Pigment dispersion occurring postoperatively may also be due to the forward movement of the crystalline lens and is reported to occur up to 7% in 10 years, depending on the publication [50]. This seems to occur much less frequently in AC-pIOLs and is only described in isolated cases in the literature [43].

Chronic Inflammation and Uveitis

Similar to pigment dispersion, chronic inflammation may also result from the local proximity of the pIOL to the iris with consecutive irritation. The incidence is 3.1% to 8.7% in AC-pIOL [4, 44, 60] and may require explantation of the AC-pIOL if this cannot be controlled conservatively. Careful postoperative control of the inflammatory response is also necessary with IF-pIOL, as fixation may cause shear forces on the iris. Synechiae that develop a few weeks after implantation are also possible. The incidence of iritis is also variable and ranks in the low single digits according to the literature [53, 67]. In pIOL, a chronic inflammatory reaction does not seem to occur.

Keypoint

Consider explantation of the pIOL in cases of chronic uveitis or pigment abrasion with a intraocular pressure increase.

Pupil Ovalization and Iris Retraction

Especially with AC-pIOLs, ovalization—caused by the placement of the haptics in the chamber angle with consecutive deformation of the anatomy—seems to occur (Fig. 1). In addition to the cosmetic appearance, glare may also occur. The incidence is reported in the literature to range from 1.3% to 38.1% [5, 7, 60] and sometimes leads to explantation of the lens [4]. In IF-pIOL, enclavation may cause ovalization in the early postoperative course, but this may be regressive [46, 70]. Consecutively, asymmetric fixation may result in optic decentration. For example, Menezo et al showed decentration above 0.5 mm in 13.5% [51] and Perez-Santonia in 43% of cases [61]. In pHKL, iris retraction or ovalization seems to occur only in isolated cases.

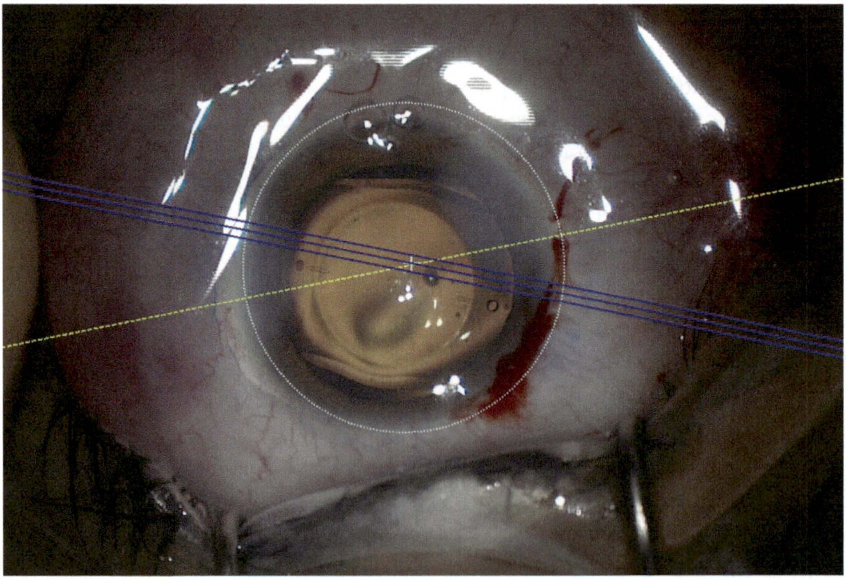

Fig. 1 Intraoperative alignment of a toric ICL The intended axis is marked by the blue lines

Pressure Increase and Pupillary Block

An increase in pressure after pIOL implantation can be attributed etiologically to different causes. In pIOL, it may occur due to pigment dispersion or as a steroid response based on postoperative local therapy. Pupillary block may occur due to forward movement of the iris, based on the retropupillary position of pIOL. In this regard, precautions should be taken by laser iridotomy or surgical iridectomy. In the current version of the myopic Visian ICL, this problem has been mitigated by the central opening (aquaport) in the optic [56] which seems to prevent postoperative IOP rise without the need for iridectomie [62]. At this point, it should be noted to educate the patient that positive dysphotopsia may occur due to the central aquaport in the early postoperative period [24] but the visual performance, higher order aberrations, and contrast sensitivity seems to be similar in eyes with and without aquaport [68]. In hyperopic ICL, iridotomy/ectomy is still mandatory due to the lack of an aquaport. If an iridectomy is displaced by the haptics of the pIOL (especially PRL), a second one can be performed at a 90° angle. If necessary, this can be done intraoperatively. In IF-pIOL, pressure elevation and pupillary block do not appear to be lens-related [17]. Possible postoperative pressure increases have been described but attributed to residual viscoelastic substance.

With AC-pIOLs, the problem of pupillary block and an increase in pressure is known [42]. Accordingly, the creation of an iridectomy or iridotomy intra- or preoperatively is obligatory. The growth of the crystalline lens may further increase the risk.

Lens Rotation, as Well as Lens Power and Position

Postoperative rotation of AC-IOLs seems to occur in a large proportion of eyes and rates of 40% to 80% within two years have been described [7, 9, 60]. However, this is not necessarily visually relevant [43]. With sufficient enclavation, rotation seems to be extremely rare in IF-pIOLs [9, 72]. For this reason, they are quite suitable as toric implants. In the case of a pIOL, lens rotation occurs mainly when a diameter too small for the eye has been selected [26]. The diameter should be determined depending on the WTW distance of the IOL master [10, 29]. However, in individual cases, this WTW measurement does not directly correlate with the sulcus diameter, so a second imaging procedure to estimate the sulcus diameter is recommended. Nevertheless one has to acknowledge that interdevice correlation and repeatability of WTW was observed to be rather low [27]. Therefore some authors prefer using the angle to angle distance measured by swept-source OCT since ATA was shown to be more reproducible using the Casia 2 SS-OCT (Tomey corparation, Japan) [31].

A measurement specific to the pIOL is the vault—the distance between the back of the pIOL and the crystalline lens. A hypervault (>750 μm) can be caused by a too large lens diameter and result in residual refractive error, halos, pigment

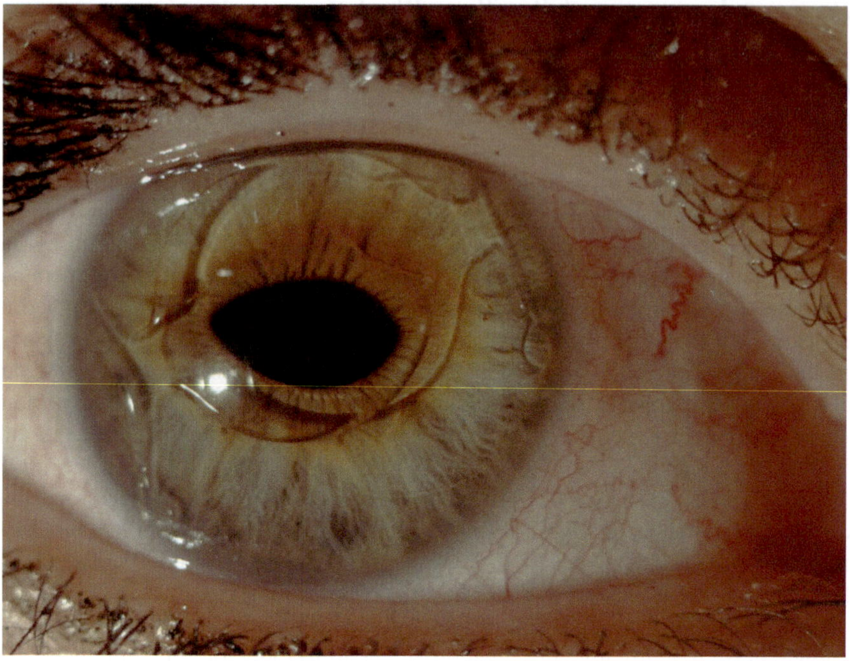

Fig. 2 Pupil ovalization 5 years postoperatively after implantation of a phakic, chamber angle-supported intraocular lens ("cat's eye")

abrasion or angle block (Fig. 2). As described by Biermann et al. in many cases, the sulcus has a higher diameter vertically than the horizontal sulcus [11], rotation of the ICL by 90 degrees from the horizontal to the vertical position postoperatively can be an alternative to ICL exchange in non-toric ICL implants to reduce the hypervault [48]. Hypovault occurs when the distances is <250 µm and can lead to accelerated cataract formation in particular. In this case, it is additionally important to consider the growth of the crystalline lens so that the ideal vault is between 500 and 750 µm [66]. In the presence of a stable hypovault without detectable opacification of the crystalline lens, it is recommended to wait with an ICL exchange after implantation of a myopic V4c model. Since the estimated postop vault is one of the important preoperative measurements for lens selection a paper on vault prediction using machine learning was published recently which could lead to a significant improvement in postop results [38]. However, this needs to be validated by real world data first. A paper by Jadidi et al. showed that over a long-term follow-up period after myopic ICL implantation, there was no opacification of the crystalline lens in any of these eyes despite a postoperative vault of 39 to 150 µm [33] (Fig. 3).

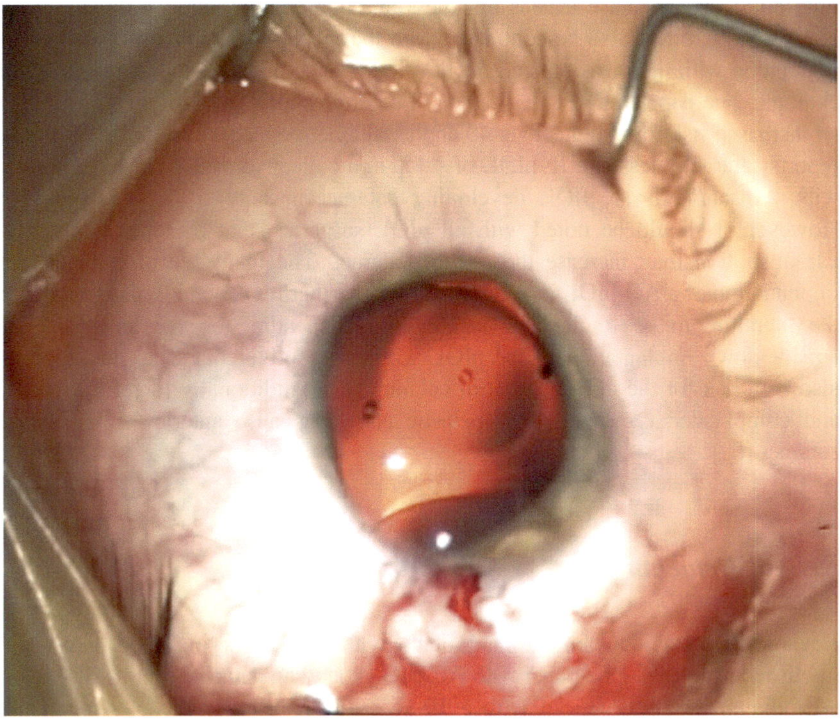

Fig. 3 Intraoperative situs during explantation of an ICL due to a Hpyervault

Keypoint

The success of the operation depends on the correct choice of lens size. It not only influences the postoperative refraction, but can also cause serious complications.

Cataract Formation

Cataractogenesis is, after the loss of endothelial cells, one of the main postoperative problems after implantation of a pIOL. This is underlined by a study showing that the main reason for explantation of pIOLs was cataract formation [79]. Phakic posterior chamber lenses were shown to have a prevalence of 3.6–25.7%, depending on the type (ICL 8.5%, PRL 3.6%). The overall prevalence in a study of 1210 eyes was 9.6% [16]. The development of new models with Aquaport has particularly helped to reduce cataract formation. Current studies show an incidence of only 0.6% for ICL V4 and 0% for V4c after 6 years (albeit with only 6 months of follow-up for V4c) [3]. An overall incidence of 0.49% at 13 months in 617 eyes from 11 studies in [56] meta-analysis seems to confirm this low risk of ICL with Aquaport. However, it should be emphasized that the risk of cataract increases over time due to the increase in lens thickness and consecutive reduction of the vault. However, this must also be contrasted with the increased likelihood of the patient population with high myopia and the development of premature lens opacities. For example, one paper found a 3% cataract rate after implantation of an IF-pIOL and an increased risk for patients over 40 and axial length over 30 mm [50]. Other work reports cataract rates with IF-pIOL of 1.1% in a collective of 2781 eyes, with eyes with Artisan/Verisyse pIOL developing cataract in only 0.3% of cases [16]. However, it should be noted with all pIOL surgeries, that postoperative steroid administration may increase the risk of cataract. The incidence of cataract after implantation of a AC-pIOL is in line with that of other pIOLs and is also reported in the literature to be in the low single digits depending on the lens [16, 41]. Upside-down implantation of the pIOL with consecutive contact to the lens may also be a risk for the development of cataract [42]. Additionally forceful irrigation and complicated removal of viscoelastic can also cause anterior sub- capsular cataract [69]

Retinal Detachment

Regarding retinal detachment in patients with pIOL, varying risks have been published (Table 1). One paper with AC-pIOL found an detachment rate of 4.8% in 44 months, whereas a paper with a 10-year follow-up after cachet implantation reported no detachment in the patient population [3, 42]. Detachment rates <1% have also been reported for IF-pIOL and pIOL [13, 28, 70] "United States Food and Drug Administration clinical trial of the Implantable Collamer Lens (ICL) for moderate to high myopia: three-year follow-up.—PubMed—NCBI" n.d.). A 2015 study reported a cumulative risk of 0.7% for the ICL and 0% for the Artisan/Verisys at 2 years [1]. However, in general, selection bias based on preoperative fundus examinations in mydriasis is also be possible, as in the patient population which is usually highly myopic there is already a 0.68% annual risk of rhegmatogenous retinal detachment in patients above –10.0dpt [58]. For this reason, thorough pre-operative and postoperative fundus checkups in mydriasis is obligatory (Table 2).

Further Complications

Other, rare complications as after any intraocular surgery include endopthalmitis, Urrets-Zavalia syndrome, or toxic anterior segment syndrome ([2, 55], "Post-cataract surgery endophthalmitis: Brief literature review.—PubMed—NCBI" n.d.; "Toxic anterior segment syndrome after Verisyse iris-supported phakic intraocular lens implantation.—PubMed—NCBI" n.d.; "Toxic anterior segment syndrome following phakic posterior chamber IOL: a rarity.—PubMed—NCBI" n.d.). However, here the incidences are overall very low or limited to single case reports.

Table 1 Endothelial cell loss of different phakic IOLs with follow up of at least 2 years

Trial	pIOL	Follow-up	Cell loss
Senthil S, IJO 2006	Artisan	2 years	6.4%
Benedetti S, JCRS 2007	Artisan	5 years	9,0%
Moshirfar M, JCRS 2007	Artisan	2 years	6.2%
Stulting RD, Ophthalmol 2008	Artisan/Verisyse	3 years	4.8%
Guell JL, Ophthalmol 2008	Artisan/Verisyse	4 years	5.1%
Silva RA, Arch Ophthalmol 2008	Artisan	5 years	14.1%
Dick HB, Ophthalmol 2009	Artiflex	2 years	1.1%
Qasem Q, Ophthalmologica 2010	Artisan	5 years	0%
Jonker SMR, Ophthalmol 2018	Artisan	10 years	16.6%
Jonker SMR, Ophthalmol 2018	toric Artisan	10 years	21.5%
Tang Y, J Ophthalmology 2020	Artisan /Verisyse	12 years	29%
Kamiya K, Arch Ophthalmol 2009	ICL	4 years	3.7%
Lee, Clin Exp Ophthalmol 2016	ICL	5 years	7.8%
Torun N, JCRS 2013	PRL	7 years	6.4%
Lu Y, AJO 2017	ICL	5 years	11%

Table 2 Frequency of rhegmatogenous retinal detachments after implantation of phakic intraocular lenses

Study	Phake IOL	Spherical equivalent	Cumulative incidence	Follow-up (years)
Ruiz-Moreno et al. [64]	ZB5M	–18.6 dpt	4.8%	2–7
Javaloy et al. [34]	ZB5M	–17.2 dpt	0%	12
Kohnen et al. [43]	AcrySof	–10.4 dpt	0%	7–10
Budo et al. [13]	Artisan	–13.0 dpt	0,8%	0.5–3
Stulting et al. [70]	Artisan	–12.3 dpt	0,5%	3
Güell et al. [28]	Artisan	–12.6 dpt	0.25%	4
Al Abdullah et al. [1]	Artisan	–12.4 dpt	0%	2
Jonker et al. [35]	Artisan/toric Artisan	–12.7 dpt/–6.5 dpt	0.26%	10
ICL ITM Study Group [65]	ICL	–10.1 dpt	0,6%	3
Donoso et al. [20]	PRL	–17.3 dpt	1.9%	1
Chang & Meau [15]	ICL	–14.5 dpt	1.6%	1
Torun et al. [73]	PRL	–12.2 dpt	3.8%	7
Al Abdullah et al. [1]	ICL	–12.4 dpt	0.7%	2
Perkins [58]	Myopes >10 dpt in spontaneous course		0.68% per year	

In IF-pIOLs, iris hemorrhage or perforation through the haptics would also be possible. In pIOLs, there are isolated reports of pIOLs luxating into the vitreous, predominantly due to zonular defects [22, 30, 47]. Malignant glaucoma three days after ICL insertion has been described once in the literature [40].

Conclusion

Phakic intraocular lenses offer a high level of efficiency and safety, with good predictability and stability. They provide sufficient correction of refractive error even in highly myopic patients, with a moderate to low risk of complications. Particular attention should be paid to regular monitoring of endothelial cell counts, education about glare sensitivity, and reduction of cataract risk through preoperative patient selection. Care should also be paid to pupil ovalization and chronic inflammation, especially with IF-pIOLs. The risk of retinal detachment appears to be unaffected by pIOL, despite a "high-risk" ccohort.

References

1. Al-Abdullah AA, Al-Falah MA, Al-Rasheed SA, Khandekar R, Suarez E, Arevalo JF. Retinal complications after anterior versus posterior chamber phakic intraocular lens implantation in a myopic cohort. J Refract Surg (Thorofare, N.J.: 1995). 2015;31(12):814–9. https://doi.org/10.3928/1081597X-20151111-05.
2. Al-Abdullah AA, Al-Falah M, Al-Rashaed S, Khandekar R, Arevalo JF. Endophthalmitis caused by rhizobium radiobacter after posterior chamber phakic intraocular lens implantation to correct myopia. J Refract Surg (Thorofare, N.J.: 1995). 2015;31(8):561–3. https://doi.org/10.3928/1081597X-20150728-02.
3. Alfonso JF, Lisa C, Fernández-Vega L, Almanzar D, Pérez-Vives C, Montés-Micó R. Prevalence of cataract after collagen copolymer phakic intraocular lens implantation for myopia, hyperopia, and astigmatism. J Cataract Refract Surg. 2015;41(4):800–5. https://doi.org/10.1016/j.jcrs.2014.07.039.
4. Alió JL, Abdelrahman AM, Javaloy J, Iradier MT, Ortuño V. Angle-supported anterior chamber phakic intraocular lens explantation causes and outcome. Ophthalmology 2006;113(12):2213–20. https://doi.org/10.1016/j.ophtha.2006.05.057.
5. Alió JL, de la Hoz F, Pérez-Santonja JJ, Ruiz-Moreno JM, Quesada JA. Phakic anterior chamber lenses for the correction of myopia: a 7-year cumulative analysis of complications in 263 cases. Ophthalmology 1999;106(3):458–66. https://doi.org/10.1016/S0161-6420(99)90103-3.
6. Alió JL, Mulet ME, Shalaby AMM. Artisan phakic iris claw intraocular lens for high primary and secondary hyperopia. J Refract Surg (Thorofare, N.J.: 1995). 2002;18(6):697–707.
7. Allemann N, Chamon W, Tanaka HM, Mori ES, Campos M, Schor P, Baïkoff G. Myopic angle-supported intraocular lenses: two-year follow-up. Ophthalmology 2000;107(8):1549–54. https://doi.org/10.1016/s0161-6420(00)00221-9.
8. Awadein A, Habib AE. ICL versus Veriflex phakic IOL for treatment of moderately high myopia: randomized paired-eye comparison. J Refract Surg (Thorofare, N.J.: 1995). 2013;29(7):445–52. https://doi.org/10.3928/1081597X-20130617-02.

9. Baumeister M, Bühren J, Kohnen T. Position of angle-supported, iris-fixated, and ciliary sulcus-implanted myopic phakic intraocular lenses evaluated by Scheimpflug photography. Am J Ophthalmol. 2004;138(5):723–31. https://doi.org/10.1016/j.ajo.2004.06.009.
10. Baumeister M, Terzi E, Ekici Y, Kohnen T. Comparison of manual and automated methods to determine horizontal corneal diameter. J Cataract Refract Surg. 2004;30(2):374–80. https://doi.org/10.1016/j.jcrs.2003.06.004.
11. Biermann J, Bredow L, Boehringer D, Reinhard T. Evaluation of ciliary sulcus diameter using ultrasound biomicroscopy in emmetropic eyes and myopic eyes. J Cataract Refract Surg. 2011;37(9):1686–93. https://doi.org/10.1016/j.jcrs.2011.03.048.
12. Bourne WM, Nelson LR, Hodge DO. Central corneal endothelial cell changes over a ten-year period. Invest Ophthalmol Vis Sci. 1997;38(3):779–82.
13. Budo C, Hessloehl JC, Izak M, Luyten GP, Menezo JL, Sener BA, et al. Multicenter study of the Artisan phakic intraocular lens. J Cataract Refract Surg. 2000;26(8):1163–71. https://doi.org/10.1016/s0886-3350(00)00545-9.
14. Castro de Luna G, Ramos-López D, Castaño Fernández AB, Cuevas Santamaría D. Artiflex foldable lens for myopia correction results of 10 years of follow-up. Eye (Lond). 2019;33(10):1564–9. https://doi.org/10.1038/s41433-019-0446-7.
15. Chang JS, Meau AY. Visian Collamer phakic intraocular lens in high myopic Asian eyes. J Refract Surg (Thorofare, N.J.: 1995). 2007;23(1):17–25. https://doi.org/10.3928/1081-597X-20070101-05.
16. Chen L-J, Chang Y-J, Kuo JC, Rajagopal R, Azar DT. Metaanalysis of cataract development after phakic intraocular lens surgery. J Cataract Refract Surg. 2008;34(7):1181–200. https://doi.org/10.1016/j.jcrs.2008.03.029.
17. Coullet J, Guëll J-L, Fournié P, Grandjean H, Gaytan J, Arné J-L, Malecaze F. Iris-supported phakic lenses (rigid vs foldable version) for treating moderately high myopia: randomized paired eye comparison. Am J Ophthalmol. 2006;142(6):909–16. https://doi.org/10.1016/j.ajo.2006.07.021.
18. Dick HB, Alió J, Bianchetti M, Budo C, Christiaans BJ, El-Danasoury MA, et al. Toric phakic intraocular lens: European multicenter study. Ophthalmology 2003;110(1):150–62. https://doi.org/10.1016/s0161-6420(02)01447-1.
19. Domínguez-Vicent A, Ferrer-Blasco T, Pérez-Vives C, Esteve-Taboada JJ, Montés-Micó R. Optical quality comparison between 2 collagen copolymer posterior chamber phakic intraocular lens designs. J Cataract Refract Surg. 2015;41(6):1268–78. https://doi.org/10.1016/j.jcrs.2014.09.050.
20. Donoso R, Castillo P. Correction of high myopia with the PRL phakic intraocular lens. J Cataract Refract Surg 2006;32(8):1296–1300. https://doi.org/10.1016/j.jcrs.2006.03.035.
21. Edelhauser HF, Sanders DR, Azar R, Lamielle H. ICL in treatment of myopia study group. Corneal endothelial assessment after ICL implantation. J Cataract Refract Surg. 2004;30(3):576–83. https://doi.org/10.1016/j.jcrs.2003.09.047.
22. Eleftheriadis H, Amoros S, Bilbao R, Teijeiro M-A. Spontaneous dislocation of a phakic refractive lens into the vitreous cavity. J Cataract Refract Surg. 2004;30(9):2013–6. https://doi.org/10.1016/j.jcrs.2004.04.060.
23. Eom Y, Kim DW, Ryu D, Kim J-H, Yang SK, Song JS, et al. Ring-shaped dysphotopsia associated with posterior chamber phakic implantable collamer lenses with a central hole. Acta Ophthalmol. 2017;95(3):e170–8. https://doi.org/10.1111/aos.13248.
24. Eppig T, Spira C, Tsintarakis T, El-Husseiny M, Cayless A, Müller M, et al. Ghost-image analysis in phakic intraocular lenses with central hole as a potential cause of dysphotopsia. J Cataract Refract Surg. 2015;41(11):2552–9. https://doi.org/10.1016/j.jcrs.2015.05.034.
25. Faron N, Hoekel J, Tychsen L. Visual acuity, refractive error, and regression outcomes in 169 children with high myopia who were implanted with Ophtec-Artisan or Visian phakic IOLs. Journal of AAPOS: the official publication of the American Association for Pediatric Ophthalmology and Strabismus. 2021. https://doi.org/10.1016/j.jaapos.2020.09.011.

26. García-Feijoó J, Alfaro IJ, Cuiña-Sardiña R, Méndez-Hernandez C, Del Castillo JMB, García-Sánchez J. Ultrasound biomicroscopy examination of posterior chamber phakic intraocular lens position. Ophthalmology 2003;110(1):163–72. https://doi.org/10.1016/s0161-6420(02)01449-5.
27. Guber I, Bergin C, Perritaz S, Majo F. Correcting interdevice bias of horizontal white-to-white and sulcus-to-sulcus measures used for implantable collamer lens sizing. Am J Ophthalmol. 2016;161:116–125.e1. https://doi.org/10.1016/j.ajo.2015.09.037.
28. Güell JL, Morral M, Gris O, Gaytan J, Sisquella M, Manero F. Five-year follow-up of 399 phakic Artisan-Verisyse implantation for myopia, hyperopia, and/or astigmatism. Ophthalmology 2008;115(6):1002–12. https://doi.org/10.1016/j.ophtha.2007.08.022.
29. Güell JL, Morral M, Kook D, Kohnen T. Phakic intraocular lenses part 1: historical overview, current models, selection criteria, and surgical techniques. J Cataract Refract Surg. 2010;36 (11):1976–93. https://doi.org/10.1016/j.jcrs.2010.08.014.
30. Hoyos JE, Cigales M, Hoyos-Chacón J. Zonular dehiscence two years after phakic refractive lens (PRL) implantation. J Refract Surg (Thorofare, N.J.: 1995). 2005;21(1):13–7.
31. Igarashi A, Shimizu K, Kato S, Kamiya K. Predictability of the vault after posterior chamber phakic intraocular lens implantation using anterior segment optical coherence tomography. J Cataract Refract Surg. 2019;45(8):1099–104. https://doi.org/10.1016/j.jcrs.2019.02.020.
32. Initial results of endothelial cell counts after Artisan lens for phakic eyes: an evaluation of the United States Food and Drug Administration Opht... - PubMed - NCBI. (o. J.). https://www.ncbi.nlm.nih.gov/pubmed/15019381. Zugegriffen: 5. Mai 2020.
33. Jadidi K, Mosavi SA, Nejat F, Mohammadi N, Aghamolaei H, Daryabari S-H, et al. Use of low-vault posterior chamber collagen copolymer phakic intraocular lenses for the correction of myopia: a 3-year follow-up. Graefe's Archive for Clinical and Experimental Ophthalmology = Albrecht Von Graefes Archiv Fur Klinische Und Experimentelle Ophthalmologie. 2019;257(7):1555–60. https://doi.org/10.1007/s00417-019-04336-9.
34. Javaloy J, Alió JL, Iradier MT, Abdelrahman AM, Javaloy T, Borrás F. Outcomes of ZB5M angle-supported anterior chamber phakic intraocular lenses at 12 years. J Refract Surg (Thorofare, N.J.: 1995). 2007;23(2):147–158. https://doi.org/10.3928/1081-597X-20070201-07.
35. Jonker SMR, Van Averbeke AAC, Berendschot TTJM, Saelens IEY, Nuijts RMMA. Risk factors for explantation of iris-fixated phakic intraocular lenses. J Cataract Refract Surg. 2019;45(8):1092–8. https://doi.org/10.1016/j.jcrs.2019.03.009.
36. Jonker SMR, Berendschot TTJM, Ronden AE, Saelens IEY, Bauer NJC, Nuijts RMMA. long-term endothelial cell loss in patients with Artisan myopia and Artisan toric phakic intraocular lenses: 5- and 10-year results. Ophthalmology 2018;125(4):486–494. https://doi.org/10.1016/j.ophtha.2017.08.011.
37. Kamiya K, Shimizu K, Igarashi A, Kitazawa Y, Kojima T, Nakamura T, et al. Posterior chamber phakic intraocular lens implantation: comparative, multicentre study in 351 eyes with low-to-moderate or high myopia. Br J Ophthalmol. 2018;102(2):177–81. https://doi.org/10.1136/bjophthalmol-2017-310164.
38. Kamiya K, Ryu IH, Yoo TK, Kim JS, Lee IS, Kim JK, et al. Prediction of phakic intraocular lens vault using machine learning of anterior segment optical coherence tomography metrics: phakic lens vault prediction using machine learning. Am J Ophthalmol. 2021. https://doi.org/10.1016/j.ajo.2021.02.006.
39. Kamiya K, Shimizu K, Igarashi A, Hikita F, Komatsu M. Four-year follow-up of posterior chamber phakic intraocular lens implantation for moderate to high myopia. Arch Ophthalmol (Chicago, Ill.: 1960). 2009;127(7):845–50. https://doi.org/10.1001/archophthalmol.2009.67.
40. Kodjikian L, Gain P, Donate D, Rouberol F, Burillon C. Malignant glaucoma induced by a phakic posterior chamber intraocular lens for myopia. J Cataract Refract Surg. 2002;28 (12):2217–21. https://doi.org/10.1016/s0886-3350(02)01213-0.
41. Kohnen T, Kook D, Morral M, Güell JL. Phakic intraocular lenses: part 2: results and complications. J Cataract Refract Surg. 2010;36(12):2168–94. https://doi.org/10.1016/j.jcrs.2010.10.007.

42. Kohnen T, Knorz MC, Cochener B, Gerl RH, Arné J-L, Colin J, et al. AcrySof phakic angle-supported intraocular lens for the correction of moderate-to-high myopia: one-year results of a multicenter European study. Ophthalmology 2009;116(7):1314–21, 1321.e1–3. https://doi.org/10.1016/j.ophtha.2009.01.041.
43. Kohnen T, LaFontaine L, Andrew R, Study investigators. Long-term safety follow-up of an anterior chamber angle-supported phakic intraocular lens. J Cataract Refract Surg. 2017;43 (9):1163–70. https://doi.org/10.1016/j.jcrs.2017.06.035.
44. Leccisotti A. Iridocyclitis associated with angle-supported phakic intraocular lenses. J Cataract Refract Surg. 2006;32(6):1007–10. https://doi.org/10.1016/j.jcrs.2006.02.030.
45. Liu T, Linghu S, Pan L, Shi R. Effects of V4c-ICL implantation on myopic patients' vision-related daily activities. J Ophthalmol. 2016;2016:5717932. https://doi.org/10.1155/2016/5717932.
46. Maloney RK, Nguyen LH, John ME. Artisan phakic intraocular lens for myopia: short-term results of a prospective, multicenter study. Ophthalmology 2002;109(9):1631–41. https://doi.org/10.1016/s0161-6420(02)01170-3.
47. Martínez-Castillo V, Elies D, Boixadera A, García-Arumí J, Mauricio J, Cavero L, Coret A. Silicone posterior chamber phakic intraocular lens dislocated into the vitreous cavity. J Refract Surg (Thorofare, N.J.: 1995). 2004;20(6):773–7.
48. Matarazzo F, Day AC, Fernandez-Vega Cueto L, Maurino V. Vertical implantable collamer lens (ICL) rotation for the management of high vault due to lens oversizing. Int Ophthalmol. 2018;38(6):2689–92. https://doi.org/10.1007/s10792-017-0757-2.
49. Menezo JL, Cisneros AL, Rodriguez-Salvador V. Endothelial study of iris-claw phakic lens: four year follow-up. J Cataract Refract Surg. 1998;24(8):1039–49. https://doi.org/10.1016/s0886-3350(98)80096-5.
50. Menezo JL, Peris-Martínez C, Cisneros AL, Martínez-Costa R. Phakic intraocular lenses to correct high myopia: Adatomed, Staar, and Artisan. J Cataract Refract Surg. 2004;30(1):33–44. https://doi.org/10.1016/j.jcrs.2003.11.023.
51. Menezo JL, Aviño JA, Cisneros A, Rodriguez-Salvador V, Martinez-Costa R. Iris claw phakic intraocular lens for high myopia. J Refract Surg (Thorofare, N.J.: 1995). 1997;13 (6):545–55.
52. Menezo JL, Peris-Martínez C, Cisneros-Lanuza AL, Martínez-Costa R. Rate of cataract formation in 343 highly myopic eyes after implantation of three types of phakic intraocular lenses. J Refract Surg (Thorofare, N.J.: 1995). 2004;20(4):317–24.
53. Moshirfar M, Holz HA, Davis DK. Two-year follow-up of the Artisan/Verisyse iris-supported phakic intraocular lens for the correction of high myopia. J Cataract Refract Surg. 2007;33 (8):1392–7. https://doi.org/10.1016/j.jcrs.2007.04.009.
54. Moya T, Javaloy J, Montés-Micó R, Beltrán J, Muñoz G, Montalbán R. Implantable collamer lens for myopia: assessment 12 years after implantation. J Refract Surg (Thorofare, N.J.: 1995). 2015;31(8):548–6. https://doi.org/10.3928/1081597X-20150727-05.
55. Oum BS, Lee JS, Choi HY, Lee JE, Kim SJ, Lee J-E. Endophthalmitis caused by pseudomonas aeruginosa after phakic posterior chamber intraocular lens implantation to correct high myopia. Acta Ophthalmol. 2011;89(2):e209–210. https://doi.org/10.1111/j.1755-3768.2009.01782.x.
56. Packer M. The implantable collamer lens with a central port: review of the literature. Clin Ophthalmol (Auckland, N.Z.). 2018;12:2427–38. https://doi.org/10.2147/OPTH.S188785.
57. Park SC, Kwun YK, Chung E-S, Ahn K, Chung T-Y. Postoperative astigmatism and axis stability after implantation of the STAAR Toric Implantable Collamer Lens. J Refract Surg (Thorofare, N.J.: 1995). 2009;25(5):403–9. https://doi.org/10.3928/1081597X-20090422-01.
58. Perkins ES. Morbidity from myopia. The Sight-Saving Rev. 1979;49(1):11–19.
59. Post-cataract surgery endophthalmitis: Brief literature review. - PubMed - NCBI. (o. J.). https://www.ncbi.nlm.nih.gov/pubmed/27579452. Zugegriffen: 6. Mai 2020.
60. Pérez-Santonja JJ, Alió JL, Jiménez-Alfaro I, Zato MA. Surgical correction of severe myopia with an angle-supported phakic intraocular lens. J Cataract Refract Surg. 2000;26(9):1288–302. https://doi.org/10.1016/s0886-3350(00)00543-5.

61. Pérez-Santonja JJ, Bueno JL, Zato MA. Surgical correction of high myopia in phakic eyes with Worst-Fechner myopia intraocular lenses. J Refract Surg (Thorofare, N.J.: 1995). 1997;13(3):268–281; discussion 281–284.
62. Repplinger B, Kohnen T. Intraocular pressure after implantation of an ICL with aquaport: development of intraocular pressure after implantation of an ICL (model V4c) with aquaport without iridotomy. Der Ophthalmologe: Zeitschrift Der Deutschen Ophthalmologischen Gesellschaft 2018;115(1):29–33. https://doi.org/10.1007/s00347-017-0556-1.
63. van Rijn GA, Gaurisankar ZS, Ilgenfritz AP, Lima JEE, Haasnoot GW, Beenakker J-WM, et al. Middle- and long-term results after iris-fixated phakic intraocular lens implantation in myopic and hyperopic patients: a meta-analysis. J Cataract Refract Surg. 2020;46(1):125–37. https://doi.org/10.1097/j.jcrs.0000000000000002.
64. Ruiz-Moreno JM, Alió JL, Pérez-Santonja JJ, de la Hoz F. Retinal detachment in phakic eyes with anterior chamber intraocular lenses to correct severe myopia. Am J Ophthalmol. 1999:127(3):270–275. https://doi.org/10.1016/s0002-9394(98)00412-7.
65. Sanders DR, Doney K, Poco M. ICL in treatment of myopia study group. United States food and drug administration clinical trial of the Implantable Collamer Lens (ICL) for moderate to high myopia: three-year follow-up. Ophthalmology 2004;111(9):1683–1692. https://doi.org/10.1016/j.ophtha.2004.03.026.
66. Schmidinger G, Lackner B, Pieh S, Skorpik C. Long-term changes in posterior chamber phakic intraocular collamer lens vaulting in myopic patients. Ophthalmology. 2010;117(8):1506–11. https://doi.org/10.1016/j.ophtha.2009.12.013.
67. Senthil S, Reddy KP, Ravisankar S. A retrospective analysis of the first Indian experience on Artisan phakic intraocular lens. Indian J Ophthalmol. 2006;54(4):251–255. https://doi.org/10.4103/0301-4738.27950.
68. Shimizu K, Kamiya K, Igarashi A, Shiratani T. Intraindividual comparison of visual performance after posterior chamber phakic intraocular lens with and without a central hole implantation for moderate to high myopia. Am J Ophthalmol. 2012;154(3):486–494.e1. https://doi.org/10.1016/j.ajo.2012.04.001.
69. Steinwender G, Varna-Tigka K, Shajari M, Kohnen T. Anterior subcapsular cataract caused by forceful irrigation during implantation of a posterior chamber phakic intraocular lens with a central hole. J Cataract Refract Surg. 2017;43(7):969–74. https://doi.org/10.1016/j.jcrs.2017.03.045.
70. Stulting RD, John ME, Maloney RK, Assil KK, Arrowsmith PN, Thompson VM, U.S. Verisyse study group. Three-year results of Artisan/Verisyse phakic intraocular lens implantation. Results of the United States food And drug administration clinical trial. Ophthalmology 2008;115(3):464–72.e1. https://doi.org/10.1016/j.ophtha.2007.08.039.
71. Tang Y, Xu J, Chen J, Lu Y. Long-term destiny of corneal endothelial cells in anterior chamber intraocular lens-implanted eyes. J Ophthalmol. 2020;2020:5967509. https://doi.org/10.1155/2020/5967509.
72. Tehrani M, Dick HB, Schwenn O, Blom E, Schmidt AH, Koch H-R. Postoperative astigmatism and rotational stability after artisan toric phakic intraocular lens implantation. J Cataract Refract Surg. 2003;29(9):1761–6. https://doi.org/10.1016/s0886-3350(03)00014-2.
73. Torun N, Bertelmann E, Klamann MKJ, Maier A-K, Liekfeld A, Gonnermann J. Posterior chamber phakic intraocular lens to correct myopia: long-term follow-up. J Cataract Refract Surg. 2013;39(7):1023–8. https://doi.org/10.1016/j.jcrs.2013.01.041.
74. Toxic anterior segment syndrome after Verisyse iris-supported phakic intraocular lens implantation. - PubMed - NCBI. (o. J.). https://www.ncbi.nlm.nih.gov/pubmed/16857515. Zugegriffen: 6. Mai 2020.
75. Toxic anterior segment syndrome following phakic posterior chamber IOL: a rarity. - PubMed - NCBI. (o. J.). https://www.ncbi.nlm.nih.gov/pubmed/30567159. Zugegriffen: 6. Mai 2020.
76. United States Food and Drug Administration clinical trial of the Implantable Collamer Lens (ICL) for moderate to high myopia: three-year follow-up. - PubMed - NCBI. (o. J.). https://www.ncbi.nlm.nih.gov/pubmed/15350323. Zugegriffen: 6. Mai 2020.

77. Vasavada V, Srivastava S, Vasavada SA, Sudhalkar A, Vasavada AR, Vasavada VA. Safety and efficacy of a new phakic posterior chamber IOL for correction of myopia: 3 years of follow-up. J Refract Surg (Thorofare, N.J.: 1995). 2018;34(12):817–23. https://doi.org/10.3928/1081597X-20181105-01.
78. Yaşa D, Ürdem U, Ağca A, Yildirim Y, Kepez Yildiz B, Kandemir Beşek N, et al. Early results with a new posterior chamber phakic intraocular lens in patients with high myopia. J Ophthalmol. 2018;2018:1329874. https://doi.org/10.1155/2018/1329874.
79. Yildirim TM, Khoramnia R, Son H-S, Mayer CS, Łabuz G, Munro DJ, Auffarth GU. Reasons for explantation of phakic intraocular lenses and associated perioperative complications: cross-sectional explant registry analysis. BMC Ophthalmol. 2021;21(1):80. https://doi.org/10.1186/s12886-021-01847-0.

Other sources:

80. a: Staar Surgical. Patient Survey; Visian ICLTM (Implantable Collamer Lens) For Nearsightedness; Facts You Need To Know About STAAR Surgical's Visian ICL; Surgery; Patient Information Booklet. Available from: https://staar.com/file/Patient-Information-Booklet-MKT-0125-Rev-2-9.7.17.pdf (Accessed May 6th, 2020).

Index

M. Shajari et al. (eds.), *Cataract and Lens Surgery*,
https://doi.org/10.1007/978-3-031-05394-8

D

E

Z

GPSR Compliance

The European Union's (EU) General Product Safety Regulation (GPSR) is a set of rules that requires consumer products to be safe and our obligations to ensure this.

If you have any concerns about our products, you can contact us on ProductSafety@springernature.com

In case Publisher is established outside the EU, the EU authorized representative is:

Springer Nature Customer Service Center GmbH
Europaplatz 3
69115 Heidelberg, Germany

Batch number: 10726129

Printed by Printforce, the Netherlands